Obesity: Concerns and Challenges

Obesity: Concerns and Challenges

Editor: Edgar Warren

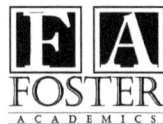

FA

FOSTER
ACADEMICS

www.fosteracademics.com

www.fosteracademics.com

FA
FOSTER
ACADEMICS

Cataloging-in-Publication Data

Obesity : concerns and challenges / edited by Edgar Warren.
    p. cm.
Includes bibliographical references and index.
ISBN 978-1-63242-650-5
1. Obesity. 2. Metabolism--Disorders. I. Warren, Edgar.
RC628 .O24 2019
616.3--dc23

Foster Academics,
118-35 Queens Blvd., Suite 400,
Forest Hills, NY 11375, USA

ISBN 978-1-63242-650-5 (Hardback)

Contents

Preface

A medical condition in which fat accumulates in the human body to such a degree that it starts to exert a negative influence on overall health and functioning is called obesity. It is characterized by a BMI (body mass index) of over 30 kg/m^2. It can lead to various diseases and illnesses and also to death. Increase in the average energy consumed, through high carbohydrate consumption and fat consumption and our sedentary lifestyles with mechanized transportation and labor saving technology have increased the incidence of obesity worldwide. More than 41 genes have been linked to the development of obesity so far. Certain mental and physical illnesses and the pharmaceutical drugs used for their treatment also increase the risk of obesity. Illnesses, which are genetic syndromes such as Bardet-Biedl syndrome, Prader-WIlli syndrome, MOMO syndrome and Cohen syndrome, as well as congenital and acquired conditions like growth hormone deficiency, hypothyroidism, Cushing's syndrome and eating disorders, are associated with obesity. Medications such as insulin, thiazolidinediones, sulfonylureas, steroids, antidepressants, etc. may also lead to changes in body composition or weight gain. The objective of this book is to give a general view of the different clinical aspects of obesity including major concerns and challenges. It is a compilation of chapters that discuss the most significant concepts and emerging trends in the study of obesity. It is a vital tool for all researching and studying this field.

The researches compiled throughout the book are authentic and of high quality, combining several disciplines and from very diverse regions from around the world. Drawing on the contributions of many researchers from diverse countries, the book's objective is to provide the readers with the latest achievements in the area of research. This book will surely be a source of knowledge to all interested and researching the field.

In the end, I would like to express my deep sense of gratitude to all the authors for meeting the set deadlines in completing and submitting their research chapters. I would also like to thank the publisher for the support offered to us throughout the course of the book. Finally, I extend my sincere thanks to my family for being a constant source of inspiration and encouragement.

Editor

1

Complex patterns of direct and indirect association between the transcription Factor-7 like 2 gene, body mass index and type 2 diabetes diagnosis in adulthood in the Hispanic Community Health Study/ Study of Latinos

Lindsay Fernández-Rhodes[1,2*†], Annie Green Howard[2,3†], Mariaelisa Graff[1], Carmen R. Isasi[4], Heather M. Highland[1], Kristin L. Young[1], Esteban Parra[5], Jennifer E. Below[6], Qibin Qi[4], Robert C. Kaplan[4], Anne E. Justice[7], George Papanicolaou[8], Cathy C. Laurie[9], Struan F. A. Grant[10], Christopher Haiman[11], Ruth J. F. Loos[12] and Kari E. North[1]

Abstract

Background: Genome-wide association studies have implicated the *transcription factor 7-like 2* (*TCF7L2*) gene in type 2 diabetes risk, and more recently, in decreased body mass index. Given the contrary direction of genetic effects on these two traits, it has been suggested that the observed association with body mass index may reflect either selection bias or a complex underlying biology at *TCF7L2*.

Methods: Using 9031 Hispanic/Latino adults (21–76 years) with complete weight history and genetic data from the community-based Hispanic Community Health Study/Study of Latinos (HCHS/SOL, Baseline 2008–2011), we estimated the multivariable association between the additive number of type 2 diabetes increasing-alleles at *TCF7L2* (rs7903146-T) and body mass index. We then used structural equation models to simultaneously model the genetic association on changes in body mass index across the life course and estimate the odds of type 2 diabetes per *TCF7L2* risk allele.

(Continued on next page)

* Correspondence: fernandez-rhodes@unc.edu

The views expressed in this manuscript are those of the authors and do not necessarily represent the views of the National Heart, Lung, and Blood Institute; the National Institutes of Health; or the U.S. Department of Health and Human Services.

†Lindsay Fernández-Rhodes and Annie Green Howard contributed equally to this work.

[1]Department of Epidemiology, UNC Gillings School of Global Public Health, University of North Carolina at Chapel Hill, 123 W Franklin St, Building C, Chapel Hill, NC, USA

[2]Carolina Population Center, University of North Carolina at Chapel Hill, 123 W Franklin St, Building C, Chapel Hill, NC, USA

Full list of author information is available at the end of the article

(Continued from previous page)

Results: We observed both significant increases in type 2 diabetes prevalence at examination (independent of body mass index) and decreases in mean body mass index and waist circumference across genotypes at rs7903146. We observed a significant multivariable association between the additive number of type 2 diabetes-risk alleles and lower body mass index at examination. In our structured modeling, we observed non-significant inverse direct associations between rs7903146-T and body mass index at ages 21 and 45 years, and a significant positive association between rs7903146-T and type 2 diabetes onset in both middle and late adulthood.

Conclusions: Herein, we replicated the protective effect of rs7930146-T on body mass index at multiple time points in the life course, and observed that these effects were not explained by past type 2 diabetes status in our structured modeling. The robust replication of the negative effects of TCF7L2 on body mass index in multiple samples, including in our diverse Hispanic/Latino community-based sample, supports a growing body of literature on the complex biologic mechanism underlying the functional consequences of TCF7L2 on obesity and type 2 diabetes across the life course.

Keywords: TCF7L2, Genetics, Obesity, Diabetes, Hispanic/Latinos

Background

Hispanic/Latino adults in the United States (US) are disproportionately affected by obesity and it consequences such as type 2 diabetes (T2D) [1] and this disparity is widening as compared to non-Hispanic Whites [2]. The *transcription factor-7 like 2 gene* (*TCF7L2*) was the first locus to be associated with T2D in genome-wide association studies (GWAS) and has been consistently associated with T2D [3, 4], *TCF7L2* (previously known as *TCF4*) encodes a transcription factor that is an effector of the Wnt signaling pathway [5]. Although the underlying biological mechanisms of *TCF7L2* remain unclear [6], the consistent association between the *TCF7L2* locus and T2D has been generalized to many diverse populations including Hispanic/Latinos [7, 8]. Indeed, the associated risk allele, rs7903146-T, harbored within the fourth intron of *TCF7L2* has the largest effect on T2D risk of all GWAS-identified T2D loci reported to date [8]. In Hispanic/Latinos each risk-allele has been associated with a 40% increased odds of T2D [7, 9].

The T2D-increasing allele at *TCF7L2* has also been associated with lower body mass index (BMI) [3, 10–12], resulting in a subsequent call for future research [13] given the strong epidemiologic correlation between increasing BMI and risk of T2D [14]. This association has been attributed to a T2D-related ascertainment bias, mainly due to the observation that the strongest and most significant *TCF7L2* associations with BMI are seen in T2D cases/controls, as compared to population-based studies [15–17].

There is mounting evidence of a complex biologic story for *TCF7L2*, explained in part by the bidirectional action of *TCF7L2* that may be cell, tissue or metabolically dependent [5]. Functional studies indicate that the rs7903146 variant may act in a cell or tissue-specific manner [18], by influencing alternative splicing of the *TCF7L2* [19–21], or by binding affinity of complex transcriptional machinery at an open chromatin region

specific to human pancreatic islets [22–25] to modulate pancreatic islet cell insulin production and secretion [17], action in adipose tissue [26], hepatic glucose output [27] or intestinal tissue differentiation [28]. Observational studies indicate that the T2D risk allele at *TCF7L2* associates with decreases insulin secretion [29–31]. Thus, we may expect individuals with the T allele have lower BMI values on average, and perhaps a differential pattern of insulin resistance.

Due to the mounting evidence on potential selection bias and the multi-faceted action of *TCF7L2* variation on insulin and glucose biology [5, 6, 18], we aimed 1) to replicate the multivariable association between *TCF7L2* T2D risk alleles and lower BMI in a population-based study of US Hispanic/Latinos accounting for key covariates, and 2) to model the structured pathways between rs7903146, at *TCF7L2*, BMI over time, and age of diabetes diagnosis. We performed these analyses in 9031 self-identified Hispanic/Latino adults (21–76 years of age at examination) residing in four US urban centers, who consented to genotyping and provided weight history and T2D diagnosis information the Hispanic Community Health Study/Study of Latinos (HCHS/SOL) baseline examination (2008–2011).

Methods

Study participants

We used data from the HCHS/SOL study, a multi-center, longitudinal, household-based cohort study of 16,415 Hispanic/Latino adults, aged 18–76 years in 2008–2011, who were sampled using a two-stage probability design from four US urban communities (The Bronx, NY; Chicago, IL; Miami, FL; San Diego, CA), as described previously in detail [32, 33]. Briefly, the complex sampling design allowed researchers to 1) over-sample individuals ≥45 years of age who were most likely to experience cardiometabolic disease outcomes either by the baseline examination or during follow up, while 2) capturing the varied socioeconomic and demographic composition of Hispanic/Latino households (as per the 2000 Census block group proportion of residents ≥25 years old with at least a high school education and the proportion Hispanic/Latino residents) and efficiently estimating cardiometabolic disease across the four Hispanic/Latino communities under study. Centrally-trained study personnel conducted the screening and baseline examinations in either English or Spanish based on participant preference.

Body mass index

As part of the HCHS/SOL baseline examination [32], current body weight was self-reported (in whole lb. or kg) and measured (to a tenth of a kg) and height was measured (to whole cm) on participants who were able to stand on both feet. As described previously [34], the accuracy and reliability of the self-reported weights were good (mean difference$_{\text{self-report−measured}}$ = 0.23 kg, r^2 = 0.97; inter-rater reliability coefficients, 0.93 and 0.97). Waist circumference was measured in cm at the umbilicus using a tape measure, and body fat percentage estimated by a Tanita Body Composition Analyzer.

Additionally, a weight history questionnaire was used to collect self-reported body weights (in whole lb. or kg, while not pregnant) at 21, 45, and 65 years of age, for individuals 21 years or older at baseline. If participants indicated that they could not remember their exact weight, personnel were instructed to inquire about their best guess. The quality control procedures and data cleaning are described in the Appendix. We converted each weight from the weight histories to kg and rounded each weight to the whole unit, to eliminate measurement error by unit of report (e.g. lb. or kg).

We excluded all weights from women who reported currently being pregnant at baseline or individuals with limb amputations that otherwise did not limit their ability to stand (Additional file 1: Figure S2 and Table S1). Using measured height at baseline, we calculated two baseline BMI measures (kg/m^2) and up to three BMIs from the weight histories of individuals at least 21 years of age (corresponding to 21, 45, and 65 years). We further excluded any BMI that was less < 16 or > 70 kg/m^2. As measured height is an imperfect proxy of an individual's height at various times in the past, all models of BMI from the weight histories (at 21, 45, and 65 years) also accounted for the age at baseline as a measure of age at time of recall.

Type 2 diabetes assessment

HCHS/SOL participants were asked to bring in the medications they were currently taking, during the baseline examination. Individuals were also asked to report if a "doctor ever said that you have diabetes (high sugar in blood or urine)" and the age when this diagnosis was received. Participants were asked to fast overnight (> 8 h)

and their glucose was measured in the entire sample, and 2-h post-oral glucose tolerance tests was measured among those who reported never having received a diabetes diagnosis. Impaired fasting glucose among non-diabetics was defined as a fasting glucose 100-125 mg/dL or 140-199 mg/dL after oral glucose challenge. We used the American Diabetes Association definition to identify T2D cases at examination based on fasting glucose (≥126 mg/dL), an oral glucose tolerance test (OGTT, ≥200 mg/dL), percent Glycated Hemoglobin (HbA1C ≥6.5%), or diabetes medications [35]. Controlled diabetes was further defined as % HbA1C < 7%.

Type of diabetes was not reported in HCHS/SOL. Therefore, we used information on age at diabetes diagnosis to create age period-specific T2D diagnosis indicators. If an individual was younger than 45 or 65 years at the baseline examination, then the classification of T2D diagnosis of the incomplete age period was set to missing (e.g. for a 50-year-old, T2D diagnosis for the period of 22–45 years could be yes/no, but would be set to missing for 46–65 years).

Genetic information

Venous blood samples were collected and for all fully consenting participants (i.e. those agreeing to genotyping and sharing of information with HCHS/SOL investigators, those not affiliated with HCHS/SOL, and specialized laboratories) and were analyzed using the MetaboChip (Illumina, Inc., San Diego, CA) (N = 12,209 or 74% of the cohort). The MetaboChip array contains approximately 200,000 single nucleotide polymorphisms (SNPs) at 257 genomic regions previously associated with cardiometabolic traits, including the *TCF7L2* region that includes 258 SNPs across over 76,159 bp [36]. HCHS/SOL participants used in this study were genotyped at the Human Genetics Center of the University of Texas-Houston (Houston, TX) and passed person-level quality control filters (< 95% call rate, sex discordance or duplicate).

Based on previous trans-ethnic fine-mapping studies with T2D [37] and BMI [15], we selected rs7903146 as our presumed functional variant of interest at *TCF7L2* as it was in strong linkage disequilibrium with several other variants in the area (Additional file 1: Figure S1). In HCHS/SOL, this SNP also had satisfactory quality control measures [38], was in Hardy-Weinberg-Equilibrium (P value = 0.10), and available in the entire sample that passed genetic quality control procedures (n = 12,117). We created an additive score of the number of T2D risk alleles [7, 8] per individual at rs7903146 (e.g. CC = 0, CT = 1, TT = 2). To aid in the interpretability of adjustments for population stratification, we adjusted for continental ancestry proportions, which as reported on previously [39] were designed to represent four a priori-selected ancestral populations using a supervised analysis (K = 4; unrelated

1000 Genomes references representing European: CEU; African: YRI; Northern: MXL; Caribbean/Southern Native American Ancestry: PUR, CLM) in the program ADMIX-TURE [40] on a pruned set of more than 45,000 MetaboChip SNPs in low linkage disequilibrium in our sample ($r^2 < 0.5$). Lastly, we also adjusted for the 'genetic analysis group' variable from the multidimensional clustering of self-reported Hispanic/Latino background and principal components from genome-wide data on a majority-overlapping sample of 12,803 HCHS/SOL participants (> 99% call rate), as described previously [39].

Statistical analyses

As shown in Fig. 1, of the entire HCHS/SOL baseline cohort of 16,415 participants, 16,322 individuals had self-reported and measured weight values that passed quality control (additional information provided as part of Additional file 1: Figure S2 and Table S1). Of the 12,209 individuals providing their full informed consent for genotyping and data sharing, 12,117 passed genetic quality control, as described above. The union of these

two quality controlled data sets included 12,073 individuals (Fig. 1), from which we excluded 87 individuals who reported diabetes diagnosis prior to 22 years of age, to restrict our analysis to those for which a diabetes diagnosis was more likely to be T2D, and 1054 individuals that did not have both a measured current height or at least one self-reported weight at 21, 45 or 65 years and who were therefore unable to contribute to our structural equation modeling. Individuals with missing covariate information, such as missing genetic analysis group ($N = 122$) or information on their highest education level achieved (categorized as less than or at least a high school diploma or equivalency) ($N = 14$), were excluded. Lastly, as described previously in HCHS/SOL we used an identity-by-descent analysis in PLINK [41] to identify close relatives (e.g. 0.35 < π < 0.98) [42], and exclude the individual in each pair with the least weight measurements ($N = 1765$). A total of 9031 individuals remained in the final analytic dataset used for all analyses, and we described their characteristics using descriptive statistics such as means, 95% confidence intervals (CIs), and frequencies.

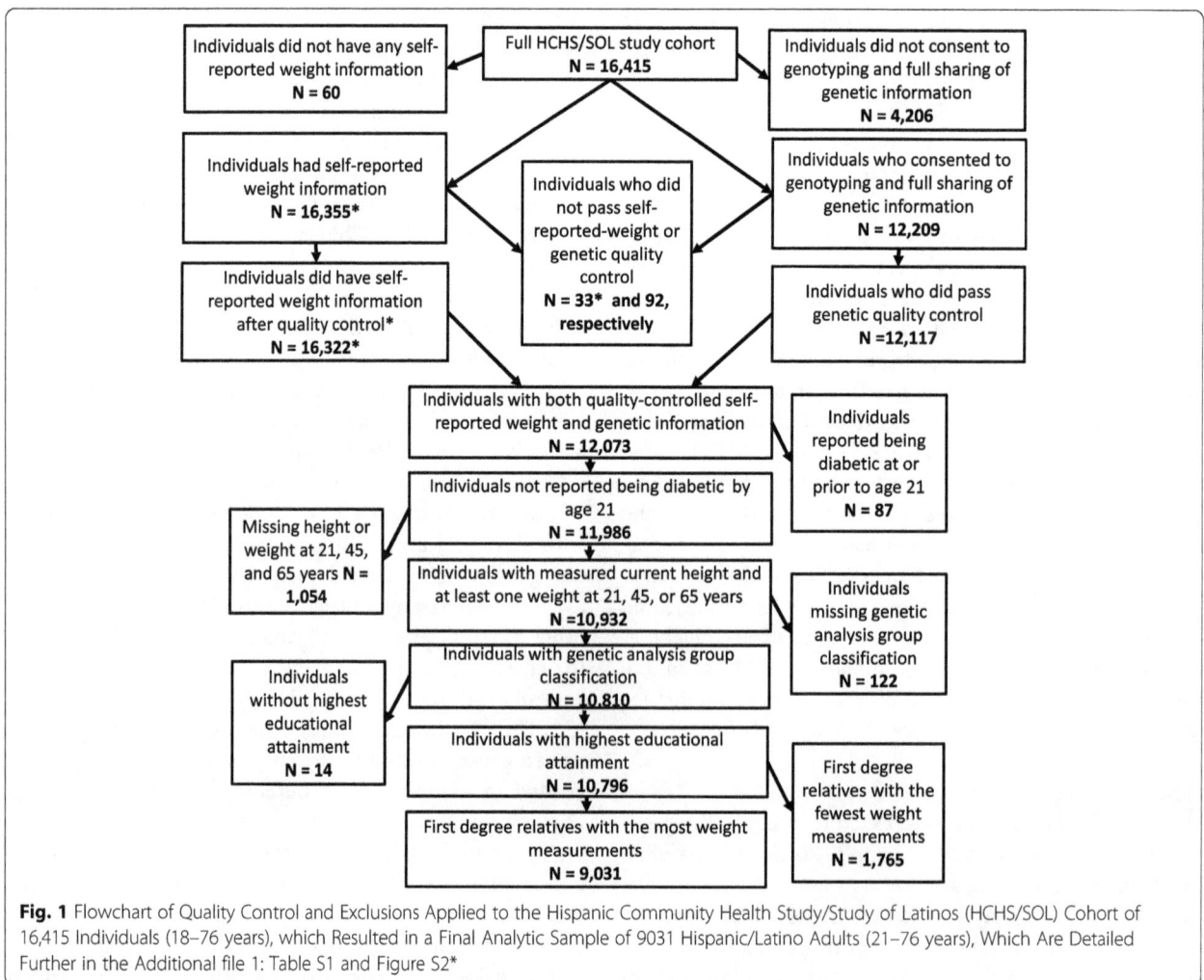

Fig. 1 Flowchart of Quality Control and Exclusions Applied to the Hispanic Community Health Study/Study of Latinos (HCHS/SOL) Cohort of 16,415 Individuals (18–76 years), which Resulted in a Final Analytic Sample of 9031 Hispanic/Latino Adults (21–76 years), Which Are Detailed Further in the Additional file 1: Table S1 and Figure S2*

Next, we modeled the association between the additive number of rs7903146-T alleles with multiple BMI measures using multivariable models (e.g. measured and self-reported BMI at baseline, as well as BMI for ages 21, 45 and 65 years), controlling for age at examination, sex, educational attainment, admixture proportions, and genetic analysis group. As an exploratory analysis, we also examined the multivariable associations with the measured BMI stratified by previous diabetes diagnosis, as well as glucose tolerance and diabetic medication at examination.

Using structural equation models, we then examined an a priori-specified set of pathways (Additional file 1: Figure S3) between the additive number of rs7903146-T alleles, BMI (at age 21, 45 and 65), and self-reported T2D status (between ages 22–45 and between ages 46–65). BMI was assumed to be directly associated with T2D status in the period immediately after the BMI measurement (between ages 22–45 or 46–65). Similarly, T2D status during the period of time immediately preceding a given BMI (e.g. T2D between 22 and 45 years and 45-year-old weight) was assumed to be directly associated with the BMI at that time. Direct pathways between rs7903146 to BMIs and T2D measurements were also included. BMI at the previous age was assumed to be directly related to BMI at the following age. Age at baseline examination (age at time of recall), sex, education level, admixture proportions and genetic analysis group, and were included in all pathways to BMI and T2D.

All analyses accounted for the HCHS/SOL complex sampling design, including primary sampling unit, strata and sampling weights, yielding valid estimates of the disease distribution in the source population. Descriptive statistics were estimated using SAS 9.3 (Research Triangle Park, NC). All multivariable and structural equation models were estimated using Mplus 7.11 software [43], using full-information maximum likelihood methods to account for missing outcome data. Additionally, we identified our analysis subpopulation ($N = 9031$), or the subpopulation of interest in any stratified models, and used the complex sampling information on the entire cohort in the variance calculations to ensure valid estimates for the source population of HCHS/SOL.

Results
Our weighted sample included women (50%) and men, an average age of 44 years at baseline examination (Table 1). Five percent of those who were at least 45 years old (unweighted $n = 5605$) received a T2D diagnosis by age 45 (Table 1). In the subsample of participants who were at least 65 years of age ($n = 729$), 23% reported received a diabetes diagnosis by age 65, with 3% being diagnosed by age 45 and 20% diagnosed between ages 46–65 years. Average BMIs increased across age of recalled weight (24 kg/m^2 at 21 years to 29 kg/m^2 at 65 years).

The number of T2D-risk alleles at rs7903146 associated with an increase in T2D prevalence by 7% (P value = 0.0002) and decreased obesity prevalence by 3–5%, based on either the use of measured or self-reported weights (P value < 0.04, Table 2). Mean BMI and waist circumference at examination showed similar quantitative decreases by $0.5–0.6 \text{ kg/m}^2$ and 1.1 cm as the number of T2D-risk allele increased (P values < 0.1). Additionally, among the subsample without a past diagnosis of T2D, at examination mean OGTT glucose levels increased by (4 mg/dL difference; P value = 0.06) and HOMA Index of Beta Cell function decreased (12 point difference; P value = 0.07). Other T2D-related measures, such as fasting glucose, insulin, and HbA1C exhibited similar trends across genotypes, but these trends were not statistically significant (P values ≥ 0.1). Further stratification of BMIs by T2D status/age at examination suggested that both increased age and T2D status corresponded to higher average BMIs, regardless of the timing of T2D diagnosis (Table 3). The subset of participants > 65 years at examination self-reported weights corresponding to a mean BMI increase of 2.8 kg/m^2 between 45 and 65 years of age among those without T2D at baseline, and of up to 3.4 kg/m^2 among those that were diagnosed with T2D after age 65.

Multivariable association analyses
We observed an association between the rs7903146 T2D-increasing allele and lower BMI, after adjustment for age, sex, education level, admixture proportions, and genetic analysis group. Specifically, we found that each T allele associated with lower BMI at examination (21–76 years), based on either measured or self-reported weight (Table 4). As described previously [15], we also observed significant inverse associations between each rs7903146-T allele and BMI ($- 0.37 \text{ kg/m}^2$, 95% CI: -0.69, $- 0.06$). Additionally, we also observed non-significant multivariable associations between rs7903146-T and lower BMIs at 21, and 45 years of age, and non-significant increases in BMI at 65 years of age.

Using data from the baseline examination, we also ran these BMI models stratified by previous diabetes diagnosis, glucose tolerance and medication status at the baseline examination (Additional file 1: Table S2). Weaker effects per allele on BMI were estimated among participants who reported having diabetes at examination as compared to those without diabetes, regardless of the use of measured or self-reported BMI at examination ($- 0.30$ to $- 0.17$ versus $- 0.45$ to $- 0.48 \text{ kg/m}^2$ per allele). Compared to our significant protective effect on BMI among all individuals without a prior diabetes diagnosis ($- 0.45 \text{ kg/m}^2$ per allele), the subset of individuals who had impaired fasting glucose or undiagnosed T2D at the examination ($N = 4284$) appeared to have an even stronger protective estimated effect on BMI ($- 0.66$ and $- 0.85 \text{ kg/m}^2$, respectively).

Table 1 Weighted Descriptive Statistics of Hispanic Community Health Study/Study of Latinos Baseline (2008–2011) Analytic Sample of 9031 Adults (21–76 years) from Four Urban United States Centers: The Bronx, NY; Chicago, IL; Miami, FL; San Diego, CA

Unweighted Analytic Sample Size and Weighted Frequency or Means (95% Confidence Interval)		
Female (%)	$n = 5187$	50%
Mean (95% CI) Age at Baseline Examination	$n = 9031$	43.67 (43.12, 44.21)
Has High School Diploma or Equivalency (%)	$n = 5768$	69%
Genetic Analysis Group (%)	South American ($n = 676$)	6%
	Central American ($n = 1069$)	8%
	Cuban ($n = 1764$)	27%
	Dominican ($n = 797$)	9%
	Mexican ($n = 3169$)	33%
	Puerto Rican ($n = 1556$)	17%
rs7903146 Genotype Frequency (%)	CC ($n = 5040$)	55%
	CT ($n = 3373$)	38%
	TT ($n = 618$)	7%
Mean (95% CI) BMI (kg/m^2)	At 21 Years ($n = 8759$)	23.77 (23.61, 23.93)
	At 45 Years ($n = 5605$)	27.48 (27.30, 27.66)
	At 65 Years ($n = 729$)	28.99 (28.46, 29.53)
% with Self-Reported Diabetes Diagnosis	Between the Ages of 22 and 45 Years	5%
	Between the Ages of 46 and 65 Years	23%

Abbreviations: *BMI* body mass index, *95% CI* 95% confidence interval

No significant effects were seen for individuals taking diabetes medication at examination.

Structured association analyses

In a structural equation model, we noted that each T allele at rs7903146 was directly associated with a 1.32 (95% CI: 1.05, 1.67) higher odds of T2D diagnosis between the ages of 22 and 45 years, and a 1.67 (95% CI: 1.15, 2.42) higher odds of T2D diagnosis between 22 and 65 years of age. We did not find any significant direct associations between the rs7903146-T and BMI at any age; however, the direction of estimated effect was inverse on BMI at 21 and 45 years (Fig. 2). Furthermore, we found no evidence of indirect associations between rs7903146 and either BMI or T2D at any time point (Additional file 1: Table S3). Similarly, the indirect association between rs7903146 and BMI at 45 and 65 years, as mediated through a previous T2D diagnosis, was negative but non-significant (Additional file 1: Table S4).

Discussion

In this study we successfully replicated the previously-reported association between T2D risk alleles at *TCF7L2* (rs7903146-T) and decreased BMI [3, 10–12], within a population-based cohort of US Hispanic/Latino adults of multiple background groups living in four urban communities (21–76 years of age at examination). We also observed consistently protective, albeit non-significant, associations on BMI at 21 and 45 years. In contrast,

among the subset of individuals 65 years or older, the non-significant association between T2D-risk variants and BMI at 65 years of age was positive.

Next, we employed a structural equation model to examine the direct and indirect pathways between rs7903146, T2D and BMI, which revealed that this suggestive protective effect between T2D-risk variants and BMI at 21 and 45 years of age remained even after controlling for earlier BMI. These results collectively suggest that there may be a persistent independent protective effect of *TCF7L2* T2D risk alleles on BMI across most of adulthood. In contrast to a previous cross-sectional study of 1235 Hispanic/Latinos, which estimated a larger effects of T2D-risk alleles at *TCF7L2* on BMI by adjusting for concurrent T2D status (– 0.3 to – 1.1 kg/m^2 for rs12255372-T) [12], our large and diverse study of US Hispanic/Latinos estimated more modest effects of T2D-risk alleles on BMI (– 0.4 kg/m^2 for rs7903146-T; unadjusted for T2D status) and leveraged information on weight and T2D histories collected during the HCHS/SOL baseline examination to further decompose the complex relationships between prior BMI and T2D (Effect of each T2D-risk allele on BMI ranged from – 0.2 to 0.2 kg/m^2 at 21 and 65 years of age, respectively).

Our findings shed light on the two predominant hypotheses put forth to explain the inverse direction of association between T2D and BMI at *TCF7L2*, as captured by variation in rs7903146. First, it has been suggested that case ascertainment bias [17] may drive the association of

Table 2 Anthropometric Measures (Body Mass Index; Weight; Height; Waist Circumference; Overall and Abdominal Obesity; Percentage Body Fat), Fasting Insulin and Glucose, Post-Oral Glucose Tolerance Test Response, and Diabetic Control Characteristics Weighted Means (Standard Deviations) or Frequencies across rs7903146 Genotypes ($n = 9031$) at the Hispanic Community Health Study/Study of Latinos Baseline Examination

	CC	CT	TT	P-value
Unweighted total analytic sample size	$n = 5040$	$n = 3373$	$n = 618$	
Measured BMI[a] (kg/m^2)	29.74 (0.17)	29.26 (0.13)	29.21 (0.28)	0.06
Self-Reported BMI[a] (kg/m^2)	29.81 (0.17)	29.34 (0.13)	29.23 (0.27)	0.05
Measured Weight (kg)	80.09 (0.52)	78.71 (0.39)	78.58 (0.79)	0.1
Self-Reported Weight (kg)	80.29 (0.53)	78.94 (0.39)	78.69 (0.76)	0.1
Measured Height (cm)	163.93 (0.18)	163.83 (0.19)	163.94 (0.32)	0.9
% Overall Measured Obesity ($\geq$30 kg/m^2 Measured BMI)	42.43%	37.89%	38.55%	0.03
% Overall Self-Reported Obesity ($\geq$30 kg/m^2 Self-Reported BMI)	43.29%	38.85%	37.66%	0.03
Waist Circumference (cm)	98.41 (0.40)	97.37 (0.31)	97.34 (0.65)	0.09
% Abdominal Measured Obesity ($\geq$120 cm for men; $\geq$88 cm for women)	56.1%	55.2%	57.1%	0.7
% Body Fat	33.58 (0.21)	32.96 (0.19)	33.18 (0.4)	0.08
% Identified as Diabetic Before or at Baseline Examination[b]	14.77%	18.24%	21.01%	0.0002
Unweighted non-diabetic subsample	$n = 4107$	$n = 2586$	$n = 454$	
Fasting Insulin (mU/L)	11.98 (0.2)	11.96 (0.19)	11.53 (0.47)	0.7
Fasting Glucose (mg/dL)	93.78 (0.18)	94.12 (0.23)	94.67 (0.51)	0.2
HOMA Index of Beta Cell Function	145.17 (2.59)	140.81 (2.33)	133.28 (4.81)	0.07
HOMA Index of Insulin Resistance	2.82 (0.05)	2.84 (0.05)	2.75 (0.12)	0.8
post OGTT Insulin (mU/L)[c]	78.06 (1.81)	81.09 (1.84)	75.39 (3.2)	0.2
post OGTT, Glucose (mg/dL)[c]	112.25 (0.78)	114.23 (0.85)	115.85 (1.6)	0.06
Glycated Hemoglobin (mmol/mol)	35.77 (0.1)	35.99 (0.1)	35.72 (0.22)	0.2
% Glycated Hemoglobin	5.42 (0.01)	5.44 (0.01)	5.41 (0.02)	0.2
Unweighted diabetic[b] subsample	$n = 933$	$n = 787$	$n = 164$	
Glycated Hemoglobin (mmol/mol)	57.55 (1.25)	57.79 (0.94)	60.06 (2.06)	0.6
% Glycated Hemoglobin	7.42 (0.11)	7.44 (0.09)	7.64 (0.19)	0.6
% Controlled Diabetes (< 7% Glycated Hemoglobin)	26.1%	31.2%	35.3%	0.1

All weighted means and standard deviations (or percentages) for anthropometric measures (weight, height, body mass index, waist circumference, fat percentage, overall and abdominal obesity) were estimated from regression models, which accounted for the complex sampling design and age, sex, and ancestry proportions. Additionally, all other weighted means and standard deviations (or percentages) were adjusted for body mass index (BMI) at examination. rs7903146 genotypes were modeled dis-jointly (i.e. no additive model was assumed)

[a]Measured and self-reported BMI values at baseline were based off of measured weight and height, and self-reported weight and measured height, respectively
[b]The diabetes subsample included individuals reporting having received a previous diabetes diagnosis at baseline examination, or being identified as diabetic at the baseline examination
[c]2-h Oral Glucose Tolerance Test (OGTT) was conducted in only individuals who did not report having had a previous diabetes diagnosis

TCF7L2 T2D risk alleles and lower BMI, as previous GWAS have shown attenuated effects of TCF7L2 on BMI among population-based samples as compared to the effect sizes in samples of T2D cases [15]. Specifically, collider stratification may bias the TCF7L2-BMI association downwards when the ratio T2D cases to controls has been distorted to over-represent cases, or cases with more favorable insulin resistance profiles [44]. The active HCHS/SOL community engagement, household sampling, and location of clinic sites in the local community all served to minimize selection bias.

The consistent negative association between T2D risk alleles and BMI in early and mid-adulthood seen in this and previous work [3, 10, 11] may point to another explanation. A growing body of literature implicates pleiotropy at TCF7L2 in both T2D and BMI [5]. We observed protective associations on BMI at 21 and 45 years of age, which were not explained by accounting for indirect pathways through T2D or earlier BMI in our structured modeling. This work leverages detailed weight history data to provide further evidence for a complex mechanism underlying TCF7L2 action across the life course that may explain its associations

Table 3 Weighted Mean Body Mass Indices at 45 and 65 years by Categories of Baseline Examination and Diabetes Diagnosis Ages in the Hispanic Community Health Study/Study of Latinos among Participants > 45 Years of Age ($n = 5643$)

	Unweighted Sample Size	BMI (95% CI) at Age 45 (kg/m^2)	BMI (95% CI) at Age 65 (kg/m^2)
Between 46 and 65 Years of Age ($n = 4,914$)			
No Diabetes Diagnosis Reporting at Baseline Examination[a]	$n = 4094$	27.49 (27.29, 27.69)	–
Diagnosed Between 22 and 45	$n = 318$	30.36 (29.53, 31.19)	–
Diagnosed Between 46 and Age at Examination	$n = 502$	29.30 (28.68, 29.93)	–
Between 66 and 76 Years of Age ($n = 729$)			
No Diabetes Diagnosis Reported at Baseline Examination[a]	$n = 502$	25.67 (25.16, 26.18)	28.43 (27.72, 29.14)
Diagnosed Between 22 and 45	$n = 26$	26.51 (25.03, 27.99)	29.71 (27.56, 31.86)
Diagnosed Between 46 and 65	$n = 153$	27.75 (27.06, 28.45)	30.65 (29.53, 31.77)
Diagnosed Between 66 and Age at Examination	$n = 48$	25.89 (24.71, 27.07)	29.32 (27.58, 31.07)

Abbreviations: *BMI* body mass index, *95% CI* 95% confidence interval
[a]This categorization includes individuals who were first diagnosed at the baseline clinic visit

with both T2D and BMI [3, 10–12], or the apparent statistical interaction between *TCF7L2* genotype and adiposity on T2D related traits seen in previous cross-sectional studies of US Hispanic/Latinos [31]. Yet, clearly future functional or longitudinal analyses in population-based samples are required to substantiate our study's findings.

Herein, we were also able to explore for the first time to our knowledge, what might be the direct effect of T2D diagnosis on subsequent BMI in the context of *TCF7L2* genetic effects. The receipt of a T2D diagnosis between 22 and 45 years of age was significantly associated with an average increase in BMI at 45 years, as compared to those that never received a diagnosis during this time (Fig. 2). We did observe a similar, but non-significant association of T2D diagnosis between 46 and 65 years on BMI at 65 years. This indicates that the possible impact of pre-diagnosis metabolic dysfunction, T2D-related lifestyle counseling, or medical intervention also does not fully explain the apparent negative association between the *TCF7L2* T2D risk allele and BMI [15]. This was further supported by our non-significant *TCF7L2* associations on

BMI at the examination among T2D individuals concurrently taking medications (Additional file 1: Table S2).

This current analysis is additionally strengthened by its focus on adults of varied Hispanic/Latino backgrounds [45]. Our sampling weights accounted for non-response and our statistical modeling approach also allowed us to account for missing data under the assumption of non-informative missingness and to base our variance calculations on information on the full population-based sample. In our dataset, missingness for age-specific BMIs was primarily determined by one's age (BMI at 45 and 65 years of age would be missing for a 35-year-old participant).

Even though a previous study, which did not genotype rs7903146 directly, has posited that their best marker SNP at *TCF7L2* (rs12255372, $r^2 = 0.7$ in AMR with rs7903146) may capture a secondary BMI signal in Hispanic/Latinos [12], subsequent trans-ethnic fine-mapping studies of BMI and T2D including diverse Hispanic/Latino samples [8, 46] and large Hispanic/Latino studies have not supported the presence of multiple signals [47]. This gives us confidence

Table 4 Adjusted Parameter Estimates[a] between rs7903146-T and Body Mass Indices[b] at the Hispanic Community Health Study/Study of Latinos Baseline Examination Representing 9031 Individuals (21–76 Years of Age), and at Several Ages Across the Lifecourse

	Sample Size[c]	Estimated Change in kg/m^2 (95% CI) per T2D risk allele	P-value
Measured BMI at Examination	$n = 9012$	−0.37 (− 0.69, − 0.06)	0.019
Self-reported BMI at Examination	$n = 8921$	−0.38 (− 0.69, − 0.08)	0.015
Self-reported BMI at 21 Years	$n = 8759$	−0.20 (− 0.45, 0.04)	0.109
Self-reported BMI at 45 Years	$n = 5605$	− 0.18 (− 0.43, 0.06)	0.134
Self-reported BMI at 65 Years	$n = 729$	0.01 (− 0.82, 0.84)	0.980

Abbreviations: *BMI* Body mass index, *T2D* Type 2 diabetes, *95% CI* 95% confidence interval
[a]Corresponding to the additive number of T2D risk alleles at *TCF7L2* (rs7903146-T) and then adjusted for age, sex, education level, genetic ancestry group and ancestry proportions
[b]Body mass index (BMI) was based on self-reported or measured weight in kg, and divided by squared measured height at examination in meters (kg/m^2)
[c]Unweighted sample size differences were a result of individuals missing certain weight measurements. For example, only individuals that were had reached 21, 45 or 65 years of age were asked to provide their weight for that particular age

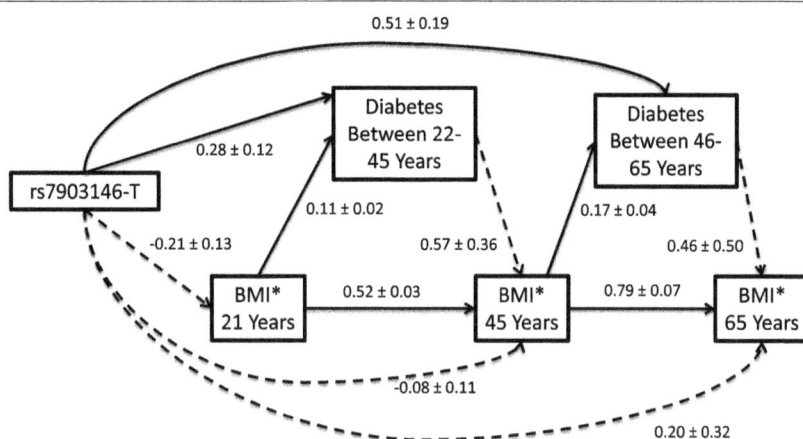

Fig. 2 Illustration of structured pathways (effect estimates and standard errors) between the additive number of rs7903146-T alleles, diabetes, and Body Mass Index (BMI), showing paths with P values < 0.05 in solid lines

that rs7903146, the lead variant for the single T2D signal observed in HCHS/SOL [48], is the best available SNP marker to simultaneously investigate allelic effects on BMI and T2D diagnosis within a structural equation modeling framework. Nonetheless, we do acknowledge that our current results do not capture all possible sources of pleiotropy at the *TCF7L2* locus, which warrants further study.

Our structural equation results are also limited by our reliance on self-reported age of diabetes diagnosis, instead of repeated quantitative measures of T2D or its successful control. Among Hispanic/Latinos 15–19 year old, less than two thirds of diabetes cases may be Type 1, but the type distribution of cases steadily trends towards more T2D cases into early adulthood [49]—a period captured in HCHS/SOL. For this reason, we excluded a small number of individuals reporting early onset (< 22 years, $N = 87$) of diabetes. In HCHS/SOL, an additional $N = 344$ individuals reported a diabetes diagnosed between 22 and 45 years of age, only 30% of which were taking insulin by the baseline examination. Without medical or medication histories, we were unable to validate if these were T2D, or Latent Autoimmune Diabetes in Adults cases who would be expected to be leaner on average [50]. Nonetheless we take confidence in the observation that the association of *TCF7L2* T2D-risk alleles and BMI was stronger among those without previous T2D diagnosis. In fact, individuals with impaired glucose tolerance and undiagnosed diabetes at examination had the greatest protective effect on BMI of T2D-risk alleles at *TCF7L2*. Forthcoming HCHS/SOL, or other prospective cohort follow up data will allow future investigators to explore the contemporaneous and interacting relationships between *TCF7L2*, BMI and T2D status across the adult life course.

Similarly, our structural equation modeling was notably limited by its reliance on self-reported weight histories,

and height measured at the baseline examination to approximate the BMIs at 21, 45 and 65 years of age. Nonetheless this study cohort self-reported their current weight with good accuracy and reliability at baseline [34], and we robustly replicated our unstructured *TCF7L2* associations with BMI at examination (21–76 years) using both measured and self-reported current weights. Lastly, we cannot rule out the role of birth cohort or healthy immigrant effects in shaping the characteristics of our sample of predominantly foreign-born middle-aged adults, especially among the subset of older adults in HCHS/SOL (e.g. ≥65 years of age) who were healthy enough to be community-dwelling at the time of recruitment, and willing to participate in the extensive baseline examination. Our structured modeling sheds light on this survival bias, as T2D-risk alleles were non-significantly associated with an increased BMI at 65 years of age, independent of earlier BMIs and T2D statuses.

Conclusions

Our significant population-based associations between T2D risk alleles at *TCF7L2* (rs7903146) and lower BMI do not support selection bias as the sole explanation of the *TCF7L2*-BMI association. This work contributes to a mounting body of literature reporting consistent protective effects of T2D risk alleles at *TCF7L2* and BMI, which points to a complex mechanistic structure underlying the functional consequences of *TCF7L2* on both T2D and BMI. Yet, future functional work is needed to describe the specific cell or tissue types that are most relevant to the observed *TCF7L2* action. Observational analyses may be particularly useful for estimating causal effects at this genetic locus and pinpointing windows of susceptibility for future public health interventions in populations, like US Hispanic/Latinos, which carry disproportionate burdens of both T2D and obesity.

Appendix

Between 2008 and 2011, up to 15 participants per site were invited to repeat the Hispanic Community Health Study/ Study of Latinos (HCHS/SOL) examination, including the weight history questionnaire, one to three months after their initial baseline examination without additional reimbursement of their time ($N = 56$). A total of 52 participants reported body weights a median of 40 days after their initial baseline examination (range: 0 to 107 days). The mean differences of the 21 and 45-year old self-reported weight were -0.9 kg (-2.7, 1.0) and -1.3 kg (-3.8, 1.1) resulting in good reliabilities and low coefficients of variation (21-year recall: ICC = 0.89, CV = 7.7% $n = 52$; 45-year recall: 0.86, 6.7%, $n = 29$). Only two participants, ≥ 65 years of age, recalled their 65-year old weight twice, which precluded reliability calculations for 65-year old weights.

HCHS/SOL personnel (requiring a minimum of 5 practice subjects with 0.5 kg weight and 0.5 cm height agreement between a trainee and expert) measured height (cm) and weight (kg) during the anthropometric examination of the full HCHS/SOL cohort using a fixed (wall mounted) stadiometer (inspected daily) and a digital scale (scales zero balanced daily and calibrated weekly) on all participants that were able to stand on both feet while wearing a scrub suit or examination gown and no shoes [34]. Currently pregnant women were rescheduled for the HCHS/SOL baseline examination approximately 3 months after their delivery. The validity of self-reported weight, and inter-rater reliability of self-reported weight, measured weight and height have been reported to be good for the HCHS/SOL baseline examination [34].

HCHS/SOL study personnel were centrally trained and periodically observed. In addition we applied a data quality control protocol, as described previously for self-reported current weight collected as part of the anthropometric examination [34] to 1) minimize potential instances of unit confusion in the self-report (lb versus kg) or 2) exclude self-reported weights during pregnancy reported during the baseline examination, self-reported or measured weights made by individuals with past limb amputation or when scaled by measured baseline height that correspond to extreme underweight (< 16 kg/m^2) or obesity (> 70 kg/m^2). However, herein, we extended this protocol to also include recalled weights at 21, 45, or 65 years of age. We first flagged entire weight histories with either a ≥ 15 kg difference between current self-reported and measured weight, or at least two ≥ 15 kg pairwise fluctuations in weight (Additional file 1: Figure S1 and Table S1). Of the entire set of 16,355 individuals with at least one self-reported weight in adulthood (40,525 observations) and based on our staged quality control protocol, we recoded a total of 54 observations, and excluded an additional 541 observations (Additional file 1: Table S1). Only six self-reported weights from the anthropometric examination (age range 27–

64 years) were recoded and retained in our final analytic sample.

Abbreviations
BMI: Body Mass Index; GWAS: Genome-wide Association Study; HCHS/ SOL: Hispanic Community Health Study/Study of Latinos; OGTT: Oral Glucose Tolerance Test; HbA1C: Glycated Hemoglobin; SNP: Single Nucleotide Polymorphism; T2D: Type 2 Diabetes; TCF7L2: Transcription Factor 7-like 2; US: United States

Acknowledgements
The authors thank the staff and participants of HCHS/SOL for their important contributions.

Funding
This work was supported by the National Institute of Diabetes and Digestive and Kidney Diseases (Grant 5R01DK101855). LFR was supported by the Eunice Kennedy Shriver National Institute of Child Health and Human Development (T32-HD007168) and the Carolina Population Center (P2C-HD050924). Additionally, the Hispanic Community Health Study/Study of Latinos was carried out as a collaborative study supported by contracts from the National Heart, Lung, and Blood Institute to the University of North Carolina (Grant N01-HC65233), University of Miami (Grant N01-HC65234), Albert Einstein College of Medicine (Grant N01-HC65235), Northwestern University (Grant N01-HC65236), and San Diego State University (Grant N01-HC65237). The following Institutes/Centers/Offices contributed to the HCHS/SOL through a transfer of funds to the NHLBI: National Center on Minority Health and Health Disparities, the National Institute of Deafness and Other Communications Disorders, the National Institute of Dental and Craniofacial Research, the National Institute of Diabetes and Digestive and Kidney Diseases, the National Institute of Neurological Disorders and Stroke, and the Office of Dietary Supplements.

Authors' contributions
The coauthors of this work have collectively contributed to the manuscript the following ways: LFR conceived of the study's aims, conducted all data quality control measures, and oversaw the statistical analyses, which were conducted by AGH using genetic variables generated by MG and CCL. LFR and AGH then drafted the manuscript jointly. CRI, HMH, KLY, ES, JEB, QQ, AEJ, SFG, CH, RJFL, and KEN have contributed to the content of the final manuscript. CRI, RCK, and GP participated in the design of the HCHS/SOL. SFG, CH, RJFL, and KEN each contributed substantially to the background and discussion of our study findings. All authors read and approved the final manuscript.

Competing interests
The authors declare that they have no competing interests.

Author details
[1]Department of Epidemiology, UNC Gillings School of Global Public Health, University of North Carolina at Chapel Hill, 123 W Franklin St, Building C, Chapel Hill, NC, USA. [2]Carolina Population Center, University of North Carolina at Chapel Hill, 123 W Franklin St, Building C, Chapel Hill, NC, USA. [3]Department of Biostatistics, UNC Gillings School of Global Public Health, University of North Carolina at Chapel Hill, Chapel Hill, NC, USA. [4]Department of Epidemiology and Population Health, Albert Einstein College of Medicine, Bronx, NY, USA. [5]Department of Anthropology, University of Toronto at Mississauga, Mississauga, ON, Canada. [6]Department of Medicine, Vanderbilt University Medical Center, Nashville, TN, USA. [7]Biomedical and Translational Informatics Institute, Geisinger Health System, Danville, PA, USA. [8]Epidemiology Branch, National Heart Lung and Blood Institute, Bethesda, MD, USA. [9]Department of Biostatistics, School of Public Health, University of Washington, Seattle, WA, USA. [10]Divisions of Human Genetics and Endocrinology, Children's Hospital of Philadelphia Research Institute, Philadelphia, PA, USA. [11]Department of Preventive Medicine, Norris Comprehensive Cancer Center, Keck School of Medicine, University of Southern California, Los Angeles, CA, USA. [12]Charles R. Bronfman Instituted for Personalized Medicine, Icahn School of Medicine at Mount Sinai, New York, NY, USA.

References
1. Davidson JA, Kannel WB, Lopez-Candales A, Morales L, Moreno PR, Ovalle F, Rodriguez CJ, Rodbard HW, Rosenson RS, Stern M. Avoiding the looming Latino/Hispanic cardiovascular health crisis: a call to action. J Cardiometab Syndr. 2007;2(4):238–43.
2. Bhupathiraju SN, Hu FB. Epidemiology of obesity and diabetes and their cardiovascular complications. Circ Res. 2016;118(11):1723–35.
3. Grant SF, Thorleifsson G, Reynisdottir I, Benediktsson R, Manolescu A, Sainz J, Helgason A, Stefansson H, Emilsson V, Helgadottir A, et al. Variant of transcription factor 7-like 2 (TCF7L2) gene confers risk of type 2 diabetes. Nat Genet. 2006;38(3):320–3.
4. Sladek R, Rocheleau G, Rung J, Dina C, Shen L, Serre D, Boutin P, Vincent D, Belisle A, Hadjadj S, et al. A genome-wide association study identifies novel risk loci for type 2 diabetes. Nature. 2007;445(7130):881–5.
5. Jin T. Current understanding on role of the Wnt signaling pathway effector TCF7L2 in glucose homeostasis. Endocr Rev. 2016:er20151146.
6. McCarthy MI, Rorsman P, Gloyn AL. TCF7L2 and diabetes: a tale of two tissues, and of two species. Cell Metab. 2013;17(2):157–9.
7. Williams AL, Jacobs SB, Moreno-Macias H, Huerta-Chagoya A, Churchhouse C, Marquez-Luna C, Garcia-Ortiz H, Gomez-Vazquez MJ, Burtt NP, Aguilar-Salinas CA, et al. Sequence variants in SLC16A11 are a common risk factor for type 2 diabetes in Mexico. Nature. 2014;506(7486):97–101.
8. Mahajan A, Go MJ, Zhang W, Below JE, Gaulton KJ, Ferreira T, Horikoshi M, Johnson AD, Ng MC, Prokopenko I, et al. Genome-wide trans-ancestry meta-analysis provides insight into the genetic architecture of type 2 diabetes susceptibility. Nat Genet. 2014;46(3):234–44.
9. Parra EJ, Cameron E, Simmonds L, Valladares A, McKeigue P, Shriver M, Wacher N, Kumate J, Kittles R, Cruz M. Association of TCF7L2 polymorphisms with type 2 diabetes in Mexico City. Clin Genet. 2007;71(4):359–66.
10. Cauchi S, Meyre D, Dina C, Choquet H, Samson C, Gallina S, Balkau B, Charpentier G, Pattou F, Stetsyuk V, et al. Transcription factor TCF7L2 genetic study in the French population: expression in human beta-cells and adipose tissue and strong association with type 2 diabetes. Diabetes. 2006;55(10):2903–8.
11. Florez JC, Jablonski KA, Bayley N, Pollin TI, de Bakker PI, Shuldiner AR, Knowler WC, Nathan DM, Altshuler D. Diabetes prevention program research G: TCF7L2 polymorphisms and progression to diabetes in the diabetes prevention program. N Engl J Med. 2006;355(3):241–50.
12. Salinas YD, Wang L, DeWan AT. Multiethnic genome-wide association study identifies ethnic-specific associations with body mass index in Hispanics and African Americans. BMC Genet. 2016;17(1):78.
13. Zeggini E, McCarthy MI. TCF7L2: the biggest story in diabetes genetics since HLA? Diabetologia. 2007, 50(1):1–4.
14. Gustafson B, Hedjazifar S, Gogg S, Hammarstedt A, Smith U. Insulin resistance and impaired adipogenesis. Trends Endocrinol Metab. 2015;26(4):193–200.
15. Locke AE, Kahali B, Berndt SI, Justice AE, Pers TH, Day FR, Powell C, Vedantam S, Buchkovich M, Consortium G. Genetic studies of body mass index yield new insights for obesity biology. Nature. 2015;518:197–206.
16. Helgason A, Palsson S, Thorleifsson G, Grant SF, Emilsson V, Gunnarsdottir S, Adeyemo A, Chen Y, Chen G, Reynisdottir I, et al. Refining the impact of TCF7L2 gene variants on type 2 diabetes and adaptive evolution. Nat Genet. 2007;39(2):218–25.
17. Timpson NJ, Lindgren CM, Weedon MN, Randall J, Ouwehand WH, Strachan DP, Rayner NW, Walker M, Hitman GA, Doney AS, et al. Adiposity-related heterogeneity in patterns of type 2 diabetes susceptibility observed in genome-wide association data. Diabetes. 2009;58(2):505–10.
18. Bailey KA, Savic D, Zielinski M, Park SY, Wang LJ, Witkowski P, Brady M, Hara M, Bell GI, Nobrega MA. Evidence of non-pancreatic beta cell-dependent roles of Tcf7l2 in the regulation of glucose metabolism in mice. Hum Mol Genet. 2015;24(6):1646–54.
19. Prokunina-Olsson L, Welch C, Hansson O, Adhikari N, Scott LJ, Usher N, Tong M, Sprau A, Swift A, Bonnycastle LL, et al. Tissue-specific alternative splicing of TCF7L2. Hum Mol Genet. 2009;18(20):3795–804.
20. Mondal AK, Das SK, Baldini G, Chu WS, Sharma NK, Hackney OG, Zhao J, Grant SF, Elbein SC. Genotype and tissue-specific effects on alternative splicing of the transcription factor 7-like 2 gene in humans. J Clin Endocrinol Metab. 2010;95(3):1450–7.
21. Pradas-Juni M, Nicod N, Fernandez-Rebollo E, Gomis R. Differential transcriptional and posttranslational transcription factor 7-like regulation among nondiabetic individuals and type 2 diabetic patients. Mol Endocrinol. 2014;28(9):1558–70.
22. Xia Q, Deliard S, Yuan CX, Johnson ME, Grant SF. Characterization of the transcriptional machinery bound across the widely presumed type 2 diabetes causal variant, rs7903146, within TCF7L2. Eur J Hum Genet. 2015;23(1):103–9.
23. Gaulton KJ, Nammo T, Pasquali L, Simon JM, Giresi PG, Fogarty MP, Panhuis TM, Mieczkowski P, Secchi A, Bosco D, et al. A map of open chromatin in human pancreatic islets. Nat Genet. 2010;42(3):255–9.
24. Gaulton KJ, Ferreira T, Lee Y, Raimondo A, Magi R, Reschen ME, Mahajan A, Locke A, Rayner NW, Robertson N, et al. Genetic fine mapping and genomic annotation defines causal mechanisms at type 2 diabetes susceptibility loci. Nat Genet. 2015;47(12):1415–25.
25. Zhou Y, Oskolkov N, Shcherbina L, Ratti J, Kock KH, Su J, Martin B, Oskolkova MZ, Goransson O, Bacon J, et al. HMGB1 binds to the rs7903146 locus in TCF7L2 in human pancreatic islets. Mol Cell Endocrinol. 2016;430:138–45.
26. Kaminska D, Kuulasmaa T, Venesmaa S, Kakela P, Vaittinen M, Pulkkinen L, Paakkonen M, Gylling H, Laakso M, Pihlajamaki J. Adipose tissue TCF7L2 splicing is regulated by weight loss and associates with glucose and fatty acid metabolism. Diabetes. 2012;61(11):2807–13.
27. Lyssenko V, Lupi R, Marchetti P, Del Guerra S, Orho-Melander M, Almgren P, Sjogren M, Ling C, Eriksson KF, Lethagen AL, et al. Mechanisms by which common variants in the TCF7L2 gene increase risk of type 2 diabetes. J Clin Invest. 2007;117(8):2155–63.
28. Korinek V, Barker N, Moerer P, van Donselaar E, Huls G, Peters PJ, Clevers H. Depletion of epithelial stem-cell compartments in the small intestine of mice lacking Tcf-4. Nat Genet. 1998;19(4):379–83.
29. Loos RJ, Franks PW, Francis RW, Barroso I, Gribble FM, Savage DB, Ong KK, O'Rahilly S, Wareham NJ. TCF7L2 polymorphisms modulate proinsulin levels and beta-cell function in a British Europid population. Diabetes. 2007;56(7): 1943–7.
30. Palmer ND, Lehtinen AB, Langefeld CD, Campbell JK, Haffner SM, Norris JM, Bergman RN, Goodarzi MO, Rotter JI, Bowden DW. Association of TCF7L2 gene polymorphisms with reduced acute insulin response in Hispanic Americans. J Clin Endocrinol Metab. 2008;93(1):304–9.

31. Watanabe RM, Allayee H, Xiang AH, Trigo E, Hartiala J, Lawrence JM, Buchanan TA. Transcription factor 7-like 2 (TCF7L2) is associated with gestational diabetes mellitus and interacts with adiposity to alter insulin secretion in Mexican Americans. Diabetes. 2007;56(5):1481–5.

32. Sorlie PD, Avilés-Santa LM, Wassertheil-Smoller S, Kaplan RC, Daviglus ML, Giachello AL, Schneiderman N, Raij L, Talavera G, Allison M, et al. Design and implementation of the Hispanic community health study/study of Latinos. Ann Epidemiol. 2010;20(8):629–41.

33. LaVange LM, Kalsbeek WD, Sorlie PD, Avilés-Santa LM, Kaplan RC, Barnhart J, Liu K, Giachello A, Lee DJ, Ryan J, et al. Sample design and cohort selection in the Hispanic community health study/study of Latinos. Ann Epidemiol. 2010;20(8):642–9.

34. Fernandez-Rhodes L, Robinson WR, Sotres-Alvarez D, Franceschini N, Castaneda SF, Buelna C, Moncrieft A, Llabre M, Daviglus ML, Qi Q, et al. Accuracy of self-reported weight in Hispanic/Latino adults of the Hispanic community health study/study of Latinos. Epidemiology. 2017;28(6):847–53.

35. American Diabetes A. Diagnosis and classification of diabetes mellitus. Diabetes Care. 2010;33(Suppl 1):S62–9.

36. Voight BF, Kang HM, Ding J, Palmer CD, Sidore C, Chines PS, Burtt NP, Fuchsberger C, Li Y, Erdmann J, et al. The metabochip, a custom genotyping array for genetic studies of metabolic, cardiovascular, and anthropometric traits. PLoS Genet. 2012;8(8):e1002793.

37. Maller JB, McVean G, Byrnes J, Vukcevic D, Palin K, Su Z, Howson JM, Auton A, Myers S, Morris A, et al. Bayesian refinement of association signals for 14 loci in 3 common diseases. Nat Genet. 2012;44(12):1294–301.

38. Buyske S, Wu Y, Carty CL, Cheng I, Assimes TL, Dumitrescu L, Hindorff LA, Mitchell S, Ambite JL, Boerwinkle E, et al. Evaluation of the metabochip genotyping array in African Americans and implications for fine mapping of GWAS-identified loci: the PAGE study. PLoS One. 2012;7(4):e35651.

39. Conomos MP, Laurie CA, Stilp AM, Gogarten SM, McHugh CP, Nelson SC, Sofer T, Fernandez-Rhodes L, Justice AE, Graff M, et al. Genetic diversity and association studies in US Hispanic/Latino populations: applications in the Hispanic community health study/study of Latinos. Am J Hum Genet. 2016;98(1):165–84.

40. Alexander DH, Novembre J, Lange K. Fast model-based estimation of ancestry in unrelated individuals. Genome Res. 2009;19(9):1655–64.

41. Purcell S, Neale B, Todd-Brown K, Thomas L, Ferreira MA, Bender D, Maller J, Sklar P, de Bakker PI, Daly MJ, et al. PLINK: a tool set for whole-genome association and population-based linkage analyses. Am J Hum Genet. 2007;81(3):559–75.

42. Lin DY, Tao R, Kalsbeek WD, Zeng D, Gonzalez F 2nd, Fernandez-Rhodes L, Graff M, Koch GG, North KE, Heiss G. Genetic association analysis under complex survey sampling: the Hispanic community health study/study of Latinos. Am J Hum Genet. 2014;95(6):675–88.

43. Muthen B, Muthen L. Mplus User's Guide. Seventh ed. Los Angeles, CA: Muthén & Muthén; 1998-2012.

44. Yaghootkar H, Bancks MP, Jones SE, McDaid A, Beaumont R, Donnelly L, Wood AR, Campbell A, Tyrrell J, Hocking LJ, et al. Quantifying the extent to which index event biases influence large genetic association studies. Hum Mol Genet. 2017;26(5):1018–30.

45. Daviglus ML, Talavera GA, Aviles-Santa ML, Allison M, Cai J, Criqui MH, Gellman M, Giachello AL, Gouskova N, Kaplan RC, et al. Prevalence of major cardiovascular risk factors and cardiovascular diseases among Hispanic/Latino individuals of diverse backgrounds in the United States. JAMA. 2012;308(17):1775–84.

46. Fernandez-Rhodes L, Gong J, Haessler J, Franceschini N, Graff M, Nishimura KK, Wang Y, Highland HM, Yoneyama S, Bush WS, et al. Trans-ethnic fine-mapping of genetic loci for body mass index in the diverse ancestral populations of the population architecture using genomics and epidemiology (PAGE) study reveals evidence for multiple signals at established loci. Hum Genet. 2017;136(6):771–800.

47. Acosta JL, Hernandez-Mondragon AC, Correa-Acosta LC, Cazanas-Padilla SN, Chavez-Florencio B, Ramirez-Vega EY, Monge-Cazares T, Aguilar-Salinas CA, Tusie-Luna T, Del Bosque-Plata L. Rare intronic variants of TCF7L2 arising by selective sweeps in an indigenous population from Mexico. BMC Genet. 2016;17(1):68.

48. Qi Q, Stilp AM, Sofer T, Moon JY, Hidalgo B, Szpiro AA, Wang T, Ng MCY, Guo X, ME-aotDiAA C, et al. Genetics of type 2 diabetes in U.S. Hispanic/Latino individuals: results from the Hispanic community health study/study of Latinos (HCHS/SOL). Diabetes. 2017;66(5):1419–25.

49. Pettitt DJ, Talton J, Dabelea D, Divers J, Imperatore G, Lawrence JM, Liese AD, Linder B, Mayer-Davis EJ, Pihoker C, et al. Prevalence of diabetes in U.S. youth in 2009: the SEARCH for diabetes in youth study. Diabetes Care. 2014;37(2):402–8.

50. Cervin C, Lyssenko V, Bakhtadze E, Lindholm E, Nilsson P, Tuomi T, Cilio CM, Groop L. Genetic similarities between latent autoimmune diabetes in adults, type 1 diabetes, and type 2 diabetes. Diabetes. 2008;57(5):1433–7.

2

Abdominal obesity in type 1 diabetes associated with gender, cardiovascular risk factors and complications, and difficulties achieving treatment targets: a cross sectional study at a secondary care diabetes clinic

Eva O. Melin[1,2,3*], Hans O. Thulesius[2,3,4], Magnus Hillman[5], Mona Landin-Olsson[1,5,6] and Maria Thunander[1,2,7]

Abstract

Background: Abdominal obesity is linked to cardiovascular diseases in type 1 diabetes (T1D). The primary aim was to explore associations between abdominal obesity and cardiovascular complications, metabolic and inflammatory factors. The secondary aim was to explore whether achieved recommended treatment targets differed between the obese and non-obese participants.

Methods: Cross sectional study of 284 T1D patients (age 18–59 years, men 56%), consecutively recruited from one secondary care specialist diabetes clinic in Sweden. Anthropometrics, blood pressure, serum-lipids and high-sensitivity C-reactive protein (hs-CRP) were collected and supplemented with data from the patients' medical records and from the Swedish National Diabetes Registry. Abdominal obesity was defined as waist circumference men/women (meters): $\geq 1.02/\geq 0.88$. Hs-CRP was divided into low-, moderate-, and high-risk groups for future cardiovascular events (< 1, 1 to 3, and > 3 to ≤ 8.9 mg/l). Treatment targets were blood pressure $\leq 130/\leq 80$, total cholesterol ≤ 4.5 mmol/l, LDL: ≤ 2.5 mmol/l, and HbA1c: ≤ 5 2 mmol/mol ($\leq 6.9\%$). Different explanatory linear, logistic and ordinal regression models were elaborated for the associations, and calibrated and validated for goodness of fit with the data variables.

Results: The prevalence of abdominal obesity was 49/284 (17%), men/women: 8%/29% ($P < 0.001$). Women (adjusted odds ratio (AOR) 6.5), cardiovascular complications (AOR 5.7), HbA1c > 70 mmol/mol ($> 8.6\%$) (AOR 2.7), systolic blood pressure (per mm Hg) (AOR 1.05), and triglycerides (per mmol/l) (AOR 1.7), were associated with abdominal obesity. Sub analyses ($n = 171$), showed that abdominal obesity (AOR 5.3) and triglycerides (per mmol/l) (AOR 2.8) were associated with increasing risk levels of hs-CRP. Treatment targets were obtained for fewer patients with abdominal obesity for HbA1c (8% vs 21%, $P = 0.044$) and systolic blood pressure (51% vs 68%, $P = 0.033$). No patients with abdominal obesity reached all treatment targets compared to 8% in patients without abdominal obesity.

(Continued on next page)

* Correspondence: eva.melin@kronoberg.se; eva.o.melin@gmail.com
[1]Department of Clinical Sciences, Section Endocrinology and Diabetes, Lund University, Lund, Sweden
[2]Department of Research and Development, Region Kronoberg, Box 1223, SE-35112 Växjö, Sweden
Full list of author information is available at the end of the article

(Continued from previous page)

Conclusions: Significant associations between abdominal obesity and gender, cardiovascular disease, and the cardiovascular risk factors low-grade inflammation, systolic blood pressure, high HbA1c, and triglycerides, were found in 284 T1D patients. Fewer patients with abdominal obesity reached the treatment targets for HbA1c and systolic blood pressure compared to the non-obese.

Keywords: Abdominal obesity, Cardiovascular complications, Diabetes mellitus type 1, Gender, Glycemic control, Hyperlipidemia, Hypertension, Inflammation, Treatment targets

Background

Both women and men with type 1 diabetes mellitus (T1D) have increased cardiovascular and all-cause mortality compared to persons without T1D, and the risk for premature death is increasing with increasing HbA1c levels [1]. Women with T1D are described to be at particular risk for both coronary artery calcification and for cardiovascular death across all age groups [1, 2]. The introduction of intensified insulin therapy for patients with type 1 diabetes mellitus (T1D) has led to decreased prevalence of diabetic retinopathy, nephropathy and neuropathy [3]. Intensive insulin therapy has however two major side effects, weight gain and increased frequency of severe episodes of hypoglycaemia [3]. Excess weight gain in T1D is associated with abdominal obesity, insulin resistance, dyslipidaemia, higher blood pressure, and atherosclerosis [4]. Particularly girls/women with T1D are at risk for developing overweight and obesity [5]. The prevalence of obesity is increasing globally [6]. When this study was conducted in 2009, the prevalence of general obesity (BMI ≥ 30 kg/m^2) was 11% in men, and 10% in women in the general population in Sweden [7].

There is evidence that low-density lipoprotein (LDL) is both an indicator of future cardiovascular risk and a causal agent in the atherothrombotic process [8]. Raised triglycerides have been associated with low-grade inflammation, artery calcification, cardiovascular disease and all-cause mortality, and there is evidence that triglycerides are causal in the atherosclerosis process [9–12]. Common causes of raised triglycerides are obesity and high alcohol intake [9]. Impaired glycemic control has been linked to raised triglycerides in type 2 diabetes (T2D) [9]. Low levels of high-density lipoprotein (HDL) are strong predictors of atherosclerosis and cardiovascular disease [13]. However the causal relation between HDL and atherosclerosis is uncertain [13]. Lipid-lowering drugs are associated with a reduced risk of cardiovascular disease and death in T1D [14].

Chronic low-grade inflammation has been associated with obesity, insulin resistance, hypertension, hyperglycemia, acute hypoglycemia, dyslipidaemia, cardiovascular disease, and smoking [15–18]. One of the most frequently used markers of low-grade inflammation is high

sensitivity C-reactive protein (hs-CRP), which is atherogenic, and a strong predictor of future cardiovascular events [15, 19]. Hs-CRP might be involved in mediating atherothrombotic disease through activation of complement pathways and immune cells [20].

In line with both international and Swedish national guidelines for diabetes, indications for lipid-lowering drugs at the clinic in 2009 were total cholesterol (TC) > 4.5 mmol/l or LDL > 2.5 mmol/l, in addition to dietary interventions and increased physical activity [21–23]. Indications for anti-hypertensive drugs were systolic blood pressure > 130 mmHg, or diastolic blood pressure > 80 mmHg [18, 21–24].

We have recently found that alexithymia, which is characterized by impaired capacity to identify and describe feelings, was associated with abdominal obesity [25]. We have also previously found that abdominal obesity, depression and smoking were independently associated with inadequate glycemic control [26].

The primary aim was to explore links between abdominal obesity, metabolic and inflammatory factors and cardiovascular complications in persons with T1D. The secondary goal was to explore whether obtained treatment targets for HbA1c, blood pressure, TC and LDL differed between the obese and non-obese participants.

Methods
Participants and procedures

This study had a cross sectional design and was one of four baseline analyses [25–27] for a randomized controlled trial (ClinicalTrials.gov: NCT01714986) where "Affect School with Script Analysis" was tried against "Basic Body Awareness Therapy" for persons with diabetes, inadequate glycemic control and psychological symptoms [28, 29]. The participants were outpatients, consecutively recruited by specialist diabetes physicians or diabetes nurses, at regular follow up visits during the period 03/25/2009 to 12/28/2009. They were recruited from one secondary care specialist diabetes clinic, with a catchment population of 125,000 in southern Sweden. In this study 284 persons with T1D were included, 66% of the eligible patients (Fig. 1). Exclusion criteria were cancer, hepatic failure, end-stage renal disease, stroke with cognitive deficiency, psychotic disorder, bipolar disorder,

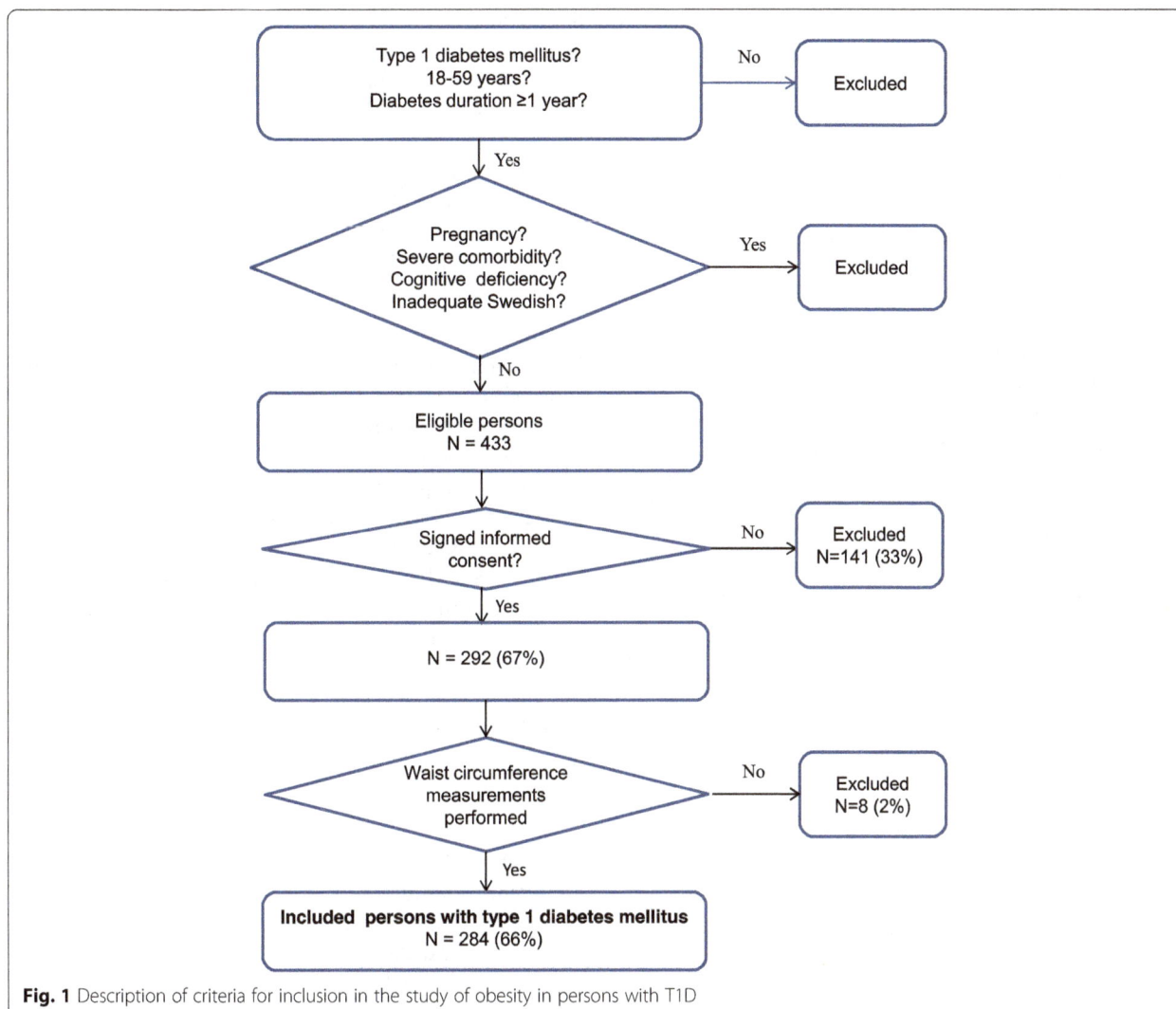

Fig. 1 Description of criteria for inclusion in the study of obesity in persons with T1D

severe personality disorder, severe substance abuse, or mental retardation. Anthropometrics, blood pressure and blood samples were collected. Data were collected from computerized medical records and the Swedish national diabetes register (S-NDR) [1, 23].

Medication
Diabetes specific treatment was divided into three groups: multiple daily insulin injections (MDII), continuous subcutaneous insulin infusion (CSII), and MDII combined with oral antidiabetic agents (OAA) (ATC code A10BA02). The indications for OAA prescription in addition to insulin were obesity and insulin resistance.

Anti-hypertensive drugs were calcium antagonists (ATC codes C08CA01–02); angiotensin-converting enzyme (ACE) inhibitors (ATC codes C09AA-BA), angiotensin II antagonists (ATC codes C09CA-DA; diuretics (ATC code C03A); selective beta-adrenoreceptor antagonists (ATC code C07AB).

Lipid-lowering drugs were HMG CoA-reductase inhibitors (statins) (C10AA).

Anthropometrics and blood pressure
Waist circumference (WC), weight, length and blood pressure were measured according to standard procedures by a nurse. Abdominal obesity was defined as WC men/women (meters): $\geq 1.02/> 0.88$ [30–32]. General obesity was defined as Body Mass Index (BMI): ≥ 30 kg/m^2 for both genders [31].

HbA1c, serum-lipids and hs-CRP
HbA1c and serum lipids analyses were performed at the department of Clinical Chemistry, Växjö Central Hospital.

Venous HbA1c was analyzed with high pressure liquid chromatography, HPLC - variant II, Turbo analyzer (Bio – Rad®, Hercules, CA, USA). HbA1c >70 mmol/mol (> 8.6%) corresponds to the 75th percentile in the whole population sample [26].

After an overnight fast, blood samples were collected and serum-lipids were were measured directly [8], using the enzymatic colour test (Olympus AU®, Tokyo, Japan). High TC was defined as > 4.5 mmol/l, high LDL as > 2.5 mmol/l, high triglycerides as ≥1.7 mmol/l; low HDL as < 1.04 mmol/l for men, and as < 1.29 mmol/l for women [33].

Samples for hs-CRP were collected, centrifuged, and stored at − 70 C Celsius until analyzed with spectrophotometry on a Roche Cobas C501 at the diabetes laboratory, Lund University Hospital, Lund. Hs-CRP was 0.54 ± 0.02 mg/l in healthy subjects according to previous research [16]. Hs-CRP < 1, 1 to 3, and > 3 to ≤10 mg/l correspond to low-, moderate- and high-risk groups for future cardiovascular events [19]. Samples with hs-CRP ≥10 mg/l were excluded as recommended in previous research [19]. Samples stored > 1 year were excluded. Hs-CRP was available for 171 (60%) participants.

Treatment targets according to the Swedish National Guidelines for diabetes in 2009
The treatment targets recommend by the Swedish National Board of Health and Welfare were for T1D patients: 1) glycemic control: HbA1c ≤52 mmol/mol; 2) systolic/diastolic blood pressure: ≤130/≤80 mmHg; 3) serum-lipids: TC ≤4.5 and LDL ≤2.5 mmol/l [22].

Hypoglycemia episodes
A severe hypoglycemia episode was defined as needing help from another person. Episodes during the last 6 months prior to recruitment were registered.

Smoking and physical inactivity
Smokers were defined as having smoked any amount of tobacco during the last year.

Physical inactivity was defined as moderate activities, such as 30 min of walking, less than once a week.

Cardiovascular complications
Cardiovascular complications were defined as ischemic heart disease or stroke/TIA.

Statistical analysis
Analysis of data distribution using histograms revealed that age, diabetes duration, hs-CRP, triglycerides, BMI and WC were not normally distributed. Data were presented as median values (quartile $(q)_1$, q_3; range), and analyses were performed with Mann-Whitney U test. Fisher's exact test (two-tailed) and Linear-by-Linear Association (two-tailed) were used to analyze categorical data. Crude odds ratios (CORs) were calculated, variables with $P \le 0.10$, and age independent of P-value, were entered in multiple logistic regression analyses (Backward: Wald). The Hosmer and Lemeshow test for goodness-of-

fit and Nagelkerke R^2 were used to evaluate each multiple logistic regression analysis model. Ordinal regression analysis (stepwise forward) was performed with 3 risk levels of hs-CRP as dependent variables. Variables with P-values ≤0.10 in simple linear regression analyses were entered into multiple linear regression analyses (Backward). Confidence intervals (CIs) of 95% were used. $P < 0.05$ was considered statistically significant. SPSS® version 18 (IBM, Chicago, Illinois, USA) was used for statistical analyses.

Results
In this population based cross sectional study of persons with T1D ($n = 284$, age 18–59 years, men 56%), persons with abdominal obesity ($n = 49$) were compared with non-obese persons ($n = 235$). Baseline data including comparisons between men and women are presented in Table 1. The women, compared with the men, had higher prevalence of both abdominal obesity (29% vs 8%, $P < 0.001$) and general obesity (18% vs 7%, $P = 0.005$). The men had higher systolic and diastolic blood pressure (both $P < 0.001$) and lower HDL ($P = 0.002$). The percentage that reached the recommended treatment targets were for HbA1c: 19%; TC: 48%; LDL: 36%; systolic blood pressure: 65%; diastolic blood pressure: 95%. Only 7% reached all treatment targets.

Comparisons between patients with and without abdominal obesity
Results of comparisons between 49 persons with abdominal obesity and 235 persons without abdominal obesity are presented in Table 2. Persons with abdominal obesity had higher prevalence of HbA1c > 70 mmol/mol (> 8.6%) ($P < 0.001$), lipid-lowering drugs ($P = 0.012$) and cardiovascular complications ($P = 0.016$); and had higher median values of hs- CRP ($P < 0.001$), triglycerides ($P < 0.001$), systolic blood pressure ($P = 0.004$), LDL ($P = 0.021$) and TC ($P = 0.047$). Fewer patients with abdominal obesity compared to the non-obese reached the recommended treatment targets for HbA1c (8% vs 21%, $P = 0.044$) and systolic blood pressure (51% vs 68%, $P = 0.033$). No patients with abdominal obesity reached all risk factor treatment targets for blood pressure, TC, LDL and HbA1c compared to 8% in the non-obese.

Comparisons between users and non-users of anti-hypertensive and lipid-lowering drugs
Persons treated with anti-hypertensive drugs had higher prevalence of high systolic blood pressure (62% vs 22%, $P < 0.001$), and cardiovascular complications ($P = 0.018$) (Table 2). Patients treated with lipid-lowering drugs had significantly higher median triglycerides ($P = 0.014$), higher prevalence of cardiovascular complications ($P = 0.$

Table 1 Baseline characteristics and comparisons between men and women for 284 persons with T1D

	All patients	Men	Women	p [a]
N	284	159 (56)	125 (44)	
Age (years)	42 (32, 51; 18–59)	43 (32, 52)	41 (30, 50)	0.12 [b]
Diabetes duration (years)	20 (11, 30; 1–55)	21 (11–32)	19 (11, 29)	0.26 [b]
WC (meters)	–	0.88 (0.82, 0.95; 0.65–1.33)	0.79 (0.75, 0.90; 0.63–1.25)	–
Abdominal obesity [c]	49 (17)	13 (8)	36 (29)	< 0.001
General obesity [d]	34 (12)	11 (7)	23 (18)	0.005
HbA1c > 52 mmol/mol (> 6.9%)	230 (81)	130 (82)	100 (80)	0.76
HbA1c > 70 mmol/mol (> 8.6%)	39 (24)	39 (24)	39 (31)	0.23
TC (mmol/l)	4.6 (4.1, 5.2; 2.1–10.9)	4.5 (4.0, 5.1)	4.7 (4.1, 5.4)	0.069 [b]
High TC (> 4.5 mmol/l)	149 (52)	78 (49)	71 (57)	0.23
LDL (mmol/l)	2.8 (2.4, 3.3; 0.6–8.3)	2.8 (2.4, 3.3)	2.9 (2.4, 3.4)	0.51 [b]
High LDL (> 2.5 mmol/l)	182 (64)	102 (64)	80 (64)	> 0.99
Triglycerides (mmol/l)	0.9 (0.7, 1.3; 0.6–5.9)	0.9 (0.7, 1.3)	0.8 (0.6, 1.3)	0.47 [b]
High triglycerides (≥ 1.7 mmol/l)	34 (12)	16 (10)	18 (14)	0.28
HDL (mmol/l)	1.5 (1.3, 1.8; 0.8–2.7)	1.4 (1.2, 1.7)	1.6 (1.4, 1.8)	0.002 [b]
Low HDL (M/W: < 1.04/< 1.29 mmol/l/)	32 (11)	17 (11)	15 (12)	0.85
Hs-CRP [e] (mg/l)	0.6 (0.3, 1.7; 0.03–8.9)	0.5 (0.2, 1.4)	0.9 (0.4, 2.5)	0.008 [b]
SBP [f] (mm Hg)	120 (111, 130; 100–160)	125 (120, 130)	120 (110, 130)	< 0.001 [b]
High SBP [f] (> 130 mmHg)	100 (35)	67 (42)	33 (26)	0.006
DBP [h] (mm Hg)	70 (70, 75; 55–100)	70 (70, 80)	70 (65, 75)	< 0.001 [b]
High DBP [g] (> 80 mmHg)	13 (5)	10 (6)	3 (2)	0.16
Hypoglycemia (severe episodes)	13 (5%)	7 (4)	6 (5)	> 0.99
Smoking [h]	28 (10)	18 (12)	10 (8)	0.42
Physical inactivity [h] (< 1/week)	31 (11)	18 (12)	13 (11)	0.85
CV [i] complications	10 (4)	6 (4)	4 (3)	> 0.99
LLD [j]	133 (47)	77 (48)	56 (45)	0.55
AHD [k]	95 (34)	61 (38)	34 (27)	0.057
MDII [l] and OAD [m]	17 (6)	6 (4)	11 (9)	0.15
CSII [n]	26 (9)	13 (8)	13 (10)	
MDII [l]	241 (85)	140 (88)	101 (81)	
Reached all treatment targets [o]	19 (7)	11 (7)	8 (6)	> 0.99

Data are n (%) or median (q$_1$, q$_3$; min-max)
[a] Fisher's exact test unless otherwise indicated. [b] Mann-Whitney U test. [c] WC: men/women ≥1.02/≥0.88 m. [d] BMI ≥30 kg/m^2. [e] N = 171, missing values for men/women: n = 54/59. [f] Systolic blood pressure. [g] Diastolic blood pressure. [h] Missing values men/women: n = 6/6. [i] Cardiovascular. [j] Lipid-lowering drugs. [k] Anti-hypertensive drugs. [l] Multiple daily insulin injections. [m] Oral antidiabetic drugs. [n] Continuous subcutaneous insulin infusion. [o] Blood pressure ≤ 130/≤ 80, TC ≤ 4.5, LDL ≤ 2.5 and HbA1c ≤ 52

007), and lower prevalence of high LDL (P = 0.006) than non-users of lipid-lowering drugs (Table 2).

Factors associated with abdominal obesity

Women (adjusted odds ratio (AOR) 6.5), systolic blood pressure (per mm Hg) (AOR 1.05), HbA1c > 70 mmol/mol (> 8.6%) (AOR 2.7), triglycerides (per mmol/l) (AOR 1.7), and cardiovascular complications (AOR 5.7) were associated with abdominal obesity (Table 3). Gender analyses showed that diastolic blood pressure (per mm Hg) (AOR 1.13) and anti-hypertensive drugs (AOR 5.3)

were associated with abdominal obesity in men. Triglycerides (per mmol/l) (AOR 2.1), lipid-lowering drugs (AOR 3.1), and HbA1c > 70 mmol/mol (> 8.6%) (AOR 2.9), were associated with abdominal obesity in women.

Factors associated with high-, moderate- and low-risk hs-CRP levels in 171 persons

Abdominal obesity (AOR (CI) 5.3 (2.1–13.6)) and triglycerides (per mmol/l) (AOR (CI) 2.82 (1.68–4.93)) were associated with increasing risk levels of hs-CRP (Table 4).

Table 2 Comparisons between obese and non-obese, users and non-users of antihypertensive and lipid-lowering drugs

	Abdominal obesity			Anti-hypertensive drugs			Lipid-lowering drugs		
	Yes	No	P [a]	Yes	No	P [a]	Yes	No	P [a]
N	49 (17)	235 (83)		95 (33)	189 (67)		133 (47)	151 (53)	
Age	45 (35, 53)	42 (31, 51)	0.11 [b]	49 (42, 56)	39 (28, 56)	< 0.001 [b]	49 (42, 54)	34 (27, 44)	< 0.001 [b]
Diabetes duration	22 (14, 28)	20 (11, 31)	0.64[b]	29 (20, 35)	16 (9, 25)	< 0.001 [b]	26 (14, 34)	17 (9, 24)	< 0.001 [b]
Abdominal obesity	49 (100)	0		22 (23)	27 (14)	0.069	31 (23)	18 (12)	0.012
HbA1c > 52 mmol/mol (> 6.9%)	45 (92)	185 (79)	0.044	79 (83)	151 (80)	0.63	114 (86)	116 (77)	0.069
HbA1c > 70 mmol/mol (> 8.6%)	24 (49)	54 (23)	< 0.001	29 (30)	49 (26)	0.48	40 (30)	38 (25)	0.42
TC (mmol/l)	4.7 (4.2, 5.8)	4.6 (4.1, 5.1)	0.047 [b]	–	–	–	4.5 (4.0, 5.2)	4.6 (4.1, 5.2)	0.32 [b]
High TC (> 4.5 mmol/l)	29 (59)	120 (51)	0.35	–	–	–	63 (47)	86 (57)	0.12
Triglycerides (mmol/l)	1.2 (0.8, 1.9)	0.9 (0.7, 1.1)	< 0.001 [b]	–	–	–	1.0 (0.7, 1.3)	0.8 (0.7, 1.1)	0.014 [b]
High triglycerides (≥ 1.7 mmol/l)	14 (29)	20 (8)	< 0.001	–	–	–	21 (16)	13 (9)	0.070
HDL (mmol/l)	1.5 (1.3, 1.7)	1.5 (1.3, 1.8)	0.47 [b]	–	–	–	1.5 (1.3, 1.8)	1.5 (1.3, 1.8)	0.48 [b]
Low HDL (m/w:< 1.04/1.29 mmol/l)	5 (10)	27 (11)	> 0.99	–	–	–	12 (9)	20 (13)	0.35
LDL (mmol/l)	3.2 (2.5, 3.8)	2.8 (2.4, 3.3)	0.021 [b]	–	–	–	2.7 (2.3, 3.3)	3.0 (2.5, 3.4)	0.058 [b]
High LDL (> 2.5 mmol/l)	36 (74)	146 (62)	0.14	–	–	–	74 (56)	108 (72)	0.006
Hs-CRP [c] (mg/l)	2.5 (0.6, 4.6)	0.6 (0.2, 1.4)	< 0.001 [b]	0.6 (0.3, 1.7)	0.7 (0.3, 1.9)	0.87	0.6 (0.3, 1.8)	0.8 (0.3, 1.7)	0.97
SBP (mm Hg)	130 (120, 132)	120 (110, 130)	0.004 [b]	130 (125, 135)	120 (110, 125)	< 0.001 [b]	–	–	–
High SBP (> 130 mmHg)	24 (49)	76 (32)	0.033	59 (62)	41 (22)	< 0.001	–	–	–
DBP (mm Hg)	70 (70, 78)	70 (65, 75)	0.051 [b]	70 (70, 78)	70 (65, 75)	0.011 [b]	–	–	–
High DBP (> 80 mmHg)	5 (10)	8 (3)	0.054	7 (7)	6 (3)	0.14	–	–	–
Hypoglycemia (severe episodes)	3 (6)	10 (4)	0.48	–	–	–	–	–	–
Smoking	4 (9)	24 (11)	0.80	6 (6)	22 (12)	0.20	13 (10)	15 (10)	> 0.99
Physical inactivity (< 1/week)	9 (19)	22 (10)	0.084	10 (11)	21 (12)	> 0.99	11 (8)	20 (14)	0.18
CV complications	5 (10)	5 (2)	0.016	7 (7)	3 (2)	0.018	9 (7)	1 (1)	0.007
LLD	31 (63)	102 (43)	0.012	62 (65)	71 (38)	< 0.001	–	–	–
AHD	22 (45)	73 (31)	0.069	–	–	–	62 (47)	33 (22)	< 0.001
MDII and OAD	13 (27)	4 (2)	< 0.001	–	–	–	–	–	–
CSII	1 (2)	25 (10)		–	–	–	–	–	–
MDII	35 (71)	206 (88)		–	–	–	–	–	–
Reached all treatment targets	0	19 (8)	0.052	–	–	–	–	–	–

Data are n (%) or median (q1, q3)
[a] Fisher's exact test unless otherwise indicated. [b] Mann-Whitney U test. [c] Missing values for abdominal obesity/no abdominal obesity: $N = 27$ (55%)/86 (37%)

Factors associated with gender, high HbA1c, systolic blood pressure and cardiovascular complications

Positive associations with women were found for abdominal obesity AOR 8.6 (3.9–19.0), $P < 0.001$; and HDL (per mmol/l) AOR 6.1 (2.7–13.6), $P < 0.001$. Negative associations with women were found for diastolic blood pressure (per mm Hg) AOR 0.91 (0.87–0.95), $P < 0.001$; and age (per year) AOR 0.97 (0.94–0.99), $P = 0.005$. Systolic blood pressure, TC and anti-hypertensive drugs were not associated with women (all $P > 0.21$). Nagelkerke R Square: 0.277. Hosmer and Lemeshow Test: 0.034.

The associations with HbA1c > 70 mmol/mol (> 8.6%) were for abdominal obesity AOR 2.7 (1.4–5.4), $P = 0.004$; triglycerides (per mmol/l) AOR 1.7 (1.1–2.5), $P = 0.010$;

and for diastolic blood pressure (per mm Hg) AOR 1.04 (1.00–1.08), $P = 0.090$. HDL, TC, age, physical inactivity, and LDL were not associated with HbA1c > 70 mmol/mol (all $P > 0.16$). Nagelkerke R Square: 0.137. Hosmer and Lemeshow Test: 0.782.

The B-coefficients for the associations with systolic blood pressure were for age 0.24 (0.13–0.34), $P < 0.001$; anti-hypertensive drugs 6.5 (3.9–9.2), $P < 0.001$; triglycerides (per mmol/l) 2.0 (0.4–3.6), $P = 0.014$; men 4.0 (1.6–6.4), $P = 0.001$; and for abdominal obesity 4.0 (0.8–7.3), $P = 0.014$. Lipid-lowering drugs ($P = 0.73$) and diabetes duration ($P = 0.99$) were not associated with systolic blood pressure. Adjusted R Square 0.276, $P < 0.001$.

Associations with cardiovascular complications were for age (per year) AOR 1.18 (1.05–1.32), $P = 0.006$;

Table 3 Associations with abdominal obesity in patients with T1DM, presented for all and gender specified

| | Abdominal obesity | | | | | | | |
| | Both genders N = 284 [a] | | | | Men N = 158 | | Women N = 119 | |
	COR	P	AOR	P [b]	AOR	P [b]	AOR	P [b]
Gender (women)	4.5 (2.3–9.0)	< 0.001	6.5 (2.9–14.5)	< 0.001	–	–	–	–
Age (per year)	1.02 (1.00–1.05)	0.11	1.01 (0.97–1.06)	0.54	1.03 (0.97–1.10)	0.31	1.01 (0.96–1.06)	0.78
Diabetes duration (per year)	1.00 (0.98–1.03)	0.77	–	–	–	–	–	–
HbA1c > 70 mmol/mol (> 8.6%)	3.2 (1.7–6.1)	< 0.001	2.7 (1.3–5.7)	0.009	1.9 (0.5–7.1)	0.36	2.9 (1.2–7.2)	0.022
TC	1.2 (0.9–1.6)	0.15	–	–	–	–	–	–
Triglycerides (per mmol/l)	1.9 (1.3–2.8)	< 0.001	1.7 (1.1–2.6)	0.010	1.0 (0.5–2.0)	> 0.99	2.1 (1.2–3.7)	0.011
HDL (per mmol/l)	0.7 (0.3–1.6)	0.34	–	–	–	–	0.4 (0.1–1.7)	0.24
LDL (per mmol/l)	1.4 (1.0–1.9)	0.072	1.0 (0.7–1.70)	0.86	–	–	1.0 (0.56–1.98)	0.88
SBP (per mm Hg)	1.04 (1.01–1.07)	0.004	1.05 (1.01–1.08)	0.005	1.01 (0.94–1.10)	0.72	1.03 (0.99–1 .07)	0.20
DBP (per mm Hg)	1.04 (1.00–1.09)	0.045	1.02 (0.96–1.09)	0.47	1.13 (1.03–1.24)	0.007	–	–
Hypoglycemia	1.5 (0.4–5.5)	0.57	–	–	–	–	–	–
Smoking [c]	0.8 (0.3–2.4)	0.66	–	–	–	–	–	–
Physical inactivity	2.1 (0,9–4.8)	0.083	1.7 (0.5–5.2)	0.36	–	–	3.4 (0.8–14.4)	0.10
CV complications	5.2 (1.5–18.9)	0.011	5.7 (1.1–28.9)	0.035	–	–	–	–
LLD	2.2 (1.2–4.2)	0.013	1.9 (0.9–4.1)	0.096	–	–	3.1 (1.3–7.6)	0.014
AHD	1.8 (1.0–3.4)	0.064	1.1 (0.5–2.6)	0.79	5.3 (1.3–20.7)	0.018	–	–

[a] Unless indicated. [b] Multiple logistic regression analysis (Backward: Wald). [c] Missing values: n = 12. All/men/women: Hosmer and Lemeshow: Test 0.039/0.799/0.471; Nagelkerke R Square 0.335/0.234/0.250

abdominal obesity AOR 5.5 (1.4–22.0), P = 0.017; and for LDL (per mmol/l) AOR 0.3 (0.1–1.1), P = 0.071. Lipid-lowering drugs, anti-hypertensive drugs and diabetes duration were not associated with cardiovascular complications (all P > 0.34). Nagelkerke R Square: 0.309. Hosmer and Lemeshow Test: 0.978.

Comparisons of patients with and without CRP measurements – A response analysis
The prevalence of abdominal obesity was lower in the 171 patients with hs-CRP measurements than in the patients without hs-CRP measurements (13% vs 24%, P = 0.024). Otherwise, they did not differ by medians for age (P = 0.10), diabetes duration (P = 0.52), diastolic blood pressure (P = 0.52), systolic blood pressure (P = 0.66), HDL (P = 0.49), LDL (P = 0.50), triglycerides (P = 0.70), TC (P = 0.79); or by prevalence of anti-hypertensive drugs (P = 0.124), physical inactivity (P = 0.33), severe hypoglycemia episodes (P = 0.38), HbA1c >70 mmol/mol (P = 0.48), lipid-lowering drugs (P = 0.72), cardiovascular complications (P = 0.74), or smoking (P = 0.84).

Discussion
In this cross-sectional study of abdominal obesity in 284 persons with T1D, age 18–59 years, consecutively recruited from one secondary care specialist diabetes clinic, we found that cardiovascular complications, women, increasing risk levels of hs-CRP, systolic blood pressure, marked inadequate glycemic control (HbA1c > 70 mmol/mol), and triglycerides were independently associated with abdominal obesity. Inadequate glycemic control, systolic blood pressure, increasing risk levels of hs-CRP, were in addition to abdominal obesity, also associated with triglycerides. Less patients with abdominal obesity reached the treatment targets recommended by the Swedish National Board of Health and Welfare for glycemic control (HbA1c ≤ 52 mmol/mol) and systolic blood pressure (≤ 130 mmHg), and no patients with abdominal obesity reached all treatment targets for TC, LDL, and blood pressure [22].

Strengths of our study are first that the population of patients with T1D was well-defined, since persons with severe comorbidities and severe substance abuse were excluded. Second, hs-CRP levels above 10 mg/l were excluded, and the CRP values were divided into 3 groups with low-, moderate- or high-risk for future cardiovascular events, as have been recommended in previous research [19]. Also, we performed a response analysis and explored whether persons with and without hs-CRP measurements differed. The patients with hs-CRP measurements had lower prevalence of abdominal obesity, otherwise they did not differ for any variable included in this study. Third, we explored interactions between the included metabolic variables.

Table 4 Associations with low-, moderate- and high-risk hs-CRP levels

	All (With CRP)	Hs-CRP risk levels Low (< 1 mg/l)	Moderate (1 to ≤3 mg/l)	High (> 3.0 to ≤ 8.9 mg/l)		Increasing hs-CRP risk levels			
	$N = 171$	$N = 107$	$N = 44$	$N = 20$		$N = 171$			
	N (%) or median (q_1, q_3)				p^a	COR (CI)	p^b	AOR (CI)	p^b
Gender Women	66 (39)	35 (33)	19 (43)	12 (60)	0.017	2.0 (1.1–3.8)	0.023	–	NS
Men	105 (61)	72 (67)	25 (57)	8 (40)					
Age	42 (30, 50)	42 (31, 50)	40 (27, 51)	42 (29, 53)	0.73 ^{c}	1.00 (0.97–1.02)	0.72	–	NS
Abdominal obesity	22 (13)	7 (6)	5 (11)	10 (50)	< 0.001	7.0 (2.8–17.9)	< 0.001	5.3 (2.1–13.6)	< 0.001
HbA1c > 70 mmol/mol	51 (30)	27 (25)	11 (25)	13 (65)	0.004	2.2 (1.2–4.3)	0.016	–	NS
TC (mmol/l)	4.6 (4.1, 5.2)	4.5 (4.0, 5.1)	4.8 (4.1, 5.4)	4.8 (4.4, 6.0)	0.035 ^{c}	1.5 (1.2–2.0)	0.002	–	NS
Triglycerides (mmol/l)	0.9 (0.7, 5.2)	0.8 (0.6, 1.1)	1.0 (0.7, 1.4)	1.3 (0.9, 2.4)	< 0.001 ^{c}	3.2 (1.9–5.7)	< 0.001	2.82 (1.68–4.93)	< 0.001
HDL (mmol/l)	1.5 (1.3, 1.8)	1.6 (1.3, 1.8)	1.6 (1.3, 1.7)	1.4 (1.1, 1.7)	0.32 ^{c}	0.6 (0.2–1.4)	0.21	–	NS
LDL (mmol/l)	2.9 (2.3, 3.3)	2.7 (2.2, 3.2)	2.9 (2.4, 3.6)	3.2 (2.8, 3.6)	0.010 ^{c}	1.7 (1.2–2.4)	0.002	–	NS
SBP (mm Hg)	120 (115, 130)	120 (115, 130)	120 (110, 130)	128 (120, 134)	0.16 ^{c}	1.02 (0.99–1.05)	0.15	–	NS
DBP (mm Hg)	70 (70, 75)	70 (65, 75)	70 (66, 80)	75 (70, 78)	0.036 ^{c}	1.07 (1.02–1.12)	0.003	–	NS
LLD	82 (48)	50 (47)	21 (48)	11 (55)	0.55	1.2 (0.6–2.2)	0,60	–	NS
AHD	51 (30)	31 (29)	14 (32)	6 (30)	0.82	1.1 (0.6–2.1)	0.78	–	NS
Smoking ^{d}	18 (10)	11 (10)	5 (12)	2 (10)	0.96	–	–	–	–
Physical inactivity ^{e}	22 (13)	10 (10)	10 (23)	2 (10)	0.28	–	–	–	–
CV complications	7 (4)	4 (4)	0	3 (15)	0.16	2.3 (0.4–12.1)	0.30	–	NS

NS Non-significant
^{a} Linear-by-linear Association (Exact 2-sided) unless indicated. ^{b} Ordinal regression analyses. ^{c} Kruskal-Wallis test. Missing values: ^{d} $n = 2$; ^{e} $n = 3$. $^{d, e}$ Not included in the ordinal regression analyses

The main limitation of our study was the rather small number of obese persons, particularly when gender sub analyses were performed. There are several possible type 2 errors. The association between the use of lipid-lowering drugs and abdominal obesity did not reach significance. The prevalence of both lipid-lowering drugs and anti-hypertensive drugs in patients with cardiovascular complications was high, but the associations were not significant. Second, the number of hs-CRP values measurements was limited, as we decided not to include hs-CRP measurements stored for more than 1 year. Despite the limited number of hs-CRP measurements and the lower prevalence of obesity in persons with hs-CRP measurements, the moderate and high-risk-levels of hs-CRP were strongly associated with abdominal obesity and triglyceride levels.

We have previously shown an association between alexithymia and abdominal obesity in this sample of patients with T1D [25]. In this study, we demonstrated the impact of abdominal obesity in T1D by the associations with cardiovascular complications, marked impaired glycemic control, low-grade inflammation, systolic blood pressure and triglycerides, all risk factors for future cardiovascular complications [1, 8–12, 14, 18]. We found a link between impaired glycemic control and raised triglycerides, which is in accordance with findings in patients with T2D [9]. Women with T1D are at a higher risk for atherosclerosis and cardiovascular death than men [1, 2]. One explanatory factor might be the noticeably higher prevalence of abdominal obesity in the women compared to the men with T1D, demonstrated in this study and in previous research [5, 25]. The prevalence of general obesity was almost twice as high in the women with T1D compared to women in the general Swedish population [7]. The reasons for the excessive abdominal obesity prevalence in women with T1D were not explained by this study, and further research of this subject is suggested. Apart from abdominal obesity, the only positive association with women was higher HDL, which is not a risk factor for cardiovascular disease according to previous research [13].

Another gender difference noted was that the men had higher blood pressure than the women, which is in accordance with previous research [34]. The prevalence of high systolic blood pressure (> 130 mmHg) was significantly higher in patients using anti-hypertensive drugs than in non-users, and the treatment target for systolic blood pressure was not obtained for a large proportion of persons using anti-hypertensive drugs. Weight reduction might help to reduce systolic blood pressure [35]. There is evidence that low-density lipoprotein (LDL) is a causal agent in the atherothrombotic process [8]. The use of lipid-lowering drugs is associated with a lower risk for cardiovascular disease and death [14]. Patients in this study using lipid-lowering drugs were successful in reaching the treatment goals for LDL more often than non-users. Improved treatment with lipid-lowering drugs is therefore suggested for patients with T1D and high LDL, in addition to weight reduction.

Due to the described detrimental effects of obesity in T1D, it is necessary to try new ways to both prevent and treat obesity. Reports of beneficial effects on weight and HbA1c have been reported for sodium-glucose cotransporter (SGLT2) inhibitors and glucagon-like peptide-1 (GLP-1) analogues [36]. Structured nutrition therapy, including reduced energy intake, lower total carbohydrate intake, and carbohydrates with lower glycemic index, has been recommended in combination with aerobic and resistance exercises [37]. As alexithymia was associated with abdominal obesity [25], psychoeducation aiming at increased emotional awareness could also be tried [28].

Conclusions

Significant associations between abdominal obesity and both cardiovascular disease and cardiovascular risk factors were found in 284 patients with T1D. Low-grade inflammation, increased systolic blood pressure, inadequate glycemic control, and increased triglycerides were linked with abdominal obesity. The obesity prevalence was particularly high in women. Action against obesity is urgent to prevent cardiovascular complications in patients withT1D.

Abbreviations

AHD: Anti-hypertensive drugs; AOR: Adjusted odds ratio; BMI: Body mass index; CI: Confidence interval; COR: Crude odds ratio; CSII: Continuous subcutaneous insulin infusion; GLP-1: Glucagon-like peptide-1; HDL: High-density lipoprotein; LDL: Low-density lipoprotein; LLD: Lipid-lowering drugs; MDII: Multiple daily insulin injections; OAA: Oral antidiabetic agents; SGLT2: Sodium-glucose cotransporter-2; T1D: Type 1 diabetes mellitus; TC: Total cholesterol; WC: Waist circumference

Acknowledgments

We are grateful to Anna Lindgren, PhD, Lund University, Centre of Mathematics, Lund, Sweden, for her statistical skills.

Funding

This research was supported by the Research and Development Fund of Region Kronoberg, Växjö, Sweden, and by the Research Council of South Eastern Sweden (FORSS), Linköping, Sweden. The funding sources were not involved in the collection, analysis and interpretation of data, in the writing of the report, or in the decision to submit the article for publication.

Authors' contributions

EOM, MT, MH, HOT, and ML-O participated as investigators and reviewed, edited, and approved of the manuscript. All authors contributed to the study design, implementation and analysis. EOM was the initiator of this study, wrote the statistical methods and the manuscript, and is the guarantor of this work and, as such, had full access to all the data in the study and takes responsibility for the integrity of the data and the accuracy of the data analysis.

Authors' information

EOM is PhD, medical doctor, specialist in paediatrics and general practice. EOM works at the Department of Research and Development, and as a GP in primary care in Växjö, and is affiliated with the Department of Clinical Sciences, Section of Endocrinology and Diabetes, Lund University, Lund. HOT is PhD, associate professor, medical doctor, specialist in general practice, and works at the department of Research and Development, and as a GP in primary care in Växjö, and is affiliated with the Department of Clinical Sciences, Section of Family Medicine, Lund University, Malmö. Magnus Hillman is PhD and works at the Department of Clinical Sciences, the Diabetes Research Laboratory, Lund University, Lund. ML-O is PhD, medical doctor, professor at the Department of Clinical Sciences, Section of Endocrinology and Diabetes, Lund University, Lund, and works at Skane University Hospital, Lund. MT is PhD, medical doctor, specialist in internal medicine and endocrinology, and works at the department of Research and Development, and at the Central Hospital, Växjö, and is affiliated with the Department of Clinical Sciences, Section of Endocrinology and Diabetes, Lund University, Lund. All Sweden.

Competing interests

The authors declare that they have no competing interests.

Author details

[1]Department of Clinical Sciences, Section Endocrinology and Diabetes, Lund University, Lund, Sweden. [2]Department of Research and Development, Region Kronoberg, Box 1223, SE-35112 Växjö, Sweden. [3]Primary Care, Region Kronoberg, Växjö, Sweden. [4]Department of Clinical Sciences, Section of Family Medicine, Lund University, Malmö, Sweden. [5]Department of Clinical Sciences, Diabetes Research Laboratory, Faculty of Medicine, Lund University, Lund, Sweden. [6]Department of Endocrinology, Skane University Hospital, Lund, Sweden. [7]Department of Internal Medicine, Central Hospital, Växjö, Sweden.

References

1. Lind M, Svensson A-M, Kosiborod M, Gudbjörnsdottir S, Pivodic A, Wedel H, et al. Glycemic control and excess mortality in type 1 diabetes. N Engl J Med. 2014;371:1972–82.
2. Colhoun HM, Rubens MB, Underwood SR, Fuller JH. The effect of type 1 diabetes mellitus on the gender difference in coronary artery calcification. J Am Coll Cardiol. 2000;36:2160–7.
3. Diabetes Control and Complications Trial Research Group. The effect of intensive treatment of diabetes on the development and progression of long-term complications in insulin-dependent diabetes mellitus. N Engl J Med. 1993;329:977–86.

4. Purnell JQ, Hokanson JE, Cleary PA, Nathan DM, Lachin JM, Zinman B, et al. The effect of excess weight gain with intensive diabetes treatment on cardiovascular disease risk factors and atherosclerosis in type 1 diabetes: results from the diabetes control and complications trial / epidemiology of diabetes interventions and complications study (DCCT/EDIC) study. Circulation. 2013;127 https://doi.org/10.1161/CIRCULATIONAHA.111.077487.

5. Fröhlich-Reiterer EE, Rosenbauer J, Bechtold-Dalla Pozza S, Hofer SE, Schober E, Holl RW, et al. Predictors of increasing BMI during the course of diabetes in children and adolescents with type 1 diabetes: data from the German/Austrian DPV multicentre survey. Arch Dis Child. 2014;99:738–43.

6. Ng M, Fleming T, Robinson M, Thomson B, Graetz N, Margono C, et al. Global, regional, and national prevalence of overweight and obesity in children and adults during 1980–2013: a systematic analysis for the global burden of disease study 2013. Lancet. 2014;384:766–81.

7. SCB. Undersökningarna av levnadsförhållanden år 2009. [internet]. 2017 Apr. Available from: www.scb.se/ulf.

8. Ridker PM. LDL cholesterol: controversies and future therapeutic directions. Lancet. 2014;384:607–17.

9. Nordestgaard BG. Triglyceride-rich lipoproteins and atherosclerotic cardiovascular disease. Circ Res. 2016;118:547–63.

10. Nordestgaard BG, Varbo A. Triglycerides and cardiovascular disease. Lancet. 2014;384:626–35.

11. Langsted A, Freiberg JJ, Tybjaerg-Hansen A, Schnohr P, Jensen GB, Nordestgaard BG. Nonfasting cholesterol and triglycerides and association with risk of myocardial infarction and total mortality: the Copenhagen City heart study with 31 years of follow-up. J Intern Med. 2011;270:65–75.

12. Bjornstad P, Maahs DM, Wadwa RP, Pyle L, Rewers M, Eckel RH, et al. Plasma triglycerides predict incident albuminuria and progression of coronary artery calcification in adults with type 1 diabetes: the coronary artery calcification in type 1 diabetes study. J Clin Lipidol. 2014;8:576–83.

13. Rader DJ, Hovingh GK. HDL and cardiovascular disease. Lancet. 2014;384: 618–25.

14. Hero C, Rawshani A, Svensson A-M, Franzén S, Eliasson B, Eeg-Olofsson K, et al. Association between use of lipid-lowering therapy and cardiovascular diseases and death in individuals with type 1 diabetes. Diabetes Care. 2016;39:996–1003.

15. Wellen KE, Hotamisligil GS. Inflammation, stress, and diabetes. J Clin Invest. 2005;115:1111–9.

16. Saito M, Ishimitsu T, Minami J, Ono H, Ohrui M, Matsuoka H. Relations of plasma high-sensitivity C-reactive protein to traditional cardiovascular risk factors. Atherosclerosis. 2003;167:73–9.

17. Esser N, Legrand-Poels S, Piette J, Scheen AJ, Paquot N. Inflammation as a link between obesity, metabolic syndrome and type 2 diabetes. Diabetes Res Clin Pract. 2014;105:141–50.

18. De Ferranti SD, De Boer IH, Fonseca V, Fox CS, Golden SH, Lavie CJ, et al. Type 1 diabetes mellitus and cardiovascular disease. Circulation. 2014;130: 1110–30.

19. Ridker PM. Clinical application of C-reactive protein for cardiovascular disease detection and prevention. Circulation. 2003;107:363–9.

20. Mold C, Gewurz H, Du Clos TW. Regulation of complement activation by C-reactive protein. Immunopharmacology. 1999;42:23–30.

21. Casagrande SS, Fradkin JE, Saydah SH, Rust KF, Cowie CC. The prevalence of meeting A1C, blood pressure, and LDL goals among people with diabetes, 1988–2010. Diabetes Care. 2013;36:2271–9.

22. The National Board of Health and Welfare. Swedish National Guidelines for diabetes. 2009.

23. Eeg-Olofsson K, Cederholm J, Nilsson PM, Gudbjörnsdóttir S, Eliasson B. Glycemic and risk factor control in type 1 diabetes. Diabetes Care. 2007;30: 496–502.

24. Chobanian AV, Bakris GL, Black HR, Cushman WC, Green LA, Izzo Jr JL, et al. The seventh report of the joint national committee on prevention, detection, evaluation, and treatment of high blood pressure: the JNC 7 report. JAMA. 2003;289:2560–71.

25. Melin EO, Svensson R, Thunander M, Hillman M, Thulesius HO, Landin-Olsson M. Gender, alexithymia and physical inactivity associated with abdominal obesity in type 1 diabetes mellitus: a cross sectional study at a secondary care hospital diabetes clinic. BMC Obes. 2017;4:21.

26. Melin EO, Thunander M, Svensson R, Landin-Olsson M, Thulesius HO. Depression, obesity and smoking were independently associated with inadequate glycemic control in patients with type 1 diabetes. Eur J Endocrinol. 2013;168:861–9.

27. Melin EO, Thunander M, Landin-Olsson M, Hillman M, Thulesius HO. Depression, smoking, physical inactivity and season independently associated with midnight salivary cortisol in type 1 diabetes. BMC Endocr Disord. 2014;14:75.

28. Melin EO, Svensson R, Gustavsson S-Å, Winberg A, Denward-Olah E, Landin-Olsson M, et al. Affect school and script analysis versus basic body awareness therapy in the treatment of psychological symptoms in patients with diabetes and high HbA1c concentrations: two study protocols for two randomized controlled trials. Trials. 2016;17:221.

29. Melin E. Thesis. Psychosomatic aspects on diabetes and chronic pain alexithymia, depression and salivary cortisol the affect school and script analysis therapy. Lund: Lund University; 2014.

30. Klein S, Allison DB, Heymsfield SB, Kelley DE, Leibel RL, Nonas C, et al. Waist circumference and Cardiometabolic risk: a consensus statement from shaping America's health: Association for Weight Management and Obesity Prevention; NAASO, the Obesity Society; the American Society for Nutrition; and the American Diabetes Association. Obesity. 2007;15:1061–7.

31. Tanamas SK, Permatahati V, Ng WL, Backholer K, Wolfe R, Shaw JE, et al. Estimating the proportion of metabolic health outcomes attributable to obesity: a cross-sectional exploration of body mass index and waist circumference combinations. BMC Obes. 2016;3:4.

32. Jacobsen BK, Aars NA. Changes in waist circumference and the prevalence of abdominal obesity during 1994–2008 - cross-sectional and longitudinal results from two surveys: the Tromsø study. BMC Obes. 2016;3:41.

33. Ford ES, Giles WH, Dietz WH. Prevalence of the metabolic syndrome among US adults: findings from the third National Health and nutrition examination survey. JAMA. 2002;287:356–9.

34. Maranon R, Reckelhoff JF. Sex and gender differences in control of blood pressure. Clin Sci. 2013;125:311–8.

35. Neter JE, Stam BE, Kok FJ, Grobbee DE, Geleijnse JM. Influence of weight reduction on blood pressure. Hypertension. 2003;42:878–84.

36. Bode BW, Garg SK. The emerging role of adjunctive noninsulin antihyperglycemic therapy in the management of type 1 diabetes. Endocr Pract. 2015;22:220–30.

37. Mottalib A, Kasetty M, Mar JY, Elseaidy T, Ashrafzadeh S, Hamdy O. Weight Management in Patients with type 1 diabetes and obesity. Curr Diab Rep. 2017;17:92.

3

In-school adolescents' weight status and blood pressure profile in South-western Nigeria: urban-rural comparison

Akinlolu Gabriel Omisore[1], Bridget Omisore[2], Emmanuel Akintunde Abioye-Kuteyi[2,3], Ibrahim Sebutu Bello[2] and Samuel Anu Olowookere[3*]

Abstract

Background: Obesity is a risk factor for hypertension. The study observed the relationship between adolescent weight status and blood pressure (BP) and the determinants of the BP pattern in urban and rural areas.

Methods: This was a cross-sectional study of 1000 randomly selected respondents (500 from urban and 500 from rural areas) who had anthropometry and BP measurements done. The pattern of BP measurements based on the weight status by location was observed. Statistical inferences were drawn via Chi-square and logistic regression.

Results: The mean age for all the respondents was 13.73 years ±2.04 (13.63 ± 2.05 for urban and 13.82 ± 2.03 for rural). Systolic and diastolic BP generally increased with increasing respondents' age, with mean pressures higher in urban areas. About 3% were obese, while 7.7% were overweight. The overall prevalence of high BP was 4.1%, with two-thirds coming from urban areas. On logistic regression analysis, the significant variables associated with high BP include being female (AOR 2.067, 95%CI1.007–4.243, $p = 0.048$), overweight (AOR 5.574, 95%CI 2.501–12.421, $p = 0.0001$) and obese (AOR 12.437, 95%CI 4.636–33.364, p = 0.0001).

Conclusion: High BP was associated with being female, overweight and obesity in both urban and rural areas. Urgent measures are needed to address increasing prevalence of overweight and obesity among adolescents and consequent high blood pressure.

Keywords: Blood pressure, Body mass index (BMI), Obesity, Urban, Rural

Background

Obesity had previously been regarded as a problem of the developed world and that of adults, however current statistics indicate that overweight and obesity are increasingly common in developing countries and among children and adolescents [1–3]. Obesity accounts for the rising incidence of hypertension among adolescents worldwide and hypertension among adolescents is frequently predictive of future adult hypertension, with its attendant morbidity and mortality and reduced life expectancy [4]. Lifestyle diseases or chronic Non-Communicable Diseases (NCDs) like hypertension, diabetes mellitus, coronary artery diseases and stroke in

adults have been related to the preponderance of risk factors in childhood and adolescence [5].

Of all the NCDs, hypertension is the most prevalent and commonest cause of morbidity and mortality [6]. It is also the commonest risk factor for cardiovascular disease (CVD) [7]. Hypertension occasionally begins in adolescence or childhood and tracks into adulthood [8]. The increasing prevalence of obesity among adolescents and children worldwide has been associated with increased prevalence of hypertension. However, more evidence on the relationship between adolescent weight status and blood pressure (BP) patterns is required despite studies done previously in Nigeria [9–11].

Previously adult obesity and high BP definitions have been used for adolescents but such are no longer recommended. The BMI changes during childhood differ between boys and girls, so age and sex-specific reference

* Correspondence: sanuolowookere@yahoo.com
[3]Department of Community Health, Obafemi Awolowo University Ile-Ife, Ile-Ife, Nigeria
Full list of author information is available at the end of the article

data (centile cut off points on charts) such as that of the International Obesity Task Force (IOTF) are necessary to interpret the measurement [12]. Similarly, the Fourth Report on the Diagnosis, Evaluation, and Treatment of High BP in Children and Adolescents recommends age-, sex-, and height-specific values that are at >95th percentile of normative systolic and diastolic BP values as diagnostic of high BP in childhood [13].

Apart from using International reference standards to measure obesity and high BP, an additional contribution to knowledge being made by this study is that it was conducted in both urban and rural areas. Few studies have attempted to look at adolescent weight status and relate it to the BP pattern and predictors among urban and rural adolescents in Nigeria. Since the relationship between increasing weight status and high BP has been established, [7, 10] and that BP during childhood and adolescence is a recognized predictor of adulthood BP, leading to increased CVD mortality, [14] it becomes imperative to study the weight status and BP profile of adolescents who are gradually moving into adulthood not only in semi-urban or urban areas where more studies have been done but also in rural areas [9, 10, 15]. Because of the different characteristics of urban and rural dwellers in terms of family values, dietary pattern, physical activity and exposure to social amenities, the pattern of obesity/hypertensive range blood pressure is expected to be different between the two areas. Thus, it is expected that the prevalence and determining factors of obesity/ hypertensive range blood pressure may differ between rural and urban areas, hence the comparative nature of this study. This is a very important consideration in determining intervention strategies to apply to both rural and urban settings. This study, therefore, aims to examine in-school adolescents' weight status and relate it to the BP profile in both urban and rural areas of Osun State, South Western Nigeria as well as identify probable predictors for the BP pattern.

Methods

The study was carried out in Osun State, one of the six states in south-western Nigeria in the year 2012 and primary data was independently collected by the authors. The State has three senatorial districts, each with two health zones and 10 local government areas (LGA). Osun East senatorial district was selected by simple random sampling out of the three senatorial districts. The minimum sample size was determined by using the formula for calculating sample size for the comparison of two independent proportions using urban and rural prevalence of 20.9% and 11.9% respectively from a previous study [16]. The study population included 500 students from urban and 500 from rural areas making a

total population of 1000 students from eight schools (four schools from urban areas and four from rural areas) across two health zones in the Osun East senatorial district selected by a multi-stage sampling method. Two communities, one urban and one rural, were chosen by simple random sampling from each of the two health zones in the Osun East senatorial district and two co-education schools were then chosen by simple random sampling from each community. The students in selected schools were stratified by arm and sex and a sample proportionate to the school population and the male-female distribution was studied from each arm. Pre-tested and pre-coded structured questionnaires were completed by the selected 1000 respondents and anthropometry (height and weight) and BP measurements were done.

The weight was measured to the nearest 0.1 kg with a bathroom weighing scale of the United Nation Children Fund (UNICEF) type and the height was measured to the nearest 0.5 cm using a stadiometer. The weight and height were measured with the respondents in light clothing. [16, 17] The BP measurements were taken with Accoson mercury sphygmomanometers with appropriate size cuff. The BP was measured with the adolescent in a sitting position, with the arm at the level of the heart. The cuff was inflated to a level at which the distal arterial pulse was not palpable. It was then deflated at a rate of 2–3 mmHg per second. Systolic blood pressure (SBP) was recorded on hearing the first sound (phase I), while Diastolic blood pressure (DBP) was taken on complete disappearance of Korotkoff sounds phase V [18]. Two measurements were taken with the patient in sitting position by the same (two) trained members of the research team and the average of the two was taken as the final measurement. In cases where there were differences of up to 10 mmHg in either of the systolic or diastolic readings, a third and final measurement was taken by the lead researcher and this was taken as the final measurement. Adolescents were classified as having normal BP, Pre-Hypertension and Hypertension corresponding to less than 85th percentile, 85th -95th percentile and above 95th percentile according to the Fourth Report on the Diagnosis, Evaluation, and Treatment of High BP in Children and Adolescents [13].

From the height and weight measurement, the Body Mass Index (BMI) of each respondent was calculated. The BMI was calculated using the formula- Weight (kg)/ Height (m2). The calculated BMI for each of the respondent in the study was compared with the IOTF age and sex-specific values before any of the study respondents were classified as normal weight, overweight or obese. The research team was made up of qualified and trained research assistants consisting of medical doctors, nurses, medical students and laboratory personnel. They were trained adequately on the study instruments and procedures prior to data collection.

The data obtained were entered and analysed using SPSS 16. Relevant descriptive and inferential statistics were done. Chi-square test and binary logistic regression were used for bivariate analysis. Multivariate analysis using binary logistic regression was used to evaluate variables that were independently associated with high BP. Criteria for inclusion of variables in the logistic regression model was a p-value of < 0.2 in the bivariate. Odds ratios (OR) and 95% confidence intervals (CI) were presented and used as measures of association. p-value < 0.05 was regarded as statistically significant.

The main outcome measures were the systolic and diastolic BP of participants as well as the BMI using the IOTF age and sex specific cut off points. Physical activity was derived from a standardised instrument recommended for adolescents [19]. The Moderate to Vigorous Physical Activity (MVPA) measure of the instrument was used for this study [19]. The measure assessed the number of days' subjects had accumulated 60 min of MVPA during the past 7 days and for a typical week. The measure defined physical activity broadly as "one that at least increases your heart rate and makes you get out of breath some of the time". An average of the 2 weeks (last 7 days plus a typical week) yielded a score of days per week the adolescent had at least 60 min of MVPA per day. Five or more days per week met the guideline of being physically active. Socio-economic status (SES) was classified into two (high and low SES) based on a modified wealth index approach [20]. The modified wealth index approach used in this study was based on an eight-item index of household assets including means of mobility such as the possession of motorcycles and cars. House type (size and whether rented or owned) and type of walls/floor materials, as well as toilet facilities available, were taken into consideration. The estimated pocket/feeding money given to the adolescents were also considered. The minimum and maximum obtainable score from the modified index was 0–20, with a mean as well as a median score of 14.00 indicating a normally distributed sample. Respondents who had a score above 14 were regrouped as belonging to high socio-economic class while those who had a score of 14 and below were regrouped as belonging to low socio-economic class (SES) based on the average score (20).

Results

Table 1 shows the socio-demographic characteristics of respondents. Most of the respondents in both urban and rural schools were in the age group 10–13 (early adolescence) and 14–16 years (middle adolescence). The mean age (SD) for all the respondents was 13.73 (2.04) years;

for urban 13.63 (2.05) and for rural 13.82 (2.03) years. Male respondents were 51.0% in both urban and rural schools. Of the 1000 respondents, higher proportions were from more highly educated parents (paternal 65.1%, maternal 60.6%) compared with their respective counterparts. The table also shows that significantly higher proportions of respondents in urban schools were in private schools and from more highly educated parents and high socioeconomic status compared with their rural counterparts.

A significantly greater proportion of urban respondents were obese and overweight (5.4% and 11.4% respectively) compared to rural respondents (0.4% and 4.0% respectively). Similarly, more females were comparatively overweight and obese (10.2% and 3.9%) than males (5.3% and 2.0%) and more respondents who had high SES were overweight and obese (11.5% and 5.4%) compared to those with low SES (4.1% and 0.6%). The proportion of physically inactive respondents who were obese (3.8%) was almost twice those who were physically active (2.0%) and more physically inactive respondents were also overweight. A significantly higher proportion of those who have increased BP was also overweight and obese (26.8% and 19.5% respectively) compared to those who did not have increased BP (6.9% and 2.2% respectively). Similarly, there were more obese and overweight respondents among children whose parents were of high educational status compared to those whose parents had low educational status as shown in Table 2.

The mean systolic BP gradually increased across ages 10–19 (from 93.4 to 110.5 mmHg) in rural schools and the pattern in urban schools was similar from age 10–14. The mean diastolic BP gradually increased from age 10–18 (59.0–73.2 mmHg) in rural schools but did not follow any particular trend in urban schools as there were variations across ages. The mean systolic BP for all ages combined was higher in schools located in urban than rural areas, 104.1 ± 14.71 mmHg versus 101.7 ± 12.36 mmHg. A similar result was obtained for and diastolic BP (66.8 ± 10.43 against 65.1 ± 9.30 respectively) as shown in Table 3.

A greater proportion of respondents in rural areas (52.3% and 52.4%) had normal systolic and diastolic BP compared to those in urban areas (47.7% and 47.6%) respectively. The reverse was the case with systolic and diastolic pre-hypertension and hypertension in which respondents from urban areas had higher figures than those from rural areas. For instance, out of those who had any form of systolic hypertension, whether singly or combined with diastolic hypertension, 72% were from urban areas compared to 28.0% from rural areas. Figures for diastolic hypertension were 59.1% and 40.9% respectively. Overall, 41 respondents (4.1%) had hypertension with

Table 1 Socio-demographic characteristics of respondents

Variable	Urban $N = 500$ (%)	Rural $N = 500$ (%)	Total $N = 1000$ (%)	Remark
Age Group				
10–13 Years	230(46.0%)	225(45.0%)	455(45.5%)	$\chi^2 = 1.56$, $p = 0.459$
14–16 Years	233(46.6%)	227(45.4%)	460(46.0%)	
17–19 Years	37(7.4%)	48(9.6%)	85(8.5%)	
Sex				
Male	255(51.0%)	255(51.0%)	510(51.0%)	$\chi^2 = 0.001$, $p = 1.00$
Female	245(49.0%)	245(49.0%)	490(49.0%)	
Ethnicity				
Yoruba	458(91.6%)	477(95.4%)	935(93.5%)	$\chi^2 = 14.32$, $p = 0.003$
Igbo	38(7.6%)	14(2.8%)	52(5.2%)	
Hausa	1(0.2%)	4(0.8%)	5(0.5%)	
Others	3(0.6%)	5(1.0%)	8(0.8%)	
Father's Educational Status				
Low[a]	60(12.0%)	115(23.0%)	175(17.5%)	$\chi^2 = 20.97$, $p < 0.001$
High[b]	348(69.6%)	303(60.6%)	651(65.1%)	
Unknown	92(18.4%)	82(16.4%)	174(17.4%)	
Mother's Educational Status				
Low[a]	79(15.8%)	140(28.0%)	219(21.9%)	$\chi^2 = 23.34$, $p < 0.001$
High[b]	334(66.8%)	272(54.4%)	606(60.6%)	
Unknown	87(17.4%)	88(17.6%)	175(17.5%)	
Socioeconomic Status				
Low	209(41.8%)	307(61.4%)	516(51.6%)	. $\chi^2 = 38.45$, $p < 0.001$
High	291(58.2%)	193(38.6%)	484 (48.4%)	
School Type				
Public	212 (42.4%)	276(55.2%)	488(48.8%)	$\chi^2 = 16.39$, $p < 0.001$
Private	288 (57.6%)	224(44.8%)	512(51.2%)	

[a]Low- No formal education to incomplete secondary education
[b]High- completed secondary education to tertiary education. #- Likelihood ratio/Fisher exact test used because at least one cell has an expected value less than five

65.8% of them coming from urban areas and the remaining 34.2% coming from rural areas (Table 4).

When the BP profiles of urban and rural respondents were compared with socio-demographic and other characteristics, respondents' BMI showed statistically significant relationships in both urban and rural areas. In urban schools, a significantly higher proportion of obese respondents (25.9%) had high BP compared to 2.9% of those with normal weight and 14.0% of those with overweight. The situation was similar in rural schools where a significantly higher proportion of obese respondents (50.0%) had high BP compared to 2.1% of those with normal weight and 15.0% of those with overweight. In both urban and rural schools, obese respondents had the highest proportion of those with high BP followed by those with overweight. A greater proportion of females (7.3%) had high BP in urban areas compared to males (3.5%), corresponding figures for rural areas were 4.5% and 1.2%. The variables "father and mother's educational

status" only showed statistically significant difference between those of low and high status in urban areas while there was no difference in rural areas. The variable sex showed a statistically significant relationship with BP in rural areas only while age-group, socio-economic status and physical activity level did not show a statistically significant difference with BP in both urban and rural areas (Table 5).

Table 6 reported findings on binary regression analysis. Among urban-based residents, significant variables associated with high BP include being overweight (OR 5.497, 95%CI 2.142–14.106, $p = 0.0001$) and obese (OR 11.783, 95%CI 4.187–33.159, p = 0.0001) while among rural residents, being females (OR 3.949, 95%CI 1.088–14.330, $p = 0.037$), overweight (OR 8.259, 95%CI 2.082–32.762, $p = 0.003$) and obese (OR 46.800, 95%CI 2.730–802.382, $p = 0.008$).

On multivariate regression analysis, the significant variables associated with high BP include being female

Table 2 Weight status and selected variables of total respondents

Variable	Category of Variable	Normal Wt (%) n = 894 (89.4)	Overweight (%) n = 77(7.7)	Obese (%) n = 29 (2.9)	Total (%) N = 1000	Remark
Location	Urban	416 (83.2)	57(11.4)	27 (5.4)	500 (100.0)	$x^2 = 43.63$
	Rural	478 (95.6)	20 (4.0)	2 (0.4)	500 (100.0)	$p < 0.001^a$
Sex	Male	473 (92.7)	27 (5.3)	10 (2.0)	510 (100.0)	$x^2 = 12.29$
	Female	421 (85.9)	50 (10.2)	19 (3.9)	490 (100.0)	$p = 0.002^a$
Age-group	Early Adolescence	403(88.5)	34(7.5)	18(4.0)	455 (100.0)	$x^2 = 3.85^b$
	Mid Adolescence	413(89.8)	37(8.0)	10(2.2)	460 (100.0)	$p = 0.426$
	Late Adolescence	78(91.7)	6(7.1)	1(1.2)	85 (100.0)	
Socio-Economic Status (SES)	Low SES	492 (95.3)	21(4.1)	3(0.6)	516 (100.0)	$x^2 = 42.23$
	High SES	402 (83.1)	56(11.5)	26(5.4)	484 (100.0)	$p < 0.001^a$
Physical Activity (MVPA +)	Physically Inactive	443(87.0)	47(9.2)	19(3.8)	509 (100.0)	$x^2 = 6.30$
	Physically Active	451(91.9.)	30(6.1)	10(2.0)	491 (100.0)	$p = 0.043^a$
High Blood Pressure	No	872 (90.9)	66 (6.9)	21 (2.2)	959 (100.0)	$x^2 = 67.11^b$
	Yes	22 (53.7)	11 (26.8)	8 (19.5)	41 (100.0)	$p < 0.001^a$
Father's Educational Status n = 826 #	Low	171(97.7)	3(1.7)	1(0.6)	175(100.0)	$x^2 = 19.85^b$
	High	571(87.7)	59(9.1)	21(3.2)	651(100.0)	$p < 0.001^a$
Mother's Educational Status n = 825 #	Low	210(95.9)	7(3.2)	2(0.9)	219(100.0)	$x^2 = 16.96^b$
	High	525(86.6)	59(9.7)	22(3.7)	606(100.0)	$p < 0.001^a$

[a]Statistically significant
[b]Likelihood ratio/Fisher exact test used because at least one cell has an expected value < 5. #- Respondents who did not know parental educational status were excluded from analysis. + MVPA = Moderate to Vigorous Physical Activity (typical plus last seven days prior to interview)

(AOR 2.067, 95%CI1.007–4.243, p = 0.048), overweight (AOR 5.574, 95%CI 2.501–12.421, p = 0.0001) and obese (AOR 12.437, 95%CI 4.636–33.364, p = 0.0001) (Table 7).

Discussion

This study assessed the weight status of adolescents (normal weight, overweight and obese) and related it to their blood pressure profile and confirmed that in both urban and rural areas, the weight status has a relationship with the blood pressure. Most of the overweight and obese respondents were from urban areas. The study population was chosen by multi-stage sampling across a randomly chosen senatorial district, out of three present in the State, with both rural and urban areas and private and public schools

Table 3 Descriptive Statistics of Respondents' Blood Pressures by Age and Location

Age	Urban(%)	Rural(%)	Mean Systolic Blood Pressure (mmHg) ± Std Deviation Urban	Rural	Mean Diastolic Blood Pressure (mmHg) ± Std Deviation Urban	Rural
10	39(7.8)	27(5.4)	94.5 ± 13.80	93.4 ± 8.80	60.8 ± 11.21	59.0 ± 7.87
11	53(10.6)	38(7.6)	96.4 ± 13.25	95.5 ± 11.58	61.4 ± 9.67	61.1 ± 9.05
12	54(10.8)	77(15.4)	100.6 ± 14.42	98.1 ± 11.64	54.7 ± 94.94	62.6 ± 9.04
13	84(16.8)	83(16.6)	105.0 ± 14.39	99.1 ± 10.99	66.8 ± 10.43	64.1 ± 7.86
14	98(19.6)	81(16.2)	108.4 ± 13.15	103.4 ± 12.00	70.3 ± 8.70	65.1 ± 9.10
15	72(14.4)	94(18.8)	105.0 ± 13.14	104.3 ± 12.36	68.6 ± 9.58	66.2 ± 9.43
16	63(12.6)	52(10.4)	109.6 ± 15.54	106.8 ± 12.29	70.0 ± 10.32	68.2 ± 8.97
17	24(4.8)	26(5.2)	104.5 ± 15.50	108.0 ± 11.87	64.2 ± 11.45	70.5 ± 8.73
18	11(2.2)	18(3.6)	105.4 ± 15.73	109.4 ± 11.10	67.3 ± 11.04	73.2 ± 7.58
19	2(0.4)	4(0.8)	110.0 ± 0.00	110.5 ± 13.20	75.0 ± 7.07	70.0 ± 14.14
Total	500(100.0)	500(100.0)	104.1 ± 14.71	101.7 ± 12.36	66.8 ± 10.43	65.1 ± 9.30

For the blood pressure measurements, total here refers to the mean score of all the score for the various ages

Table 4 Blood pressure distribution of respondents

Blood Pressure category	Urban (%)	Rural (%)	Total (%)
Normal Systolic BP	386 (47.7)	424 (52.3)	810(100.0)
Normal Diastolic BP	392 (47.6)	432 (52.4)	824 (100.0)
"Pre-Hypertension" (Systolic)	96 (58.2)	69 (41.8)	165 (100.0)
"Pre-Hypertension" (Diastolic)	95 (61.7)	59 (38.3)	154 (100.0)
"Hypertension" (Systolic)	18 (72.0)	7 (28.0)	25 (100.0)
"Hypertension" (Diastolic)	13 (59.1)	9 (40.9)	22 (100.0)
Total respondents with high BP (either systolic or diastolic or both)[a]	27 (65.8)	14 (34.2)	41 (100.0)

[a]Out of the 41 respondents who had "hypertension", 19 had isolated systolic "hypertension", 16 had isolated diastolic "hypertension" and six had both systolic and diastolic "hypertension"

taken into consideration and thus the findings can be confidently stated as generalizable.

Both SBP and DBP generally increased with age in both urban and rural areas but especially in urban areas. This is in keeping with previous studies [21–23]. The age-specific systolic and DBP were generally higher for urban areas especially among early and mid-adolescents and the respondents in urban schools also had a significantly higher mean SBP and DBP than those in rural schools. In terms of actual prevalence of "hypertension", respondents in urban areas constituted two-thirds of the high BP cases compared to a third from rural schools. In a Nigerian study done among adolescents the prevalence of point-hypertension was 4.6% in a semi-urban area

compared to 17.5% in an urban area [10]. In another rural-urban Nigerian study, the prevalence of high BP in the urban community (9.5%) was higher than the rural community (6.3%) [24]. The rural-urban disparity has been attributed to the difference in lifestyle between urban and rural populations [10].

The combined proportion of respondents who were either overweight or obese (10.6%) showed that at least one out of every ten adolescents was either overweight or obese. The proportion of people who were overweight and/or obese is slightly higher in this study compared to similar previous studies done over the last few years in Nigeria in which the prevalence was generally less than 10 % [25, 26]. This might imply that overweight and obesity are on the increase in Nigeria as it is in most other countries of the world.

Both overweight and obesity were common in urban areas than rural areas in this study- This finding is in keeping with previous studies done in Nigeria that showed that obesity was commoner in urban schools [26, 27]. In a study done in Lagos, the prevalence rates of overweight and obesity in the urban and rural areas of Eti-osa LGA among 1504 in-school adolescents were 3.7% and 0.4%, and 3.0% and 0.0% respectively, showing a slight preponderance in urban schools [26]. In a study done earlier in rural and urban schools in Osun state, the same state as this study, using the WHO cut off points values for classifying obesity and overweight, the

Table 5 High blood pressure and selected variables of urban and rural respondents

Socio-demographic /other variables	Category	Urban n = 500 High BP		χ_r^2 (p value)	Rural n = 500 High BP		χ_r^2 (p value)
		YES(%)	NO (%)		YES (%)	NO (%)	
Sex	Male	9(3.5)	246(96.5)	3.565 (0.059)	3(1.2)	252(98.8)	5.040 (0.025[a])
	Female	18(7.3)	227(92.7)		11(4.5)	234(95.5)	
Age	Early adolescence	14(6.1)	216(93.9)	4.327[b] (0.115)	8(3.6)	217(96.4)	1.755[b] (0.416)
	Mid adolescence	13(5.6)	220(94.4)		4(1.8)	223(98.2)	
	Late adolescence	0(0.0)	37(100.0)		2(4.2)	46(95.8)	
BMI (Weight Status)	Normal weight	12(2.9)	404(97.1)	24.24[b] (< 0.001[a])	10(2.1)	468(97.9)	10.91[b] (0.004[a])
	Overweight	8(14.0)	49(86.0)		3(15.0)	17(85.0)	
	Obese	7(25.9)	20(74.1)		1(50.0)	1(50.0)	
Socio-economic Status	Low	12(5.7)	197(94.3)	0.082 (0.775)	7(2.3)	300(97.7)	0.790 (0.374)
	High	15(5.2)	276(94.8)		7(3.6)	186(96.4)	
Physical activity level	Physically inactive	15(6.2)	226(93.8)	0.618 (0.432)	10(3.7)	258(96.3)	1.841 (0.175)
	Physically active	12(4.6)	247(95.4)		4(1.7)	228(98.3)	
Father's Educational Status n = 826 #	Low	0(0.0)	60(100.0)	7.212[b] (0.007)[a]	5(4.3)	110(95.7)	1.241 (0.265)
	High	22(6.3)	326(93.7)		7(2.3)	296(97.7)	
Mother's Educational Status n = 825 #	Low	1(1.3)	78(98.7)	4.257[b] (0.039)[a]	4(2.9)	136(97.1)	0.432[b] (0.511)
	High	21(6.3)	313(93.7)		5(1.8)	267(98.2)	

[a]Statistically significant at $p < 0.05$. Likelihood Ratio used because at least one cell has an expected value less than 5
[b]Likelihood ratio/Fisher exact test used because at least one cell has an expected value < 5. #- Respondents who did not know parental educational status were excluded from analysis

Table 6 Binary regression analysis of variables predicting high blood pressure among urban and rural based respondents

Variable	OR, 95%CI, p-value
Urban	
Sex (vs male)	
Female	2.167, 0.954–4.922, 0.065
Body Mass Index (vs normal)	
Obese	11.783, 4.187–33.159, 0.0001
Overweight	5.497, 2.142–14.106, 0.0001
Physically activity (vs physically inactive)	
Physically active	0.732, 0.335–1.597, 0.433
Rural	
Sex (vs male)	
Female	3.949, 1.088–14.330, 0.037
Body Mass Index (vs normal)	
Obese	46.800, 2.730–802.382, 0.008
Overweight	8.259, 2.082–32.762, 0.003
Physically activity (vs physically inactive)	
Physically active	0.453, 0.140–1.463, 0.185

overall prevalence of overweight amongst 450 respondents was 3.2% with 4.1% prevalence in urban schools and 1.5% in rural schools while 0.5% of urban students were obese and no obesity was recorded in rural areas, thus overweight and obesity were commoner in urban areas [27]. Results of rural-urban studies done beyond the shores of Nigeria revealed that overweight and obesity are common in urban areas for developed/developing economies in Asia [28–30], but for western nations overweight and obesity are now commoner in rural areas [31, 32].

Both overweight and obesity were commoner in girls than boys in this study and this was statistically

Table 7 Multivariate regression analysis of variables predicting high blood pressure among respondents

Variable	Crude OR, 95%CI, p-value	Adjusted OR, 95%CI, p-value
Sex (vs male)		
Female	2.611, 1.317–5.177, 0.006	2.067, 1.007–4.243, 0.048
Body Mass Index (vs normal)		
Obese	15.100, 6.031–37.801, 0.0001	12.437, 4.636–33.364, 0.0001
Overweight	6.606, 3.072–14.208, 0.0001	5.574, 2.501–12.421, 0.0001
Physically activity (vs physically inactive)		
Physically active	1.533, 0.808–2.909, 0.191	0.891, 0.451–1.759, 0.739
Residence (vs rural)		
Urban	1.982, 1.026–3.925, 0.042	1.189, 0.576–2.453, 0.639

significant. This is in keeping with some studies that have been done previously in some developing countries [27, 28]. However, some studies have also reported a higher prevalence of overweight and obesity in boys compared to girls [16, 30]. The higher prevalence of overweight and obesity in females in this study might be due to physiological changes such as hormonal variations with respect to their age; girls tend to grow and develop secondary sexual characteristics a bit earlier than boys of the same age. This is, in fact, more likely to be true since the greater percentage of overweight and obese respondents in this study are in the early adolescent group aged 10–13 years as reported in a previous study in urban Cameroon [3]. This may be because a lot of pubertal growth spurt takes place in females during this period however further research is required.

Majority of those who were overweight and obese in this study were from high socio-economic background and parents' having high educational status. This is in conformity with other studies that showed that overweight and obesity are common within young people in higher socio-economic group in developing countries [30, 33, 34] unlike in developed countries where it is commoner among the low socio-economic group in both urban and rural areas [35]. Similarly, more respondents who were physically active were less overweight and obese compared to physically inactive. This is in keeping with other studies which have shown that physical activity is associated with overweight and obesity, [32, 35, 36] with little or no physical activity being a predisposing factor to overweight and obesity. Overweight and obesity were found to be associated with higher systolic and diastolic BP in this study as has been found in some other studies [37–40].

From previous studies, the higher the BMI the greater the BP and this has been found in both urban and rural areas [10, 11, 41]. In a study done in Lagos, an urban area of Nigeria, higher BMI was significantly associated with hypertensive range systolic and diastolic BP [22]. Although the precise mechanisms of the positive correlation between BMI and BP are not entirely understood, factors that have been attributed include sedentariness, excessive sodium intake, hyperactivity of the renin-angiotensin and sympathetic nervous systems, insulin resistance and abnormalities in vascular structure and function [42, 43].

More females were obese and consequently had high BP than males. Unlike the finding in this study, more males had high BP in both urban and rural areas than females in a study done in Slovakia. [44] However, similar to this study, Slovakian males also had statistically higher mean values of BMI than females, thus, stressing the fact that the BP level often corresponds to the weight status. Using multi-variate analysis, the BMI (weight status) was predictive of BP in both urban and rural areas, further, confirming the association of BP with the BMI.

This study is limited in being a cross-sectional survey as no cause-effect relationship could be established. Also, some respondents did not know their parents' educational status hence, were excluded from some analyses. However, the study findings add to the body of knowledge more information linking obesity and hypertension among in-school adolescents.

Conclusion

BP generally increased with age with the mean systolic and diastolic BP for all ages combined higher in schools located in urban than rural areas. A little over 10 % of the respondents were either overweight or obese. A greater proportion of respondents who were overweight or obese were females, from urban areas, physically inactive, of high socioeconomic status and had high BP. The overall prevalence of high BP was 4.1%, with almost two-thirds coming from urban areas and the remaining third from rural areas. More females had high BP than males and this was significant in rural areas. BMI was significantly associated with high BP in both rural and urban areas. In both areas, especially in rural areas respondents with normal weight were less likely to have high BP compared with those who were obese.

The already documented effects of increasing weight and rising BP have been demonstrated again in this study, but this among adolescents in both rural and urban areas of a developing country. Since overweight and obesity are increasing globally, urgent measures are needed to address their increasing prevalence and the consequent high BP.

Abbreviations
AOR: Adjusted Odd Ratio; BMI: Body Mass Index; BP: Blood pressure; CVD: Cardiovascular disease; DBP: Diastolic blood pressure; IOTF: International Obesity Task Force; LGA: Local government area; MVPA: Moderate to Vigorous Physical Activity; NCDs: Non Communicable Diseases; OAUTHC: Obafemi Awolowo University Teaching Hospitals Complex; SBP: Systolic blood pressure; SD: Standard deviation; SES: Socio-economic status; UNICEF: United Nation Children Fund

Acknowledgements
The authors wish to acknowledge the Permanent Secretary, Ministry of Education, Osun State and the Local Inspectorate of education, Principals, Teachers as well as Students involved in the project. We also appreciate health workers and students involved in the data collection process.

Funding
Funding was essentially provided by the authors as no grant was received for this research.

Authors' contributions
AGO: Conceptualization of the study, study design, data collection, data analysis and interpretation, discussion and editing/ review of the final draft for publication. BO: Conceptualization of the study, study design, data collection, discussion and editing/ review of the final draft for publication. EAA: General oversight/supervision of the entire work, discussion and editing/ review of the final draft for publication. ISB: Data collection, discussion and editing/ review of the final draft for publication. SAO: Data collection, data analysis, draft write up, discussion and editing/review of the final draft for publication. All authors read and approved the final manuscript.

Authors' information
A.G Omisore is a Senior Lecturer and Consultant Public Health Physician. His research interest is mainly focussed on public health issues, especially epidemiology of Non Communicable Diseases. B. Omisore is a Consultant Family Physician. Her research interest is mainly focussed on family medicine, in particular, lifestyle medicine as it affects the family. E. A. Abioye-Kuteyi is a Professor of Family Medicine. His research areas include family medicine and population health. I. S. Bello is a Consultant Family Physician. His research interest is mainly focussed on family medicine and preventive care. S. A. Olowookere is a Senior Lecturer and Consultant Family Physician. His research interest is mainly focussed on family medicine and public health.

Competing interests
The authors declare that we have no financial or personal relationships which may have inappropriately influenced us in reaching the conclusions in this paper.

Author details
[1]Department of Community Medicine, Osun State University, Osogbo, Nigeria. [2]Department of Family Medicine, Obafemi Awolowo University Teaching Hospitals Complex, Ile-Ife, Nigeria. [3]Department of Community Health, Obafemi Awolowo University Ile-Ife, Ile-Ife, Nigeria.

References
1.   World Health Organization. Obesity: preventing and managing the global epidemic; report of a WHO consultation on obesity. Geneva: WHO; 2000.
2.   Hothan KA, Alasmari BA, Alkhelaiwi OK, Althagafi KM, Alkhaldi AA, Alfityani AK, et al. Prevalence of hypertension, obesity, hematuria, proteinuria amongst healthy adolescents living in western Saudi Arabia. Saudi Med J. 2016;37:1120–6.
3.   Choukem S, Kamdeu-Chedeu J, Leary SD, Mboue-Djieka Y, Nebongo DN, Akazong C, et al. Overweight and obesity in children aged 3-13 years in urban Cameroon: a cross-sectional study of prevalence and association with socio-economic status. BMC Obesity. 2017;4:7.
4.   Franks W, Hanson RL, Knowler WC, Sievers ML, Bennett PH, Looker HC. Childhood obesity, other cardiovascular risk factors and premature death. N Engl J Med. 2010;362:485–93.
5.   Malhotra K, Nistane RH. Study of obesity and hypertension in adolescents and their relationships with anthropometric indices. Int J Contemp Pediatr. 2016;3:1014–21.
6.   World Health Organization. World Health Report. Reducing risks, promoting healthy life. Geneva: World Health Organization; 2002.
7.   Bo S, Gambino R, Gentile L, Pagano G, Rosato R, Saracco GM, et al. High-normal blood pressure is associated with a cluster of cardiovascular and metabolic risk factors: a population based study. J Hypertens. 2009;27:102–8.

8. Raja D, Vinoth R. A study of relationship between BMI and hypertension among adolescents in Kancheepuram districts, Kamil Nadu. International Journal of Applied Research. 2015;1:8–12.

9. Ejike CE, Ugwu C. Hyperbolic relationship between blood pressure and body mass index in a Nigerian adolescent population. Webmed Central HYPERTENSION. 2010;1:WMC00797.

10. Ejike CE, Ugwu CE, Ezeanyika LUS. Variations in the prevalence of point (pre)hypertension in a Nigerian school-going adolescent population living in a semi-urban and an urban area. BMC Pediatr. 2010;10:13. doi:https://doi.org/10.1186/1471-2431-10-13.

11. Eberechukwu LE, Eyam ES, Nsan E. Types of obesity and its effect on blood pressure of secondary school students in rural and urban areas of Cross River state, Nigeria. IOSR Journal of Pharmacy. 2013;3:60–6.

12. Cole TJ, Bellizzi MC, Flegal KM, Dietz WH. Establishing a standard definition for child overweight and obesity worldwide: international survey. BMJ. 2000;320:1240–3.

13. National High Blood Pressure Education Program Working Group on High Blood Pressure in Children and Adolescents. The fourth report on the diagnosis, evaluation, and treatment of high blood pressure in children and adolescents. Pediatrics. 2004;114:555–76.

14. Li S, Chen W, Srinivasan SR, Berenson GS. Childhood blood pressure as a predictor of arterial stiffness in young adults: the Bogalusa heart study. Hypertension. 2004;43:541–6.

15. Uwaezuoke SN, Okoli CV, Ubesie AC, Ikefuna AN. Primary hypertension among a population of Nigerian secondary school adolescents: prevalence and correlation with anthropometric indices: a cross-sectional study. Niger J Clin Pract. 2016;19:649–54.

16. Unnithan AG, Syamakumari S. Prevalence of overweight, obesity and underweight among school going children in rural and urban areas of Thiruvananthapuram Educational District, Kerala state, India. Internet J Nutr Wellness. 2008;6:2.

17. McCarthy HD, Ellis SM, Cole TJ. Central overweight and obesity in British youth aged 11-16 years: cross sectional surveys of waist circumference. BMJ. 2003;326:624.

18. Taksande A, Chaturvedi P, Vilhekar K, Jain M. Distribution of blood pressure in school going children in rural area of Wardha district, Maharashatra. India Ann Pediatr Cardiol. 2008;1:101–6.

19. Prochaska JJ, Sallis JF, Long B. A physical activity screening measure for use with adolescents in primary care. Arch Pediatr Adolesc Med. 2001;155:554.

20. Isiugo-Abanihe U, Oyediran K. Household socio-economic status and sexual behaviour among Nigerian female youth. Afr Popul Stud. 2004;19:81–98. Available at: http://www.bioline.org.br/pdf?ep04005. Accessed 29 Apr 2012

21. Al Salloum AA, El Mouzan MI, Al Herbish AS, Al Omar AA, Qurachi MM. Blood pressure standards for Saudi children and adolescents. Ann Saudi Med. 2009;29:173–8. Available at: http://www.ncbi.nlm.nih.gov/pubmed/19448364. Accessed 26 Apr 2012

22. Oduwole AA, Ladapo TA, Fajolu BI, Ekure EN, Adeniyi OF. Obesity and elevated blood pressure among adolescents in Lagos, Nigeria: a cross-sectional study. BMC Public Health. 2012;12:616. doi:https://doi.org/10.1186/1471-2458-12-616.

23. Agyemang C, Redekop WK, Owusu-Dabo E, Bruijnzeels MA. Blood pressure patterns in rural, semi-urban and urban children in the Ashanti region of Ghana, West Africa. BMC Public Health. 2005;5:114.

24. Obika LF, Adedoyin MA, Olowoyeye JO. Pattern of paediatric blood pressure in rural, semi-urban and urban communities in Ilorin, Nigeria. Afr J Med Med Sci. 1995;24:371–7.

25. Akinpelu O, Oyewole OO, Oritogun KS. Overweight and obesity: does it occur in Nigerian adolescents in an urban community? International Journal of Biomedical and Health sciences. 2008;4:11–7.

26. Ben-Bassey UP, Oduwole AO, Ogundipe OO. Prevalence of overweight and obesity in Eti-Osa LGA, Lagos, Nigeria. Obes Rev. 2007;8:475–9.

27. Olumakaiye MF. Prevalence of underweight: a matter of concern among adolescents in Osun state, Nigeria. Pak J Nutr. 2008;7:503–8.

28. Saraswathi YS, Najafil M, Gangadhar MR, Malinil SS. Prevalence of childhood obesity in school children from rural and urban areas in Mysore, Karnataka, India. J Life Sci. 2011;3:51–5. Available at: http://www.krepublishers.com/02-Journals/JLS/JLS-03-0-000-11. Accessed 26 Apr 2012

29. Ghosh A. Rural–urban comparison in prevalence of overweight and obesity among children and adolescents of Asian Indian origin. Asia Pac J Public Health. 2011;23:928–35. doi:https://doi.org/10.1177/1010539511428697.

30. Chen TJ, Modin B, Ji CY, Hjern A. Regional, socioeconomic and urban-rural disparities in child and adolescent obesity in China: a multilevel analysis. Acta Paediatr. 2011;100:1583–9.

31. Tai-Seale T, Chandler C. Nutrition and overweight concerns in rural areas. In: Gamm L, Hutchison L, Dabney B, Dorsey A, editors. Rural healthy people: a companion document to healthy people 2010, vol. volume 2. College Station: South-west rural health research centre; 2003. p. 115–30. Available at: http://srph.tamhsc.edu/centers/rhp2010/09Volume1nutrition%20.htm. Accessed 23 June 2017.

32. Patterson D, Moore CG, Probst JC, Shinogle JA. Obesity and physical activity in rural America. J of Rural Health (Spring). 2004;2004:151–9.

33. Laxmaiah A, Nagalla B, Vijayaraghavan K, Nair M. Factors affecting prevalence of overweight among 12- to 17-year-old urban adolescents in Hyderabad, India. Obesity. 2007;15:1384–90. doi:https://doi.org/10.1038/oby.2007.165.

34. Nagwa MA, Elhussein AM, Azza M, Abdulhadi NH. Alarming high prevalence of overweight/obesity among Sudanese children. Eur J Clin Nutr. 2011;65:409–11.

35. Liu J, Bennett KJ, Harun N, Zheng X, Probst JC, Pate RR. Overweight and physical inactivity among rural children aged 10–17: a national and state portrait. South Carolina rural Health Research Center. 2007. Available at- http://rhr.sph.sc.edu/report/SCRHRC_KF_ObesityChartbook.pdf. Accessed 23 Apr 2017.

36. Hohepa M, Schofield G, Kolt G. Adolescent obesity and physical inactivity. N Z Med J. 2004;117:1207.

37. Hvidt KN. Blood pressure and arterial stiffness in obese children and adolescents. Effect of weight reduction. Dan Med J. 2015;62:1–22.

38. Itagi V, Patil R. Obesity in children and adolescents and its relationship with hypertension. Turk J Med Sci. 2011;14:259–66.

39. Salvadori M, Sontrop JM, Garg AX, Truong J, Suri RS, Mahmud FH, et al. Elevated blood pressure in relation to overweight and obesity among children in a rural Canadian community. Pediatrics. 2008;122:821–7.

40. Senbanjo IO, Oshikoya KA. Obesity and blood pressure levels of adolescents in Abeokuta, Nigeria. Cardiovascular Journal of Africa. 2012;23:260–4. doi: https://doi.org/10.5830/CVJA-2011-037.

41. Ejike ECC, Ugwu CE, Ezeanyika LUS, Olayemi AT. Blood pressure patterns in relation to geographic area of residence: a cross-sectional study of adolescents in Kogi state, Nigeria. BMC Public Health. 2008;8:411. doi:https://doi.org/10.1186/1471-2458-8-411.

42. Sorof J, Daniels S. Obesity hypertension in children: a problem of epidemic proportions. Hypertension. 2002;40:441–7.

43. Mohan B, Kumar N, Aslam N, Rangbulla A, Kumbkami S, Sood NK, et al. Prevalence of sustained hypertension and obesity in urban and rural school going children in Ludhiana. Indian Heart J. 2004;56:310–4.

44. Hujova Z, Lesniakova M. Anthropometric risk factors of artherosclerosis: difference between urban and rural east Slovakian children and adolescents. Bratisl Lek Listy. 2011;112:491–6.

4

Television exposure and overweight/obesity among women in Ghana

Derek Anamaale Tuoyire

Abstract

Background: Although the public health importance of the association between television (TV) viewing and obesity and/or related outcomes have been demonstrated in both cross-sectional and prospective studies elsewhere, similar studies are lacking within the African region. With the view to fill this gap in the literature, the current study explored the association between TV exposure and overweight/obesity among Ghanaian women.

Methods: Based on a sample of 4158 women, descriptive statistics and binary logistic regression were applied to data on TV ownership, TV viewing frequency, and body mass index (BMI) measures from the 2014 Ghana Demographic and Health Survey (GDHS) to explore the association between TV exposure and overweight/obesity among Ghanaian women.

Results: Despite controlling for other factors (age educational level, marital status, wealth quintile, occupation, type of locality, and parity), the results show that women with TV in their households, and with high TV exposure were significantly ($P < 0.05$) more likely (OR = 1.39, 95% CI = 1.002, 1.923) to be overweight/obese compared to those with no TV in their households, and no TV exposure.

Conclusion: The study demonstrates that increased TV exposure is significantly associated with overweight/obesity among women in Ghana even after adjusting for other factors. Interventions aimed at tackling obesity in Ghana should focus on encouraging the uptake of more physically demanding pastime activities in place of TV "sit time".

Keywords: Television exposure, Obesity, Overweight, Women, Ghana

Background

There is growing concern about the rising global prevalence of overweight and obesity, as well as their associated adverse health implications [1–3]. One feature of this global problem is the fast pace at which developing countries are being affected compared to the developed countries. For example, while the number of people affected by overweight or obesity increased 1.7 times between 1980 and 2008 in developed countries, those affected in developing countries more than tripled from around 250 million people to 904 million over the same period [4].

As in many developing countries, the prevalence of overweight and obesity in Ghana has consistently increased over the last few decades, disproportionately affecting women than men. For instance, the Ghana Demographic and Health Survey (GDHS) estimated the prevalence of overweight or obesity among women (40%) aged 15–49 years to be more than twice that of men (16%) [5]. Specifically, the prevalence among women was estimated to have increased by 27% between 1993 and 2014 [5]. Further, the prevalence of overweight or obesity in Ghana affects more urban than rural residents, and increases with household wealth and level of education [5].

Although overweight and obesity result from energy imbalance (consuming more calories than are equivalently expended in physical activity), studies have found a variety of factors to be associated with the phenomenon. Various associations, in terms of magnitude and direction have been reported between overweight and obesity, and a number of factors including age [6, 7], gender [8, 9], socioeconomic status [10, 11], marital status [12, 13], education [14, 15], occupation [6, 15], ethnicity [6, 14], genetics [16], dietary [17, 18] and physical activity patterns [19]. For instance, contrary to developed countries, the wealthier,

Correspondence: d.anamaale@uccsms.edu.gh
Department of Community Medicine, School of Medical Sciences, College of Health and Allied Sciences, University of Cape Coast, Cape Coast, Ghana

more educated and urban populations are more at risk of overweight and obesity in developing countries [10, 11, 20]. Prior studies [6, 21, 22] in Ghana have found overweight and obesity to be positively associated with age, household wealth, education, being married, and parity among others.

Engaging in sedentary behaviours, such as television (TV) viewing has been implicated among the multiplicity of the factors underlying the increasing prevalence of overweight and obesity observed in many populations around the world [23, 24]. A number of theoretical propositions about the possible mechanisms through which TV viewing affects overweight and obesity have been advanced. It is hypothesized that, TV viewing displaces participation in high-intensity discretionary physical activity, reduces resting energy expenditure compared to other activities, and increases sleep deprivation [19, 25]. Nonetheless, studies exploring this hypothesis have found a weak relationship between TV viewing and physical activity [19, 25].

An alternatively hypothesis posited is that TV viewing leads to an increase in overall energy intake either indirectly through exposure to advertising and consequent intake of foods commonly advertised on TV, or directly through the consumption of high calorie foods and beverages while viewing TV [17, 18]. Indeed studies involving both children and adults have found a positive association between TV viewing and intake of high calorie foods such as soda, pizza, and high-energy snacks [17, 18, 23]. In an experimental study involving children, Blass et al. [26] found children's energy intake to be higher when viewing TV than in control conditions when the TV is switched off.

Beyond exploring the possible mechanisms between TV viewing and physical activity or calorie intake, positive associations between TV viewing and obesity and/or related indicators have consistently been observed across space and time. Studies in the United States (US) have found that men and women viewing the most TV have an increased risk of obesity compared with those viewing the least TV [27–29]. In Australia, women who viewed TV for more than three hours a day were found to have a higher prevalence of severe abdominal obesity; while men who viewed TV for the same amount of time had a higher prevalence of moderate abdominal obesity [23]. More recently, a worldwide cross-sectional study across low, middle, and high income countries involving 207,672 adolescents from 37 countries and 77,003 children from 18 countries found increased TV viewing hours to be positively associated with body mass index (BMI) [30].

Although the public health importance of the association between TV viewing and obesity or related outcomes have been demonstrated in both cross-sectional and prospective studies involving children, adolescent and adult samples in other regions of the world, similar studies are rare within the African region. Nonetheless, while examining the relationship between ownership of different types of household assets and BMI among Ghanaian women, Dake and Fuseini [31] tangentially observed that women who reported viewing TV almost every day were likely to have obesity compared to those who did not. Taking cue from Dake and Fuseini [31], this study explored the association between TV exposure and overweight/obesity in Ghana with the view to contributing to the discourse on TV viewing and obesity, particularly in the African region.

In Ghana, TV ownership has been increasing since the inception of Television broadcasting in 1965. The sixth Ghana Living Standard Survey (GLSS) [32] estimated TV ownership to have increased between 1998/99 and 2012/13 from 40 to 75% and from 12 to 34% in urban and rural households, respectively. Indeed, hardly would one pass by a street, shop, bar, restaurant, bus station or even an office in most cities, towns and villages in Ghana without seeing a TV streaming. The screening of foreign telenovelas (soap operas) during primetime has become a means for competing stations to attract large audience, particularly women [33]. Telenovelas seem to have gone "viral" to the extent that TV stations screen them almost simultaneously with people – mostly women – seated and viewing for considerable hours each day. Some TV stations translate telenovelas into the local language (Twi) which makes it the more attractive for those who would otherwise have been deterred by language barriers.

With TV viewing considerably a part of life in Ghana today, this study explored the relationship between TV viewing and overweight/obesity among Ghanaian women using data from the 2014 GDHS. The study focused on women mainly because of the disproportionately high and rapid rates of overweight/obesity among Ghanaian women, compared to men [5]. In addition, Ghanaian women have also been found to report low levels of vigorous physical activity, which could increase their risk of developing overweight/obesity [34, 35]. This study would be useful in broadening our understanding of some of the drivers of obesity in Ghana or Africa, as well as at-risk groups for designing interventions.

Methods

Data source

The data used for the current study is the 2014 GDHS by Ghana Statistical Service (GSS), Ghana Health Service (GHS), and Inner City Fund (ICF) International. Specifically, the women's dataset was used given that they constituted the population of interest in this study. The GDHS collected the data using a two-staged stratified random sampling procedure. At the initial stage, clusters were selected using systematic random sampling. The sampling frame for selection of the clusters was an updated list of enumeration areas used in the 2010 Ghana Population and Housing Census. This was then followed with the selection of households in each cluster through a systematic random sampling procedure. Eligible women who provided signed written consent to participate in the survey were interviewed.

The GDHS collected anthropometric measures of all eligible women. To this end, a SECA 874 digital scale was used to measure their weight in 0.01 kg, while a Shorr height board was used to measure their height to the nearest 0.1 cm. Additional information regarding protocols used for taking these anthropometric measurements can be found in the MEASURE DHS Biomaker field manual [36]. The total sample for this study, excluding all pregnant women and lactating mothers was 4158. Permission was obtained from MEASURE DHS to download the 2014 GDHS raw data from http://dhsprogram.com/data/available-datasets.cfm for the purpose of the current study.

Study variables

The outcome variable in this study was generated from BMI scores of the women. A binary outcome variable was generated guided by the standard World Health Organisation's (WHO) BMI cut-off points (underweight, < 18.5 kg/m^2; normal weight, 18.5–25 kg/m^2; overweight, 25.0–29.9 kg/m^2; obese, ≥ 30.0 kg/m^2). Hence, for the purpose of this study and consistent with prior studies [5, 6, 21, 37], a BMI of 25.0 kg/m^2 or more was categorised as overweight/obese while a BMI lower than 25.0 kg/m^2 was categorised otherwise.

The key independent variable for this study was generated from two variables. The first variable assessed whether there was a TV in the household of respondents, with two response options: yes and no. The second variable assessed respondent's frequency of viewing TV, with three response options: not at all, less than once a week (moderate), and at least once a week (high). For the purpose of this study, not at all, less than once a week, and at least once a week were considered as: no exposure, moderate exposure, and high exposure, respectively. Based on these two variables, another categorical variable (TV exposure) was generated

out of possible outcomes of the presence of TV in a household and the frequency of TV viewing and coded with the following options: "no TV in household, no TV exposure" = 0; "no TV in household, moderate TV exposure" = 1; "no TV in household, high TV exposure" = 2; "TV in household, no TV exposure" = 3; "TV in household, moderate TV exposure" = 4; and "TV in household, high TV exposure" = 5.

This categorisation of TV exposure as presented in Fig. 1 is meant to demonstrate the scenarios of TV exposure in Ghana. In Ghana, it is typical for people who do not have TV sets in their household to spend time in neighbouring homes or nearby shops viewing TV. Communal TV viewing is also a common phenomenon in Ghana – where those who own TV sets take them outdoors for other community members to join in viewing. Any of these forms constitutes a certain level of TV exposure with possible implications on physical activity, calorie intake and general health of the involved.

Other explanatory variables in this study included age (15–24, 25–34, 40–44, and 45+); educational level (no education, primary, middle/junior secondary school (JSS)/junior high school (JHS), and secondary/higher); marital status (never married, married, cohabiting, and (divorced/widowed/separated); occupation (not working, professional/managerial, sales/trade, agricultural and manual labour); wealth quintile (poorest, poorer, middle, rich and richest); type of locality (rural, and urban); and parity (zero, one, two, three, four, five, six, and seven or more). Parity was included as proxy to account for the potential effect of childbearing on women's weight as noted in the literature [38, 39].

Statistical analysis

Both descriptive and inferential statistics were applied in estimating the association between TV exposure and overweight/obesity using STATA 11.0 software. The descriptive analysis used percentages to estimate the prevalence of TV exposure and overweight/obesity in relation to the characteristics of women in the study (Table 1). In the second level of analysis, two binary logistic regression models were conducted to estimate the effect of TV exposure on

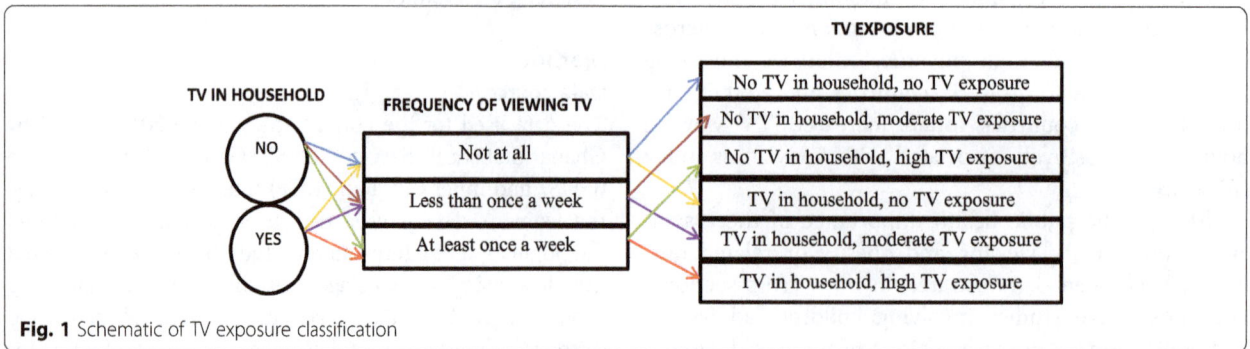

Fig. 1 Schematic of TV exposure classification

Table 1 Television exposure and overweight/obesity prevalence by background characteristics of women in Ghana, GDHS: 2014

Characteristic	No TV in household, no TV exposure (n = 824) %	No TV in household, moderate TV exposure (n = 367) %	No TV in household, high TV exposure (n = 345) %	TV in household, no TV exposure (n = 183) %	TV in household, moderate TV exposure (n = 693) %	TV in household, high TV exposure (n = 1746) %	Overweight/ obesity %	Total No.
Age group (years)								
15–24	19.0	10.3	11.1	5.0	14.4	40.3	17.6	1445
25–34	17.4	7.6	7.3	3.0	17.9	46.8	48.4	1242
35–44	21.4	8.8	6.1	4.9	17.9	41.0	56.2	1062
45+	25.9	7.8	6.8	5.7	17.7	36.0	52.6	410
Total	19.8	8.8	8.3	4.4	16.7	42.0	40.1	4158
Educational level								
No education	44.2	10.3	7.6	5.1	11.7	21.1	26.8	794
Primary	24.1	14.3	9.5	4.6	13.4	34.0	37.4	765
Middle/JHS	14.3	8.2	9.6	4.7	20.0	43.1	42.8	1710
Secondary/higher	4.8	4.0	5.4	3.0	17.5	65.4	49.2	889
Total	19.8	8.8	8.3	4.4	16.7	42.0	40.1	4158
Marital status								
Never married	16.1	9.7	11.1	4.5	15.8	42.8	22.1	1408
Married	22.6	6.8	4.4	4.5	18.3	43.4	50.1	1699
Cohabiting	19.1	9.4	7.5	4.8	13.8	45.4	40.8	585
Wid/div/sep	21.5	12.9	15.0	3.2	17.1	30.2	57.4	466
Total	19.8	8.8	8.3	4.4	16.7	42.0	40.1	4158
Wealth quintile								
Poorest	62.9	12.1	8.7	3.6	4.9	7.8	12.6	696
Poorer	37.3	19.0	14.6	4.1	8.6	16.4	24.8	709
Middle	11.5	13.0	15.8	7.1	18.0	34.6	38.6	863
Richer	1.3	3.6	3.8	4.5	24.5	62.3	52.5	925
Richest	1.0	0.2	1.0	2.7	22.4	72.6	60.6	967
Total	19.8	8.8	8.3	4.4	16.7	42.0	40.1	4158
Occupation								
Not working	18.6	9.4	8.7	4.8	14.8	43.8	23.8	968
Prof/managl/cleric	3.9	3.6	5.3	2.0	22.5	62.8	58.6	348
Sales/trade	10.9	7.0	7.5	4.7	20.7	49.2	54.6	1535
Agric	47.3	13.1	9.7	3.9	8.8	17.2	19.7	780

Table 1 Television exposure and overweight/obesity prevalence by background characteristics of women in Ghana, GDHS: 2014 (*Continued*)

Characteristic	No TV in household, no TV exposure (n=824) %	No TV in household, moderate TV exposure (n=367) %	No TV in household, high TV exposure (n=345) %	TV in household, no TV exposure (n=183) %	TV in household, moderate TV exposure (n=693) %	TV in household, high TV exposure (n=1746) %	Overweight/obesity %	Total No.
Manual	18.0	10.6	9.8	5.3	16.1	40.1	45.7	523
Total	19.8	8.8	8.3	4.4	16.7	41.9	40.1	4153
Type of locality								
Urban	6.0	5.6	7.4	4.1	18.5	58.3	49.2	2289
Rural	36.7	12.8	9.3	4.8	14.4	22.0	28.9	1869
Total	19.8	8.8	8.3	4.4	16.7	42.0	40.1	4158
Parity								
Zero	15.4	9.0	10.2	4.3	15.0	46.0	23.7	1327
One	12.3	9.3	10.7	4.0	16.9	46.9	39.2	531
Two	15.0	6.6	7.5	2.7	18.8	49.3	55.1	567
Three	18.5	8.4	7.3	4.2	18.3	43.3	55.4	495
Four	21.4	9.8	3.8	6.1	18.8	40.1	50.6	405
Five	28.0	6.3	8.2	5.2	22.5	29.8	43.1	319
Six	28.9	14.9	6.9	6.0	12.6	30.7	49.8	237
Seven or more	47.6	8.5	6.2	4.5	10.6	22.6	35.4	278
Total	19.8	8.8	8.3	4.4	16.7	42.0	40.1	4158
TV exposure								
No TV in household, no TV exposure							20.7	824
No TV in household, moderate TV exposure							25.9	367
No TV in household, high TV exposure							29.2	345
TV in household, no TV exposure							30.3	183
TV in household, moderate TV exposure							50.7	694
TV in household, high TV exposure							51.2	1746
Total							40.1	4158

overweight/obesity. In this regard, there was a bivariate model (Model I) consisting of only TV exposure, and a multivariate model (Model II) in which the other aforementioned explanatory variables were included. The GDHS survey design and weighting factors were taken into consideration in all analyses. To test for fitness of the models, the Hosmer- Lemeshow goodness-of-fit test was used.

Results

Table 1 shows the distribution of background characteristics of women in relation to TV exposure and prevalence of overweight/obesity. In general, TV exposure ranged from about 4% among those with TV in their households, but with no TV exposure to 42% among those with TV in their households, and with high TV exposure. This is further illustrated in Fig. 2. TV exposure varied across the various age cohorts considered in this study. For example, while slightly more than a quarter (26%) of those with no TV in their households, and no TV exposure were 45 years or older, 47% of those with TV in their households, and with high TV exposure were within the 25–35 year cohort.

TV exposure also varied by educational status. The proportion of those with no TV in their households, and with no TV exposure decreased as level of education increased (from about 44% among those with no education to approximately 5% among those with secondary/higher education). In contrast, the proportion of those with TV in their households, and with high TV exposure seemed to increase with each higher level of educational. This ranged from about 21% among those without education to about 65% among those with secondary/higher education. The results on marital status show that 15% of women without TV in their households, but with high TV exposure were in the widowed/divorced/separated category; while approximately 45% of their counterparts with TV in their households and with high TV exposure were cohabiting.

More than two-thirds of those in the poorest wealth quintile had no TV in their households, and no TV ex-

posure. However, the proportion of women with TV in their households, and with high TV exposure increased along with wealth quintile from about 8% in the poorest quintile to about 73% in the richest quintile. With regards to occupation, a greater proportion of those with TV in their households, and with moderate TV exposure (23%), and those with TV in their households, and with high TV exposure (63%) were engaged in professional/managerial/clerical occupations. The results also show differences in TV exposure by type of locality. For instance, while more rural (9%) than urban (7%) women had no TV in their households, but had high TV exposure; more urban (58%) than rural (22%) women had TV in their households, and had high TV exposure.

The prevalence of overweight/obesity among the women in this study was 40%, with some variations observed in relation to their TV exposure and background characteristics (Table 1). Overweight/obesity ranged from about 21% among those with no TV in their households, and no TV exposure to about 51% among those with TV in their households, and with high TV exposure. Regarding the other characteristics of women, the prevalence of overweight/obesity increased with age, educational level, and wealth quintile. Overweight/obesity was highest among widowed/divorced/separated (57%) women, those in professional/managerial/clerical (59%) occupations, urban (49%) dwellers, and those with three children (55%).

The logistic regression results on the association between TV exposure and overweight/obesity is presented in Table 2. The results in Model I show that the likelihood of developing overweight/obesity was significantly higher among women across all the categories of TV exposure, except for those with no TV in their households, but with moderate TV exposure. Specifically, women who had TV in their households, and with high TV exposure had the highest likelihood (OR = 4.01, 95% CI = 3.214, 4.999) of overweight/obesity compared with the other categories of TV exposure.

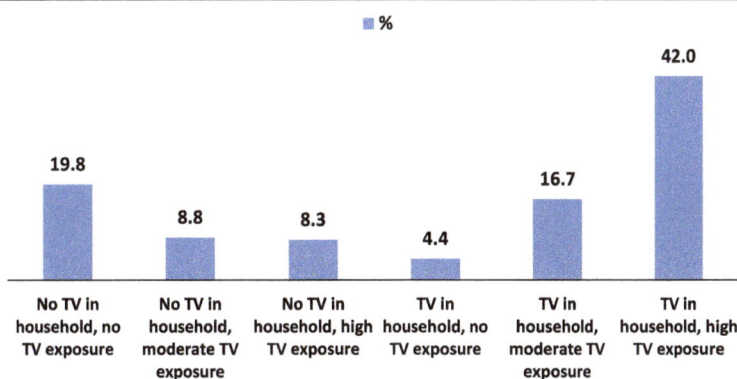

Fig. 2 Percentage distribution of TV exposure classification

Table 2 Logistic regression results on television exposure and overweight/obesity among women in Ghana, GDHS: 2014

	Model I		Model II	
Characteristic	OR	95% CI	OR	95% CI
TV exposure				
No TV in household, no TV exposure				
No TV in household, moderate TV exposure	1.338	[0.963,1.860]	0.987	[0.670,1.454]
No TV in household, high TV exposure	1.578**	[1.130,2.203]	1.219	[0.833,1.784]
TV in household, no TV exposure	1.662*	[1.088,2.537]	0.751	[0.436,1.293]
TV in household, moderate TV exposure	3.933**	[3.004,5.151]	1.364	[0.956,1.946]
TV in household, high TV exposure	4.008**	[3.214,4.999]	1.388*	[1.002,1.923]
Age group (years)				
15–24				
25–34			2.447**	[1.819,3.294]
35–44			3.790**	[2.642,5.436]
45+			3.568**	[2.312,5.505]
Educational level				
No education				
Primary			1.493**	[1.122,1.985]
Middle/JHS			1.489**	[1.133,1.958]
Secondary/higher			2.045**	[1.412,2.962]
Marital status				
Never married				
Married			1.746**	[1.211,2.519]
Cohabiting			1.365	[0.929,2.006]
Wid/div/sep			2.033**	[1.335,3.097]
Wealth quintile				
Poorest				
Poorer			1.914**	[1.386,2.643]
Middle			3.087**	[2.143,4.447]
Richer			4.948**	[3.212,7.622]
Richest			7.124**	[4.437,11.44]
Occupation				
Not working				
Prof/managl/cleric			1.560*	[1.063,2.290]
Sales/trade			1.447**	[1.120,1.870]
Agriculture			0.610**	[0.437,0.852]
Manual			1.459*	[1.059,2.010]
Type of locality				
Urban				
Rural			1.335*	[1.048,1.702]
Parity				
Zero				
One			1.169	[0.807,1.692]
Two			1.817**	[1.205,2.741]
Three			1.791*	[1.138,2.818]
Four			1.317	[0.820,2.114]

Table 2 Logistic regression results on television exposure and overweight/obesity among women in Ghana, GDHS: 2014 *(Continued)*

Characteristic	Model I		Model II	
	OR	95% CI	OR	95% CI
Five			1.275	[0.778,2.090]
Six			2.156**	[1.260,3.690]
Seven or more			1.807*	[1.053,3.099]
Wald x^2	210.81 (5)		652.95 (30)	
Prob. $> x^2$	0.0000		0.0000	
Hosmer-Lemeshow X^2 (d.f)	0.000 (4)		4.53 (8)	
Prob. $> x^2$	1.0000		0.8068	

OR Odds Ratios; 95% confidence intervals in brackets
* $p < .05$, ** $p < .01$

From the multivariate results (Model II), however, it was observed that only those with TV in their households, and with high TV exposure were significantly more likely (OR = 1.39, 95% CI = 1.002, 1.923) to have overweight/obesity, compared to those with no TV in their households, and no TV exposure. With the exception of marital status and parity, significant associations were observed between overweight/obesity and all the other background characteristics included in the multivariate model.

Discussion

This study sought to explore the association between TV exposure and overweight/obesity among Ghanaian women. Despite the attenuation of the association between TV exposure and overweight/obesity after adjusting for other factors, the results show that women who had TV in their households, and had high TV exposure were significantly more likely to have developed overweight/obesity than their counterparts with no TV in their households, and no TV exposure. This finding resonates with previous studies [23, 30, 31, 40] on the association between TV viewing and obesity, irrespective of the fact that such studies have reported varied magnitudes of association, depending on the covariates studied and how TV viewing and obesity were measured and categorized.

The cross-sectional nature of this study limits the possibility of drawing direct cause-and-effect conclusions based on the results. Nonetheless, a number of plausible explanations for the findings could be surmised, particularly in the light of existing body of knowledge on the subject. First, it is possible that women who have TV in their households, inherently spend a lot of time viewing TV in place of engaging in exercise or other forms of rigorous physical activities (for example, traditional dancing or wrestling competitions among others), resulting in an overall decrease in energy expenditure and the subsequent development of overweight/obesity [17, 18, 23, 40].

There is evidence of reduced physical activity globally, which is attributable to gradual shifts from outdoor leisure-time physical activities to sedentary types of activity such as viewing television [41]. In the developing world for instance, Ng and Popkin [42] report high declines in physical activity and a shift towards sedentary activity in domestic domains aided by greater access to home appliances including TV and computers. Hence, it might as well be the case that women with overweight/obesity resort to TV viewing as their main form of recreation rather than engaging in more physically demanding recreational activities such as sports.

An alternative explanation is that the more time such women spend viewing TV, the more they are likely to be inundated with the dozens of commercials and programmes which promote the consumption of high calorie foods [17, 18, 43]. Indeed, commercials on food and beverages (both alcoholic and non-alcoholic) seem to dominate in all the TV stations available in Ghana. Besides the potential of TV commercials to influence dietary patterns and risk of overweight/obesity among Ghanaian women, there is equally the tendency that such women have the habit of consuming high calorie food or drinks simultaneously while viewing TV without realising the quantities being consumed [17, 18].

Overall, a cycle of mutual interaction and reinforcement between TV viewing, physical activity, and dietary patterns could be at play [41], leading to an increased risk of overweight/obesity among Ghanaian women. Thus, as more time is spent viewing TV, less time is spent engaging in physical activities, while the consumption of high caloric food increases, leading to the development of overweight/obesity. And with the onset of overweight/obesity, the drive to substitute more active pastime activities for passive ones such as TV viewing increases, and the cycles continues on.

The positive effect of TV exposure on overweight/obesity could equally be a function of other confounders as prior studies [17, 18] have noted. Indeed the strong association found between the control variables in the present study and overweight/obesity, and their effect on the link between TV exposure and overweight/obesity demonstrate this possibility. In particular, the strong positive effect of education and wealth on overweight/ obesity in this study highlight the consistent effect of socioeconomic status on the risk of developing overweight/obesity typically observed in developing countries such as Ghana [6, 22], in contrast to developed countries [10, 11]. In developing countries, including Ghana, socioeconomic development has been found to be associated with changes in dietary and physical activity patterns such that Western type foods and energy saving devices replace traditional (healthier) staple foods and ways of doing things [31, 44].

Apart from the socioeconomic dimensions which seem to be playing out in this study, socio-cultural interpretations are equally plausible. Some Ghanaian women might still hold on to the historic Ghanaian perceptions that large-bodied women are beautiful, healthier and more prestigious, and may therefore be engaging in fattening dietary and physical activity patterns [45, 46]. Contrary to the reported protection that residing in a rural locality provides against overweight/obesity, this study found women in rural localities to be at risk of developing overweight/obesity. As Tuoyire et al. [6] noted, this could be the result of the gradual exposure of rural residents to obesogenic risks commonly seen in urban areas.

Much as the study provides some useful insights for interventions to remedy the problem of overweight/ obesity in Ghana, the results need to be interpreted with caution in the light of some limitations. As already alluded to in the preceding section, the study cannot directly establish cause-and-effect relationship between TV exposure and overweight/obesity due to the fact that the data was collected based on a cross-sectional design. Nonetheless, the associations established in this study are to a large extent consistent with prior prospective [27] and cross-sectional studies [23, 30] that have demonstrated connections between TV exposure/viewing/ watching and the development of overweight/obesity. Secondly, due to lack of data, the study could not control for other potential mediators of the relationship between TV exposure and overweight/obesity, most importantly dietary behaviour, physical activity and genetic factors. In a related development, the measurement of TV exposure as used in this study could not account for specific duration of TV viewing; neither could it account for the content of the messages to which study participants were exposed. Perhaps, the temporal amount and content of exposure to TV messages is one research area that needs to be explored further.

These limitations notwithstanding, the current study is about the first to specifically examine the relationship between TV exposure and overweight/obesity in Ghana and Africa where overweight/obesity and associated non-communicable diseases are increasing rather rapidly. An additional strength of this study is that the findings can be generalised to a large extent, since national level GDHS data with a high response rate (98.5%) was used. Further, the study contributes to the TV-obesity discourse and broadens our knowledge on some of the potential drivers of overweight/obesity in Ghana and perhaps the rest of the African region.

Conclusion

The study demonstrates that increased TV exposure is significantly associated with overweight/obesity among women in Ghana even after adjusting for other factors. Interventions aimed at tackling obesity in Ghana should focus on encouraging the uptake of more physically demanding pastime activities (such as brisk-walking and dancing) in place of TV "sit time". More importantly, intervention planners should consider using the TV as an important means to channel tailored behavioural change communication messages that seek to promote healthy dietary and physical activity behaviours.

Abbreviations
BMI: Body Mass Index; DHS: Demographic and Health Survey; GDHS: Ghana Demographic and Health Survey; GHS: Ghana Health Service; GSS: Ghana Statistical Service; ICF: Inner City Fund; JHS: Junior High School; JSS: Junior Secondary School; WHO: World Health Organization

Acknowledgements
The author wishes to acknowledge Measure DHS for granting permission to use the data.

Funding
No sources of funding were used to assist in the preparation of this manuscript.

Author's contributions
DAT conceived of the study and designed the analytical approach, performed the data analyses and produced the first and final drafts.The author read and approved the final manuscript.

Competing interests
All authors declare that they have no competing interests.

References
1. World World Health Organization (WHO). Obesity and overweight. WHO. 2015. Accessed 21 Feb 2016 from http://www.who.int/mediacentre/ factsheets/fs311/en/ .
2. Bogers R, Bemelmans W, Hoogenveen R, Boshuizen H, Woodward M, Knekt P, et al. Association of overweight with increased risk of coronary heart disease partly independent of blood pressure and cholesterol levels: a meta-analysis of 21 cohort studies including more than 300 000 persons. Arch Intern Med Am Med Assoc. 2007;167(16):1720.

3. Howard RA, Freedman D, Park Y, Hollenbeck A. Physical activity, sedentary behavior, and the risk of colon and rectal cancer in the NIH-AARP diet and health study. Cancer Causes Control. 2008;19(9):939–53.

4. Stevens GA, Singh GM, Lu Y, Danaei G, Lin JK, Finucane MM, et al. National, regional, and global trends in adult overweight and obesity prevalences. Popul Health Metr. 2012;10(1):22.

5. Ghana Statistical Service (GSS). Ghana health service (GHS) and ICF international. Ghana demographic and health survey. Rockville: GSS, GHS, and ICF International. 2014, 2015. p. 175.

6. Tuoyire DA, Kumi-Kyereme A, Doku DT. Socio-demographic trends in overweight and obesity among parous and nulliparous women in Ghana. BMC Obes. 2016;3(1):44.

7. Zafon C. Oscillations in total body fat content through life: an evolutionary perspective. Obes Rev. 2007;8(6):525–30.

8. Finucane MM, Stevens GA, Cowan MJ, Danaei G, Lin JK, Paciorek CJ, et al. National, regional, and global trends in body-mass index since 1980: systematic analysis of health examination surveys and epidemiological studies with 960 country-years and 9.1 million participants. Lancet. 2011; 377(9765):557–67.

9. Flegal KM. Prevalence of obesity and trends in the distribution of body mass index among us adults, 1999-2010. JAMA J Am Med Assoc. 2012; 307(5):491.

10. Dinsa GD, Goryakin Y, Fumagalli E, Suhrcke M. Obesity and socioeconomic status in developing countries: a systematic review. Obes Rev. 2012;13(11): 1067–79.

11. McLaren L. Socioeconomic status and obesity. Epidemiol Rev. 2007; 29(1):29–48.

12. Tzotzas T, Vlahavas G, Papadopoulou SK, Kapantais E, Kaklamanou D, Hassapidou M. Marital status and educational level associated to obesity in Greek adults: data from the National Epidemiological Survey. BMC Public Health. 2010;10(1):732.

13. Sobal J, Hanson KL, Frongillo EA. Gender, ethnicity, marital status, and body weight in the United States. Obesity. 2009;17(12):2223–31.

14. Sidik SM, Rampal L. The prevalence and factors associated with obesity among adult women in Selangor, Malaysia. Asia Pac Fam Med. 2009;8(1):2.

15. Abdulai A. Socio-economic characteristics and obesity in underdeveloped economies: does income really matter? Appl Econ. 2010;42(2):157–69.

16. Stanley JC. The regulation of energy balance. Lipid Technol. 2009;21(5–6): 124–6.

17. Maher C, Olds T, Eisenmann J, Dollman J. Screen time is more strongly associated than physical activity with overweight and obesity in 9-to 16-year-old Australians. Acta Paediatr. 2012;101(11):1170–4.

18. Rey-López JP, Vicente-Rodríguez G, Biosca M. Sedentary behaviour and obesity development in children and adolescents. Nutr Metab. 2008; 18(3):242–51.

19. Bennett GG, Wolin KY, Viswanath K, Askew S, Puleo E, Emmons KM. Television viewing and pedometer-determined physical activity among multiethnic residents of low-income housing. Am J Public Health. 2006; 96(9):1681–5.

20. Neuman M, Kawachi I, Gortmaker S, Subramanian SV. Urban-rural differences in BMI in low- and middle-income countries: the role of socioeconomic status. Am J Clin Nutr. 2013;97(2):428–36.

21. Doku DT, Neupane S. Double burden of malnutrition: increasing overweight and obesity and stall underweight trends among Ghanaian women. BMC Public Health. 2015;15(1):670.

22. Dake FA, Tawiah EO, Badasu DM. Sociodemographic correlates of obesity among Ghanaian women. Public Health Nutr. 2011;14(7):1285–91.

23. Cleland VJ, Schmidt MD, Dwyer T, Venn AJ. Television viewing and abdominal obesity in young adults : is the association mediated by food

and beverage consumption during viewing time or reduced leisure-time physical activity ? Am J Clin Nutr. 2008;87:1148–55.

24. Prentice A, Jebb S. Obesity in Britain: gluttony or sloth? BMJ Br Med J. 1995; 311(7002):437.

25. Hu F, Li T, Colditz G, Willett W, Manson J. Television watching and other sedentary behaviors in relation to risk of obesity and type 2 diabetes mellitus in women. JAMA. 2003;289(14):1785–91.

26. Blass E, Anderson D, Kirkorian H, Pempek T. On the road to obesity: television viewing increases intake of high-density foods. Physiol. 2006;88(4): 597–604.

27. Chen CY, Pereira MA, Kim KH, Erickson D, Jacobs DR, Zgibor JC, et al. Fifteen-year prospective analysis of television viewing and adiposity in African-American and Caucasian men and women. SAGE Open. 2015;5(3): 215824401560048.

28. He K, Hu FB, Colditz G. A, Manson JE, Willett WC, Liu S. Changes in intake of fruits and vegetables in relation to risk of obesity and weight gain among middle-aged women. Int J Obes Relat Metab Disord. 2004;28(12):1569–74.

29. Tucker LA, Bagwell M. Television viewing and obesity in adult females. Am J Public Health. 1991;81(7):908–11.

30. Braithwaite I, Stewart AW, Hancox RJ, Beasley R, Murphy R, Mitchell EA. The worldwide association between television viewing and obesity in children and adolescents: cross sectional study. PLoS One. 2013;8(9):e74263.

31. Dake FA, Fuseini K. Recreation, transportation or labour saving? Examining the association between household asset ownership and body mass index among Ghanaian women. BMC Obes. 2015;2(1):45.

32. Ghana Statistical Service. Ghana living standards survey round 6: poverty profile in Ghana 2005–2013. Accra: Ghana Statistical Service; 2014. p. 12–6.

33. Adia E. Programme element importance: an analysis of telenovelas in the Ghanaian media. Int J ICT Manag. 2014;2(1):96–101.

34. Tagoe HA, Dake FA. Healthy lifestyle behaviour among Ghanaian adults in the phase of a health policy change. Glob Health. 2011;7(1):7.

35. Dake FA. Obesity among Ghanaian women: past prevalence, future incidence. Public Health Elsevier. 2013;127(6):590–2.

36. ICF International. Biomarker field manual: demographic and health surveys methodology. Calverton: ICF International; 2012. p. 11–22.

37. WHO. Physical status: the use and interpretation of anthropometry. Report of a WHO expert committee. World Health Organ Tech Rep Ser. 1995;854:1–452.

38. Robinson WR, Cheng MM, Hoggatt KJ, Sturmer T, Siega-Riz AM. Childbearing is not associated with young women's long-term obesity risk. Obesity. 2014;22(4):1126–32.

39. Gunderson EP. Childbearing and obesity in women: weight before, during, and after pregnancy. Obstet Gynecol Clin N Am. 2009;36(2):317–32.

40. Tucker L, Bagwell M. Television viewing and obesity in adult females. Am J Public. 1991;81(7):908-11.

41. Misra A, Khurana L. Obesity and the metabolic syndrome in developing countries. J Clin Endocrinol Metab. 2008;93(11 Suppl 1):S9–30.

42. Ng SW, Popkin BM. Time use and physical activity: a shift away from movement across the globe. Obes Rev. 2012;13(8):659–80.

43. Strasburger V. Children, adolescents, obesity, and the media. Pediatrics. 2011;128(1):201–8.

44. Steyn N, Mchiza Z. Obesity and the nutrition transition in sub-Saharan Africa. Ann New York Acad. 2014;1311(1):88–101.

45. Renzaho A, Mellor D. Applying socio-cultural lenses to childhood obesity prevention among African migrants to high-income western countries: the role of acculturation, parenting and family functioning. Int J Migr Heal Soc Care. 2010;6(1):34–42.

46. Mavoa H, Kumanyika S, Renzaho A. Socio-c ultural i ssues and b ody i mage. Prev child Obes. Chichester: Wiley-Blackwell; 2010. p. 138–46.

5

The association between high-sensitivity C-reactive protein and metabolic risk factors in black and white South African women: a cross-sectional study

Cindy George[1][*] [iD], Juliet Evans[2], Lisa K. Micklesfield[3,4], Tommy Olsson[5] and Julia H. Goedecke[1,4]

Abstract

Background: High-sensitivity C-reactive protein (hsCRP) is associated with metabolic risk, however it is unclear whether the relationship is confounded by racial/ethnic differences in socioeconomic status (SES), lifestyle factors or central adiposity. The aims of the study was, (1) to investigate whether hsCRP levels differ by race/ethnicity; (2) to examine the race/ethnic-specific associations between hsCRP, HOMA-IR and serum lipids [total cholesterol (TC), triglycerides (TG), high-density lipoproteins (HDL-C) and low-density lipoproteins (LDL-C)]; and (3) to determine whether race/ethnic-specific associations are explained by SES, lifestyle factors or waist circumference (WC).

Methods: The convenience sample comprised 195 black and 153 white apparently health women, aged 18–45 years. SES (education, assets and housing density) and lifestyle factors (alcohol use, physical activity and contraceptive use) were collected by questionnaire. Weight, height and WC were measured, and fasting blood samples collected for hsCRP, glucose, insulin, and lipids.

Results: Black women had higher age- and BMI-adjusted hsCRP levels than white women ($p = 0.047$). hsCRP was associated with HOMA-IR ($p < 0.001$), TG ($p < 0.001$), TC ($p < 0.05$), HDL-C ($p < 0.05$), and LDL-C ($p < 0.05$), independent of age and race/ethnicity. The association between hsCRP and lipids differed by race/ethnicity, such that hsCRP was positively associated with TG and LDL-C in white women, and inversely associated with HDL-C in black women. Higher hsCRP was also associated with higher TC in white women and lower TC in black women. Furthermore, when adjusting for SES and lifestyle factors, the associations between hsCRP, and TC and TG, remained, however the associations between hsCRP, and HDL-C and LDL-C, were no longer significant.

Conclusion: Although circulating hsCRP may identify individuals at increased metabolic risk, the heterogeneity in these associations between racial/ethnic groups highlights the need for prospective studies investigating the role of hsCRP for risk prediction in different populations.

Keywords: High-sensitivity C-reactive protein, Race/ethnicity, Metabolic risk, Women

* Correspondence: cindy.george@mrc.ac.za
[1]Non-Communicable Diseases Research Unit, South African Medical Research Council, Francie van Zijl Drive, Parow Valley, PO Box 19070, Cape Town, South Africa
Full list of author information is available at the end of the article

Background

The prevalence and incidence of non-communicable diseases (NCDs), such as type 2 diabetes (T2D) and cardiovascular disease (CVD), are different for black and white women. Several studies and global reports have shown that T2D disproportionately burdens black women [1, 2], while CVD is more prevalent amongst white women [3]. Obesity and central body fat is linked to increased metabolic risk, including insulin resistance and elevated serum lipid levels [4]. Indeed, visceral adipose tissue (VAT) is associated with a greater risk of metabolic complications [5, 6]. However, for the same level of body fatness, black women have less VAT than white women [5, 6], have a lower prevalence of the metabolic syndrome [7, 8] due to their more "favourable" lipid profile [7, 9], but are more insulin resistant than white women [10, 11]. The reason for this paradox may be that different racial/ethnic groups have a different inflammatory response to obesity and that the differential effects of body fat and body fat distribution on metabolic risk may be partially mediated via inflammatory pathways [12].

C-reactive protein (CRP), an acute-phase protein secreted by the liver in response to interleukin-6 (IL-6) and tumor necrosis factor (TNF)-α [13], is a well-characterized marker of inflammation, and increased circulating levels have been shown to be associated with obesity and increased metabolic risk [14]. Interestingly, marked racial/ethnic differences in high-sensitivity CRP (hsCRP) concentrations have been reported, with black women having higher levels compared to white women, independent of adiposity [4, 12, 15]. These findings are however not consistent, as some studies do not show racial/ethnic differences in hsCRP levels after adjusting for body fat [16, 17]. In addition to the racial/ethnic differences in adiposity, inflammation and metabolic risk, there are inherent racial/ethnic differences in socioeconomic status (SES) and lifestyle factors, which also influence metabolic risk and outcome [18]. Indeed, studies have shown that lower SES is associated with a higher inflammatory profile [19, 20], possibly due to negative health behaviours, as well as a higher prevalence of NCDs, including T2D and CVD [21, 22]. Currently, it is not known whether the association between hsCRP levels and metabolic risk factors for T2D and CVD differ between black and white South African women, and whether SES and lifestyle factors influence the association, or whether the relationship may be explained by racial/ethnic differences in central adiposity.

Accordingly, the aims of this study were, 1) to investigate whether hsCRP levels differ by race/ethnicity in South African women; 2) to examine the race/ethnic-specific associations between hsCRP, insulin resistance (HOMA-IR) and serum lipids (total cholesterol (TC), triglycerides (TG), high-density lipoproteins (HDL-C) and

low-density lipoproteins (LDL-C)); and 3) to determine whether the race/ethnic-specific associations between hsCRP and the metabolic risk factors may be explained by differences in SES, lifestyle factors and/or central adiposity between black and white South African women.

Methods

Participants

This cross-sectional study consisted of a convenience sample of 194 black and 153 white apparently healthy, premenopausal, South African women, as previously described [23]. Race/ethnicity was self-reported. Participants were recruited from church groups, community centers and universities, in urban settings around Cape Town, South Africa. Women were included in the study if they were between 18 and 45 years of age, with no known diseases and not taking medication that may alter metabolism, were not currently pregnant, lactating or postmenopausal (self-reported). Women with hsCRP > 10 μg/ml ($n = 59$) were also excluded from the study, as this can be indicative of acute inflammation.

Approval was obtained from the Health Sciences Research Ethics Committee of the University of Cape Town and written informed consent was obtained from all subjects prior to participation.

Socio-economic status and lifestyle factors

A questionnaire was administered that included measures of SES, lifestyle factors and family history of disease [24]. Three indicators of SES were assessed, namely, level of education, number of assets per household (asset index) and housing density. Level of education was categorized as not completed high school, completed high school and post-high school (tertiary) education. The asset index score was based on indoor access to running water and/or flushing toilet, electricity and ownership of 12 household amenities, which included a television, radio, motor vehicle, fridge, oven/stove, washing machine, telephone, video machine, microwave, computer, cellular telephone and paid television channels (e.g. DSTV). Housing density was calculated as the number of persons per household divided by the number of rooms in the household. Participants were classified as non-smokers, if they had never smoked, ex-smokers if they were smokers but stopped smoking prior to the time of the interview, and current smokers if they smoked more than 1 cigarette per day at the time of the interview. Alcohol consumption was based on an average weekly intake of alcohol and participants were categorized as a non-drinker if they did not consume any alcohol, a moderate drinker if they consumed ≤7 drinks/week (≤1 drink/day), and a heavy drinker if they consumed > 7 drinks/week. Physical activity levels were determined using the Global Physical Activity Questionnaire (GPAQ) [25], and moderate-to-vigorous intensity physical activity ≥150 min/week was categorized as sufficiently active and moderate-to-vigorous intensity physical activity < 150 min/week was categorized as insufficiently active. Contraceptive use was self-reported and was categorized as none, oral contraceptives or injectable contraceptives. Participants were also asked whether they had a family history of T2D and/or CVD.

Anthropometry and blood pressure measures
Standard anthropometric procedures [26] were used to measure weight, height and waist circumference (WC), measured at the level of the umbilicus. Blood pressure measurements were taken in a seated position after 5 min of seated rest. The systolic and diastolic blood pressure (SBP and DBP, respectively) were recorded three times at 1-min intervals, using an appropriately sized cuff and an automated blood pressure monitor (Omron 711, Omron Health Care, Hamburg, Germany). An average of the last two readings was used in the analyses.

Biochemical analysis
Blood samples were drawn after an overnight fast (10–12 h) for plasma glucose, determined by the glucose oxidase method (Glucose Analyzer 2, Beckman Instruments, Fullerton, CA, USA), serum insulin, determined by a Microparticle Enzyme Immunoassay (MEIA) (AxSym Insulin Kit, Abbot, IL, USA), TC, HDL-C, and TG, analyzed using the Roche Modular auto analyzer and enzymatic colorimetric assays, and LDL-C calculated using the Friedewald formula [27]. Homeostatic model assessment (HOMA-IR) was estimated from fasting insulin and glucose levels as previously described [28]. Serum concentrations of hsCRP (Immun Diagnostik AG, Bensheim, Germany) were analyzed using commercially available ELISA kits according to the manufacturer's protocols.

Statistical analysis
All statistical analyses were performed using STATA version 13 (Statcorp, College Station, TX) and statistical significance was based on a p-value < 0.05. Normally distributed data are presented as mean ± standard deviation (SD) and skewed variables, as median and interquartile range (IQR). Racial/ethnic differences in SES and lifestyle factors, anthropometry and metabolic risk factors were compared using chi-squared analysis for categorical variables, and Student-t test and Wilcoxon rank-sum test for normally and not normally distributed continuous variables, respectively. Analysis of covariance (ANCOVA), adjusting for age and BMI, was used to compare means of serum-associated metabolic risk factors (HOMA-IR, TG, TC, HDL-C and LDL-C) between black and white women. The non-normally distributed

metabolic risk factors were logarithmically transformed and Pearson correlation analysis (continuous variables) and ANOVA (categorical variables) were used to determine which SES and lifestyle factors were significantly associated with the different metabolic risk factors (outcome variables). Based on the results of these bivariate associations (data not shown), multivariate linear regression analyses were used to examine the associations between hsCRP and the metabolic risk factors, with the following models: Model 1: age + race/ethnicity + interaction term (interaction between race/ethnicity and hsCRP); Model 2: Model 1 + SES and lifestyle factors; Model 3: Model 2 + WC.

Results
Participant characteristics
The general characteristics of the study population are presented in Table 1 and the age and BMI-adjusted blood-based metabolic risk factors are presented in Table 2. Black women were younger (24 vs. 31 years; $p < 0.0001$) and had a higher BMI (30.4 vs 24.5 kg/m^2; $p = 0.0003$) than white women. Of the total sample, 55.2% of the black women and 44.4% of the white women were overweight or obese (BMI ≥25 kg/m^2). Although there was no significant difference in plasma glucose concentrations between the racial/ethnic groups, black women had higher serum insulin concentrations and HOMA-IR, and lower TC, TG, HDL-C and LDL-C concentrations than white women, before and after adjusting for differences in age and BMI. High-sensitivity CRP did not differ by race/ethnicity ($p = 0.9605$), but after adjusting for age and BMI, black women had higher hsCRP levels than white women ($p = 0.047$). Black and white women also had similar systolic and diastolic blood pressure. Family history of T2D (21.1 vs. 13.7%, $p = 0.117$) and CVD (25.8 vs. 24.2%, $p = 0.698$) were not different between black and white women. There were also significant racial/ethnic differences in SES between the groups, such that the black women had lower levels of education ($p < 0.0001$) and asset index ($p < 0.0001$), and greater housing density ($p < 0.0001$) than white women. Black women were less likely to smoke ($p < 0.0001$) and drink alcohol ($p < 0.0001$), and more likely to meet physical activity guidelines ($p < 0.0001$) than white women. Approximately a third of the women reported using contraceptives, with white women primarily using oral contraceptives, and black women primarily using injectable contraceptives.

Association between serum hsCRP and metabolic risk factors, accounting for the potential effect of SES, lifestyle factors and central adiposity
Based on the results of the bivariate associations between the metabolic risk factors and the different SES and lifestyle factors, multivariate linear regression models were

Table 1 General characteristics of sample population

Variables	Black women (n = 194)	White women (n = 153)	p-value
Age (years)	24 (21–30)	31 (24–38)	< 0.0001
Anthropometry			
Height (m)	1.6 ± 0.1	1.7 ± 0.1	< 0.0001
Weight (cm)	74.9 (58.9–90.6)	69.3 (61.0–85.1)	0.5368
BMI (kg/m²)	30.4 (23.0–36.0)	24.5 (21.7–30.8)	0.0003
WC (cm)	86.5 (74.0–103.5)	85.0 (77.0–96.0)	0.6503
Blood pressure			
Systolic blood pressure (mmHg)	101.5 (101.5–118.0)	102.5 (102.5–116.0)	0.523
Diastolic blood pressure (mmHg)	68.0 (68.0–80.5)	67.5 (67.5–81.5)	0.6211
SES factors			
Education (%)			< 0.0001
Have not completed high school	43.3	3.3	
Completed high school	39.7	18.3	
Tertiary education	17	78.4	
Housing density (persons/room)	1.0 (0.6–1.5)	0.4 (0.3–0.6)	< 0.0001
Asset index (amenities/house)	7.0 (5.0–10.0)	12.0 (11.0–14.0)	< 0.0001
Lifestyle factors			
Smoking status (%)			< 0.0001
Current smoker	7.2	15.7	
Ex-smoker	2.6	15.7	
Non-smoker	90.2	68.6	
Alcohol use (%)			< 0.0001
Non-drinker	70.7	20.5	
Moderate drinker	16	46.6	
Heavy drinker	13.3	32.9	
Physical activity (%)			< 0.0001
Insufficiently active (< 150 min/week)	64.7	84	
Sufficiently active (≥150 min/week)	35.3	16	
Contraceptive use (%)			< 0.0001
None	68.6	68.6	
Oral	4.6	25.5	
Injection	26.8	5.9	

Data presented as mean ± SD and median (interquartile range) or percentages. *BMI* body mass index, *WC* waist circumference, *HOMA-IR* homeostasis model of insulin resistance, *TC* total cholesterol, *TG* triglycerides, *HDL-C* high-density lipoprotein cholesterol, *LDL-C* low-density lipoprotein cholesterol, *hsCRP* high sensitivity C-reactive protein

used to examine the association between the metabolic risk factors and hsCRP, adjusting for age, race/ethnicity and the interaction between hsCRP and race/ethnicity (Model 1), and accounting for SES and lifestyle factors (Model 2), and WC (central adiposity) (Model 3). The truncated models are presented in Table 3, with the full models presented as supporting information (Additional file 1: Table S1, Additional file 2: Table S2, Additional file 3: Table S3, Additional file 4: Table S4, Additional file 5: Table S5).

High-sensitivity CRP was positively associated with HOMA-IR in the combined sample of black and white

women (Model 1), independent of SES and lifestyle factors (Model 2). When further adjusting for WC, hsCRP was no longer associated with HOMA-IR, but age was inversely associated with HOMA-IR, whereas injectable contraceptive use and WC were positively associated with HOMA-IR (Model 3).

In contrast to HOMA-IR, there were race/ethnic-specific associations between hsCRP and serum lipid levels. High-sensitivity CRP was associated with TG, independent of age (Model 1), SES, lifestyle factors (Model 2) and WC (Model 3) in the white women only (Fig. 1, A1, A2

Table 2 Unadjusted and age and BMI-adjusted blood-based metabolic risk factors of black and white South African women

Variables	Unadjusted			Adjusted values		
	Black women	White women	p-value	Black women	White women	p-value
Glucose (mmol/l)	4.4 (4.1–4.8)	4.6 (4.4–4.9)	0.068	4.4 (4.3–4.6)	4.5 (4.5–4.7)	0.966
Insulin (mU/l)	8.0 (5.0–15.4)	6.1 (4.4–9.9)	0.0003	9.0 (6.5–12.4)	6.6 (5.0–8.7)	< 0.0001
HOMA-IR (units)	1.6 (1.0–3.1)	1.2 (0.9–2.1)	0.006	1.8 (1.2–2.6)	1.4 (1.0–1.9)	0.0003
TC (mmol/l)	3.9 ± 0.8	4.7 ± 1.0	< 0.0001	3.8 ± 0.2	4.6 ± 0.2	< 0.0001
TG (mmol/l)	0.7 ± 0.3	0.9 ± 0.5	< 0.0001	0.7 ± 0.1	0.8 ± 0.1	< 0.0001
HDL-C (mmol/l)	1.3 ± 0.4	1.7 ± 0.4	< 0.0001	1.3 ± 0.2	1.6 ± 0.1	< 0.0001
LDL-C (mmol/l)	2.2 ± 0.7	2.6 ± 0.9	< 0.0001	2.1 ± 0.2	2.5 ± 0.2	< 0.0001
hsCRP (µg/ml)	2.3 (1.0–5.1)	2.3 (0.8–5.2)	0.9605	2.5 (1.1–3.9)	2.0 (1.4–3.3)	0.047

Data presented as mean ± SD or median (interquartile range). P-values are presented as unadjusted and adjusted for age and BMI. *HOMA-IR* homeostasis model of insulin resistance, *TC* total cholesterol, *TG* triglycerides, *HDL-C* high-density lipoprotein cholesterol, *LDL-C* low-density lipoprotein cholesterol, *hsCRP* high sensitivity C-reactive protein

and A3, respectively). There was also a race/ethnic-specific association between hsCRP and TC levels independent of age (Model 1), such that hsCRP was associated with higher TC in the white women, but lower TC in the black women (Fig. 1, B1). These associations were independent of SES and lifestyle factors (Model 2) for both black and white women (Fig. 1, B2). When including WC in the model, the association between hsCRP and TC was no longer significant in the white women, but the relationship remained in the black women (Fig. 1, B3). In this model, higher age and higher SES (represented by having completed high school) as well as oral contraceptive use were associated with higher TC levels. High-sensitivity CRP was also inversely associated with HDL-C, independent of age (Model 1) in the black women only (Fig. 1, C1). When adjusting for SES and lifestyle factors, the inverse association between hsCRP and HDL-C remained, but there was no longer a significant interaction between hsCRP and race/ethnicity (Model 2; Fig. 1, C2). In this model, higher SES (represented by having a tertiary education and lower housing density), consuming less than one drink per day and oral contraceptive use were associated with higher HDL-C levels. Conversely, injectable contraceptive use was associated with lower HDL-C levels. When including WC in the model, hsCRP was no longer significantly associated with HDL-C in the combined sample (Model 3), but the relationship between hsCRP and HDL-C remained in the black women. High-sensitivity CRP was positively associated with LDL-C levels, independent of age (Model 1), in the white women only (Fig. 1, D1). When including SES and lifestyle factors in the model the relationship between hsCRP and LDL-C remained, however there was no longer an interaction between hsCRP and race/ethnicity (Model 2). In this model, higher age, completing high school and a higher housing density were associated with higher LDL-C levels. Conversely, consuming less that one alcoholic drink per day was

associated with lower LDL-C levels. When further adding WC to the model, hsCRP was no longer significantly associated with LDL-C levels (Model 3; Fig. 1, D3).

Discussion

In this cross-sectional study of apparently healthy, premenopausal, South African women, we have shown that black women have higher hsCRP levels when adjusted for age and BMI, compared to white women. In addition, hsCRP levels were significantly associated with HOMA-IR, a measure of insulin resistance, and lipid levels in the combined sample, however except for TG, this was not independent of central adiposity. The novel findings in this study were that the association between hsCRP and the lipid markers differed by race/ethnicity, and that SES and lifestyle factors accounted for the association between hsCRP and the lipoproteins (HDL-C and LDL-C), but not for the association with TC and TG.

Our study corroborates the findings of other studies that black women have higher hsCRP levels compared to white women. Our study also lends support to the existing understanding that increased hsCRP is associated with an adverse metabolic profile, including increased HOMA-IR and a more atherogenic lipid profile, characterized by higher TG, TC and LDL-C, and lower HDL-C concentrations [14, 29]. Accordingly, hsCRP concentrations seems a likely candidate to identify individuals at increased metabolic risk. Therefore, based on our findings, it could be assumed that the higher hsCRP in the black women is associated with metabolic risk in this population. However, we and others have consistently shown that black women have a higher HOMA-IR [10, 11], but a more "favourable" lipid profile [7, 9], compared to white women. Consequently, the association between hsCRP and metabolic risk may be different in persons of differing race/ethnicities. We further hypothesized that these race/ethnic-specific associations could be mediated, either directly or indirectly, by differences

Table 3 Adjusted associations between log-transformed metabolic risk factors, insulin resistance [HOMA-IR (units)] and serum lipids (TG, TC, HDL-C and LDL-C (mmol/l)), and hsCRP (µg/ml) in black and white South African women

Variables	Model 1	Model 2	Model 3
ln(HOMA-IR)	β [95% CI]	β [95% CI]	β [95% CI]
hsCRP	0.09 [0.05; 0.13]**	0.10 [0.06; 0.14]**	0.03 [−0.01; 0.07]
Age	−0.01 [−0.02; 0.00]	−0.01 [−0.02; 0.00]	−0.02 [−0.03; −0.01]**
Race/ethnicity	0.26 [0.03; 0.48]*	0.00 [−0.27; 0.27]	−0.00 [−0.23; 0.23]
hsCRPxrace/ethnicity	−0.02 [−0.07; 0.04]	−0.04 [−0.09; 0.02]	−0.02 [−0.07; 0.02]
Adjusted-R²	*0.11** *	*0.15** *	*0.38** *
ln(TG)	β [95% CI]	β [95% CI]	β [95% CI]
hsCRP	0.07 [0.05; 0.10]**	0.06 [0.04; 0.09]**	0.04 [0.02; 0.07]**
Age	0.01 [0.00; 0.01]*	0.01 [0.00; 0.02]*	0.01 [−0.00; −0.00]
Race/ethnicity	−0.04 [−0.18; 0.10]	−0.14 [−0.30; 0.03]	−0.14 [−0.30; 0.02]
hsCRPxrace/ethnicity	−0.05 [−0.09; −0.02]*	−0.05 [−0.08; −0.01]*	−0.04 [−0.08; −0.01]*
Adjusted-R²	*0.18** *	*0.20** *	*0.26** *
ln(TC)	β [95% CI]	β [95% CI]	β [95% CI]
hsCRP	0.02 [0.01; 0.03]*	0.02 [0.00; 0.03]*	0.01 [−0.00; 0.02]
Age	0.00 [0.00; 0.01]*	0.01 [0.00; 0.01]**	0.01 [0.00; 0.01]**
Race/ethnicity	−0.05 [−0.11; 0.02]	−0.04 [−0.12; 0.03]	−0.04 [−0.12; 0.03]
hsCRPxrace/ethnicity	−0.04 [−0.06; −0.03]**	−0.03 [−0.05; −0.02]**	−0.03 [−0.05; −0.01]**
Adjusted-R²	*0.26** *	*0.29** *	*0.30** *
ln(HDL-C)	β [95% CI]	β [95% CI]	β [95% CI]
hsCRP	−0.01 [−0.03; −0.01]*	−0.02 [−0.03; −0.00]*	−0.00 [−0.02; 0.01]
Age	−0.00 [−0.01; 0.00]	−0.00 [−0.00; 0.00]	0.00 [−0.00; 0.01]
Race/ethnicity	−0.16 [−0.25; −0.07]**	−0.01 [−0.12; 0.09]	−0.03 [−0.13; 0.08]
hsCRPxrace/ethnicity	−0.03 [−0.05; −0.01]*	−0.02 [−0.04; 0.01]	−0.02 [−0.04; 0.00]
Adjusted-R²	*0.22** *	*0.34** *	*0.39** *
ln(LDL-C)	β [95% CI]	β [95% CI]	β [95% CI]
hsCRP	0.03 [0.01; 0.05]*	0.02 [−0.00; 0.04]*	0.01 [−0.02; 0.03]
Age	0.01 [−0.00; 0.01]	0.01 [0.00; 0.12]*	0.01 [−0.00; 0.01]
Race/ethnicity	−0.02 [−0.14; 0.09]	−0.14 [−0.29; 0.01]	−0.13 [−0.27; 0.02]
hsCRPxrace/ethnicity	−0.04 [−0.07; −0.01]*	−0.03 [−0.06; 0.00]	−0.03 [−0.06; 0.00]
Adjusted-R²	*0.08** *	*0.15** *	*0.19** *

Data represents β-coefficients [95% confidence interval] and adjusted-R². Model 1: hsCRP + age + race/ethnicity + (hsCRP x race/ethnicity interaction); Model 2: (Model 1) + SES + lifestyle factors; Model 3: (Model 2) + WC. hsCRP, C-reactive protein; interaction term, interaction between hsCRP and race/ethnicity; ln(HOMA-IR), ln(TG), natural log of triglycerides; natural log of homeostatic model assessment; ln(TC), natural log of total cholesterol; ln(HDL-C), natural log of high-density lipoprotein cholesterol; ln(LDL-C), natural log of low-density lipoprotein cholesterol. *p < 0.05 and **p < 0.001

in SES, lifestyle factors or central adiposity; factors known to alter hsCRP levels and influence metabolic risk and outcome [18]. Certainly, some studies have shown that a higher inflammatory profile is linked to a lower SES [20], as well as greater central body fat [30], both of which are characteristic of black South African women.

Indeed, we found that higher hsCRP levels were associated with higher levels of HOMA-IR in both racial/ethnic groups, however despite hsCRP being associated with a more atherogenic lipid profile, the relationship differed by race/ethnicity, such that hsCRP was positively associated with TG and LDL-C in the white

women only, and inversely associated with HDL-C in the black women only. An interesting finding in this study, which has not been described before, was the inverse association between hsCRP and TC in the black women, in direct contrast to the association found in the white women. However, contrary to our hypothesis, SES, lifestyle factors and central adiposity had no mediatory effect on the race/ethnic-specific relationship between hsCRP, TG and TC. Though the exact mechanism underlying this disparate relationship is still unknown, other lifestyle factors such as dietary intake, not measured in this study, might have had a more significant

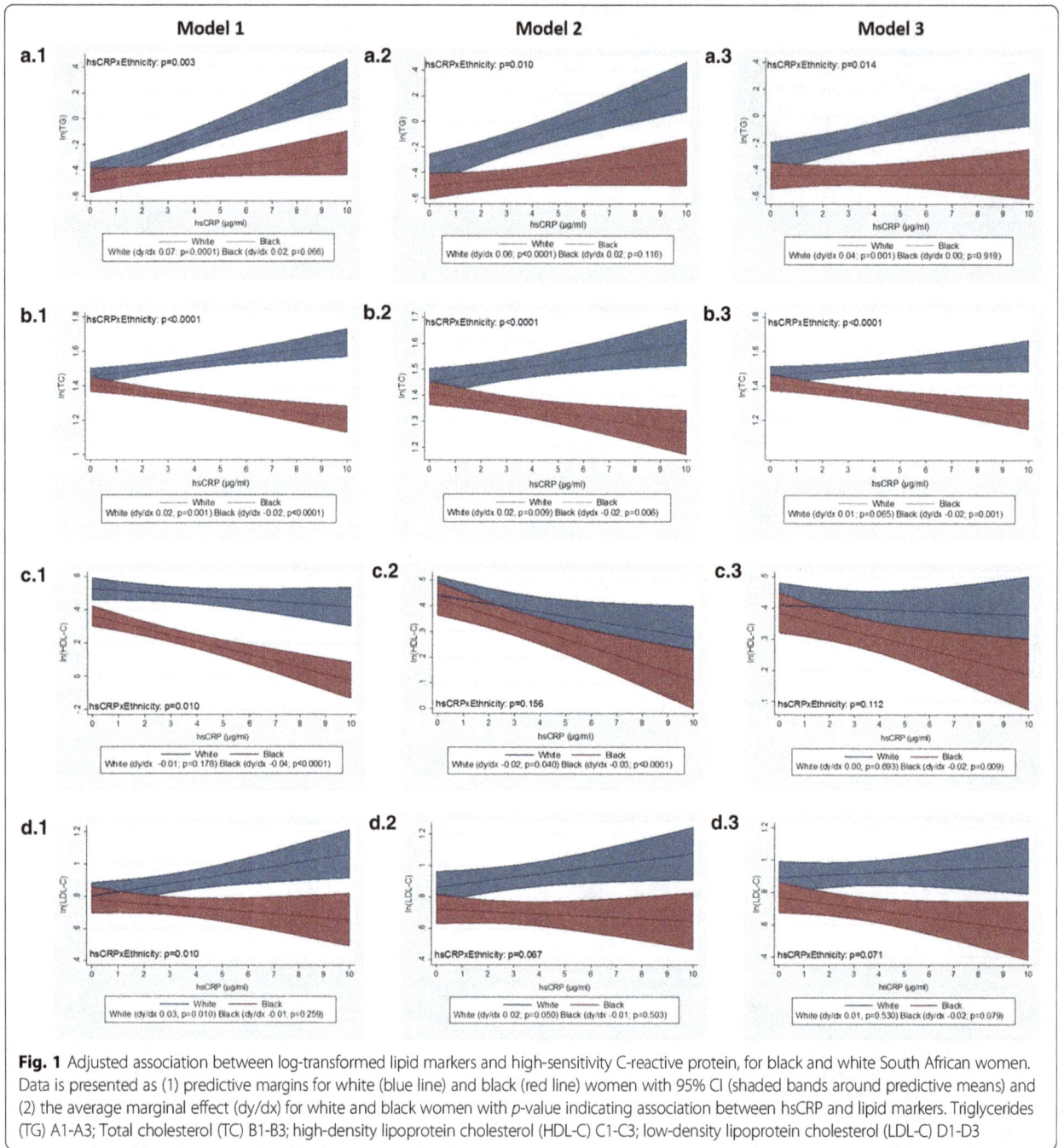

Fig. 1 Adjusted association between log-transformed lipid markers and high-sensitivity C-reactive protein, for black and white South African women. Data is presented as (1) predictive margins for white (blue line) and black (red line) women with 95% CI (shaded bands around predictive means) and (2) the average marginal effect (dy/dx) for white and black women with *p*-value indicating association between hsCRP and lipid markers. Triglycerides (TG) A1-A3; Total cholesterol (TC) B1-B3; high-density lipoprotein cholesterol (HDL-C) C1-C3; low-density lipoprotein cholesterol (LDL-C) D1-D3

race/ethnic-specific mediatory effect on the association between hsCRP and lipid levels. Indeed, various studies have reported a positive association between inflammation and fatty acids, glucose, lipids, and an inverse association with fibre, fruits, and vegetables [31]. In the context of South Africa, the black population have been shown to display an eating pattern reflecting a higher consumption of fat and calories, and lower consumption of fruits and vegetables [32]. Furthermore, previous studies have also shown a stronger association between TG, TC and VAT depots compared to SAT [33], because VAT is more lipolytically active than SAT, owing to higher β-adrenoreceptor-mediated catecholamine-induced lipolysis and greater resistance to the antilipolytic activity of insulin [34]. Thus, the race/ethnic-specific association might be mediated via abdominal fat depots, as opposed to WC, which is a general measure of central adiposity. This could also explain why hsCRP was positively associated with TG and TC in the white women, as white women have a greater abdominal VAT depot compared to black women, who present with greater SAT [5, 6]. Further studies are however needed to explore these race/ethnic-specific associations in further detail.

In contrast, the race/ethnic-specific association between hsCRP and the lipoproteins (HDL-C and LDL-C) were explained by racial/ethnic differences in SES, alcohol consumption and contraceptive use. Indeed, as shown in other studies, we have shown that higher SES [35], depicted by a higher level of education, and lower housing density, as well as moderate alcohol use [36] were associated with higher LDL-C and lower HDL-C concentrations, independent of hsCRP. Within the South African context, SES influences contraceptive use [37], which we show here to be independently associated with HDL-C levels. In our study, most of the black women using contraceptives reported using injectable contraceptives. These injectable contraceptives are most likely the progestin-based injectable contraceptives (depot medroxyprogesterone acetate), which has been associated with a reduction in HDL-C [38]. Conversely, oral contraceptives, predominantly used by the white women in this study, have been associated with higher HDL-C [39]. With that said, there is still a great need for research to better understand what influences SES and lifestyle factors have on inflammation within different racial/ethnic groups.

Some limitations of this study must be considered. Firstly, due to the cross-sectional nature of the study, data cannot be used to investigate the causal relationship between hsCRP and metabolic risk. Furthermore, this study has a relatively small sample size and consists of a relatively homogenous population of apparently healthy, predominantly overweight and obese, premenopausal women, and therefore it is not appropriate to generalize the findings to the general population. Though we have studied a convenience sample, they are representative of the general black and white South African adult female population, in terms of the level of obesity [40]. Indeed, according to The South African National Health and Nutrition Examination Survey (SANHANES-1) the average BMI of South African women is 28.9 kg/m^2 and 39.2% of South African women are obese [40]. Similarly, the average BMI found in our sample was 28.5 kg/m^2 and 41.2% of the participants fall within the obese range. However, our sample has a higher % of tertiary educated individuals, as well as a higher rate of current smokers and alcohol consumers, compared to the general South African population [40]. The current study is also limited to only hsCRP as a marker of inflammation, thus additional markers such as TNF-α and IL-6 could be incorporated in future studies. In addition, only basic anthropometric measures of body fatness and central adiposity were used, but these have been shown to be as good as dual energy X-ray absorptiometry-derived measures of risk in this population [41]. Furthermore, HOMA-IR was used as a

proxy for insulin resistance, but it has been validated against a euglycaemic hyperinsulinamic clamp and proved to be a reliable measure of insulin resistance in this population [42]. Other limitations include, not measuring dietary intake and nutrient composition.

Conclusions

This study highlights the significant relationship between inflammation and increased metabolic risk in black and white pre-menopausal South African women. Furthermore, despite the relationship between hsCRP and HOMA-IR (a measure of insulin resistance) being independent of race/ethnicity, SES and lifestyle factors, it is not independent of central adiposity, supporting the pivotal role of body fat distribution in metabolic risk. For the first time we have shown that the association between inflammation and lipids are race/ethnic-specific. Therefore, although circulating hsCRP may identify individuals at increased metabolic risk, the heterogeneity in these associations in black and white women highlights the need for prospective studies investigating these associations in different populations, as well as which factors mediate or influence the relationship between inflammation and metabolic risk in different populations, in order to design more effective interventions.

Additional files

Additional file 1: Table S1. Adjusted associations between insulin resistance (HOMA-IR) and hsCRP in black and white South African women. Data represents β-coefficients [95% confidence interval] and adjusted-R^2. Model 1: hsCRP + age + race/ethnicity + (hsCRP x race/ethnicity interaction); Model 2: (Model 1) + SES + lifestyle factors; Model 3: (Model 2) + WC. hsCRP, C-reactive protein; hsCRP x race/ethnicity, interaction between hsCRP and race/ethnicity; WC, waist circumference; SES, socio-economic status; ln(HOMA-IR), natural log of homeostatic model assessment. *$p < 0.05$ and **$p < 0.001$ (PDF 1343 kb)

Additional file 2: Table S2. Adjusted associations between triglycerides and hsCRP in black and white South African women. Data represents β-coefficients [95% confidence interval] and adjusted-R^2. Model 1: hsCRP + age + race/ethnicity + (hsCRP x race/ethnicity interaction); Model 2: (Model 1) + SES + lifestyle factors; Model 3: (Model 2) + WC. hsCRP, C-reactive protein; hsCRP x race/ethnicity, interaction between hsCRP and race/ethnicity; WC, waist circumference; SES, socio-economic status; ln(TG), natural log of triglycerides. *$p < 0.05$ and **$p < 0.001$ (PDF 545 kb)

Additional file 3: Table S3. Adjusted associations between total cholesterol and hsCRP in black and white South African women. Data represents β-coefficients [95% confidence interval] and adjusted-R^2. Model 1: hsCRP + age + race/ethnicity + (hsCRP x race/ethnicity interaction); Model 2: (Model 1) + SES + lifestyle factors; Model 3: (Model 2) + WC. hsCRP, C-reactive protein; hsCRP x race/ethnicity, interaction between hsCRP and race/ethnicity; WC, waist circumference; SES, socio-economic status; ln(TC), natural log of total cholesterol. *$p < 0.05$ and **$p < 0.001$ (PDF 542 kb)

Additional file 4: Table S4. Adjusted associations between HDL-C and hsCRP in black and white South African women. Data represents β-coefficients [95% confidence interval] and adjusted-R^2. Model 1: hsCRP + age + race/ethnicity + (hsCRP x race/ethnicity interaction); Model 2: (Model 1) + SES + lifestyle factors; Model 3: (Model 2) + WC. hsCRP, C-reactive protein; hsCRP x race/ethnicity, interaction between hsCRP and race/ethnicity; WC, waist circumference; SES, socio-economic status; ln(HDL-C), natural log of high-density lipoprotein cholesterol. *$p < 0.05$ and **$p < 0.001$ (PDF 549 kb)

Additional file 5: Table S5. Adjusted associations between LDL-C and hsCRP in black and white South African women. Data represents β-coefficients [95% confidence interval] and adjusted-R^2. Model 1: hsCRP + age + race/ethnicity + (hsCRP x race/ethnicity interaction); Model 2: (Model 1) + SES + lifestyle factors; Model 3: (Model 2) + WC. hsCRP, C-reactive protein; hsCRP x race/ethnicity, interaction between hsCRP and race/ethnicity; WC, waist circumference; SES, socio-economic status; ln(LDL-C), natural log of low-density lipoprotein cholesterol. *$p < 0.05$ and **$p < 0.001$. (PDF 565 kb)

Acknowledgements
The authors wish to thank the research volunteers for their participation in this study, Nandipha Sinyanya for her excellent field work, Courtney Jennings, Yael Joffe and Madelaine Carstens for assisting with data collection, and Judy Belonje, Hendriena Victor and Ingegerd Söderstrom for their expert technical assistance.

Funding
This study was funded by the National Research Foundation of South Africa, the South African Medical Research Council, the International Atomic Energy Agency, Novonordisk Fonden, and the University of Cape Town, South Africa.

Authors' contributions
We acknowledge that all authors have made substantial contributions to either the conception or design of the study (JE, TO, JG), the acquisition of data (JE), or the analysis and interpretation of data (CG, LM, JG). All authors were involved in either the drafting of the article (CG, LM, JG) or revising it critically for important intellectual content (CG, JE, LM, TO, JG) and all the authors have read and approved the version to be submitted (CG, JE, LM, TO, JG).

Competing interests
The authors declare that they have no competing interests.

Author details
[1]Non-Communicable Diseases Research Unit, South African Medical Research Council, Francie van Zijl Drive, Parow Valley, PO Box 19070, Cape Town, South Africa. [2]Health Impact Assessment, Western Cape Department of Health, Cape Town, South Africa. [3]South African Medical Research Council/ University of the Witwatersrand Developmental Pathways for Health Research Unit, Department of Pediatrics, Faculty of Health Sciences, University of Witwatersrand, Johannesburg, South Africa. [4]Department of Human Biology, Division of Exercise Science and Sports Medicine, University of Cape Town, Cape Town, South Africa. [5]Department of Medicine, Umeå University, Umeå, Sweden.

References
1. International Diabetes Federation. IDF Diabetes Atlas. 2017.
2. Spanakis EK, Golden SH. Race/ethnic difference in diabetes and diabetic complications. Curr Diab Rep. 2013;13(6):814–23.
3. Benjamin EJ, Blaha MJ, Chiuve SE, Cushman M, Das SR, Deo R, et al. Heart Disease and Stroke Statistics-2017 update: a report from the American Heart Association. Circulation. 2017;135(10):e146–603.
4. Khan UI, Wang D, Sowers MR, Mancuso P, Everson-Rose SA, Scherer PE, et al. Race-ethnic differences in adipokine levels: the study of Women's health across the nation (SWAN). Metabolism. 2012;61(9):1261–9.
5. Goedecke JH, Levitt NS, Evans J, Ellman N, Hume DJ, Kotze L, et al. The role of adipose tissue in insulin resistance in women of African ancestry. J Obes. 2013;2013:952916.
6. Rush EC, Goedecke JH, Jennings C, Micklesfield L, Dugas L, Lambert EV, et al. BMI, fat and muscle differences in urban women of five ethnicities from two countries. Int J Obes. 2007;31(8):1232–9.
7. Schutte AE, Olckers A. Metabolic syndrome risk in black South African women compared to Caucasian women. Horm Metab Res. 2007;39(9):651–7.
8. Zeno SA, Deuster PA, Davis JL, Kim-Dorner SJ, Remaley AT, Poth M. Diagnostic criteria for metabolic syndrome: caucasians versus African-Americans. Metab Syndr Relat Disord. 2010;8(2):149–56.
9. Ellman N, Keswell D, Collins M, Tootla M, Goedecke JH. Ethnic differences in the association between lipid metabolism genes and lipid levels in black and white South African women. Atherosclerosis. 2015;240(2):311–7.
10. Goedecke JH, Dave JA, Faulenbach MV, Utzschneider KM, Lambert EV, West S, et al. Insulin response in relation to insulin sensitivity: an appropriate beta-cell response in black South African women. Diabetes Care. 2009;32(5):860–5.
11. Wang L, Sacks FM, Furtado JD, Ricks M, Courville AB, Sumner AE. Racial differences between African-American and white women in insulin resistance and visceral adiposity are associated with differences in apoCIII containing apoAI and apoB lipoproteins. Nutr. Metab. 2014;11(1):56.
12. Morimoto Y, Conroy SM, Ollberding NJ, Kim Y, Lim U, Cooney RV, et al. Ethnic differences in serum adipokine and C-reactive protein levels: the multiethnic cohort. Int J Obes. 2014;38(11):1416–22.
13. Emerging Risk Factors Collaboration, Kaptoge S, Di Angelantonio E, Pennells L, Wood AM, White IR, et al. C-reactive protein, fibrinogen, and cardiovascular disease prediction. N Engl J Med. 2012;367(14):1310–20.
14. Zand H, Morshedzadeh N, Naghashian F. Signaling pathways linking inflammation to insulin resistance. Diabetes & metabolic syndrome. 2017; 11(Suppl 1):S307-s9.
15. Mokhaneli MC, Fourie CM, Botha S, Mels CM. The association of oxidative stress with arterial compliance and vascular resistance in a bi-ethnic population: the SABPA study. Free Radic Res. 2016;50(8):920–8.
16. Fisher G, Hyatt TC, Hunter GR, Oster RA, Desmond RA, Gower BA. Markers of inflammation and fat distribution following weight loss in African-American and white women. Obesity (Silver Spring). 2012;20(4):715–20.
17. Goedecke JH, Keswell D, Weinreich C, Fan J, Hauksson J, Victor H, et al. Ethnic differences in hepatic and systemic insulin sensitivity and their associated determinants in obese black and white South African women. Diabetologia. 2015;58(11):2647–52.
18. Schneider M, Bradshaw D, Steyn K, Norman R, Laubscher R. Poverty and non-communicable diseases in South Africa. Scand. J. Public Health. 2009;37(2):176–86.
19. Deverts DJ, Cohen S, Kalra P, Matthews KA. The prospective association of socioeconomic status with C-reactive protein levels in the CARDIA study. Brain Behav Immun. 2012;26(7):1128–35.
20. Koster A, Bosma H, Penninx BW, Newman AB, Harris TB, van Eijk JT, et al. Association of inflammatory markers with socioeconomic status. J Gerontol A Biol Sci Med Sci. 2006;61(3):284–90.
21. Carlsson AC, Li X, Holzmann MJ, Wandell P, Gasevic D, Sundquist J, et al. Neighbourhood socioeconomic status and coronary heart disease in individuals between 40 and 50 years. Heart. 2016;102(10):775–82.
22. Walsemann KM, Goosby BJ, Farr D. Life course SES and cardiovascular risk: heterogeneity across race/ethnicity and gender. Soc. Sci. Med. (1982). 2016; 152:147–55.
23. Evans J, Micklesfield L, Jennings C, Levitt NS, Lambert EV, Olsson T, et al. Diagnostic ability of obesity measures to identify metabolic risk factors in South African women. Metab Syndr Relat Disord. 2011;9(5):353–60.
24. Goedecke JH, Levitt NS, Lambert EV, Utzschneider KM, Faulenbach MV, Dave JA, et al. Differential effects of abdominal adipose tissue distribution on insulin sensitivity in black and white South African women. Obesity (Silver Spring). 2009;17(8):1506–12.
25. Bull FC, Maslin TS, Armstrong T. Global physical activity questionnaire (GPAQ): nine country reliability and validity study. J Phys Act Health. 2009; 6(6):790–804.

26. Kengne AP, Erasmus RT, Levitt NS, Matsha TE. Alternative indices of glucose homeostasis as biochemical diagnostic tests for abnormal glucose tolerance in an African setting. Prim Care Diabetes. 2017;11(2):119–31.

27. Friedewald WT, Levy RI, Fredrickson DS. Estimation of the concentration of low-density lipoprotein cholesterol in plasma, without use of the preparative ultracentrifuge. Clin Chem. 1972;18(6):499–502.

28. Matthews DR, Hosker JP, Rudenski AS, Naylor BA, Treacher DF, Turner RC. Homeostasis model assessment: insulin resistance and beta-cell function from fasting plasma glucose and insulin concentrations in man. Diabetologia. 1985;28(7):412–9.

29. Donath MY. Targeting inflammation in the treatment of type 2 diabetes: time to start. Nat Rev Drug Discov. 2014;13(6):465–76.

30. Ridker PM, Buring JE, Cook NR, Rifai N. C-reactive protein, the metabolic syndrome, and risk of incident cardiovascular events: an 8-year follow-up of 14 719 initially healthy American women. Circulation. 2003;107(3):391–7.

31. Nettleton JA, Steffen LM, Mayer-Davis EJ, Jenny NS, Jiang R, Herrington DM, et al. Dietary patterns are associated with biochemical markers of inflammation and endothelial activation in the Multi-Ethnic Study of Atherosclerosis (MESA). Am J Clin Nutr. 2006;83(6):1369–79.

32. Mchiza ZJ, Steyn NP, Hill J, Kruger A, Schonfeldt H, Nel J, et al. A review of dietary surveys in the adult South African population from 2000 to 2015. Nutrients. 2015;7(9):8227–50.

33. Veilleux A, Caron-Jobin M, Noel S, Laberge PY, Tchernof A. Visceral adipocyte hypertrophy is associated with dyslipidemia independent of body composition and fat distribution in women. Diabetes. 2011;60(5):1504–11.

34. Lee MJ, Wu Y, Fried SK. Adipose tissue heterogeneity: implication of depot differences in adipose tissue for obesity complications. Mol Asp Med. 2013; 34(1):1–11.

35. Panagiotakos DB, Pitsavos CE, Chrysohoou CA, Skoumas J, Toutouza M, Belegrinos D, et al. The association between educational status and risk factors related to cardiovascular disease in healthy individuals: the ATTICA study. Ann Epidemiol. 2004;14(3):188–94.

36. Albert MA, Glynn RJ, Ridker PM. Alcohol consumption and plasma concentration of C-reactive protein. Circulation. 2003;107(3):443–7.

37. Cooper D, Marks AS. Community-based distribution of contraception: a pilot project in Khayelitsha, Cape Town. Urban Health Newsl. 1996;30:49–55.

38. Grossman RA, Asawasena W, Chalpati S, Taewtong D, Tovanabutra S. Effects of the injectable contraceptive depot medroxyprogesterone acetate in Thai women with liver fluke infestation: final results. Bull World Health Organ. 1979;57(5):829–37.

39. Cauci S, Di Santolo M, Culhane JF, Stel G, Gonano F, Guaschino S. Effects of third-generation oral contraceptives on high-sensitivity C-reactive protein and homocysteine in young women. Obstet Gynecol. 2008;111(4):857–64.

40. Shisana O, Labadarios D, Rehle T, Simbayi L, Zuma K, Dhansay A, et al. The South African National Health and Nutrition Examination Survey (SANHANES-1). 2013.

41. Jennings CL, Micklesfield LK, Lambert MI, Lambert EV, Collins M, Goedecke JH. Comparison of body fatness measurements by near-infrared reactance and dual-energy X-ray absorptiometry in normal-weight and obese black and white women. Br J Nutr. 2010;103(7):1065–9.

42. Otten J, Ahren B, Olsson T. Surrogate measures of insulin sensitivity vs the hyperinsulinaemic-euglycaemic clamp: a meta-analysis. Diabetologia. 2014; 57(9):1781–8.

6

Morbidity and health-related quality of life of patients accessing laparoscopic sleeve gastrectomy: a single-centre cross-sectional study in one province of Canada

Laurie K. Twells[1,2]* [iD], Shannon Driscoll[1], Deborah M. Gregory[1], Kendra Lester[1], John M. Fardy[1,3] and Dave Pace[1,3]

Abstract

Background: In Canada, severe obesity (BMI $\geq$ 35 kg/m^2) affects 5% or 1.2 million adults. Bariatric surgery is the only effective treatment for severe obesity, but the demand for publicly funded procedures is high and capacity limited. Little is known in Canada about the types of patients undergoing these procedures, especially laparoscopic sleeve gastrectomy (LSG). The study objective is to examine the socio-demographic profile, morbidity and HRQoL of patients accessing LSG in one Canadian province.

Methods: Health status and HRQoL were examined in patients ($n = 195$) undergoing LSG. HRQoL was assessed using the EQ-5D-3L, SF-12v2 and the Impact of Weight on Quality of Life-lite questionnaire.

Results: Mean age and BMI were 44 and 49 kg/m^2 and most were women (82%). Pre-surgery, comorbidities were sleep apnea (65%), dyslipidemia (48%), hypertension (47%) and osteoarthritis (44%). Patients reported impaired HRQoL with 44–67% reporting problems in mobility, usual activities, pain and anxiety/depression. Physical health was impaired more than mental health. There were few socio-demographic differences between women and men, but significant differences in comorbid conditions such as sleep apnea, dyslipidemia, hypertension and gout exist ($p < .05$). Women reported fewer problems with self-care (9.5% vs. 25.0%, $p < .05$), and better overall health (VAS 61.5 vs. 52.0, $p < .05$) and General Health (39.3 vs. 32.9, $p < .05$), but greater impairment in self-esteem (27.3 vs. 44.1, $p < .01$) and sexual life (49.2 vs. 63.6, $p < .05$).

Conclusions: Before LSG, patients reported significant morbidity and impaired HRQoL. Although baseline characteristics were similar between men and women, gender specific differences were observed in comorbid profile and HRQoL.

Keywords: Severe obesity, Laparoscopic sleeve gastrectomy, Health-related quality of life, HRQoL

Background

In Canada, severe obesity, measured as a body mass index or BMI $\geq$ 35 kg/m^2) affects on average about 5% or over 1.2 million adults and is projected to increase to 6.4% by 2019. The rate of severe obesity is slightly higher in women (5.7%) compared to men (4.6%). [1] Significant and durable weight loss can be achieved with the use of bariatric surgery as a treatment for severe obesity.

[2–4] It improves the health status and life expectancy of those affected. [5–7] The eligibility criteria for accessing bariatric surgery includes the following: 1. BMI $\geq$ 40 kg/m^2 or a BMI between 35 and 39.9 kg/m^2 with a comorbidity and 2. unsuccessful weight loss attempts [8]. North America studies indicate that women are more likely than men to access bariatric surgery [9, 10].

In Canada, the volume and provision of bariatric surgery has increased. In 2012/2013 almost 6000 procedures were performed compared to less than 1600 procedures in 2006–2007 and the number of hospitals performing bariatric procedures increased from 34 to 46 over the same time period [9]. There is a disconnect between the supply

* Correspondence: ltwells@mun.ca
[1]Faculty of Medicine, Memorial University, Medical Education Building, 300 Prince Philip Drive, St. John's, NL A1B 3V6, Canada
[2]School of Pharmacy, Memorial University, Health Sciences Centre, 300 Prince Philip Drive Newfoundland and Labrador, St. John's A1B 3V6, Canada
Full list of author information is available at the end of the article

and demand of bariatric surgery resulting in long wait times for patients that average 5 years [11–15]. There are significant regional variations in the provision of surgical services in Canada and inequities in access to surgery based on geographical and socio-economic factors [13, 16, 17]. In Canada, the percentage of patients that meet eligibility criteria for bariatric surgery is estimated to be about 1% [18]. Consequently bariatric surgery is available to very few individuals who could potentially benefit from it. This is further heightened by the absence of any universally accepted and judicious approach to triaging patients for surgery [13, 14, 19]. Laparascopic sleeve gastrectomy (LSG) is the most frequently performed bariatric surgery option in Canada. In North America, the number of LSG's increased by 244% between 2011 and 2013. Forty-three percent of all bariatric surgeries are now LSG's [20].

One of the most important patient-reported reasons for wanting to undergo bariatric surgery is reduced quality of life. [21] Measures of well-being, functioning, and health under physical, social, and psychosocial domains comprise the concept Health-Related Quality of Life (HRQoL). [22, 23] It is important to examine HRQoL in pre-surgical patients in order to analyze changes after surgery and over time. A recent publication highlights the limited number of studies available for meta-analysis for a variety of reasons (e.g., selective reporting of HRQoL, use of non-validated tools and inconsistent reporting and presentation of results) [24].

Little is known in Canada [9, 18] or internationally [25] about the types of patients undergoing these procedures. Examining data on socio-demographics, sex distribution, pre-surgery BMI, comorbid profile and patient reported quality of life will help to inform healthcare providers, payers and health practitioners about the profile of patients that seek, are referred to and access bariatric surgery in Canada. This information is critical in order to: evaluate outcomes post-surgery; aggregate and compare data across centres; include data in national or international registries.

The current study objective is to investigate the morbidity and HRQoL of patients accessing LSG at a single-centre in one Canadian province. A second objective is to determine whether differences in HRQoL exist between male and female bariatric surgery candidates.

Methods

The current study is a cross-sectional analysis of the HRQoL of patients undergoing bariatric surgery at different time points in one centre in one province of Canada. Assessment of patients undergoing LSG takes place pre-surgery and post-surgery at 1, 3, 6, 12, 18, 24 months and annually thereafter. The provincial Health Research Ethics Authority (#11.101) approved the study and subjects provided written informed consent to take part.

Setting

In response to the increasing demand for a treatment for severe obesity, Eastern Health, one of four regional health authorities established a provincial multi-disciplinary bariatric surgery program to offer bariatric surgery to its residents of Newfoundland and Labrador (~500,000, of which approximately 8% is potentially eligible for surgery) [9]. Based on surgeon preference and expertise, LSG is most often (98%) performed at this centre. The surgical technique used in the current study has been previously described [26]. Since 2011, 417 LSGs have been performed. This study examines the socio-demographic profile, morbidity and HRQoL of 200 consecutive patients accessing bariatric surgery in this newly established surgical program.

Measures of health-related quality of life

We evaluated HRQoL in patients before surgery and by sex using three validated tools: the Euroqol-5 Dimension-3 level (EQ-5D-3L) [27], the Short-Form-12 version 2 (SF-12v2) [28] and a weight specific tool, the Impact of Weight on Quality of Life-Lite (IWQOL-Lite) [29]. The EQ-5D-3L, is an indirect preference-based health survey that consists of a 5 dimension descriptive system assessing mobility, self-care, pain, usual activity and anxiety each of which can be rated at one of three levels (no problems, some problems or extreme problems). These combine to create 243 possible health states. The descriptive system is scored using a set of weights that represent the general population's preferences and allows for the calculation of a single summary preference-based utility index or score. EQ-5D-3L utility scores range between full health of 1 (where the respondent has no problems on any dimension) to the lowest score of –0.59 (where the respondent reports that they are at the bottom level of each dimension) [27]. An overall health EQ-5D-3L visual analogue scale (VAS) is also calculated. This score ranges from 0 (worst imaginable health) to 100 (perfect health) and is presented as a mean and standard deviation. The SF-12v2 is a short version of the SF-36, a validated tool used to assess quality of life. It has been validated against the SF-36 for patients with and without obesity [30]. The SF-12v2 survey contains 12 questions that assess 8 domains: physical function, role physical, bodily pain, general health, vitality, social function, role emotional and mental health. These domains are used to calculate a physical component score (PCS) and a mental health component scores (MCS) [28]. The PCS and MCS scores follow a T distribution (mean 50, SD 10), normalized for the general United States (US) population. License specific software accounts for any missing data and generates a mean score for each domain and for both component scores [28]. The IWQOL-Lite, a shorter form of the original questionnaire, assesses the impact of weight on quality of life in individuals exploring treatments for weight loss. The IWQOL-

Lite includes 31 statements that start with "Because of my weight..." with response options to each statement ranging from (1) "Never true" to (5) "Always true" that measure the impact of weight on 5 domains (i.e., physical function, self-esteem, sexual life, public distress and work life). A score is calculated for each domain for each patient that answers at least 50% of the questions in any given domain. A total score is calculated if patients have responded to at least 26 out of the 31 questions. Raw scores are converted into a T-score (0–100), with 100 representing best possible health. Mean and standard deviations are reported for each domain [29].

Statistical analysis

Descriptive analyses were performed for continuous variables that included the calculation of mean, standard deviation, standard error, median, interquartile range, minimum and maximum, and range. For categorical variables, data are presented as n and %'s. IBM SPSS version 22.0 [31] was used to analyze survey data from the EQ-5D-3L and the IWQOL-Lite surveys. The EQ-5D-3L index values were calculated using US time trade-off (TTO) data. As required, the SF-12v2 results were analyzed using licenser specific software (i.e., Health Outcomes Software version 4.5) [28]. Differences by sex in demographic and individual survey results were determined using t-tests for continuous variables and Pearson's chi-squared test for categorical variables and, where appropriate, the Fisher exact test is reported. Statistical significance was set at $p < .05$.

Results

In May 2011 when the bariatric surgery program commenced, 200 consecutive pre-surgical patients were recruited to the Newfoundland and Labrador Bariatric Surgery Study. One hundred ninety-five patients (98%) completed the baseline questionnaires. Pre-surgery socio-demographic characteristics and comorbidity profile are presented in Tables 1 and 2. Overall 82% of patients accessing bariatric surgery were women. The average age, weight and BMI were 44 ± 10 years (range 22–70 years), 135 ± 23.2 kg and 49 kg/m^2 ± 6.7, respectively. A small number of eligible patients gained weight between the initial assessment/ acceptance for surgery and actual surgery ($n = 10$) resulting in a range of BMI values between 35.2–67.2 kg/m^2. The majority of the sample had post-secondary or some post-secondary education (75%) and were in full or part-time employment (62%). The average number of comorbidities reported were 5 and 74% of the sample reported ≥4 comorbidities. Obstructive sleep apnea (OSA) (65%), dyslipidemia (48%), back pain (51%), hypertension (47%), osteoarthritis (44%), gastroesophageal reflux disease (GERD) (43%) and type 2 diabetes mellitus (T2DM) (42%) were reported most often.

According to the EQ-5D-3L, patients reported some or extreme problems in mobility (47.2%), usual activity (53.1%), pain/discomfort (67.0%) and anxiety/depression (44.1%) with few reporting problems in self-care (12.4%) (Table 3). The average EQ-5D index and VAS scores were 0.78 ± 0.01SE and 59.8 ± 18.7SD, respectively. (data not shown) According to the SF-12v2, the PCS and MCS were 36.4 and 47.8 respectively, with normative scores of 50(10) (Table 4). As the SF-12v2 provides normative data for the general US population, it is possible to calculate what percentage of the current surgical sample provided scores below, at or above the population norm (mean 50 ± 10). For the total surgical sample, the percentages of patients that scored below, at or above the population norm were 77%, 21% and 2% for PCS and 36%, 29% and 35% for MCS. According to the IWQOL-Lite questionnaire, an instrument developed to specifically assess weight-related quality of life where lower scores (0–100) indicate greater impairment, the domains most impacted by weight were self-esteem (30.4), physical function (41.9), public distress (44.1), sexual life (51.8) and work (61.0). The IWQOL-Lite total score was 43.2 ± 18.7 (Table 5).

Socio-demographic characteristics by sex

There were very few differences in baseline characteristics pre-surgery (Table 1). Women had a significantly lower weight than men (130.2kgs vs 155.8kgs, $p < .001$), although BMI was not different. Women were less likely to be partnered (69.0% vs 86.1%, $p < .05$). Women and men were similar in terms of age, income, education, employment status, ethnicity and smoking behavior.

Pre-surgical Comorbid conditions by sex

The comorbidity profiles comparing women and men were somewhat different (Table 2). Men most often presented for surgery with OSA, hypertension, dyslipidemia, GERD and T2DM, while women presented with OSA, back pain, dyslipidemia, osteoarthritis and gallbladder disease. There were some statistically significant gender differences; compared to women, men reported more OSA, dyslipidemia, hypertension, and gout, while women reported double the prevalence of gallbladder disease/gallstones compared to men pre-surgery.

Health related quality of life by questionnaire and sex

Table 3 presents the results from the EQ-5D-3L. Fewer women reported problems with self-care compared to men (9.5% vs. 25%, $p < 0.05$) and while fewer women reported problems with mobility (44.0% vs. 61.1%) and usual activities (50.6% vs 63.9%) compared to men, these differences were not significant. In contrast, more women reported problems with pain/ discomfort (69.0% vs 58.3%) and anxiety/depression (45.3% vs 38.9%) compared to men, although not significantly different. Women reported

Table 1 Baseline characteristics of total sample and by sex

	Total population n = 195		Women n = 159		Men n = 36		p-value
	Mean (SD)	Range	Mean (SD)	Range	Mean (SD)	Range	
Age (years)	44 (10)	22–70	44 (9)	22–70	46 (11)	29–66	$p = 0.110$
Weight (kg)	134.9 (23.2)	90.0–231.0	130.2 (19.8)	90.0–187.5	155.8 (25.9)	106.0–231.0	P < .001
BMI (kg/m^2)	48.8 (6.7)	35.2–67.2	48.7 (6.8)	35.2–67.2	49.6 (6.5)	37.8–60.7	$p = 0.428$
Obese Class II	16 (8.2%)		13 (8.2%)		3 (8.3%)		$p = 0.975$
Obese Class III	179 (91.8%)		146 (91.8%)		33 (91.7%)		
	n	%	n	%	n	%	
Female	159	81.5%	143		52		
Smoking							
Never	81	47.6%	65	45.5%	16	59.3%	$p = 0.188$
Former	53	31.2%	45	31.5%	8	29.6%	$p = 0.850$
Current	36	21.2%	33	23.1%	3	10.7%	$p = 0.142$
Marital Status							
Married/Common Law	140	72.2%	109	69.0%	31	86.1%	$p = 0.039$
Divorced/Separated/Single/ Never married/Widow	54	27.8%	49	31.0%	5	13.9%	
Education							
None/Some High School or diploma	47	24.6%	39	25.0%	8	22.9%	$p = 0.790$
Some post-secondary/Post-Secondary	144	75.4%	117	75.0%	27	77.1%	
Annual Income							
< $15,000	8	4.1%	7	4.4%	1	2.8%	$p = 0.877$
$15,000 - $29,999	24	12.3%	21	13.2%	3	8.3%	
$30,000 - $49,999	45	23.1%	37	23.3%	8	22.2%	
$50,000 – $79,999	38	19.5%	30	18.9%	8	22.2%	
≥ $80,000	53	27.2%	41	25.8%	12	33.3%	
Not Answered	27	13.8%	23	14.5%	4	11.1%	
Employment Status							
Full-time/Part-time	120	61.9%	98	61.6%	22	62.9%	$p = 0.893$
Other	74	38.1%	61	38.4%	13	37.1%	
Race							
Caucasian	179	95.2%	146	95.4%	33	94.3%	$p = 0.776$
Other	9	4.8%	7	4.6%	2	5.7%	
Average # of comorbidities (SD)	5.4 (2.7)	0–16	5.2 (2.8)	0–16	6.3 (2.3)	2–11	
Number of Comorbidities							
< 4	49	26.1%	45	28.8%	4	12.5%	$p = 0.055$
≥ 4	139	73.9%	111	71.2%	28	87.5%	

significantly higher scores (i.e., better self reported health) on the VAS (61.5 ± 18.5SD vs 52.0 ± 17.6SD, $p = 0.009$) compared to men, although there was no significant difference between the two on the EQ Index ($0.79 \pm .013$SE vs $0.75 \pm .031$SE) which describes the patient's health state [data not shown].

According to the SF-12v2 (Table 4), women reported significantly less impairment in General Health (39.3 vs 32.9, $p < .05$) and in the PCS (37.2 vs 33.3, $p = 0.048$). Based on the normative data for women, the percentage of the study sample whose PCS was below, at or above population norms correspond to: 75% below, 22% at, and 3% above the norm. The percentage of the study sample whose MCS was below, at or above the population norm was: 37% below, 27% at, and 36% above the population norm. For men, the PCS values corresponded

Table 2 Comorbidity profile of total sample and by sex

		Total $n = 195$ n (%)	Women $n = 159$ n (%)	Men $n = 36$ n (%)	p-value
Sleep Apnea		127 (65.1)	94 (59.1)	33 (91.7)	p < .001
	On CPAP	89 (70.1)	61 (64.9)	28 (84.8)	
Back Pain ($n = 188$)		95 (50.5)	80 (51.3)	15 (46.9)	p = 0.650
Dyslipidemia ($n = 186$)		89 (47.8)	68 (43.9)	21 (67.7)	p = 0.015
Hypertension ($n = 188$)		89 (47.3)	67 (42.9)	22 (68.8)	p = 0.008
Osteoarthritis ($n = 188$)		83 (44.1)	68 (43.6)	15 (46.9)	p = 0.733
Type 2 Diabetes		82 (42.1)	64 (40.3)	18 (50.0)	p = 0.285
Gastroesophageal Reflux Disease ($n = 189$)		81 (43.1)	64 (41.0)	17 (53.1)	p = 0.155
Gallbladder Disease/Gallstones ($n = 187$)		75 (40.1)	68 (43.6)	7 (22.6)	p = 0.029
Asthma ($n = 188$)		42 (22.3)	32 (20.5)	10 (31.3)	p = 0.184
Polycystic Ovary Syndrome ($n = 159$)		32 (20.1)	32 (20.1)	n/a	
Yeast/Fungal Infection ($n = 187$)		26 (13.9)	24 (15.5)	2 (6.3)	p = 0.169
Hypothyroidism ($n = 187$)		21 (11.2)	19 (12.3)	2 (6.3)	p = 0.327
Gout ($n = 188$)		21 (11.2)	9 (5.8)	12 (37.5)	p = 0.000

to 83%, 11% and 6% below, at or above the norm and for the MCS, 31%, 39% and 31% reported scores below, at or above the norm [data not shown].

The IWQOL-Lite scores are presented in Table 5. Women reported significantly lower scores than men for self-esteem (27.3 vs. 44.1, $p < 0.05$) and sexual life (49.2 vs. 63.6, p < 0.05) suggesting that in women, these domains were more impaired by their weight. Men and women did not differ in scores for three of five domains (i.e., physical function, public distress or work). The IWQOL-Lite total score was significantly lower for woman compared to men (42.0 vs 48.7, p < 0.05).

Discussion

Patients in this study averaged 44 years of age and had an average BMI of 49 kg/m^2. The majority of the sample were: women with post-secondary or some post-secondary education in full or part- time employment.

Health status was significantly impaired pre-surgery with patients reporting on average 5.4 comorbidities. OSA affected two thirds (65%) of the study sample while half of the sample reported having been diagnosed with hypertension (47%), dyslipidemia (48%) and back pain (51%). Almost half of the study sample reported having osteoarthritis (44%), T2DM (42%), GERD (43%) and gallbladder disease (40%). Pre-operatively, women and men did not differ significantly on select socio-demographics variables (i.e., age, income, education or employment status, although there were differences in comorbid profiles. A high prevalence of OSA was diagnosed in both sexes (65%), and rates were one third higher for men. Men also reported higher rates of dyslipidemia, hypertension and gout. In contrast, women reported double the rate of gallbladder disease/gallstones.

Pre-surgery HRQoL was significantly impaired in the study sample. Few patients reported problems with self-

Table 3 EQ-5D-3L scores for total sample and by sex

	Mobility n(%)			Self-Care* n(%)			Usual Activities n(%)			Pain/Discomfort n(%)			Anxiety/Depression n(%)		
	Total	Women	Men	Total	Women	Men	Total	Women	Men	Total	Women	Men	Total	Women	Men
No Problems	103 (52.8%)	89 (56.0%)	14 (38.9%)	170 (87.6%)	143 (90.5%)	27 (75.0%)	91 (46.9%)	78 (49.4%)	13 (36.1%)	64 (33.0%)	49 (31.0%)	15 (41.7%)	109 (55.9%)	87 (54.7%)	22 (61.1%)
Some/ Extreme Problems	92 (47.2%)	70 (44.0%)	22 (61.1%)	24 (12.4%)	15 (9.5%)	9 (25.0%)	103 (53.1%)	80 (50.6%)	23 (63.9%)	130 (67.0%)	109 (69.0%)	21 (58.3%)	86 (44.1%)	72 (45.3%)	14 (38.9%)
p-value	0.064			0.021			0.150			0.220			0.485		
Total	195	159	36	194	158	36	194	158	36	194	158	36	195	159	36

*p < .05 between men and women. T-tests were performed comparing "no problems" to "problems" (some and extreme problems were combined) between men and women

Table 4 SF-12v2 scores for total sample and by sex

Domain	Overall n = 195 Mean (SD)	Women n = 159 Mean (SD)	Men n = 36 Mean (SD)	p-value
Physical Function	37.1 (10.4)	37.3 (10.3)	36.3 (10.8)	0.618
Role Physical	39.0 (10.7)	39.6 (10.4)	36.3 (12.0)	0.095
Bodily Pain	40.9 (12.7)	40.9 (12.3)	41.0 (14.7)	0.953
General Health*	38.2 (10.6)	39.3 (10.4)	32.9 (9.8)	0.001
Vitality	43.0 (9.3)	43.5 (9.3)	41.0 (9.3)	0.158
Social Functioning	42.0 (12.1)	42.1 (12.0)	41.9 (12.3)	0.927
Role Emotional Health	44.4 (12.1)	44.2 (11.9)	45.2 (13.2)	0.645
Mental Health	47.0 (10.0)	46.6 (10.0)	48.8 (9.9)	0.229
Physical Health Component Score (PCS)*	36.4 (10.6)	37.2 (10.3)	33.3 (11.3)	0.048
Mental Health Component Score (MCS)	47.8 (10.7)	47.5 (10.9)	49.1 (9.9)	0.416

*$p < 0.05$ between men and women

care; however, between 44% and 67% of patients reported problems with anxiety/depression, mobility, usual activities and pain and discomfort. Patient perceptions of general health and physical health were impaired more than mental health.

According to the weight-specific IWQOL-Lite scale, patients reported impairment on all scales (most to least impairment): Self Esteem, Physical Function, Public Distress, Sexual Life and Work. Significant differences in HRQoL were reported by women and men on self esteem, sexual life and the IWQOL total score.

Women self-reported better General Health as evidenced by higher scores on the SF-12v2 (39.3 vs. 32.9) and the VAS (61.5 vs. 52.0) and better Physical Health (PCS 37.2 vs. 33.3). Although 10% of the total patient sample reported problems with self care on the EQ-5D-3L, women reported significantly fewer problems in this area than men (9.5% vs. 25.0%). Based on the IWQOL-Lite, women reported greater weight associated impairment than men on Self Esteem (27.3 vs. 44.1) and Sexual Life (49.2 vs. 63.6).

Our study population, the majority of whom were women, is similar to other patients seeking treatment for severe obesity [2, 18, 32–34]. Patients undergoing bariatric surgery are more often female with an average pre-

surgery weight and BMI of 124.5kgs and 46 kg/m^2, respectively [2]. With respect to socio-demographics, our sample represents a high level of socio-economic status, with over 75% having some/full post-secondary education and half in higher income brackets. Findings on the relationship between socio-economic status and access to bariatric surgery are inconsistent, although in North America it appears that access to bariatric surgery has been reserved for those of higher social standing [18, 32, 35, 36]. This finding has been supported by publications that highlight inequities in access to bariatric surgery in Canada [13, 18]. Women and men had similar baseline characteristics, with the exception that women were less likely to be in partnered relationships, a finding similar to other studies [18, 32, 33, 37].

A very high level of obesity-related comorbidity was observed in the current study sample although the comorbid profile of patients seeking obesity treatment can vary signficantly by centre [18, 33, 38, 39]. In the Alberta population-based prospective evaluation of the quality of life outcomes and economic impact of bariatric surgery (APPLES) study, Padwal et al., assessed 150 bariatric surgical patients in Alberta, Canada. Compared to the current study, the APPLES authors reported higher rates

Table 5 IWQOL-Lite scores for total sample and by sex

Domain	Overall n	Mean(SD)	Women n	Mean(SD)	Men n	Mean(SD)	p-value
Physical Function	194	41.9 (20.7)	158	42.2 (20.1)	36	40.7 (23.6)	0.705
Self Esteem**	194	30.4 (26.4)	158	27.3 (24.3)	36	44.1 (30.9)	0.004
Sexual Life*	181	51.8 (32.1)	148	49.2 (31.9)	33	63.6 (30.6)	0.019
Public Distress	193	44.1 (25.2)	157	42.5 (24.7)	36	51.5 (26.2)	0.051
Work	185	61.0 (24.7)	153	60.3 (25.3)	32	64.8 (21.6)	0.341
Total score*	193	43.2 (18.7)	157	42.0 (17.7)	36	48.7 (21.9)	0.049

*$p < 0.05$ between men and women. **$p < .01$ between men and women

of hypertension (61% vs. 47%) and dyslipidemia (60% vs. 48%) in their pre-surgery population, but similar rates of T2DM (42% vs. 44%) [38]. In contrast, compared to national Canadian data published on bariatric surgery recipients, obesity-related comorbidity was much higher in our study population with higher rates of hypertension (47% vs.13%), dyslipidemia (48% vs. 2.4%) and T2DM (42% vs. 21%) [18]. This variation may be partly explained by the fact that Newfoundland and Labrador has the highest rates of T2DM and CVD in Canada [40, 41]. Although, there may be potential under-coding of pre-existing conditions in administrative datasets when compared to prospectively collected data [18]. High levels of comorbidity may be one factor that motivates patients to seek treatment for severe obesity. [39, 42] In previous research conducted at our centre, individuals seeking treatment for severe obesity reported health concerns as the primary reason for wanting to lose weight, similar to other studies [21]. In the current study, the prevalence of comorbid conditions differed between women and men seeking treatment (e.g., OSA, dyslipidemia, hypertension, gout, and gallbladder disease/gallstones) similar to a study of over 200 patients undergoing bariatric surgery conducted in Germany from the University Hospital Heidelberg. In this study the authors examined patient expectations of surgery and collected data on baseline comorbidity. A similar prevalence of hypertension was reported with men more likely than women to be affected. Although much lower prevalences of OSA and dyslipidemia were reported, men were twice as likely to report being affected than women. [39] Gender differences in the rates of OSA and risk factors for CVD are often reported, but differences in the rates of other conditions are more inconsistent [33, 39, 43, 44].

Consistent with the results of other published studies, individuals seeking obesity treatment in the current study, demonstrated significantly impaired HRQoL compared to: the general population, individuals with overweight/obesity, or those with severe obesity not seeking surgical treatment. [23, 45–47] Studies consistently demonstrate that in individuals seeking treatment for severe obesity, physical health is impacted more than mental health [5, 32, 46, 48], although the magnitude of the impact varies. In the current study, the PCS of 36.4 is lower than the PCS of 41.5 reported by Warkentin et al., in the Canadian APPLES study [49] although the MCS score of 47.8 is more comparable to the APPLES results of 46.9. Compared to the Utah Obesity Study [50], a prospective cohort study of over 400 patients accessing Roux-en-Y Gastric Bypass (RYGB), the current study's pre-surgery HRQoL scores are higher than those reported by the authors (PCS 31.4, MCS 41.4). In a study on pre-surgical patients conducted in Germany, the authors reported a similar PCS to the

current study (34.3 versus 36.4), although the MCS was lower (42.1 versus 47.8). In both these studies the direction of the impairment remained similar in that physicial health was impacted more than mental health. [48] The EQ index of 0.78 reported in the current study is similar to that reported by the APPLES Study authors (0.79), and significantly lower than population norms (0.82). Surgical patients in the current study reported overall health (VAS 59.8) that was slightly lower than the APPLES study authors (VAS 63.6) and significantly lower than population norms (VAS 78.8) [49, 51].

Similar to other studies, patients seeking surgical treatment for severe obesity report significantly impaired weight-related HRQoL, although the level of impairment varies [23, 46, 50]. In the current study, the total IWQOL-Lite score (0–100), was 43.2, which was lower than scores reported by Padwal et al., in the APPLES study (IWQOL-Lite: 49.9) [47] or Belle et al., in the US Longitudinal Assessment of Bariatric Surgery (LABS), (IWQOL-Lite 46.8) [52] but higher than that reported by the Utah Obesity Study (IWQOL-Lite 41.8) [50]. These total scores are well below those reported by the general population (IWQOL-Lite 94.7) and lower than those reported by individuals living with severe obesity not seeking surgical treatment (IWQOL-Lite 54.9) [52]. Similar to other studies using North American data, in the current study, the domains most impacted by weight in decreasing order of impact were self-esteem, physical health, public distress, sexual life and work [37, 52], but are in contrast to data from Europe where patients report that weight impairs physical function more than self-esteem. [37, 46] It is an interesting finding that work life was reported as least impaired by weight in the current study and in other published studies [37, 52] as research suggests that absenteeism from work and more importantly presenteeism are much higher in individuals living with severe obesity compared to other BMI categories [53]. This is an area that could warrant further exploration.

Gender analysis

Significant differences were found between women and men with respect to HRQoL. Women reported better General Health on the SF-12v2 (39.3 vs. 32.9) and the EQ-5D VAS (61.5 vs. 52.0) and better Physical Health (SF-12v2: PCS 37.2 vs. 33.3). This finding is inconsistent with studies by Kolotkin et al. who found that General Health was more impaired in women than men [33] and Karlsson [6] and Belle [52] who found no gender differences in General Health or physical HRQoL. In the current study, this may be partly explained by the fnding that fewer women reported having problems with Self Care compared to men (9.5% vs. 25.0%). Accordng to the IWQOL-Lite, weight impacted self-esteem and sexual life more in women than men.

Previous research on gender differences using the IWQOL-Lite has been inconsistent, however the weight-related impairment consistently affects women more than men in the domains self-esteem and sexual life [30, 33, 37, 52, 54, 55]. Stout et al., found no gender differences on the IWQOL-Lite scores. [54] In contrast, other studies have reported differences, but not in the same domains. Kolotkin et al. [33] and Belle et al. [52] report gender differences in self-esteem, sexual life, work and total score while White et al. [55] report gender differences in physical function, self-esteem, sexual life and total score. In a study by Caxias et al., [37] assessing HRQoL in bariatric surgery treatment seeking individuals in North America, gender differences are limited to self-esteem, sexual life and total score with women reporting greater impairment than men. The consistency of study findings in this area and across numerous studies suggest that weight negatively impacts these psychosocial domains in women more than men and may be a leading reason for why women seek treatment for severe obesity four to five times more often than men in North America. Previous qualitative research has shown that women seeking bariatric surgery are more likely than men to have weight and body image concerns. [56] The gender difference in uptake of bariatric surgery may also be partly explained by the fact that women seek out health care services in general and for mental health concerns more often than men [57].

Strengths of this study include: the use of three validated instruments to assess generic and obesity-specific HRQoL; the availability of key socio-demographic variables and co-morbidity data to allows for exploration of and gender comparisons among these variables. Examining gender differences in HRQoL may provide a potential explanation for this reported imbalance of bariatric surgery seeking behaviors of women as opposed to men. This study also has some limitations. First, it is difficult to infer a causal relationship exists between severe obesity and HRQoL in a cross-sectional study. Methodological challenges of reverse causality and temporality are inherent in this study design. Second, most comorbidities were self-reported. Third, we did not have access to specific data on depression, although the EQ-5D-3L data reports that almost half the study sample reported problems with depression/anxiety, and there were no gender differences observed. Although depression is often seen as an important determinant of HRQoL, studies report varying degrees of depression in patients seeking bariatric surgery contingent on assessment type (i.e., self-report versus diagnosis by a healthcare professional) that range from one to two thirds of the population, with inconsistent results on gender differences. [33, 49, 52] Finally, as the current study took place in one Canadian province, it may lack generalizability to other populations; however, the socio-demographics, comorbid

profile and HRQoL of our patients are comparable to those in North America and other centres [9, 32, 52].

Future research should explore reasons why men are less likely to seek out bariatric surgery than women as this may signal potential sex-related disparities in access to bariatric surgery [35, 36]. For example, there may be inherent biases in referral patterns for bariatric surgery or different health-seeking behaviors between women and men. [57] A better understanding of why weight appears to impact women more than men in psychosocial areas is also warranted especially in the context of societal pressures [13, 33, 56]. In addition, the impact of surgery on HRQoL in the short, medium and specifically long term should be explored. The publication of HRQoL data 2 to 4 years after bariatric surgery for this study sample is planned.

Conclusion

Our study results demonstrate that similar to other programs in North America and elsewhere, patients living with severe obesity who access bariatric surgery tend to be women with high socio-economic status. Individuals seeking treatment report significant morbidity and impaired HRQoL. Women and men presented with substantial but significantly different pre-operative comorbid profiles. HRQoL was significantly impaired in men and women. Women compared to men reported better scores in general and physical health and fewer problems with self-care. However, weight impaired women's sexual life and self-esteem significantly more than men.

Acknowledgements

We would like to thank Kim Manning, Research Nurse and the Multidisciplinary Bariatric Program at Eastern Health as well as the bariatric surgery patients who took part in our study.

Authors' contributors

LT, DG, JF and DP conceived the study concept. SD was responsible for data entry and SD and KL performed data analyses. LT wrote the initial draft with input from all authors. All authors were involved in the interpretation of the data. DG, JF, DP contributed to, reviewed, edited and approved the final manuscript. All authors read and approved the final manuscript.

Funding

This study was funded by the Newfoundland and Labrador Centre for Applied Health Research and the Health Care Foundation.

Competing interest

The authors declare that they have no competing interests.

Author details
[1]Faculty of Medicine, Memorial University, Medical Education Building, 300 Prince Philip Drive, St. John's, NL A1B 3V6, Canada. [2]School of Pharmacy, Memorial University, Health Sciences Centre, 300 Prince Philip Drive Newfoundland and Labrador, St. John's A1B 3V6, Canada. [3]Eastern Health, Health Sciences Centre, 300 Prince Philip Drive, St. John's, NL A1B 3V6, Canada.

References
1. Twells LK, Gregory DM, Reddigan J, Midodzi W. Current prevalence and future predictions of obesity in Canada: a trend analysis. CMAJ Open. 2014;2(1):E18–26.
2. Chang SH, Stoll CR, Song J, Varela JE, et al. The effectiveness and risks of bariatric surgery: an updated systematic review and meta-analysis, 2003-2012. JAMA Surg. 2014;149(3):275–87.
3. Padwal R, Klarenbach S, Wiebe N, Hazel M, Karmali S, et al. Bariatric surgery: a systematic review of the clinical and economic evidence. J Gen Intern Med. 2011;26(10):1183–94.
4. Picot J, Jones J, Colquitt JL, Gospodarevskaya E, Loveman E, Baxter L, et al. The clinical effectiveness and cost-effectiveness of bariatric (weight loss) surgery for obesity: a systematic review and economic evaluation. Health Technol Assess. 2009;13(41):1–190, 215-357, iii-iv.
5. Driscoll S, Gregory DM, Fardy JM, Twells LK. Long-term health-related quality of life in bariatric surgery patients: a systematic review and meta-analysis. Obesity (Silver Spring). 2016;24(1):60–70.
6. Karlsson J, Taft C, Rydén A, Sjöström L, Sullivan M. Ten year trends in health-related quality of life after surgical and conventional treatment for severe obesity: the SOS intervention study. Int J Obes. 2007;38(8):1248–61.
7. Pontiroli AE, Morabito A. Long-term prevention of mortality in morbid obesity through bariatric surgery. A systematic review and meta-analysis of trials performed with gastric banding and gastric bypass. Ann Surg. 2011;253(3):484–7.
8. Lau DC, Douketis JD, Morrison KM, et al. 2006 Canadian clinical practice guidelines on the management and prevention of obesity in adults and children [summary]. CMAJ. 2007;176(suppl. 8):S1–13.
9. Canadian Institute for Health Information. Bariatric surgery in Canada. Ottawa: CIHI; 2014.
10. Samuel I, Mason EE, Renquist KE, Huang YH, Zimmerman MB, Jamal M. Bariatric surgery trends: an 18-year report from the international bariatric surgery registry. Am J Surg. 2006;192(5):657–62.
11. Christou NV, Efthimiou E. Bariatric surgery waiting times in Canada. Can J Surg. 2009;52(3):229–34.
12. Christou NV. Access to bariatric (metabolic) surgery in Canada. Can J Diabetes. 2011;35(2):123–8.
13. Gregory DM, Temple Newhook J, Twells LK. Patients' perceptions of waiting for bariatric surgery: a qualitative study. Int J Equity Health. 2013;12(86) doi: 10.1186/1475-9276-12-86.
14. Lakkoff JM, Elsmere J, Ransom T. Cause of death in patients awaiting bariatric surgery. Can J Surg. 2015;58(1):15–8.
15. Padwal RS, Sharma AM. Treating severe obesity: morbid weights and morbid waits. CMAJ. 2009;181(11):777–8.
16. Domouras AG, Saleh F, Gmora S, Anvari M, Hong D. Regional variations in the public delivery of bariatric surgery: an evaluation of the center of excellence model. Ann Surg. 2016;263(2):306–11.
17. Sharma AM. Inequalities in access to bariatric surgery in Canada. CMAJ. 2016;188(5):317–8.
18. Padwal RS, Chang H, Klarenbach S, Sharma AM, Majumder S. Characteristics of the population eligible for and receiving publicly funded bariatric surgery in Canada. Int J Equity Health. 2012;11(54) doi:10.1186/1475-9276-11-54.
19. Padwal RS, Pajewski NM, Sharma AM. Using the Edmonton obesity staging system to predict mortality in a population – representative cohort of people with overweight and obesity. CMAJ. 2011;183(14):E1059–66.
20. Angrisani L, Santonicola A, Iovino P, Formisano G, Buchwald H, Scopinaro N. Bariatric surgery worldwide 2013. Obes Surg. 2015;25(10):1822–32.
21. Price HI, Gregory DM, Twells LK. Weight loss expectations of laparoscopic sleeve gastrectomy candidates compared to clinically expected weight loss outcomes 1-year post-surgery. Obes Surg. 2013;23(12):1987–93.
22. Guyatt G, Feeny DH, Patrick DL. Measuring health-related quality of life. Ann Intern Med. 1993;118(8):622–9.
23. Kolotkin RL, Meter K, Williams GR. Quality of life and obesity. Obes Rev. 2001;2(4):19–29.
24. Andersen JR, Aasprang A, Karlsen TI, Natviq GK, Våge V, Kolotkin RL. Health-related quality of life after bariatric surgery: a systematic review of prospective long-term studies. Surg Obes Relat Dis. 2015;11(2):466–73.
25. The IFSO Global Registry. First IFSO global registry report. Oxfordshire: Dendrite Clinical Systems Ltd.; 2014.
26. Falk V, Twells LK, Gregory DM, Smith C, Boone D, Murphy R, Pace D. Laparoscopic sleeve gastrectomy at a new bariatric surgery center in Canada: 30-day complication rates using the Clavien-Dindo classification. Can J Surg. 2016;59(2):93–7.
27. EuroQol Group: EQ-5D: A standardized instrument for use as a measure of health outcomes. Available from: http://www.euroqol.org/. Accessed 16 June 2016.
28. SF-36.org. The SF-12®: An even shorter health survey. Available from http://campaign.optum.com/optum-outcomes/what-we-do/health-surveys/sf-12v2-health-survey.html. Accessed 16 June 2016.
29. Quality of Life Consulting. Impact of Weight on Quality of Life-Lite. Available from: http://www.qualityoflifeconsulting.com/iwqol-lite.html. Accessed 16 June 2016.
30. Wee CC, Davis RB, Hamel MB. Comparing the SF-12 and SF-36 health status questionnaires in patients with and without obesity. Health Qual Life Outcomes. 2008;6(11) doi:10.1186/1477-7525-6-11.
31. IBM Corp. ReleasedIBM SPSS statistics for windows, version 22.0. Armonk: IBM Corp; 2013.
32. Dreyer N, Dixon JB, Okerson T, Finkelstein EA, Globe D. Prevalence of comorbidities and baseline characteristics of LAP-BAND AP® subjects in the helping evaluate reduction in obesity (HERO) study. PLoS One. 2013;8(11) doi:10.1371/journal.pone.0078971.
33. Kolotkin RL, Crosby RD, Gress RE, Hunt SC, Engel SG, Adams TD. Health and health-related quality of life: differences between men and women who seek gastric bypass surgery. Surg Obes Relat Dis. 2008;4(5):651–8.
34. Nicke F, Schmidt L, Bruckner T, Billeter AT, Kenngott HG, Müller-Stich BP, Fischer L. Gastrointestinal quality of life improves significantly after sleeve Gastrectomy and roux-en-Y gastric bypass—a prospective cross-sectional study within a 2-year follow-up. Obes Surg. 2017;27(5):1292–7.
35. Halloran K, Padwal RS, Johnson-Stoklossa C, Sharma AM, Birch DW. Income status and approval for bariatric surgery in a publicly funded regional obesity program. Obes Surg. 2011;21(3):373–8.
36. Martin M, Beekley A, Kjorstad R, Sebesta J. Socioeconomic disparities in eligibility and access to bariatric surgery: a national population-based analysis. Surg Obes Relat Dis. 2010;6(1):8–15.
37. Caixàs A, Lecube A, Morales MJ, Calañas A, Moreiro J, Cordido F, et al. Weight-related quality of life in Spanish obese subjects suitable for bariatric surgery is lower than in their north American counterparts: a case-control study. Obes Surg. 2013;23(4):509–14.
38. Padwal RS, Rueda-Clausen CF, Sharma AM, Agborsangaya CB, Klarenbach S, Birch DW, et al. Weight loss and outcomes in wait-listed, medically managed, and surgically treated patients enrolled in a population-based bariatric program: prospective cohort study. Med Care. 2014;52(3):208–15.
39. Fischer L, Nickel F, Sander J, Ernst A, Bruckner T, Herbig B, Büchler MW, Müller-Stich BP, Sandbu R. Patient expectations of bariatric surgery are gender specific—a prospective, multicenter cohort study. Surg Obes Relat Dis. 2014;10(3):516–23.
40. Statistics Canada CANSIM Tables, "Diabetes, by sex, provinces and territories. " Available online: http://www.statcan.gc.ca/tables-tableaux/sum-som/l01/cst01/health54b-eng.htm. Accessed 16 June 2016.
41. Public Health Agency of Canada (PHAC) Chronic Disease Infobase, "Chronic disease and injury indicator framework." Available online: http://infobase.phac-aspc.gc.ca:9600/PHAC/dimensionMembers.jsp?l=en&rep=i3212B12F133F4CE88AD13DB60CA37237&s#. Accessed 16 June 2016.
42. Fischer L L, Wekerle AL, Sander J, Nickel F F, Billeter AT, Zech U, Bruckner T, Müller-Stich BP BP. Is there a reason why obese patients choose either conservative treatment or surgery? Obes Surg. 2017;2017:1–7.
43. Risidori L, García-Lorda P, Flancbaum L, Pi-Sunyer FX, Laferrère B. Prevalence of co-morbidities in obese patients before bariatric surgery: effect of race. Obes Surg. 2003;13(3):333–40.
44. Tymitz K, Kerlakian G, Engel A, Bollmer C. Gender differences in early outcomes following hand-assisted laparoscopic roux-en-Y gastric bypass

surgery: gender differences in bariatric surgery. Obes Surg. 2007;17(12): 1588–91.

45. Sarwer DB, Lavery M, Spitzer JC. A review of the relationships between extreme obesity, quality of life and sexual function. Obes Surg. 2012;22(4): 668–76.

46. van Nunen AM, Wouters EJ, Vingerhoets AJ, Hox JJ, Geenen R. The health-related quality of life of obese persons seeking or not seeking surgical or non-surgical treatment: a meta-analysis. Obes Surg. 2007;17(10):1357–66.

47. Warkentin LM, Majumdar SR, Johnson JA, Agborsangaya CB, et al. Predictors of health-related quality of life in 500 severely obese patients. Obesity (Silver Spring). 2014;22(5):1367–72.

48. Nickel F, Schmidt L, Bruckner T, Büchler MW, Müller-Stich BP, Fischer L. Influence of bariatric surgery on quality of life, body image, and general self-efficacy within 6 and 24 months-a prospective cohort study. Surg Obes Relat Dis. 2017;13(2):313–9.

49. Warkentin LM, Majumdar SR, Johnson JA, Agborsangaya CB, et al. Weight loss required by the severely obese to achieve clinically important differences in health-related quality of life: two-year prospective cohort study. BMC Med. 12:2014. doi:10.1186/s12916-014-0175-5.

50. Adams TD, Davidson LE, Litwin SE, Kolotkin RL, et al. Health benefits of gastric bypass surgery after 6 years. JAMA. 2012;308(11):1122–31.

51. Johnson JA, Pickard AS. Comparison of the EQ-5D and SF-12 health surveys in a general population survey in Alberta, Canada. Med Care. 2000;38(1):115–21.

52. Belle SH, Berk PD, Chapman WH, Christian NJ, et al. Baseline characteristics of participants in the longitudinal assessment of bariatric Surgery-2 (LABS-2) study. Surg Obes Relat Dis. 2013;9(6):926–35.

53. Finkelstein EA, DiBonaventura MD, Burgess SM, Hale BC. The costs of obesity in the workplace. J Occup Eviron Med. 2010;52(10):971–6.

54. Stout AL, Applegate KL, Friedman KE, Grant JP, Musante GJ. Psychological correlates of obese patients seeking surgical or residential behavioral weight loss treatment. Surg Obes Relat Dis. 2007;3(3):369–75.

55. White MA, O'Neil PM, Kolotkin RL, Byrne TK. Gender, race, and obesity-related quality of life at extreme levels of obesity. Obes Res. 2004;12(6):949–55.

56. Temple Newhook J, Gregory DM, Twells LK. Fat girls and 'big guys': gendered meanings of weight loss surgery. Sociol Health & Illness. 2015; 37(5):653–67.

57. Thompson AE, Anisimowicz Y, Miedema B, Hogg W, Wodchis WP, Aubrey-Bassler K. The influence of gender and other patient characteristics on health care seeking behaviour: a QUALICOPC study. BMC Fam Pract. 2016; 17(38) doi:10.1186/s12875-016-0440-0.

7

Mighty Mums – a lifestyle intervention at primary care level reduces gestational weight gain in women with obesity

Karin Haby[1,2]* ⓘ, Marie Berg[2,3], Hanna Gyllensten[2,3], Ragnar Hanas[4,5] and Åsa Premberg[1,2]

Abstract

Background: Obesity (BMI ≥30) during pregnancy is becoming an increasing public health issue and is associated with adverse maternal and perinatal outcomes. Excessive gestational weight gain (GWG) further increases the risks of adverse outcomes. However, lifestyle intervention can help pregnant women with obesity to limit their GWG. This study evaluated whether an antenatal lifestyle intervention programme for pregnant women with obesity, with emphasis on nutrition and physical activity, could influence GWG and maternal and perinatal outcomes.

Methods: The intervention was performed in a city in Sweden 2011–2013. The study population was women with BMI ≥30 in early pregnancy who received standard antenatal care and were followed until postpartum check-up. The intervention group ($n = 459$) was provided with additional support for a healthier lifestyle, including motivational talks with the midwife, food advice, prescriptions of physical activity, walking poles, pedometers, and dietician consultation. The control group was recruited from the same ($n = 105$) and from a nearby antenatal organisation ($n = 790$).

Results: In the per-protocol population, the intervention group had significantly lower GWG compared with the control group (8.9 ± 6.0 kg vs 11.2 ± 6.9 kg; $p = 0.031$). The women managed to achieve GWG < 7 kg to a greater extent (37.1% vs. 23.0%; $p = 0.036$) and also had a significantly lower weight retention at the postpartum check-up (− 0.3 ± 6.0 kg vs. 1.6 ± 6.5 kg; $p = 0.019$) compared to the first visit. The most commonly used components of the intervention, apart from the extra midwife time, were support from the dietician and retrieval of pedometers. Overall compliance with study procedures, actual numbers of visits with logbook activity, and dietician contact correlated significantly with GWG. There was no statistically significant difference in GWG (10.3 ± 6.1 kg vs. 11.2 ± 6.9 kg) between the intervention and control groups in the intention-to-treat population.

Conclusion: Pregnant women with obesity who follow a lifestyle intervention programme in primary health care can limit their weight gain during pregnancy and show less weight retention after pregnancy. This modest intervention can easily be implemented in a primary care setting.

Keywords: Pregnancy, Obesity, Lifestyle intervention, Gestational weight gain

---

* Correspondence: karin.haby@vgregion.se
[1]Primary Health Care, Research and Development Unit, Närhälsan, Region Västra Götaland, Gothenburg, Sweden
[2]Institute of Health and Care Sciences, Sahlgrenska Academy, University of Gothenburg, Gothenburg, Sweden
Full list of author information is available at the end of the article

Background

In line with rising global figures for the general population, obesity in relation to pregnancy is becoming an increasing global public health issue. Across Europe, the majority of countries in 2013 had high rates of overweight and obesity in early pregnancy; Scotland showed the highest prevalence (48%) and Slovenia the lowest (18%), with Sweden in between (38%) [1].

Of women assigned to antenatal care in Sweden in 2016, 26.6% had overweight (body mass index [BMI] ≥25) and 14.1% had obesity (BMI ≥30). The prevalence was higher in pregnant women with elementary education (vs. high school or university) and women born in foreign countries [2]. Women with lower education also had the largest BMI increase between pregnancies [3].

Living in communities with low socioeconomic standards is associated with higher BMI. Moreover, women in disadvantaged neighbourhoods are more likely to gain unhealthy weight, which supports the need for improved preconception and antenatal care [4]. The well-being of the next generation is at risk, since maternal obesity is a significant factor leading to obesity in offspring, with further negative health consequences [5, 6]. Thus, even if healthy living habits are the responsibility of the individual, potential social and environmental factors involved must also be considered, so that children, youth, and women have the possibility of living healthy lives to prevent obesity and its negative consequences [4].

According to a systematic review of 22 reviews, obesity in pregnancy was associated with increased risk of gestational diabetes, preeclampsia, gestational hypertension, depression, preterm birth, large-for-gestational-age babies, congenital anomalies, instrumental and caesarean birth, perinatal death, and surgical site infection [7]. Obesity in early pregnancy was a predictor for excessive gestational weight gain (GWG) [8] and excessive GWG per se was a predictor for postpartum weight retention [8–10]. Excessive GWG has been associated with high foetal birthweight [11] and with offspring becoming overweight or obese in childhood and adolescence [12–14]. In addition, women with excessive GWG were more likely to experience postpartum weight retention and long-term obesity [8, 15], in particular, those with first-trimester weight gain [16].

To minimise the risks of negative health consequences of both inadequate and excessive GWG, American guidelines on limiting GWG have been developed by the Institute of Medicine (IOM) [17], which are used internationally. However, these guidelines have not been systematically implemented in Sweden, since a Swedish study showed that if GWG is even lower than the IOM recommendation, the increased risk of complications for both woman and offspring can be reduced, especially among women with obesity [18, 19]. The study, with almost 300,000 pregnancies, showed that a GWG below 6 kg in obese women was associated with a lower risk of adverse maternal and neonatal outcomes [18].

Programmes are being introduced in antenatal care that address obesity to prevent excessive GWG, and there has been a tendency towards decreasing GWG in Swedish women with high BMI [2]. Diet, exercise, or both can reduce the risk of excessive GWG [20], and diet- and physical activity-based interventions during pregnancy reduce GWG and lower the odds of caesarean section [21]. On one hand, evidence suggests that exercise is a strong part of controlling GWG [20], while other studies support interventions based on diet appearing to be most effective [22]. Behavioural interventions may be effective in reducing GWG in obese women during pregnancy, but the variation in interventions that have been tested makes comparisons difficult [23]. Evaluations of interventions have yielded mixed results, and specific characteristics of effective interventions are under-reported in the literature [24]. Also, there is a demand for interventions that facilitate positive future outcomes and decreased negative effects for the offspring [25]. Routine weighing alone appears not to be effective in reducing GWG, especially in women with obesity [26, 27], and there is thus a demand for implementation of evidence-based strategies to enhance healthy lifestyle in routine antenatal care [10].

The primary aim of this study was to evaluate whether a structured antenatal lifestyle intervention at primary care level for pregnant women with obesity can result in lower mean GWG; a larger proportion of women with a GWG less than the target of 7 kg, a limit used in earlier research [28]; and lower weight at the postnatal checkup, compared with women receiving standard care. The secondary aims were to study whether the intervention had impact on maternal and child perinatal health outcomes, and to identify which subcomponents of the intervention were favoured by the participants who were successful in limiting GWG.

Methods

The Mighty Mums (MM) project was a standardised programme delivered during regular antenatal care, aiming to reduce GWG in pregnant women with obesity. Results from a pilot study have been described elsewhere [29]. Theories of empowerment [30], motivational interviewing (MI) [31], and person-centred care [32] inspired the individualised approach used in the intervention.

Study population

The study, conducted in a city area in western Sweden over 3 years (2011–2013), involved 3300 pregnant women with BMI ≥30 at the first visit to the antenatal care. Based on the organisation of the antenatal care, the intervention was conducted in the major part of the city with 2500 pregnant women having BMI ≥30. A smaller catchment area within the city with 800 pregnant women having BMI ≥30 was assigned as a control area. After informed consent, women enrolled in the intervention group ($n = 459$) and the control group ($n = 105$) were followed from the first trimester of the pregnancy until postpartum check-up, in registers and during antenatal care.

An adjacent area with 790 pregnant women with BMI ≥30 was added to the control group. Altogether, 1354 women were enrolled, 459 in the intervention and 895 in the total control group (Fig. 1). Due to clinical routines and the medical record system, BMI was rounded

off, and some women having a true BMI of less than 30 were included ($n = 37$, see Table 1).

Standard antenatal care and the intervention

All women received standard antenatal care. This comprised care by a midwife during pregnancy and the postpartum visit, usually a total of nine visits to the midwife. All women's weights were checked at the first visit, at weeks 25 and 37, and at the postnatal check-up, according to the regular antenatal programme. This also included referral to the anaesthetic unit for women with BMI ≥40 for assessment and planning of the upcoming labour and birth.

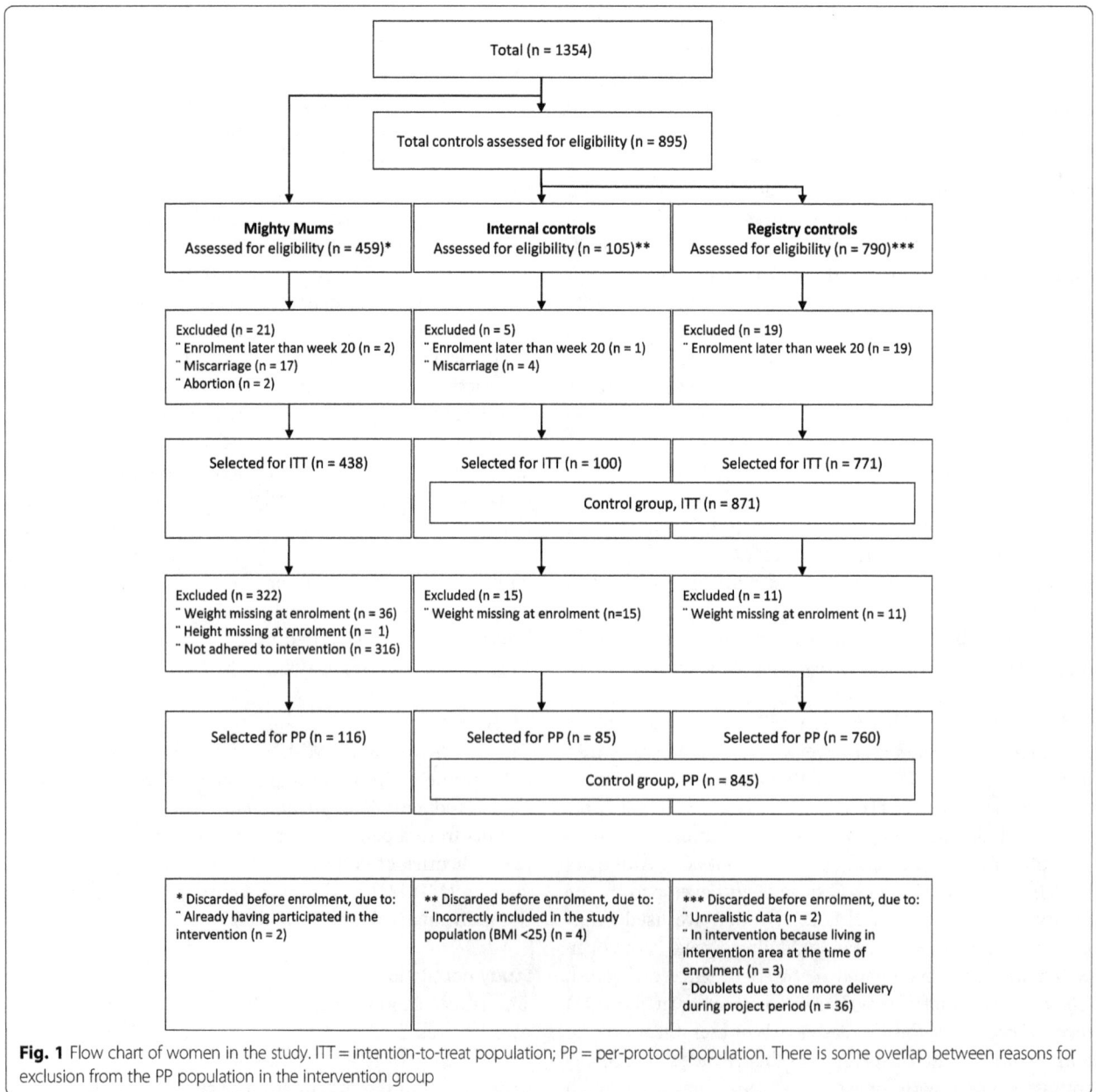

Fig. 1 Flow chart of women in the study. ITT = intention-to-treat population; PP = per-protocol population. There is some overlap between reasons for exclusion from the PP population in the intervention group

Table 1 Baseline characteristics of participants

Variable	Intention-to-treat population		Per-protocol population	
	Intervention Mean (SD) Median (range) (n = 438)	Controls Mean (SD) Median (range) (n = 871)	Intervention Mean (SD) Median (range) (n = 116)	Control Mean (SD) Median (range) (n = 845)
Weeks pregnant at first pregnancy visit	8.6 (2.5) 8.2 (3–20)	7.9 (2.3) 7.9 (5–18)	8.3 (2.1) 7.9 (4 15)	7.9 (2.3) 7.7 (5–18)
Age, years	30.9 (5.5) 30.5 (18.2–47.4)	30.7 (5.1) 30.4 (17.6–46.1)	30.7 (5.4)30.1 (20.7–47.4)	30.7 (5.1) 30.3 (17.6–46.1)
Weight at first pregnancy visit, transformed to week 15, kg	94.0 (13.9) 92.0 (63.0–152.0)	93.4 (11.5) 92.0 (69.0–153.0)	94.1 (14.7) 91.0 (67.0–152.0)	93.3 (11.3) 92.0 (69.0–144.0)
Height at first pregnancy visit, cm	165.8 (7.5) 165.0 (133.0–187.0) n = 437	166.4 (6.2) 166.0 (148.0–185.0)	165.8 (7.2) 165.0 (148.0–180.0)	166.4 (6.2) 166.0 (148.0–185.0)
BMI at first pregnancy visit, transformed to week 15	34.1 (4.0) 33.3 (27.7–57.2) n = 437	33.7 (3.2) 32.8 (29.7–50.0)	34.1 (3.7) 33.1 (29.3–49.6)	33.6 (3.1) 32.8 (29.7–47.0)
	n (%)	n (%)	n (%)	n (%)
Overweight BMI < 30.0[a]	28 (6.4)	5 (0.6)	6 (5.2)	5 (0.6)
Obese Class I BMI 30.0–34.9	271 (62.0)	611 (70.1)	74 (63.8)	596 (70.5)
Obese Class II BMI 35.0–39.9	98 (22.4)	210 (24.1)	25 (21.6)	204 (24.1)
Obese Class III BMI ≥40	40 (9.2)	45 (5.2)	11 (9.5)	40 (4.7)
Primipara	204 (46.6)	338 (38.8)	63 (54.3)	326 (38.6)
Born outside Sweden	131 (29.9)	92 (10.6)	35 (30.2)	89 (10.5)
Use of translator	46 (10.5)	17 (2.0)	14 (12.1)	17 (2.0)
Education ≤12 years[b]	269 (61.6)	564 (64.8)	68 (58.6)	545 (64.6)
Other than employed[c]	151 (34.5)	194 (22.3)	43 (37.1)	187 (22.2)
Use of nicotine	33 (7.5)	79 (11.0)	8 (6.9)	77 (11.1)

Values represent mean (SD) and median (range) for continuous variables, and n (%) for categorical variables
[a]Due to clinical routines, BMI has been rounded off and some women having a true BMI less than 30 have been included, n = 37
[b]Below university studies
[c]Being subsidised by parental leave, unemployment benefits, student loans, or social security

The MM project was designed to function in everyday practice and one of the fundaments was MI [31]. Women in the intervention group received additional care in the form of motivational talks and personalised counselling on food and physical activity, delivered by the midwife at two extra appointments, around 30 min each, during early pregnancy. Based on each participant's choice, the women were also offered individualised dietary advice from a dietician, food discussion groups with a dietician, aqua aerobics led by a physiotherapist and a midwife, prescriptions for physical activity, walking poles, pedometers, and information about community health centres offering lifestyle education and lighter exercise. Apart from the two extra appointments in early pregnancy, about 5 min of each appointment with the midwife were dedicated to the follow-up of lifestyle. The woman's weight was checked at every appointment, approximately 11 check-ups in total, including postpartum check-up.

Moreover, at one of the first visits to the midwife, food and activity habits were mapped, and a logbook was introduced. The woman and the midwife used the logbook throughout the pregnancy and at the postpartum check-up to register weight and record comments on successes and drawbacks as well as enablers and obstacles in managing the planned lifestyle changes. With the logbook it was possible for the woman and the midwife to work together in partnership with the lifestyle changes, and for the woman to take responsibility for her choices and adapt the plan to her own capacity. The activities in the programme were built on the idea that the woman should be active and take part in all decisions of the programme, which is crucial and a cornerstone in person-centred care [32].

Before the start of the project, the midwives were given education about obesity, and about current recommendations on nutrition and physical activity during pregnancy. They were also trained in MI [31] and how to use the logbook. Information on the project and advice on food and physical activity were available on the antenatal care website for the midwife to use for self-education, and to hand out to women in the intervention. A network with the surrounding community was formed, and healthcare providers and doulas (coaches for the woman during pregnancy and labour) were contacted to find areas for interaction and support. Collaboration was initiated with community health centres.

Data collection

Data were collected from the antenatal medical records and included country of birth, language, need for interpreter, educational level, employment status, smoking status, height, weight (as measured in light clothing on a digital scale in the antenatal clinic), mode of delivery and the child's weight and Apgar score (numerical summary of the health of the newborn). Information on pregnancy complications (gestational hypertension, preeclampsia, gestational diabetes) was gathered from the antenatal record. Data on the intervention were collected from the logbook. The weight measured at the first antenatal visit was used to calculate baseline BMI. The information on education was collected from the national maternity health register.

Weight at the first visit to antenatal care was transformed to week 15 using data from the national maternity health register, if first weight was measured after week 15 ($n = 11$) [33]. For missing data on postpartum weight, stochastic imputation was performed using fully conditional specifications (FCS) with seed = 4918. GWG was calculated as the difference between weight at the postpartum check-up and first visit weight.

Analyses

The main analyses were comparisons between the total intervention and control groups (intention to treat analyses, ITT), including all women and adjusted for significant confounders ($p \leq 0.05$), including weeks pregnant at first visit, height, country of birth (mother), need of translator, main occupation, and BMI at first visit transformed to 15 weeks of pregnancy. The adjusted mean differences, for GWG and secondary outcome variables, were estimated with 95% confidence intervals. Analyses

included multivariable binary logistic regression for dichotomous variables, analysis of covariance (ANCOVA) for normally distributed continuous variables, and multivariable binary logistic regression for non-normally distributed continuous variables and ordered categorical variables, respectively. Correlations for adherence to the intervention were performed using Spearman's correlation coefficient.

To address potential lack of adherence to the programme, and to the standard antenatal care, additional analyses were conducted for an identified per-protocol (PP) population. Women were included in the PP population if they had registered weight and height at first visit to antenatal care and registered last weight in pregnancy. For the women in the intervention, it was furthermore required that they had participated at a defined minimum level: adherence to activities with food and physical activity, with at least level 2 (of 1–4 where 1 is "not followed" and 4 is "followed"), according to at least three (of six possible) notifications in the logbook. The criteria for the intervention group were established before statistical analyses were performed. A composite variable was constructed, indicating the number of activities that each woman chose to participate in.

Power calculation

With 100 women in each group, the power of this study was 80% for finding a difference between groups of at least 1.1 kg at a significance level of 0.05.

Results

Characteristics of the study participants

Descriptive data for the women's baseline characteristics are given in Table 1. Significant differences were seen between the intervention group and controls, for the ITT population with regard to country of birth, need of translator, employment status, and BMI at enrolment, and for the PP population, to country of birth, use of translator, and employment. These variables were controlled for in the statistical analyses.

Gestational weight gain

The PP analysis (Table 2) showed that the women in the intervention group had a significantly lower GWG compared to controls (8.9 ± 6.0 kg vs 11.2 ± 6.9 kg; $p = 0.031$) (Fig. 2). A significantly larger number of these women managed GWG < 7 kg (37.1% vs. 23.0%; $p = 0.036$) (Fig. 3), and also had a significantly lower weight retention at postpartum check-up (-0.3 ± 6.0 kg vs. 1.6 ± 6.5 kg; $p = 0.019$) (Fig. 2). There were no significant differences for variables connected to birth size in the PP population.

Table 2 Results from the per-protocol and intention-to-treat analyses

Variable	Intention-to-treat population			Per-protocol population		
	Intervention Mean (SD) Median (range) ($n = 438$)	Controls Mean (SD) Median (range) ($n = 871$)	Adjusted p-value[a]	Intervention Mean (SD) Median (range) ($n = 116$)	Controls Mean (SD) Median (range) ($n = 845$)	Adjusted p-value[a]
Week of delivery	39.1 (2.5) 40.0 (24–42) $n = 429$	39.8 (2.0) 40.0 (23–42) $n = 866$	0.001	39.6 (1.5) 40.0 (36–42)	39.8 (2.0) 40.0 (23–42)	0.142
Weight change: from first pregnancy visit to last pregnancy visit, kg	10.3 (6.1) 10.0 (−6.0–41.0)	11.2 (6.9) 11.0 (−15.0–46.0)	0.695	8.9 (6.0) 9.00 (−6.0–28.0)	11.2 (6.9) 11.0 (−15.0–46.0)	0.031
Weight change: from first pregnancy visit to postpartum check-up, kg	1.4 (6.4) 1.0 (−19.0–23.0)	1.6 (6.5) 2.0 (−27.0–27.0)	0.731	−0.3 (6.0) −1.0 (−17.0–18.0)	1.6 (6.5) 2.00 (−27.0–27.0)	0.019
Child weight at delivery, g	3591 (594) 3605 (830–5430) $n = 420$	3695 (637) 3705 (418–5760) $n = 866$	0.037	3603 (505) 3515 (2480–5430) $n = 113$	3703 (627) 3705 (418–5760)	0.300
	n (%)	n (%)		n (%)	n (%)	
GWG < 7 kg	120 (27.4)	204 (23.4)	0.882	43 (37.1)	194 (23.0)	0.036
Macrosomia	22 (5.0)	77 (8.8)	0.017	5 (4.3)	76 (9.0)	0.172
SGA[b]	34 (7.8)	45 (5.2)	0.196	10 (8.6)	38 (4.5)	0.199

Values represent mean (SD) and median (range) for continuous variables, and n (%) for categorical variables
[a]Adjusted for weeks pregnant at enrolment, height at enrolment, country of birth (mother), translator needed, main occupation, and BMI at enrolment transformed to 15 weeks
[b]Small for gestational age

In the ITT population (Table 2) there was a slightly, but not significantly, lower GWG compared to the control group (10.3 ± 6.1 kg vs. 11.2 ± 6.9 kg) and 27.4% of women in the intervention group managed to keep GWG < 7 kg in comparison with 23.4% among controls.

Child weight was significantly higher, and macrosomia (i.e. birth weight > 4500 g) significantly more common in the control group.

Overall, the prevalence of adverse maternal outcomes (gestational diabetes, gestational hypertension, and

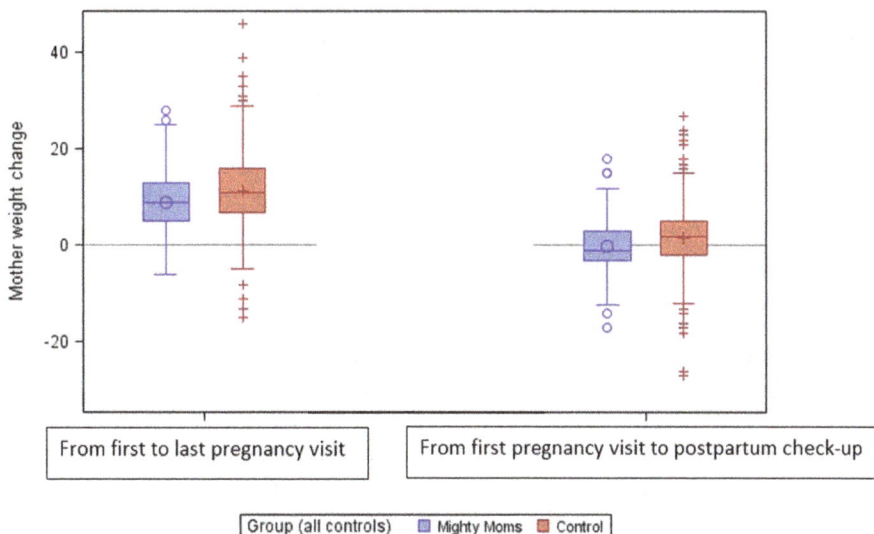

Fig. 2 Change in mothers' weight during and after pregnancy, by group (PP)

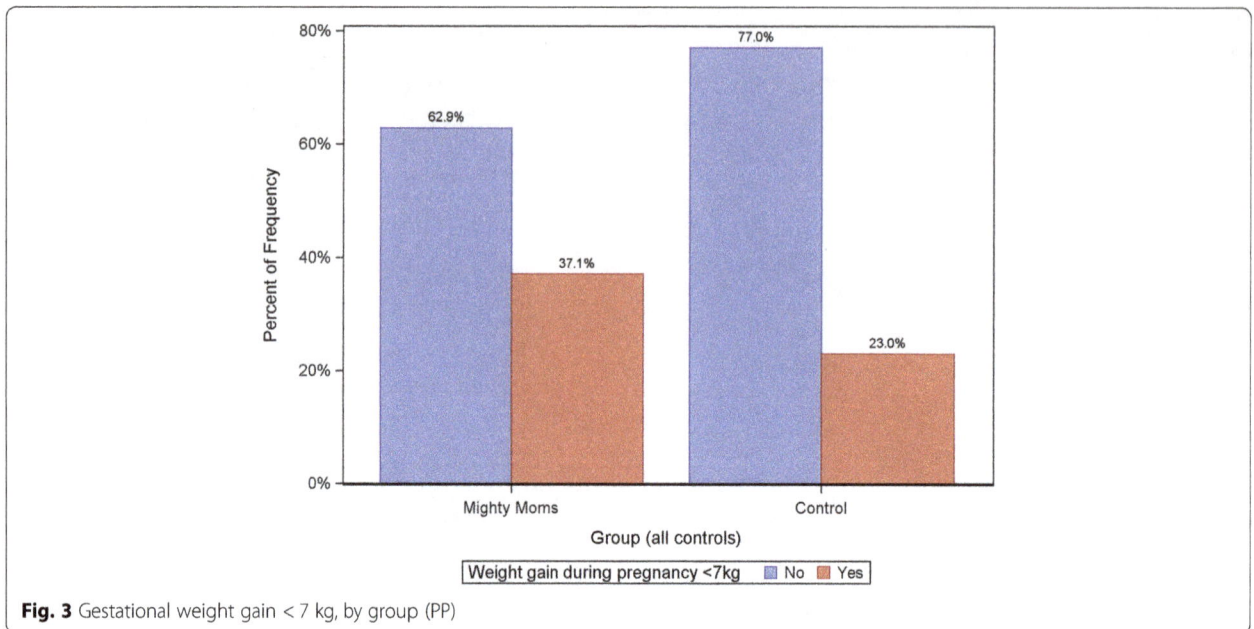

Fig. 3 Gestational weight gain < 7 kg, by group (PP)

preeclampsia) and perinatal outcomes (preterm delivery, intrauterine foetal death, caesarean delivery, Apgar) did not differ significantly between groups.

Adherence to the programme

Maximum attendance (Table 3) implied seven notifications in the logbook, corresponding to seven discussions on the topic with the midwife: one initial visit, five follow-ups throughout the pregnancy, and one at the postpartum check-up. Of the women in the intervention ($n = 438$), 27.2% ($n = 119$) fulfilled the criterion of adherence to the study protocol, that is, fulfilled the prescribed activities at level two on at least three follow-ups with the midwife during pregnancy. All extra activities were optional; 39.0% ($n = 170$) had contact with the dietician (individually or in food discussion groups), 34.7% ($n = 148$) used pedometers, 20.0% ($n = 86$) used walking poles and 16.9% ($n = 73$) participated in aqua aerobics. Most women chose to organise physical activities on their own, and the most common activity was walking, often on a level of 30 min 5–7 days a week. The mean number of visits with logbook activity was higher (6.3 ± 0.6) in the PP population than in the ITT population (4.7 ± 2.3). Dietician counselling and use of walking poles and pedometers as well as participation in aqua aerobics were more common in the PP population, and this group also had a slightly higher score concerning the composite variable for all activities (4.3 ± 1.1 vs. 3.5 ± 1.7).

Overall compliance with study procedures (number of visits with both food and physical activity on at least level 2) correlated significantly with GWG (Table 4), as did actual numbers of visits with logbook activity and having contact with the dietician. Participating in

activities with physical activity (i.e. pedometers, walking poles, and aqua aerobics) did not correlate with GWG.

The logbook gave an idea of which food advice was agreed upon and how it was discussed. Most midwives gave general food advice from the website, but it was also common to note individual advice in the logbook: "restrict carbohydrates", "eat regularly", "cut out sweets and sweet drinks", and more positively, "increase fruit and vegetables", "eat fish", and "savour the food".

Discussion

This study shows that an antenatal care programme resulted in a significantly lower GWG, significantly lower weight retention at the postnatal check-up, and significantly more women being successful in limiting GWG to less than 7 kg if they followed the individually planned lifestyle changes.

The results from this study are in line with other lifestyle studies where effect on GWG has been shown after nutritional advice alone, or in combination with advice on physical activity [28, 34–37]. Interesting findings from trials seem to be that the effect of getting information from brochures, seminars, and websites should not be underestimated [35, 37, 38], and that more intense interventions do not always give the best results [28, 36]. One explanation may be that delivery of objective information in group settings or electronically is successful, since pregnant women with BMI ≥30 have the experience of being addressed in a judgemental way about their weight, and request accurate and appropriate information about the benefits of limited gestational weight gain [39].

Table 3 Adherence to the Mighty Mums study protocol

Variable	Intention-to-treat population	Per-protocol population
	Mean (SD) Median (range) n = 438	Mean (SD) Median (range) n = 116
Food adherence[a], of all visits	2.9 (0.8) 3 (1–4) n = 346	3.2 (0.7) 3 (2–4)
Physical activity adherence[a], of all visits	2.5 (0.8) (1–4) n = 356	2.8 (0.6) 3 (2–4)
Number of logbook visits	4.7 (2.3) 6 (0–7)	6.3 (0.6) 6 (5–7)
Composite variable for all activities	3.5 (1.7) 4 (0–7)	4.3 (1.1) 4 (3–7)
	n (%)	n (%)
Adherence[a] to both food and physical activity criteria	119 (27.2)	116 (100)
Adherence[a] to food criteria	276 (63.0)	116 (100)
Adherence[a] to physical activity criteria	295 (67.4)	116 (100.0)
Use of pedometer	148 (34.7)	45 (38.8)
Use of walking poles	86 (20.0)	34 (29.3)
Contact with dietician	170 (39.0)	49 (42.2)
Participated in aqua aerobics	73 (16.9)	24 (20.7)
At least one visit with follow-up of food activities	333 (76.0)	116 (100)
At least one visit with follow-up of physical activity	317 (72.4)	116 (100)
At least one logbook visit	391 (89.3)	116 (100)
Number of logbook visits		
0–4	136 (30.9)	0 (0)
5–6	220 (50.2)	70 (60.3)
7	82 (18.7)	46 (39.7)

Values represent mean (SD) and median (range) for continuous variables, and n (%) for categorical variables
[a]Adherence = at least level 2 on at least three visits according to registration in logbook

Several reviews conclude that behavioural GWG interventions, even if successful, should be more systematically designed and evaluated, as well as based on insights from behavioural science [22, 24, 40, 41]. The MM project was designed to function in structured everyday practice, and one of the fundaments was the skill in MI that all midwives exerted, or were educated in before start of the project. The correlations between GWG and the specific activities (pedometers, walking poles, aqua aerobics) were non-significant, which is in line with

Table 4 Correlation between adherence and weight gain among women in the intervention group, ITT population

Variable	Number of observations	Spearman correlation coefficient	P-value
Adherence[a] to both food and physical activity criteria	402	−0.157	0.002
Number of visits with adherence[a] to both food and physical activity criteria	402	−0.162	0.001
Adherence[a] to food criteria	402	−0.127	0.011
Number of visits with adherence[a] to food criteria	402	−0.129	0.010
Adherence[a] to physical activity criteria	402	−0.119	0.017
Number of visits with adherence[a] to physical activity criteria	402	−0.179	< 0.001
Contact with dietician	400	−0.122	0.015
Number of logbook visits	402	−0.169	0.001

[a]Adherence = above level 1 on more than two visits according to registration in logbook

previous findings that extra activities do not always have the expected effect [28, 35–38]. The women in the MM intervention described the opportunity to set their own goals for lifestyle change as crucial, and experienced as supportive being in a group setting with other obese pregnant women [42].

An important result of the present study is that the midwives had the opportunity to develop skills for working with obesity and lifestyle issues in the everyday clinic, a topic that midwives in earlier research had expressed having difficulties with [43, 44]. The midwives thus had the opportunity of being empowered to see that their advice would make a difference, since feeling confident in giving advice on GWG is an important predictor of higher guideline adherence [45]. To feel confident and be able to accomplish an efficient and worthy handling of obesity, midwives should have access to nutrition and lifestyle expertise [4].

A strength of the MM programme is that it was population-based and that the women who were eligible for MM were from geographically as well as socio-economically similar compositions. Women with languages other than Swedish were also invited, since it was possible to use interpreters. To avoid biased results caused by an over-representation of highly motivated women, the intervention was delivered through the standard antenatal care system. MM was originally designed as a development project, and a further strength is that the midwives were not involved in the project because they had a particular interest, but were representative of the regular staff. Another strength is that the weight of the woman in the beginning of pregnancy was registered, not reported by the woman, as is often the case in similar studies.

A limitation is that the intervention was not randomised. Also, the area first selected for the control group did not recruit enough women, which led to extending to an adjacent area. However, all three areas were expected to have similar sociodemographic structures. Analyses were adjusted for socioeconomic differences on an individual level.

Another limitation is that even though the MM project was intended to reach all women with BMI ≥30 entering pregnancy, it turned out that 35% were not invited. The low contact level might have been due to midwives neglecting or forgetting to inform women, or abstaining because of a full agenda. The fact that not all midwives and staff feel comfortable in addressing women with obesity has been described elsewhere [43, 46, 47], and may explain why only 65% of the women were asked about participation. Correspondingly, the explanation for why only 62% of the women who were approached chose to participate could be that more negative attitudes towards being pregnant have been

reported by women with obesity [48], as well as more unpleasant experiences from attending health care services [43, 46].

The fact that 38% of women declined participation might be explained by their not wanting or feeling able to adhere to the intervention, or being less health literate [49]. A possible selection bias is that the most motivated women opted to join [50]. Both the midwives who invited the women and the women accepting participation (as interventions or controls) may have been more comfortable in dealing with lifestyle issues (the midwife) [45, 46] and had a higher readiness to cope with lifestyle changes (the woman) [50]. Since less than one third of the women in the intervention group fulfilled the criterion of adherence to the study protocol, the conclusions of the PP population are drawn from a rather small proportion of those eligible for participation.

On the other hand, participation in lifestyle interventions in pregnancy is reported to be low, with 40–60% of women eligible to participate declining to do so [44]. A reason for the relatively high participation rate in the Mighty Mums programme could be the possibility of exercising one's own choice regarding which areas to focus on or which activities to take part in. This in turn lowered the numbers of women participating in the separate activities, and individuals may have missed out on certain aspects of the intervention. Attracting the women to participate is thus of paramount importance, and the person-centred approach with individualised advice formed the base of Mighty Mums.

A related possible source of bias is that the women taking part in the intervention to a greater extent were born in countries other than Sweden, had higher use of interpreters, and were more often not engaged in work. Also, more women in the intervention than in the control group were in Obese Class III (BMI ≥40) and fewer were in the lowest Obese Class I (BMI 30.0–34.9). Higher BMI may have contributed to a lower GWG in the intervention group compared to controls, since GWG usually is lower in women with higher BMI [2, 19]. The challenge of counselling women with obesity and eating disorders has been described by midwives [51], and pregnant women with obesity have asked for culturally adapted programmes [52]. Being born in another country and being less fluent in Swedish may have negatively affected the ability to keep GWG below the determined limit, due to difficulties in understanding and assimilating the information and advice from the midwife. On the other hand, midwives in areas with higher socio-economic and cultural demands might have had to develop certain working skills to cope with this, since counselling women from other cultures is described as a certain challenge [51]. However, the results from this study indicate that the intervention was as relevant to women with a foreign background as to those born in Sweden, potentially due to its person-centred focus on the women's own capabilities.

Women in the control group may have been influenced by the ongoing MM project, since there is formal and informal communication between midwives, and pregnant women move between areas and voluntarily tell each other pregnancy-related health tips. Women in the control group may also have been referred to a dietician or physiotherapist, taken part in community activities related to lifestyle or other issues independent of the project, or enrolled in other health-related research studies. These circumstances could in reality have decreased the differences between women in the intervention and control groups.

Another limitation is that the intervention programme with free choice of activities makes it difficult to differentiate exactly which parts of the MM intervention contributed to the difference in GWG between the intervention and control groups. The variety in support and activities and the possibility to choose may be factors contributing to success, but it is difficult to define which measure was most effective within the current study design. The extra time with the midwife or contact with the dietician, both weakly correlating with GWG, may also be of importance. Being weighed at every visit has been described with conflicting results [26, 27], and it is unclear whether this contributed to limiting weight gain. However, women in the MM intervention reported that being weighed regularly encouraged them to continue the positive lifestyle changes [42]. Another factor influencing GWG could be the network that was formed with the surrounding community and health centres.

Two extra appointments with the midwife were planned for the intervention group. The extra time with the midwife, as such, and not the content of the intervention visits, may have helped empower the women in the intervention to succeed with the lifestyle project. In the pilot study of MM, where visits to the midwife were counted manually, there was a similar number of visits among women in the intervention and women in the control group [29]. In the full study, however, it was not possible to obtain reliable data on the number of midwife visits for all women, due to differences in routines for reporting to the register, both in time and between areas.

Also, there are concerns about how well the effect of an intervention like MM can be studied, since pregnant women choosing to enter a lifestyle intervention will have a high motivation to make healthy changes during pregnancy, regardless of being in a study or not [37].

The low participation in the MM intervention might be surprising, since pregnancy, preconception, and postnatal periods often are viewed as important and timely stages in the life course for public health intervention

[53]. Also, for the pregnant woman with obesity, the health-promoting ambition of the health care service can result in additional demands. It is likely that this is not the first time the woman is addressing concerns about her body weight. The woman's acceptance of her actual weight and lack of motivation for lifestyle change, as well as sensitivity to being scrutinised and observed for weight matters, has been suggested to negatively impact the possibility of succeeding in restricting GWG and may have hindered some women from participating [48, 54]. The fact that the public health and community services generally lack structured maternal obesity objectives aggravates the possibility of succeeding with lifestyle interventions and calls for more strategic and national support concerning evidence and guidance to plan, develop, and implement effective maternal obesity services [47].

The many barriers that exist for both women and health care providers affect the successful initiation of behavioural change during pregnancy [44]. Midwives describe pregnancy as an ideal time for interventions concerning health among pregnant women, and say that they require support and better cooperation with other healthcare professionals to be able to carry forward greater collaboration with the women they care for [55]. Person-centred care in pregnancy is sparsely studied, and the extent to which person-centred care may improve health outcomes and satisfaction with care in this population needs further research [56].

Conclusions

This study, which is based on relatively modest changes in the routine visits in primary care, shows that it is possible to guide the pregnant woman with obesity towards everyday lifestyle changes that decrease GWG and lessen weight retention after pregnancy. The number of visits with logbook activity on both food and physical activity as well as dietician consultation correlated significantly with GWG. The individual choice of level of activity and engagement, as well as the personal support and documenting in the logbook, may also be factors in success. However, measures need to be evaluated to have a larger proportion of participants taking full advantage of the programme, and future studies are warranted to put strategies in antenatal care into perspective regarding the whole health care system and society's handling of overweight and obesity in pregnant women.

Implications for clinical practice

The findings in this study suggest that a programme starting in early pregnancy, monitoring weight regularly and with an opportunity to discuss nutrition and physical activity with the midwife or other professionals throughout pregnancy, can be an important part of active antenatal care concerning lifestyle issues. Also, the postpartum check-up may be an opportunity for the woman with obesity to be addressed about her current weight and lifestyle and offered further monitoring in primary care. However, for an optimal effect, women need to receive better information on risks and advice on losing weight even before getting pregnant [57].

Activities in the intervention programme that correlated significantly with GWG (extra midwife visits, advice on food and physical activity, and dietician consultation; Table 4), together with mandatory weighing, have been picked up in regional guidelines for antenatal care. However, the implementation of guidelines and optimal antenatal care of obesity require a supportive management and a general consensus in the health care organisation that obesity and overweight are important issues. Further involvement with person-centred care may enhance the outcome of similar interventions in the future.

Abbreviations

BMI: Body mass index; GWG: Gestational weight gain; IOM: Institute of Medicine; MI: Motivational interviewing; MM: Mighty Mums

Acknowledgements

The authors wish to express their gratitude to all Mighty Mums participating in the project and to all midwives and staff engaged in carrying out the programme in their everyday busy practices. Also thanks to the local board of medical care in Gothenburg who funded the project Mighty Mums.

Funding

This study has been funded by the local Research and Development Board for Gothenburg and Södra Bohuslän, Gothenburg, Sweden, and the Centre for Person-centred Care (GPCC), University of Gothenburg, Gothenburg, Sweden.

Authors' contributions

KH designed the clinical study, with the assistance of RH and the head of the antenatal care unit, Anna Glantz. Data collection and statistical analyses were designed by HG, KH, MB, RH, ÅP. KH carried out the study and collected all data. The Statistical Consulting Group, Gothenburg (together with KH and HG), performed statistical analyses, and the data were interpreted by all authors. KH wrote the first draft, but all authors have been involved in further drafting of the manuscript and revising it critically for important intellectual content, and have given final approval of the version to be published.

Competing interests

The authors declare that they have no competing interests.

Author details

[1]Primary Health Care, Research and Development Unit, Närhälsan, Region Västra Götaland, Gothenburg, Sweden. [2]Institute of Health and Care Sciences, Sahlgrenska Academy, University of Gothenburg, Gothenburg, Sweden. [3]GPCC – University of Gothenburg Centre for Person-centred Care, Gothenburg, Sweden. [4]Department of Pediatrics, NU Hospital Group, Region Västra Götaland, Uddevalla, Sweden. [5]Institute of Clinical Sciences, Sahlgrenska Academy, University of Gothenburg, Gothenburg, Sweden.

References

1. Zeitlin J, Mohangoo A, Delnord M. European perinatal health report health and care of pregnant women and babies in Europe in 2010. Paris: INSERM Institut national de la santé et de la recherche médicale; 2010.
2. Pregnancy register, yearly report 2016. Stockholm: Quality Register Center; 2016.
3. Holowko N, Chaparro MP, Nilsson K, Ivarsson A, Mishra G, Koupil I, Goodman A. Social inequality in pre-pregnancy BMI and gestational weight gain in the first and second pregnancy among women in Sweden. J Epidemiol Community Health. 2015;69(12):1154–61.
4. Campbell EE, Dworatzek PD, Penava D, de Vrijer B, Gilliland J, Matthews JI, Seabrook JA. Factors that influence excessive gestational weight gain: moving beyond assessment and counselling. J Matern Fetal Neonatal Med. 2016;29(21):3527–31.
5. Drake AJ, Reynolds RM. Impact of maternal obesity on offspring obesity and cardiometabolic disease risk. Reproduction. 2010;140(3):387–98.
6. Stamnes Koepp UM, Frost Andersen L, Dahl-Joergensen K, Stigum H, Nass O, Nystad W. Maternal pre-pregnant body mass index, maternal weight change and offspring birthweight. Acta Obstet Gynecol Scand. 2012;91(2):243–9.
7. Marchi J, Berg M, Dencker A, Olander EK, Begley C. Risks associated with obesity in pregnancy, for the mother and baby: a systematic review of reviews. Obes Rev. 2015;16(8):621–38.
8. Begum F, Colman I, McCargar LJ, Bell RC. Gestational weight gain and early postpartum weight retention in a prospective cohort of Alberta women. J Obstet Gynaecol Can. 2012;34(7):637–47.
9. Fraser A, Tilling K, Macdonald-Wallis C, Hughes R, Sattar N, Nelson SM, Lawlor DA. Associations of gestational weight gain with maternal body mass index, waist circumference, and blood pressure measured 16 y after pregnancy: the Avon Longitudinal Study of Parents and Children (ALSPAC). Am J Clin Nutr. 2011;93(6):1285–92.
10. Goldstein R, Teede H, Thangaratinam S, Boyle J. Excess gestational weight gain in pregnancy and the role of lifestyle intervention. Semin Reprod Med. 2016;34(2):e14–21.
11. Ludwig DS, Currie J. The association between pregnancy weight gain and birthweight: a within-family comparison. Lancet. 2010;376(9745):984–90.
12. Tie HT, Xia YY, Zeng YS, Zhang Y, Dai CL, Guo JJ, Zhao Y. Risk of childhood overweight or obesity associated with excessive weight gain during pregnancy: a meta-analysis. Arch Gynecol Obstet. 2014;289(2):247–57.
13. Sridhar SB, Darbinian J, Ehrlich SF, Markman MA, Gunderson EP, Ferrara A, Hedderson MM. Maternal gestational weight gain and offspring risk for childhood overweight or obesity. Am J Obstet Gynecol. 2014;211(3):259 e251–8.
14. Leonard SA, Petito LC, Rehkopf DH, Ritchie LD, Abrams B. Weight gain in pregnancy and child weight status from birth to adulthood in the United States. Pediatr Obes. 2017;12(Suppl 1):18–25.
15. Amorim AR, Rossner S, Neovius M, Lourenco PM, Linne Y. Does excess pregnancy weight gain constitute a major risk for increasing long-term BMI? Obesity (Silver Spring). 2007;15(5):1278–86.
16. Walter JR, Perng W, Kleinman KP, Rifas-Shiman SL, Rich-Edwards JW, Oken E. Associations of trimester-specific gestational weight gain with maternal adiposity and systolic blood pressure at 3 and 7 years postpartum. Am J Obstet Gynecol. 2015;212(4):499 e491–12.
17. IOM American Institute of Medicine. Weight gain during pregnancy: reexamining the guidelines. Washington: National Academy Press; 2009.

18. Cedergren MI. Optimal gestational weight gain for body mass index categories. Obstet Gynecol. 2007;110(4):759–64.

19. Blomberg M. Maternal and neonatal outcomes among obese women with weight gain below the new Institute of Medicine recommendations. Obstet Gynecol. 2011;117(5):1065–70.

20. Muktabhant B, Lawrie TA, Lumbiganon P, Laopaiboon M. Diet or exercise, or both, for preventing excessive weight gain in pregnancy. Cochrane Database Syst Rev. 2015;6:CD007145.

21. International Weight Management in Pregnancy (i-WIP) Collaborative Group. Effect of diet and physical activity based interventions in pregnancy on gestational weight gain and pregnancy outcomes: meta-analysis of individual participant data from randomised trials. BMJ. 2017;j3119:358.

22. Thangaratinam S, Rogozinska E, Jolly K, Glinkowski S, Roseboom T, Tomlinson JW, Kunz R, Mol BW, Coomarasamy A, Khan KS. Effects of interventions in pregnancy on maternal weight and obstetric outcomes: meta-analysis of randomised evidence. BMJ. 2012;344:e2088.

23. Agha M, Agha RA, Sandall J. Interventions to reduce and prevent obesity in pre-conceptual and pregnant women: a systematic review and meta-analysis. PLoS One. 2014;9(5):e95132.

24. Gardner B, Wardle J, Poston L, Croker H. Changing diet and physical activity to reduce gestational weight gain: a meta-analysis. Obes Rev. 2011;12(7):e602–20.

25. Zhang S, Rattanatray L, Morrison JL, Nicholas LM, Lie S, McMillen IC. Maternal obesity and the early origins of childhood obesity: weighing up the benefits and costs of maternal weight loss in the periconceptional period for the offspring. Exp Diabetes Res. 2011;2011:585749.

26. Jeffries K, Shub A, Walker SP, Hiscock R, Permezel M. Reducing excessive weight gain in pregnancy: a randomised controlled trial. Med J Aust. 2009;191(8):429–33.

27. Brownfoot FC, Davey MA, Kornman L. Routine weighing to reduce excessive antenatal weight gain: a randomised controlled trial. BJOG. 2016;123(2):254–61.

28. Claesson IM, Sydsjo G, Brynhildsen J, Cedergren M, Jeppsson A, Nystrom F, Sydsjo A, Josefsson A. Weight gain restriction for obese pregnant women: a case-control intervention study. BJOG. 2008;115(1):44–50.

29. Haby K, Glantz A, Hanas R, Premberg A. Mighty Mums - an antenatal health care intervention can reduce gestational weight gain in women with obesity. Midwifery. 2015;31(7):685–92.

30. Jacobs G. "Take control or lean back?" barriers to practicing empowerment in health promotion. Health Promot Pract. 2011;12(1):94–101.

31. Rollnick S, Butler CC, Kinnersley P, Gregory J, Mash B. Motivational interviewing. BMJ. 2010;340:c1900.

32. McCormack B, McCance TV. Development of a framework for person-centred nursing. J Adv Nurs. 2006;56(5):472–9.

33. Johansson K, Hutcheon JA, Stephansson O, Cnattingius S. Pregnancy weight gain by gestational age and BMI in Sweden: a population-based cohort study. Am J Clin Nutr. 2016;103(5):1278–84.

34. Wolff S, Legarth J, Vangsgaard K, Toubro S, Astrup A. A randomized trial of the effects of dietary counseling on gestational weight gain and glucose metabolism in obese pregnant women. Int J Obes. 2008;32(3):495–501.

35. Shirazian T, Monteith S, Friedman F, Rebarber A. Lifestyle modification program decreases pregnancy weight gain in obese women. Am J Perinatol. 2010;27(5):411–4.

36. Vinter CA, Jensen DM, Ovesen P, Beck-Nielsen H, Jorgensen JS. The LiP (Lifestyle in Pregnancy) study: a randomized controlled trial of lifestyle intervention in 360 obese pregnant women. Diabetes Care. 2011;34(12):2502–7.

37. Bogaerts AF, Devlieger R, Nuyts E, Witters I, Gyselaers W, Van den Bergh BR. Effects of lifestyle intervention in obese pregnant women on gestational weight gain and mental health: a randomized controlled trial. Int J Obes (Lond). 2013;37(6):814–21.

38. Quinlivan JA, Lam LT, Fisher J. A randomised trial of a four-step multidisciplinary approach to the antenatal care of obese pregnant women. Aust N Z J Obstet Gynaecol. 2011;51(2):141–6.

39. Dencker A, Premberg A, Olander EK, McCourt C, Haby K, Dencker S, Glantz A, Berg M. Adopting a healthy lifestyle when pregnant and obese - an interview study three years after childbirth. BMC Pregnancy Childbirth. 2016;16(1):201.

40. Tanentsapf I, Heitmann BL, Adegboye AR. Systematic review of clinical trials on dietary interventions to prevent excessive weight gain during pregnancy among normal weight, overweight and obese women. BMC Pregnancy Childbirth. 2011;11:81.

41. Oteng-Ntim E, Varma R, Croker H, Poston L, Doyle P. Lifestyle interventions for overweight and obese pregnant women to improve pregnancy outcome: systematic review and meta-analysis. BMC Med. 2012;10:47.

42. Fieril DP, Olsen PF, Glantz D, Premberg DA. Experiences of a lifestyle intervention in obese pregnant women - a qualitative study. Midwifery. 2017;44:1–6.

43. Furness PJ, McSeveny K, Arden MA, Garland C, Dearden AM, Soltani H. Maternal obesity support services: a qualitative study of the perspectives of women and midwives. BMC Pregnancy Childbirth. 2011;11:69.

44. Dodd JM, Briley AL. Managing obesity in pregnancy - an obstetric and midwifery perspective. Midwifery. 2017;49:7–12.

45. Herring SJ, Platek DN, Elliott P, Riley LE, Stuebe AM, Oken E. Addressing obesity in pregnancy: what do obstetric providers recommend? J Women's Health (Larchmt). 2010;19(1):65–70.

46. Heslehurst N, Moore H, Rankin J, Ells LJ, Wilkinson JR, Summerbell CD. How can maternity services be developed to effectively address maternal obesity? A qualitative study. Midwifery. 2011;27(5):e170–7.

47. Smith SA, Heslehurst N, Ells LJ, Wilkinson JR. Community-based service provision for the prevention and management of maternal obesity in the North East of England: a qualitative study. Public Health. 2011;125(8):518–24.

48. Nyman VM, Prebensen AK, Flensner GE. Obese women's experiences of encounters with midwives and physicians during pregnancy and childbirth. Midwifery. 2010;26(4):424–9.

49. Kennen EM, Davis TC, Huang J, Yu H, Carden D, Bass R, Arnold C. Tipping the scales: the effect of literacy on obese patients' knowledge and readiness to lose weight. South Med J. 2005;98(1):15–8.

50. Tanvig M. Offspring body size and metabolic profile - effects of lifestyle intervention in obese pregnant women. Dan Med J. 2014;61(7):B4893.

51. Wennberg A: Pregnant women and midwives are not in tune with each other about dietary counselling - studies in Swedish antenatal care. Umeå University; 2015.

52. Mills A, Schmied VA, Dahlen HG. Get alongside us', women's experiences of being overweight and pregnant in Sydney, Australia. Matern Child Nutr. 2013;9(3):309–21.

53. Phelan S. Pregnancy: a "teachable moment" for weight control and obesity prevention. Am J Obstet Gynecol. 2010;202(2):135 e131–8.

54. Phelan S, Phipps MG, Abrams B, Darroch F, Schaffner A, Wing RR. Practitioner advice and gestational weight gain. J Women's Health (Larchmt). 2011;20(4):585–91.

55. Aquino MR, Edge D, Smith DM. Pregnancy as an ideal time for intervention to address the complex needs of black and minority ethnic women: views of British midwives. Midwifery. 2015;31(3):373–9.

56. Olander EK, Berg M, McCourt C, Carlstrom E, Dencker A. Person-centred care in interventions to limit weight gain in pregnant women with obesity - a systematic review. BMC Pregnancy Childbirth. 2015;15:50.

57. Forsum E, Brantsaeter AL, Olafsdottir AS, Olsen SF, Thorsdottir I. Weight loss before conception: a systematic literature review. Food Nutr Res. 2013;57. https://doi.org/10.3402/fnr.v57i0.20522. Epub 2013 Mar 13.

8

Community-based childhood obesity prevention intervention for parents improves health behaviors and food parenting practices among Hispanic, low-income parents

Laura Otterbach[1], Noereem Z. Mena[1], Geoffrey Greene[1], Colleen A. Redding[2], Annie De Groot[3] and Alison Tovar[1*]

Abstract

Background: Given the current prevalence of childhood obesity among Hispanic populations, and the importance of parental feeding behaviors, we aimed to assess the impact of the evidence-based Healthy Children, Healthy Families (HCHF) intervention on responsive food parenting practices (FPPs) in a low-income Hispanic population.

Methods: This community-based pilot study used a non-experimental pre/post within-subjects design. Parents ($n =$ 94) of children aged 3–11 years old were recruited to participate in an 8-week, weekly group-based intervention. The intervention was delivered to nine groups of parents by trained paraprofessional educators over a two-year period. Children participated in a separate curriculum that covered topics similar to those covered in the parent intervention. Parents completed self-administered pre/post surveys, which included demographic questions, seven subscales from the Comprehensive Feeding Practices Questionnaire, and the 16-item HCHF Behavior Checklist. Descriptive statistics and paired samples t-tests were used to analyze data from parents that completed the intervention.

Results: Fifty-two, primarily Hispanic (93%) parents completed the intervention (39% attrition rate). For parents who completed the intervention, there was a significant increase in one of the feeding practice subscales: encouragement of balance and variety ($p = 0.01$). There were significant improvements in several parent and child diet and activity outcomes ($p \leq 0.01$).

Conclusions: Although attrition rates were high, parents completing the study reported enjoying and being satisfied with the intervention. For parents who completed the intervention, reported 'encouragement of balance and variety', in addition to several health behaviors significantly improved. Larger studies utilizing an experimental design, should further explore the impact of the HCHF curriculum on improving certain FPPs and health behaviors that contribute to obesity.

* Correspondence: alison_tovar@uri.edu
[1]Department of Nutrition and Food Sciences, University of Rhode Island,
Fogarty Hall, 41 Lower College Rd, Kingston, RI 02881, USA
Full list of author information is available at the end of the article

Background

Prevention of childhood obesity is an ongoing public health priority. From 2011 to 2014, 17% of children and adolescents in the United States (U.S.) were obese [1], with Hispanic children experiencing a greater prevalence of obesity compared to non-Hispanic White children (22% vs. 14%, respectively) [1]. To reduce these racial/ethnic disparities, obesity prevention programs and interventions for Hispanic parents are urgently needed [1–4]. In addition, more research is needed on community-based interventions that actively engage parents around their child's healthy eating, physical activity and the home environment [4, 5]. Given that parents influence their children's health behaviors and environment early in life, involving them in childhood obesity prevention is critical [4, 6–11].

Parents influence their child's health behaviors through the home environment and their parenting practices [4, 6–18]. Food parenting practices (FPPs) are strategies used by parents to influence both the amount and types of food a child eats [11, 13, 18, 19]. It is important to teach parents about responsive feeding practices, such as role modeling healthy eating behaviors for their child; involving their child in food decisions such as grocery shopping and meal preparation; and encouraging a balanced and varied diet with their child [11–13, 15, 17–24]. These responsive FPPs have been associated with healthier diets and body mass index (BMI), while non-responsive feeding practices such as restriction and pressure have been associated with lower quality diets and higher BMIs [11–13, 15, 17–24].

Although multiple interventions aim to prevent childhood obesity [14–16, 25], few have specifically targeted the use of responsive FPPs among high-risk populations [9, 10, 14, 16], such as low-income Hispanics. *Healthy Children, Healthy Families: Parents making a difference!* (HCHF) is an evidence-based curriculum designed to be delivered to parents of children 3–11 years of age that focuses on developing healthy lifestyle behaviors [26–28]. Goals of the HCHF curriculum include increasing parent knowledge and skills surrounding implementation of healthy family habits, which ultimately impact child health behaviors [26–29]. Previous studies utilizing the HCHF curriculum reported significant improvements in several parent and child health behaviors using the 16-item HCHF Behavior Checklist (HCHF-BC) [26, 28–30]. While the checklist was developed specifically for the HCHF intervention, it does not comprehensively measure changes in FPPs using validated tools [28, 30]. Therefore, the goal of this pilot study was to assess if parents from a primarily Hispanic and low-income community, who participated in a childhood obesity intervention (HCHF) improved their responsive FPPs, specifically, 1) modeling healthy eating behaviors to their child, 2) encouraging a balanced and varied diet to their child, 3) involving children in food decisions, and 4) teaching their children about nutrition. In addition, the study aimed to assess changes in parent and child behaviors related to dietary intake and activity, using the 16-item HCHF-BC.

Methods
Study design
The pilot study utilized a non-experimental, pre/post within-subjects design in a community-based setting. The study involved a community partnership with Clinica Esperanza/Hope Clinic (CEHC), a clinic providing free healthcare services and programs to uninsured adults. The intervention was delivered by formally trained community paraprofessionals called *Navegantes*. A total of five *Navegantes* delivered the HCHF intervention to participants over the 2-year study period, with 2-3 *navegantes* teaching or facilitating each lesson at a time. All *Navegantes* were women from the surrounding community that were employed at CEHC. Over the course of 2 years (2014-2016), parents of 3-11-year-old children were recruited to participate in the study, which was framed as a community program entitled 'Niños Activos y Sanos: Healthy & Active Children'. All of the protocols in the study were approved by the University of Rhode Island Institutional Review Board.

Participants and recruitment
Both parents and primary caregivers, such as grandparents, (all referred to as 'parents' throughout this manuscript) with a child between the ages of 3-11 years were recruited. The target population were parents living in Olneyville and South Providence, Rhode Island where the median household income is $17,538, and 61% of the population is Hispanic [31].

Both in-person recruitment at different community settings (i.e. local parks, churches, community centers, events, etc.) and recruitment fliers were distributed throughout the community to recruit participants on a rolling basis from 2014 to 2016. In addition, researchers and *Navegantes* collaborated with community partners including other healthcare clinics and health-related programs to recruit parents for the study. Parents and/or primary caregivers were screened in-person or via telephone to determine eligibility. Participants were eligible to participate if they were a parent or primary caregiver of a child between 3 and 11 years of age at the beginning of enrollment and spoke English or Spanish. During the first year, 44 parents enrolled, 50 in year two ($N = 94$), with a total of nine groups of parents completing the intervention over the 2 year period. Groups occurred sequentially over the two-year study period. During the second year, the intervention was reduced by 1 week in effort to improve study retention.

Intervention

Navegantes participated in a formal 2-day training prior to delivering the HCHF curriculum, which was delivered primarily in Spanish. Based on previous evidence, the HCHF curriculum was designed to provide parents with strategies to help children adopt behaviors that promote a healthy weight [26, 27]. Through problem-solving strategies and role-playing, the HCHF intervention highlights *'paths to success'* (nutrition and physical behaviors) and *'keys to success'* (parental strategies to facilitate progress on the path to healthy behaviors in families, which highlight several responsive FPPs, and encourage parents to use these practices at home) [26, 27].

For example, paths to success include 'eating more fruits and vegetables,' 'eating fewer high-fat and high-sugar foods,' 'playing actively,' and 'limiting television and computer time' [26, 27]. Examples of keys to success include setting a good example for their child (modeling), and offering healthy choices within limits (guiding, or encouraging a balanced and varied diet) [26, 27].

Parents attended 90-min, weekly sessions of HCHF, which were conducted on Wednesday evenings, usually beginning at 5:30 pm. Written informed consent was obtained from all participants. Parents completed written informed consent forms to participate in the study and informed assent/written permission forms for their child if they were under the age of 7 years. Modified forms were used to allow children over the age of seven to better understand the study and provide written informed assent to participate. After consent was obtained from all participants, parents and children completed anthropometric measurements and parents then completed a written survey. Researchers were present during completion of consent forms and surveys to answer questions, assist parents who could not read or write, and provide clarification as needed. All study materials were available in both English and Spanish. The intervention was designed for the parents, given their role in shaping their child's environment and behaviors. During the sessions however, childcare and nutrition lessons were provided to children if parents chose to bring them. Parents then returned to CEHC weekly, for a total of eight sessions to complete the intervention. At the last session, the same procedures were repeated to collect post-intervention data (with the exception of consent forms). Parents were compensated with a $10 gift card after the first session, and a $40 gift card following the last session. Each session also included a weekly prize (such as pedometers, mixing bowls, and spatulas) for parents and their children in addition to raffle prizes (such as food prep equipment, small kitchen tools).

Measures
Anthropometrics

Standing height and weight measurements of each parent-child dyad were taken using standardized procedures [32], taken in duplicate. Parent's BMI was calculated based on their height and weight. Pre and post-intervention BMI percentiles were calculated for children using age- and sex-specific references [32, 33].

Survey

The self-administered survey consisted of 84 questions and parents answered questions as it pertained to their child that was consented to participate in the study. Parents with more than one child between ages 3-11 were instructed to base their responses on their youngest child within that age range. The decision to do this was driven by the literature on the importance of shaping health behaviors early in life given that these track into later childhood [4, 6, 7, 9, 10, 16, 21].

Parents were asked to report on the following socio-demographic characteristics: age, sex, ethnicity, race, education level, number/ages of children, marital status, if they were born in the U.S., number of years in the U.S., employment status, health insurance status, annual household income, child date of birth, and child gender.

Reported food parenting practices were assessed using seven subscales from the previously validated CFPQ [34], including modeling (4 items; $\alpha = 0.79$), involvement (3 items; $\alpha = 0.89$), encouraging balance and variety (4 items; $\alpha = 0.72$), and teaching about nutrition (3 items; $\alpha = 0.42$). Response options, ranged on a scale from disagree (1), disagree slightly (2), neutral (3), slightly agree (4), to agree (5) [34]. Subscale means were calculated for the seven subscales, with a higher score on each subscale indicating greater agreement with the corresponding practice.

To assess frequency of parent and child health behaviors, including dietary and physical activity/screen time behaviors (11 items), and home environment/parenting behaviors (5 items), parents completed the self-reported 16-item HCHF-BC [30]. Each item was assessed using a 5-point response scale from least to most frequent options in a range of frequencies appropriate to each reported behavior [30]. For example, for some of the questions response options ranged from (1) once in a while, (2) 1-2 days each week, (3) 3-4 days each week, (4) 5-6 days each week, to (5) every day or from (1) almost never, (2) 1-3 days each week, (3) 4-6 days each week, (4) once each day, to (5) 2 or more times each day. Mean scores for each item were calculated for analysis.

In addition to study objectives focused on parental feeding and diet and activity measures, a brief evaluation survey (14 questions) was provided to parents at the end of the final HCHF session, in effort to obtain their opinions and feedback on the program. Twenty participants that completed the study filled out an evaluation survey (surveys were provided in both English and Spanish).

Statistical analysis

Post-hoc analysis was completed to assess if there were significant changes between demographic variables for study completers vs. non-completers. Chi-square tests for categorical variables and an ANOVA for continuous variables were completed to compare demographics between completers and non-completers. Paired samples t-tests were performed to assess for statistically significant changes pre/post intervention for seven CFPQ subscales and the 16-item HCHF-BC. Given that this was a pilot study to assess the preliminary efficacy of the intervention, it was not adequately powered for multivariate analyses. To account for multiple comparisons, a conservative significance level was set post hoc for the t-tests at $p \leq 0.01$. The datasets used and/or analyzed during the current study are available from the corresponding author on reasonable request.

To assess parent participation, attendance was recorded at each session. Parents were considered study completers and were included in data analyses if they attended four or more of the eight sessions in year one, or three or more of the seven sessions in year two. To assess intervention fidelity (described as the extent to which the intervention is delivered as it was intended) [35], 59% of the HCHF sessions were observed by a trained research assistant using a previously-developed observation checklist. All statistical analysis was performed using SPSS version 23.

Results

Of the 94 parents who consented to participate over the 2 year study, nine did not complete baseline measurements, and were therefore excluded from analysis, leaving a total of 85 participants. Throughout the 2-year period, 33 parents dropped out of the intervention (i.e. did not return to the program sessions and/or did not complete post-intervention measures) and were therefore considered non-completers, leaving $n = 52$ participants with both baseline and post-intervention data (attrition rate of 39%). Figure 1 depicts a flow diagram showing the recruitment/consent process. Study completers were significantly older as compared to non-completers (39.9 vs. 34.4 mean years of age, respectively), ($p = 0.031$) (see Table 1).

Of the 85 parents at baseline, 94% were female and Hispanic with a mean age of 37.6 years. Less than a third

(30%) of parents had less than a high school degree, over half (64%) reported an annual household income of $15,000 or less and the majority (79%) were not born in the U.S. (Table 1). At baseline, over 75% of the parents were either overweight or obese. Of the participating children, mean age was 5.9±2.8 years, 56% were female, and almost half (49%) were either overweight or obese. Intervention fidelity was high (97%), indicating that the *Navegantes* delivered the intervention as it was intended based on the HCHF curriculum protocol.

For responsive FPPs, there was a significant increase in the frequency of reported use of encouraging balance and variety (4.5 pre, 4.63 post, $p = 0.01$; Effect size (Cohens d = 0.263). There were increases in the frequency of other responsive FPPs including modeling, involvement, and teaching about nutrition, however these changes were not statistically significant. For outcomes related to non-responsive FPPs, changes were not significant (Table 2).

For changes in parent and child behaviors related to dietary intake and physical activity, there were significant increases in frequency reported intake of fruit (2.9 pre, 3.7 post; $p < 0.001$), vegetable (2.9 pre, 3.6 post; $p < 0.001$) and low-fat dairy products for parents, (3.1 pre, 3.7 post; $p = 0.003$). Parents significantly increased the frequency of their own reported physical activity (2.5 pre, 2.9 post; $p = 0.006$) (Table 3).

There were also changes in measures related to the home food environment. Reported fruit availability significantly increased (4.3 pre, 4.6 post; $p = 0.009$), while energy dense snack availability (2.4 pre, 1.8 post; $p = 0.001$) and fast food intake (1.7 pre, 1.3 post; $p = 0.003$) significantly decreased. The changes in reported parental use of food autonomy (parent letting their child decide how much to eat), and the frequency of family meals were not significant (Table 4).

Parents who completed the evaluation survey ($n = 20$) were very satisfied with the intervention. For example, they all selected 'agree' to the following statements; 'I enjoyed coming to HCHF sessions', 'I would recommend HCHF to my friends and family', 'What I learned in

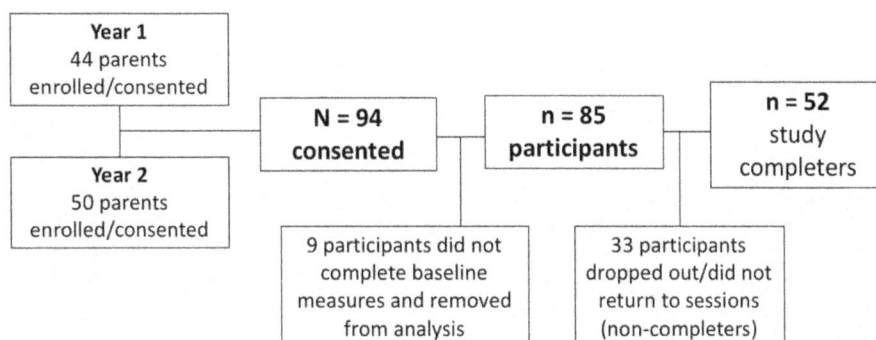
Fig. 1 Flowchart for study recruitment & completion

Table 1 Baseline characteristics of NASA participants ($n = 85$)

Participant characteristics	All parents ($n = 85$) n (%)	Study completers ($n = 52$) n (%)	Non-completers ($n = 33$) n (%)
Sex			
Female	81 (95.3)	50 (96.2)	30 (90.9)
Age (mean±SD)	37.6±11.3	39.9±10.9[a]	34.4±11.1[a]
Hispanic/Latino			
Yes	78 (91.8)	49 (94.2)	29 (87.9)
Race (check all that apply)			
White	36 (42.4)	23 (44.2)	13 (39.4)
African-American	10 (11.8)	7 (13.5)	3 (9.1)
American Indian/Alaskan Native	1 (1.2)	0 (0.0)	1 (3.0)
More than once race	9 (10.6)	5 (9.6)	4 (12.1)
Wish not to answer/don't know	10 (11.8)	4 (7.7)	6 (18.2)
Did not answer/Missing	19 (22.4)	13 (25)	6 (18.2)
Education			
Less than high school	25 (29.4)	13 (24.9)	12 (36.4)
High school graduate/GED	24 (28.2)	17 (32.7)	7 (21.2)
Post High School Trade/Technical school	9 (10.6)	7 (13.5)	2 (6.1)
Some college or higher	27 (31.7)	15 (28.9)	12 (36.4)
Living with Spouse			
No	45 (52.9)	26 (50.0)	19 (57.6)
Marital Status			
Never Married	26 (30.6)	12 (23.5)	14 (42.4)
Married	32 (37.6)	21 (41.2)	11 (33.3)
Divorced/Separated or Widowed	26 (30.6)	18 (35.3)	8 (24.3)
Born in the U.S.			
No	67 (78.8)	43 (82.7)	24 (72.7)
Years in the U.S. (mean±SD)	13.0±10.3	12.4±9.7	14.1±11.4
Employment Status			
Employed Full time (> 35 hrs/wk)	24 (28.2)	11 (21.2)	13 (39.4)
Employed Part time (< 35 hrs/wk)/Seasonally	21 (24.7)	14 (26.9)	7 (21.2)
Unemployed/Looking for work	25 (29.4)	17 (32.7)	8 (24.2)
Homemaker	13 (15.3)	10 (19.2)	3 (9.1)
Student	1 (1.2)	0 (0.0)	1 (3.0)
Health Insurance			
Yes	53 (62.4)	32 (69.6)	21 (63.6)
Annual Household Income			
$15,000 or less	43 (50.6)	29 (55.8)	14 (42.4)
$15,000 - $30,000	15 (17.6)	9 (17.3)	6 (24)
$30,000 - $45,000	8 (9.4)	3 (5.8)	5 (15.2)
More than $45,000	2 (2.4)	2 (3.8)	0 (0.0)
Parent Baseline BMI score (kg/m^2)			
Underweight (< 18.5)	0 (0.0)	0 (0.0)	0 (0.0)
Normal Weight (18.5 – 24.9)	16 (19.2)	12 (22.8)	4 (12.0)

Community-based childhood obesity prevention intervention for parents improves health...

79

Table 1 Baseline characteristics of NASA participants (n = 85) (Continued)

Participant characteristics	All parents (n = 85)	Study completers (n = 52)	Non-completers (n = 33)
	n (%)	n (%)	n (%)
Overweight (25.0 – 29.9)	25 (30)	16 (30.4)	9 (27.0)
Obese (30.0 or higher)	38 (49.4)	23 (43.7)	17 (51.0)
Child Baseline BMI Percentile			
Underweight (<5th)	1(1.2)	1 (2.3)	1 (3.8)
Normal Weight (5th – <85th)	32 (37.7)	20 (46.5)	12 (46.2)
Overweight (85th - <95th)	12 (14.1)	9 (20.9)	4 (15.4)
Obese (≥95th)	40 (47.0)	13 (30.2)	9 (34.6)
Child Age (mean±SD)	5.9±2.8	5.8±2.5	5.9±3.3
Child Gender			
Female	46 (54.1)	28 (53.8)	18 (54.5)

Values above that do not add to 100% reflect missing data
Abbreviations: NASA Ninos Activos y Sanos/Healthy & Active Children (Name of the program), SD Standard deviation, GED General Education Diploma, U.S. United States, Hrs Hours, Wk Week, BMI Body Mass Index
[a] Differences between variables for completers and non-completers were significant (p < 0.05), p = 0.031

HCHF is useful for me and my family', and 'I learned new parenting skills that help me get along better with my children.' For questions pertaining to time and location, 95% of participants agreed that the time that the sessions were held was convenient for them, while 85% agreed that the location was convenient for them. Through open-ended questions, participants shared what they liked the most of the intervention which included being able to make changes in their homes, learning about the importance of eating healthy meals and how to share them with their children, in addition to their shared experiences with other parents.

Discussion

This pilot study assessed preliminary changes in parents' use of parent-reported FPPs and diet and activity behaviors of parents and children pre/post participation in the evidenced-based HCHF intervention. Recruitment and retention of this population was a challenge. For parents that did complete the intervention, the frequency of parent-reported encouragement of balance and variety

increased. Although changes in other FPPs (both responsive and non-responsive) were not significant, trends toward improvement in most FPPs were observed. There were also improvements in reported dietary intake and physical activity measures (fruit, vegetable, and soda intake for parents, and parent-reported low-fat dairy intake and physical activity for their children). Parents also reported changes in measures related to the home food environment, including a significant increase in fruit availability and a significant decrease in energy dense snack availability and fast food availability for their children. Given the pilot nature of this work and the high rate of attrition, results should be interpreted with caution. Future studies should consider testing the effectiveness of the HCHF intervention using an experimental design and exploring FPPs as possible mediators of healthy eating and obesity.

The HCHF curriculum highlights healthy eating patterns and teaches parents ways to encourage healthy eating habits with their children. The HCHF curriculum may have had the greatest impact on encouragement of

Table 2 Parent pre/post intervention FPPs using Subscales from the CFPQ (n = 52)

CFPQ subscale	Pre		Post		95% Confidence Interval of the Difference		Effect size (Cohens d)	p-value
	Mean	SD	Mean	SD	Lower	Upper		
Modeling	4.47	0.75	4.62	0.65	−3.59	0.07	0.20	0.17
Encouragement of Balance and Variety	4.50	0.52	4.63	0.56	−0.29	0.04	0.26	0.01*
Involvement	3.90	0.97	4.03	0.99	−0.49	0.24	0.12	0.48
Teaching About Nutrition	3.73	0.72	3.87	0.58	−0.34	0.06	0.21	0.17
Restriction for Health	3.80	0.88	3.86	1.04	−0.35	0.23	0.07	0.66
Restriction for Weight Control	3.04	1.05	3.17	1.07	−0.42	0.14	0.16	0.33
Food as Reward	3.09	0.96	2.93	0.95	−0.19	0.50	0.14	0.38

* p ≤ 0.01 denoted statistically significant difference between pre/post measures from the CFPQ subscale

Table 3 Parent-reported pre/post intervention diet and physical activity outcomes from the HCHF-BC ($n = 52$)

Item on HCHF-BC	Pre		Post		95% Confidence Interval of the Difference		p-value
	Mean	SD	Mean	SD	Lower	Upper	
Parent Fruit Intake	2.98	1.48	3.74	1.17	−1.14	−0.38	0.000**
Parent Vegetable Intake	2.92	1.34	3.58	1.05	−0.97	−0.35	0.000**
Parent Soda Intake	1.72	1.17	1.45	0.90	−0.03	0.59	0.079
Parent Low-Fat Dairy Intake	3.12	1.36	3.66	1.36	−0.88	−0.20	0.003*
Parent Physical Activity	2.45	1.51	2.92	1.46	−0.80	−0.14	0.006*
Child Fruit Intake	4.04	1.03	4.10	1.13	−0.39	0.27	0.714
Child Vegetable Intake	2.88	1.38	3.18	1.20	−0.66	0.05	0.087
Child Low-Fat Dairy Intake	3.28	1.34	3.72	1.20	−0.84	−0.04	0.033
Child Soda Intake	1.55	0.89	1.55	1.10	−0.27	0.27	1.00
Child Physical Activity	2.90	1.49	3.53	1.30	−1.04	−0.22	0.003*
Child Screen Time	2.20	0.78	2.02	0.71	−0.05	0.41	0.118

*$p \leq 0.01$, **$p \leq 0.001$ denoted statistically significant difference between pre/post measures from the HCHF Behavior Checklist

balance and variety due to the intervention content and the parent's ability to implement this practice in the home. Previous studies focusing on FPPs have targeted mostly non-responsive practices; for example, one longitudinal study found that non-responsive FPPs at 6, 12, and 24 months post participation in a parent-centered childhood obesity treatment program decreased significantly at each time point [36]. The longitudinal study had a longer treatment intervention compared to the present study and also focused on non-responsive FPPs; it is possible that it is easier for parents to extinguish non-responsive FPPs versus learning about new and responsive practices [20]. Using more responsive practices however supports the development of healthy eating, favorable diet quality and weight outcomes over time [13, 18, 19, 21–24, 36, 37]. It is possible that there was not as much change as expected for several of the responsive FPPs given that they may be harder practices to operationalize in the home setting such as role modeling or involving children. The mean baseline scores for these other practices were also relatively high to begin with (mean = 3.7–4.5), creating ceiling effects for these measures. In addition, although the CFPQ is a validated tool, it has not been validated in this specific population (i.e. Hispanic, low-income), and future validation with these populations is needed [34].

The improvements seen in reported parent and child diet and activity behaviors are similar to previous studies utilizing the HCHF intervention, where significant improvements in parent-reported parent and child diet behaviors, including significant increases for fruit, vegetable, and low-fat dairy intake, and significant reductions in parent soda intake were found [28, 29]. These findings are not surprising in light of the topics thoroughly covered during the curriculum, including the importance of fruit and vegetable intake and drinking water or milk instead of sugar-sweetened beverages [26–29]. Although the targeted population was different from previously published studies, the results from this pilot study are consistent and support the possible efficacy of this intervention in improving health behavior outcomes for parents and children, particularly in low-income, Spanish-speaking populations.

Certain aspects of this study require additional comment. It is well known that participant recruitment and retention can be challenging in health-related studies and programs that aim to reach both parents and children [38–42]. In the present study, the attrition rate of parents was 40%. Furthermore, parents that completed the study were older than non-completers. Our experience is similar to that of other researchers where

Table 4 Parent-reported pre/post intervention parenting and home food environment outcomes from the HCHF-BC ($n = 52$)

Item on HCHF-BC	Pre		Post		95% Confidence Interval of the Difference		p-value
	Mean	SD	Mean	SD	Lower	Upper	
Autonomy	3.25	1.55	3.71	1.35	−1.03	0.09	0.096
Family Meals	4.08	1.28	3.78	1.40	−0.05	0.64	0.096
Fruit Availability	4.30	0.91	4.58	0.70	−0.49	−0.07	0.009*
Energy Dense Snack Availability	2.39	1.27	1.80	0.87	0.27	0.92	0.001*
Fast Food Availability	1.65	0.77	1.33	0.55	0.12	0.51	0.003*

*$p \leq 0.01$ denoted statistically significant difference between pre/post measures from the HCHF Behavior Checklist

recruiting and retaining low-income populations in health-related studies remains difficult, especially those "hardest to reach" [41, 43]. Evidence suggests that the most common barriers to recruitment and retention include socioeconomic status, education level, study location (school vs. home vs. community) and program/intervention targets (i.e. parents or children only vs. parent and children), all of which may have affected retention in the current study [39, 42]. Common reported barriers of parent participation in this study, included transportation, parents' work schedules and competing demands on family time [38]. Despite these barriers, the participants that were engaged continued to return to sessions and in fact requested additional sessions and education. To try and overcome the recruitment and retention challenges, barriers to study participation were reduced by working with a local community clinic, providing child care, healthy meals, and in some cases, transportation to the intervention. In order eliminate the health disparities experienced by low-income, ethnic minorities, continued efforts to reduce participation barriers in research studies are needed. Innovative approaches, including comprehensive policies and evidence-based strategies to improve recruitment and retention is warranted [43].

Given the funding mechanism and pilot nature of the study, an experimental design was not feasible. Findings need to be interpreted with caution given the lack of a control group and high attrition rates; significant results may be attributable to other factors and not necessarily the intervention itself. For example, participants may have been subjected to the observer-expectancy effect, as the study was described to participants as a health program for parents with the aim to improve the health of their families. In addition, behaviors were self-reported by parents, and therefore actual behaviors were not observed. Despite these limitations, the study utilized an evidence-based curriculum in a community-based setting, and was able to reach an at-risk population. By targeting a population served by a free clinic in a low-income area, the intervention was able to reach Hispanic and low-income parents of children who are disproportionately at risk for obesity [1–3, 31, 44]. Future studies should continue to explore cost-effective intervention strategies to engage low-income parents and assess long-term changes in behavior.

Conclusions

This pilot study found that participation in the HCHF intervention by a primarily low-income and Hispanic population increased the reported frequency of encouragement of balance and variety, a responsive FPP, which is associated with favorable weight status and diet habits in children [6–8, 12, 13, 21, 24].

However, the study is a pilot and would benefit from further randomized studies to examine evidence of effectiveness of this intervention in similar populations. Although there are several obesity prevention studies, few have specifically targeted or measured FPPs, and few have taken a family-based approach [4, 9, 10, 14, 16]. Interventions to prevent childhood obesity may include some information on modifying FPPs, but few have had a comprehensive focus and/or have not measured changes in these practices pre/post intervention [36, 37, 45, 46].

Future interventions should focus on improving both responsive and non-responsive FPPs [6, 11–13, 19]. The results of the current study highlight the importance of possibly targeting those responsive FPPs and parenting behaviors surrounding the home food environment in health interventions aimed at reducing childhood obesity risk. These results add to the current literature on interventions focused on FPPs in a population at higher risk for obesity, by a targeting low-income, Hispanic population.

Abbreviations

BMI: Body mass index; CEHC: Clinica Esperanza/Hope Clinic; CFPQ: Comprehensive feeding practices questionnaire; FPP: Food parenting practice; HCHF: Healthy children, healthy families; HCHF-BC: Healthy children, healthy Families behavior checklist; U.S.: United States

Acknowledgements

This research was funded by a Blue Cross Blue Shield of Rhode Island Blue Angel Community Health Grant, awarded to CEHC in partnership with the University of Rhode Island. The authors thank the *navegantes* (Damaris Rosales, Luz Betancur, Ingrid Castillo, Cindy Estrada, Brenda Veliz) and program/CEHC staff (Jacob Buckley, Erik Simpanen) and the CEHC staff/volunteers, all of who provided their time and dedication throughout the study. We also thank Noereem Mena and Fatima Tobar for delivering the child curriculum during year 1 and year 2 of the study, respectively. We thank all research assistants from the URI Community Nutrition and Childhood Obesity Prevention research group (Megan Fallon, Margaret Garcia, Maggie Tsai) for their assistance with data collection. We thank Candace Corbeil for her assistance with data analysis. We also thank Dr. Kathleen Webster for her input regarding statistical analysis. Thank you to Dr. Katherine Dickin, of Cornell University for her support during study implementation and review of this manuscript. We thank the Cornell University/creators of HCHF for creating and sharing this intervention for use in this study. We would finally like to thank all of the parents, children, and families that participated in this study.

Funding

The current study was funded by a Blue Angel Community Health Grant received Blue Cross Blue Shield of Rhode Island. This work was also supported by the USDA National Institute of Food and Agriculture, [Hatch/Tovar/ 1001894].

Authors' contributions
LO used this project to complete her Master's thesis work at the University of Rhode Island and drafted the manuscript. LO's responsibilities included overseeing the intervention delivery, communicating with *navegantes*, organizing materials, collecting and entering data and assisting with data analysis and interpretation. AT oversaw all aspects of the study and reviewed drafts of the manuscript. AD is the Medical Director of Clinica Esperanza/Hope Clinic which was the community setting for the current study, she was involved in writing the grant for this study and reviewing drafts of the manuscript. NM assisted in data collection, manuscript development, and developing and delivering the nutrition curriculum for children while their parents participated in the intervention. GG and CR contributed to the development of the overall study design (i.e. research methods and objectives/research questions), in addition manuscript development and review. All authors have given final approval of the manuscript for submission for publication.

Competing interests
The authors declare that they have no competing interests.

Author details
[1]Department of Nutrition and Food Sciences, University of Rhode Island, Fogarty Hall, 41 Lower College Rd, Kingston, RI 02881, USA. [2]Cancer Prevention Research Center and Department of Psychology, University of Rhode Island, Chafee Hall, 142 Flagg Road, Kingston, RI 02881, USA. [3]Institute for Immunology and Informatics, University of Rhode Island, Shepard Building, 80 Washington Street, Providence, RI 02903, USA.

References
1. Ogden CL, Carroll MD, Lawman HG, Fryar CD, Kruszon-Moran D, Kit BK, Flegal KM. Trends in obesity prevalence among children and adolescents in the United States, 1988-1994 through 2013-2014. JAMA. 2016;315(21):2292–9.
2. The burden of overweight and obesity in Rhode Island. In: Initiative for a healthy weight program. Providence: The Rhode Island Department of Health Initiative for a Healthy Weight Program; 2011.
3. Pratt CA, Loria CM, Arteaga SS, Nicastro HL, Lopez-Class M, de Jesus JM, Srinivas P, Maric-Bilkan C, Schwartz Longacre L, Boyington JEA, et al. A systematic review of obesity disparities research. Am J Prev Med. 2017;53(1):113–22.
4. Ash T, Agaronov A, Young T, Aftosmes-Tobio A, Davison KK. Family-based childhood obesity prevention interventions: a systematic review and quantitative content analysis. Int J Behav Nutr Phys Act. 2017;14(1):113.
5. Wang Y, Cai L, Wu Y, Wilson RF, Weston C, Fawole O, Bleich SN, Cheskin LJ, Showell NN, Lau BD, et al. What childhood obesity prevention programmes work? A systematic review and meta-analysis. Obes Rev. 2015;16(7):547–65.
6. Golan M. Parents as agents of change in childhood obesity - from research to practice. Int J Pediatr Obes. 2006;1(2):66–76.
7. Golan M, Crow S. Parents are key players in the prevention and treatment of weight-related problems. Nutr Rev. 2004;62(1):39–50.
8. Golan M, Weizman A. Familial approach to the treatment of childhood obesity: conceptual mode. J Nutr Educ. 2001;33(2):102–7.
9. Davison KK, Jurkowski JM, Lawson HA. Reframing family-centred obesity prevention using the family ecological model. Public Health Nutr. 2013; 16(10):1861–9.
10. Davison KK, Lawson HA, Coatsworth JD. The family-centered action model of intervention layout and implementation (FAMILI): the example of childhood obesity. Health Promot Pract. 2012;13(4):454–61.
11. Patrick H, Hennessy E, McSpadden K, Oh A. Parenting styles and practices in children's obesogenic behaviors: scientific gaps and future research directions. Child Obes. 2013;9(Suppl):S73–86.
12. Rodgers RF, Paxton SJ, Massey R, Campbell KJ, Wertheim EH, Skouteris H, Gibbons K. Maternal feeding practices predict weight gain and obesogenic eating behaviors in young children: a prospective study. Int J Behav Nutr Phys Act. 2013;10:24.
13. Sleddens EF, Kremers SP, Stafleu A, Dagnelie PC, De Vries NK, Thijs C. Food parenting practices and child dietary behavior. Prospective relations and the moderating role of general parenting. Appetite. 2014;79:42–50.
14. Olson S. Obesity in the early childhood years: state of the science and implementation of promising solutions: workshop in brief. National Academies of Sciences, Engineering, and Medicine; 2016.
15. Shloim N, Edelson LR, Martin N, Hetherington MM. Parenting styles, feeding styles, feeding practices, and weight status in 4-12 year-old children: a systematic review of the literature. Front Psychol. 2015;6:1849.
16. Birch LL, Ventura AK. Preventing childhood obesity: what works? Int J Obes. 2009;33(Suppl 1):S74–81.
17. Pinard CA, Yaroch AL, Hart MH, Serrano EL, McFerren MM, Estabrooks PA. Measures of the home environment related to childhood obesity: a systematic review. Public Health Nutr. 2012;15(1):97–109.
18. Vollmer RL, Mobley AR. Parenting styles, feeding styles, and their influence on child obesogenic behaviors and body weight. A review. Appetite. 2013; 71:232–41.
19. Vaughn AE, Ward DS, Fisher JO, Faith MS, Hughes SO, Kremers SP, Musher-Eizenman DR, O'Connor TM, Patrick H, Power TG. Fundamental constructs in food parenting practices: a content map to guide future research. Nutr Rev. 2016;74(2):98–117.
20. Natale RA, Messiah SE, Asfour L, Uhlhorn SB, Delamater A, Arheart KL. Role modeling as an early childhood obesity prevention strategy: effect of parents and teachers on preschool children's healthy lifestyle habits. J Dev Behav Pediatr. 2014;35(6):378–87.
21. Couch SC, Glanz K, Zhou C, Sallis JF, Saelens BE. Home food environment in relation to children's diet quality and weight status. J Acad Nutr Diet. 2014; 114(10):1569–79. e1561
22. Tschann JM, Martinez SM, Penilla C, Gregorich SE, Pasch LA, de Groat CL, Flores E, Deardorff J, Greenspan LC, Butte NF. Parental feeding practices and child weight status in Mexican American families: a longitudinal analysis. Int J Behav Nutr Phys Act. 2015;12:66.
23. Farrow CV, Haycraft E, Blissett JM. Teaching our children when to eat: how parental feeding practices inform the development of emotional eating–a longitudinal experimental design. Am J Clin Nutr. 2015;101(5):908–13.
24. Spruijt-Metz D, Li C, Cohen E, Birch L, Goran M. Longitudinal influence of mother's child-feeding practices on adiposity in children. J Pediatr. 2006;148(3):314–20.
25. Dawson-McClure S, Brotman LM, Theise R, Palamar JJ, Kamboukos D, Barajas RG, Calzada EJ. Early childhood obesity prevention in low-income, urban communities. J Prev Interv Community. 2014;42(2):152–66.
26. Dickin KL, Hill TF, Dollahite JS. The collaboration for health, activity, and nutrition in Children's environments (CHANCE): a program integrating parenting and nutrition behavioral education improves food, active play, and parenting practices in low-income families. Anaheim: Experimental Biology; 2010.
27. Healthy Children, Healthy Families: Parents Making a Difference! Food and Nutrition Education in Communities. http://fnec.cornell.edu/for-partners/curricula/hchf/. Accessed 5 Jan 2015.
28. Dickin KL, Hill TF, Dollahite JS. Practice-based evidence of effectiveness in an integrated nutrition and parenting education intervention for low-income parents. J Acad Nutr Diet. 2014;114(6):945–50.
29. Lent M, Hill TF, Dollahite JS, Wolfe WS, Dickin KL. Healthy children, healthy families: parents making a difference! A curriculum integrating key nutrition, physical activity, and parenting practices to help prevent childhood obesity. J Nutr Educ Behav. 2012;44(1):90–2.
30. Dickin KL, Lent M, Lu AH, Sequeira J, Dollahite JS. Developing a measure of behavior change in a program to help low-income parents prevent unhealthful weight gain in children. J Nutr Educ Behav. 2012;44(1):12–21.
31. Olneyville: action for a healthier community: Rhode Island Department of Health. Providence: Olneyville Housing Corportation; 2011.
32. Lohman TG. Advances in body composition, vol. 3. Champain: Human Kinetics Publishers; 1992.
33. Centers for Disease Control and Prevention. CDC Table for calculating body mass index values for selected heights and weights for ages 2 to 20. 2000. http://www.cdc.gov/growthcharts/html_charts/bmiagerev.htm. Accessed Apr 2017.
34. Musher-Eizenman D, Holub S. Comprehensive feeding practices questionnaire: validation of a new measure of parental feeding practices. J Pediatr Psychol. 2007;32(8):960–72.

Community-based childhood obesity prevention intervention for parents improves health...

83

35. Gearing RE, El-Bassel N, Ghesquiere A, Baldwin S, Gillies J, Ngeow E. Major ingredients of fidelity: a review and scientific guide to improving quality of intervention research implementation. Clin Psychol Rev. 2011;31(1):79–88.

36. Burrows T, Warren JM, Collins CE. The impact of a child obesity treatment intervention on parent child-feeding practices. Int J Pediatr Obes. 2010;5(1):43–50.

37. Johnson SL. Developmental and environmental influences on young Children's vegetable preferences and consumption. Adv Nutr. 2016;7(1): 220S–31S.

38. Axford N, Lehtonen M, Kaoukji D, Tobin K, Berry V. Engaging parents in parenting programs: lessons from research and practice. Child Youth Serv Rev. 2012;34(10):2061–71.

39. Cui Z, Seburg EM, Sherwood NE, Faith MS, Ward DS. Recruitment and retention in obesity prevention and treatment trials targeting minority or low-income children: a review of the clinical trials registration database. Trials. 2015;16:564.

40. Lucas PJ, Curtis-Tyler K, Arai L, Stapley S, Fagg J, Roberts H. What works in practice: user and provider perspectives on the acceptability, affordability, implementation, and impact of a family-based intervention for child overweight and obesity delivered at scale. BMC Public Health. 2014;14:614.

41. Probstfield JL, Frye RL. Strategies for recruitment and retention of participants in clinical trials. JAMA. 2011;306(16):1798–9.

42. Coatsworth JD, Duncan LG, Pantin H, Szapocznik J. Patterns of retention in a preventive intervention with ethnic minority families. J Prim Prev. 2006;27(2):171–93.

43. Raphael JL, Lion KC, Bearer CF. Policy solutions to recruiting and retaining minority children in research. Pediatr Res. 2017;82(2):180–2.

44. Lovasi GS, Hutson MA, Guerra M, Neckerman KM. Built environments and obesity in disadvantaged populations. Epidemiol Rev. 2009;31:7–20.

45. Holland JC, Kolko RP, Stein RI, Welch RR, Perri MG, Schechtman KB, Saelens BE, Epstein LH, Wilfley DE. Modifications in parent feeding practices and child diet during family-based behavioral treatment improve child zBMI. Obesity (Silver Spring). 2014;22(5):E119–26.

46. Vaughn AE, Tabak RG, Bryant MJ, Ward DS. Measuring parent food practices: a systematic review of existing measures and examination of instruments. Int J Behav Nutr Phys Act. 2013;10:61.

9

Avoiding exercise mediates the effects of internalized and experienced weight stigma on physical activity in the years following bariatric surgery

SeungYong Han[1]* , Gina Agostini[1], Alexandra A. Brewis[1,2] and Amber Wutich[2]

Abstract

Background: People living with severe obesity report high levels of weight-related stigma. Theoretically, this stigma undermines weight loss efforts. The objective of this study is to test one proposed mechanism to explain why weight loss is so difficult once an individual becomes obese: that weight-related stigma inhibits physical activity via demotivation to exercise.

Methods: The study focused on individuals who had bariatric surgery within the past 5 years (N = 298) and who report a post-surgical body mass index (BMI) ranging from 16 to 70. Exercise avoidance motivation (EAM) and physical activity (PA) were modeled as latent variables using structural equation modeling. Two measures of weight stigma, the Stigmatizing Situations Inventory (SSI) and the Weight Bias Internalization Scale (WBIS) were modified for people with a long history of extreme obesity for use as observed predictors.

Results: Exercise avoidance motivation (EAM) significantly mediated the association between both experienced (SSI) and internalized (WBIS) weight stigma and physical activity (PA) in this population.

Conclusion: Exercise avoidance motivation, influenced by weight stigma, may be a significant factor explaining the positive relationship between higher body weights with lower levels of physical activity.

Keywords: Obesity, Bariatric surgery, Stigma, Physical activity, Exercise

Background

Weight-related stigma is frequently reported by people living with the highest levels of obesity, and its generally negative effects on health and wellbeing are well documented [1–9]. Larger-bodied individuals more frequently endure both direct and indirect forms of felt (experienced) weight stigma in many common environments, including work, school, medical facilities, and government centers [10]. Importantly, people with severe obesity (BMI ≥ 35) are more likely than those of normal weight to internalize the weight-related stigma expressed by others (i.e., to self-stigmatize) over their life course [10, 11]. Internalized

weight stigma (sometimes termed self-stigma or self-directed stigma), is the extent to which a person reports feeling of low social value due to his or her current or former weight status. Internalized stigma arises because an individual agrees with the publicly held, usually negative, stereotypes used to characterize a group or population (e.g., overweight individuals) and adopts these negative views about the self or of his/her capabilities [12]. Internalized stigma more strongly affects both self-esteem and self-efficacy than do other forms of stigma (e.g., public stigma) across many different contexts, and, further, has long-lasting effects [13]. There is growing evidence that such stigma predicts difficulty in both reaching and maintaining a healthy weight, especially for individuals with a higher BMI. For example, higher levels of internalized weight stigma are associated with a number

* Correspondence: shan32@asu.edu
[1]Mayo Clinic/Arizona State University Obesity Solutions, 1000 Cady Mall Suite 164, Tempe, AZ 85287, USA
Full list of author information is available at the end of the article

of behavioral changes, including greater calorie consumption, demotivation to diet, and binge eating disorder, all factors that can stymie weight loss [4, 14–16]. Furthermore, individuals who report high levels of internalized weight stigma are less likely to show improvement when they do seek treatment for disordered eating [17].

Weight stigma also impacts behaviors and attitudes toward physical activity. This can manifest as a reluctance to engage in specific, public forms of activity (e.g., gyms, swimming pools, or social sports teams) or as exercise avoidance more generally [1, 10, 18, 19]. For example, Vartanian and Shaprow [20] found a significant effect of experienced weight stigma on exercise avoidance in female college students which predicted less frequent bouts of strenuous and moderate physical activity. These effects were exacerbated among those already overweight and obese, or who believed themselves to be so. In a study of adult females with a body mass index (BMI) at or over 25, Pearl, Puhl, and Dovidio [21] found a significant effect of experienced weight stigma on exercise behavior and, further, that internalized weight stigma partially mediated this association. Similarly, among males who perceived themselves as overweight or obese, internalized societal attitudes toward appearance (including anti-fat attitudes) moderated the association between experienced weight stigma and exercise avoidance, which itself was negatively associated with self-reported strenuous exercise [18]. Among health program enrollees, Mensinger et al. [22] discovered that individuals who initially reported lower internalized weight stigma also had greater enjoyment of and engagement in moderate intensity physical activity (PA) while those individuals with high levels of internalized stigma showed little change to either over 6 months. While exercise avoidance was not a specific target of this study, these more negative attitudes towards exercise may express as a general reluctance to engage in activity (i.e., exercise avoidance). In total, these studies suggest that the mechanisms fueling exercise avoidance include direct and immediate concerns of judgment or mistreatment, but also that internalized stigma may undermine self-efficacy [17, 21–23] to create a "why try" mentality when it comes to weight loss, particularly when an individual is overweight [10, 19, 21, 24–27].

To expand the evidential basis of how stigma shapes exercise avoidance, here we focus on a population of bariatric patients in the years after their surgery. This is a population where the connections between stigma, obesity, and exercise avoidance decisions should be especially apparent. Bariatric (weight loss) patients decide to have surgery after difficult and long, often lifetime, struggles with both high body weight and the stigma it engenders [28]. To qualify for surgery, patients must often have a BMI of 40 or above, or a BMI of 35 or more (technically severe obesity) with associated co-morbidities. Studies show that individuals who elect to have surgery commonly report long-term exposure to stigmatized treatment by others, such as being stared at, enduring negative statements from children or other adults, and being overlooked for certain opportunities (e.g., work promotion) [1, 28, 29]. Evidence suggests that social stigmas are more severe and more likely to manifest as internalized stigma or self-blame when an individual is deemed personally responsible for his/her stigmatizing condition (i.e., being overweight), the effects of which are long lasting and may persist even if the stigmatizing variables change. [15, 30, 31].

After surgery, clinicians set guidelines for physical activity to assist with both weight-loss and maintenance [32–34]. However, Bond et al. [35] found no significant difference in moderate-to-vigorous physical activity (MVPA) tracked via accelerometer between patients assessed at presurgical and postsurgical (6 month) windows. For individuals like bariatric surgery patients who have lost a substantial amount of weight, a high level of physical activity is crucial to maintain their reduced weight status and prevent regain [36–39]. And yet bariatric surgery patients are less likely to comply with physical activity guidelines than other guidelines, including dietary ones, with rates of exercise program noncompliance increasing after surgery [40–42]. A lack of motivation and related psychological factors have been proposed to explain these persistently low levels of physical activity [43]. Given this, connecting stigma to exercise avoidance in the years after surgery has important practical applications for understanding (and preventing) weight regain in bariatric patients, particularly given the greater success in long-term weight loss for patients who engage in even low levels of regular physical activity [33, 44].

Methods

All participants in this study were identified on the basis of age (greater than 21) and having had bariatric surgery within the previous 5 years in a single large hospital system. Final sample composition was consistent with the hospital's bariatric surgery population generally [45]: patients were primarily female (77%) and Non-Hispanic White (93%). The majority of patients reported undergoing roux-en-y gastric bypass surgery (74%), followed by a sleeve gastrectomy (17%), duodenal switch with biliopancreatic diversion (5%), and laparoscopic gastric binding (2%). Two percent of respondents were uncertain which surgical procedure they received. Patients ranged in age from 19 to 82 years and had a BMI greater than 35 at the time of surgery (see Table 1). Data were generated using paper surveys disseminated via mail in 2015 with follow-up phone calls to encourage participation and assist with completion as needed. The survey was

Table 1 Summary Statistics of Outcome, Mediator, Predictors, and Covariates

	N	N miss	Mean	S.D.	Min	Max
Physical activity (PA)						
Non-vigorous physical activity, days	285	13	4.65	2.13	0	7
Non-moderate physical activity, days	283	15	3.84	2.26	0	7
No walk > 10 mins, days	283	15	2.17	2.35	0	7
Exercise Avoidance Motivation (EAM)						
Uncomfortable going to a gym	287	11	2.20	1.68	1	7
Too many thin people at a gym	286	12	1.94	1.60	1	7
Embarrassed to use gym equipment	282	16	2.04	1.60	1	7
Embarrassed to exercise in public places	293	5	1.70	1.34	1	7
Experienced weight stigma (SSI)	219	79	4.27	7.10	0	66
Internalized weight stigma (WBIS)	283	15	2.33	0.45	1.2	3.5
Covariates						
Current BMI	291	7	30.60	6.53	16.0	70.4
Weight loss (%)	293	5	−33.36	9.96	−67.9	−1.7
Time since surgery (months)	293	5	20.92	12.44	0	60
Male	289	9	0.23	0.42	0	1
Age	288	10	53.76	12.72	19	82
University or above	295	3	0.45	0.50	0	1
Household income > $10,000	289	9	0.29	0.45	0	1

The total sample size is 298

paired with a long-term ethnographic study of bariatric patients' experiences with stigma [2, 28]. These associated qualitative interviews informed the survey tool development. All procedures were approved by the relevant university and hospital human subjects review boards. For a mail–disseminated survey of this type, the response rate of 30% (298 out of 994 patients) was excellent.

For data analysis, a structural equation model (SEM) in Mplus 7.4 was used. The visual model of the analysis is presented in Fig. 1, with ovals signifying the latent variables of exercise avoidance motivation (EAM) and physical activity (PA), and boxes reflecting observed variables (4 constructs of exercise avoidance, 3 constructs of

physical activity, as well as experienced (SSI: Stigmatizing Situations Inventory) and internalized (WBIS: Weight Bias Internalization Scale) weight stigma). This analytical approach was suitable for our data and superior to other such methods (e.g., a series of multiple logistic or ordinary least square regressions) in that (1) SEM incorporates random and systematic measurement error in the indicators of EAM and PA; (2) the indirect effects of either experienced or internalized weight stigma through exercise avoidance could be tested, each controlling for the other; and (3) a full sample ($N = 298$) could be used via the full information maximum likelihood (FIML) method to handle missing data in Mplus 7.4 [46]. In addition, to deal

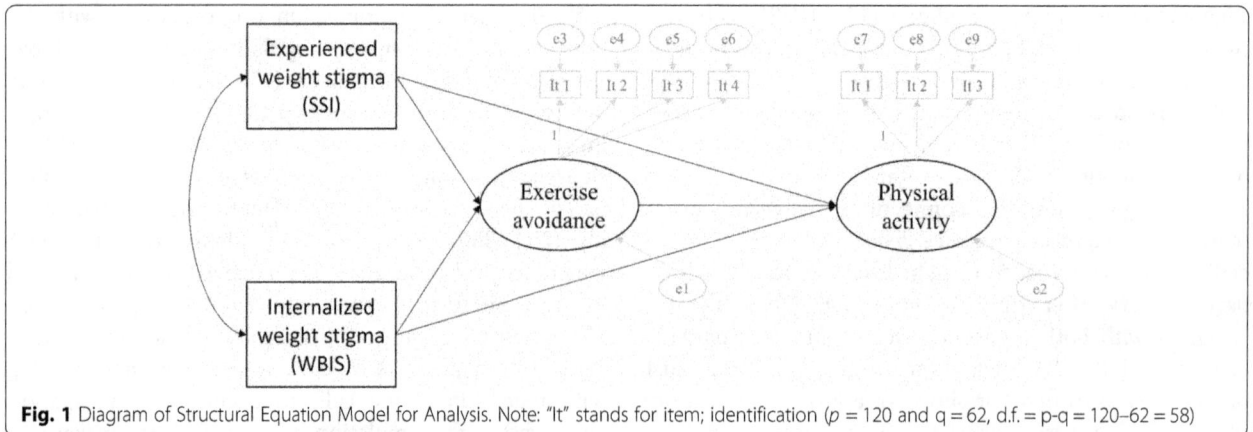

Fig. 1 Diagram of Structural Equation Model for Analysis. Note: "It" stands for item; identification ($p = 120$ and q = 62, d.f. = p-q = 120–62 = 58)

with the imbalance of confidence limits due to the non-normal distribution of the indirect effect, bias-corrected bootstrap confidence intervals after 5000 replications were used to interpret the results. The outcome, one mediator, two predictors, and seven covariates used for the SEM were measured as follows.

Physical activity as an outcome

We used a structural equation framework wherein three items of physical activity were used to construct a latent variable measuring overall physical activity: (1) the number of days of no vigorous physical activity per week, (2) the number of days of no moderate physical activity per week, and (3) the number of days not walking more than 10 min per week. Higher values, therefore, indicated lower physical activity. The associations between the latent variable and those three items are visualized in Fig. 1. This physical activity index has a medium level of internal consistency using all three items (Cronbach's alpha = .68).

Exercise avoidance as a mediator

The survey adopted eight questions from Vartanian and Shaprow [20] that were used to construct an exercise-avoidance motivation (EAM) scale. Each question was scored from zero ("not at all true") to seven ("completely true"), and patients reported on their experiences within the prior 3 months. The EAM scale has been employed previously with obese and general populations [18, 20], but has not been validated for bariatric populations specifically. In addition, despite the high level of internal consistency for the index using all eight items (Cronbach's alpha = .86), a maximum of four items are recommended to construct a latent variable [47]. Accordingly, four items were selected based on the results of a common factor analysis allowing two factors (average eigenvalue used as the criterion) to be correlated with each other (oblique PROMAX rotation, results provided upon request). The four questions asked whether a respondent felt (1) uncomfortable going to a gym, (2) that there were too many thin people at the gym, (3) embarrassed to use gym equipment, and (4) embarrassed to exercise in public places, including gyms. Contextually, all four questions refer to gyms, so theoretical internal consistency is high. The associations between the latent variable and these four items are also visualized in Fig. 1. Higher values for the latent variable, therefore, indicated a greater tendency to avoid exercise.

External and internal weight stigma measures as predictors

Two indices were used to assess a patient's level of experienced and internalized weight stigma: one focused on experiences of being stigmatized by others (SSI) while the other captured respondents' weight-related self-judgment (WBIS). The Stigmatizing Situations Inventory (SSI) measured experiences of weight-related stigma, sources of stigma (e.g., from family or strangers), and encounters with weight-related physical barriers (e.g., ill-fitting seatbelts) reported by participants. It captured how often people recognize various encounters with stigma in their everyday lives. The SSI index has been applied to both those populations seeking bariatric surgery [18] and those seeking non-surgical weight loss interventions [7]. We reduced the SSI items from 50 [1] to 29 to limit respondent burden. Each item was scored from zero ("never") to three ("several times"), and patients reported on experiences during the 3 months prior to the survey. All items were categorized into 11 stigmatizing situations, the sum of which was used to construct the SSI index. It should be noted that for one stigmatizing situation, "being physically attacked," all respondents answered the same: that they had never experienced this situation before. The SSI index was only valid if there are no missing items. The valid range of our constructed index was between 0 and 90, and the level of internal consistency (excluding "being physically attacked" due to no variance) was high (Cronbach's alpha = .82).

To assess internalized weight stigma experienced in the 3 months prior to survey, 13 questions were chosen from the original 19 questions used by Durso and Latner [48] to construct their 11-item Weight Bias Internalized Scale (WBIS). The phrasing of these questions were slightly modified so they would be more applicable to our participants, each of whom had a long history of extreme obesity. To test whether all items reflected the same construct, SAS 9.2 was used to conduct a principal component analysis with varimax rotation on the 13 items following Durso and Latner [48]. Results confirmed that these items clustered around two components (eigenvalues > 1), with component 1 explaining most of the variance (73% and eigenvalue = 3.84). Due to the low variance explained by the second component (eigenvalue = 1.58) and the single dimensionality of the hypothesized construct, Mplus 9.2 was used to conduct confirmatory factor analysis to assess whether the two components could be merged. Based on these results, six items were dropped from the constructed WBIS because of non-significant or low factor loadings (< 0.35). Therefore, an abbreviated 7-item WBIS was used to reflect internalized weight stigma for subsequent analyses (see the Additional file 1 for the description of the final questions selected) [49]. The final 7-item WBIS was only created for cases where all seven items were complete. The level of internal consistency was high (Cronbach's alpha = .87).

Covariates

Multiple covariates potentially associated with EAM and PA were controlled for. In addition to body mass index (BMI) at the time of the survey, percent weight change between the time of surgery and the time of survey completion was also controlled in the model. It should be noted that because this survey was part of a larger social science study of patient's lived experience and because medical records were not accessible, direct measurement of weight was not possible. Other covariates included age, gender, time since surgery (months), education (university educated or above), and household income (over $100,000 or not). Due to low variation within the sample, we did not include ethnicity as a covariate.

Results

Summary statistics

Moderate physical activity (PA) was more common than vigorous physical activity among patients after bariatric surgery, and patients walked at least 10 min per week for 2 days on average (see Table 1). All four items of the latent variable of exercise avoidance motivation (EAM) showed relatively low values with wide variance. Bariatric surgery patients had not experienced many stigmatizing situations (SSI) during their lives and showed a relatively low level of internalized weight stigma (WBIS). Results for covariates showed, on average, that the bariatric patients in the sample were middle aged (54 years old), primarily female, highly educated and affluent, that they lost 33% of their weight at the time of surgery, that they still had a high body mass index (BMI > 30), and that surgery was performed more than 21 months before the survey. The percent weight change was not significantly correlated with the three items measuring physical activity. However, it was significantly correlated with whether a respondent felt that there were too many thin people at the gym (coef. = 0.19, p-value = 0.0015) and

whether they were embarrassed to use gym equipment (coef. = 0.13, p-value = 0.0315).

Structural equation model results

The main results of the structural equation model are summarized in (Fig. 2, see the Additional file 2 for the full results). One of our primary interests was whether the effect of weight stigma on physical activity could be mediated by exercise avoidance. All covariates (exogenous variables omitted in Figs. 1 and 2) were allowed to correlate, and they were uncorrelated with all the errors or disturbances. The test statistic from the Chi-square test comparing the suggested model with the saturated model was 106.522 with 58 degrees of freedom (p-value = .0001), but this was likely due to the relatively large sample size (N = 298). The other fit statistics indicated good fit to the data with RMSEA close to 0.05 (=0.053 with 90% C.I. [0.037; 0.069]) and CFI and TLI larger than .90 (CFI = 0.933 and TLI = 0.904).

The unstandardized and standardized estimated direct effects are summarized in Fig. 2. Both experienced (SSI) and internalized (WBIS) weight stigma had significant and positive effects on exercise avoidance motivation (EAM) at the p-value .05 level. On the other hand, neither SSI nor WBIS showed a significant *direct* effect on physical activity (PA). Only EAM showed a marginally significant effect on PA (p-value = 0.063). The absence of a direct effect of experienced and internalized weight stigma on PA does not necessarily mean that indirect effects do not exist. The estimated direct, indirect, and total effects of each type of weight stigma after 4856 successful bootstraps (5000 attempts) are summarized in Table 2. The numbers are unstandardized estimates. The bias-corrected 95% confidence intervals confirmed that EAM significantly mediated the associations of PA with both SSI and WBIS. In detail, there was a 0.066 unit increase in the latent variable of PA through EAM for every unit increase in WBIS. The scale of a latent

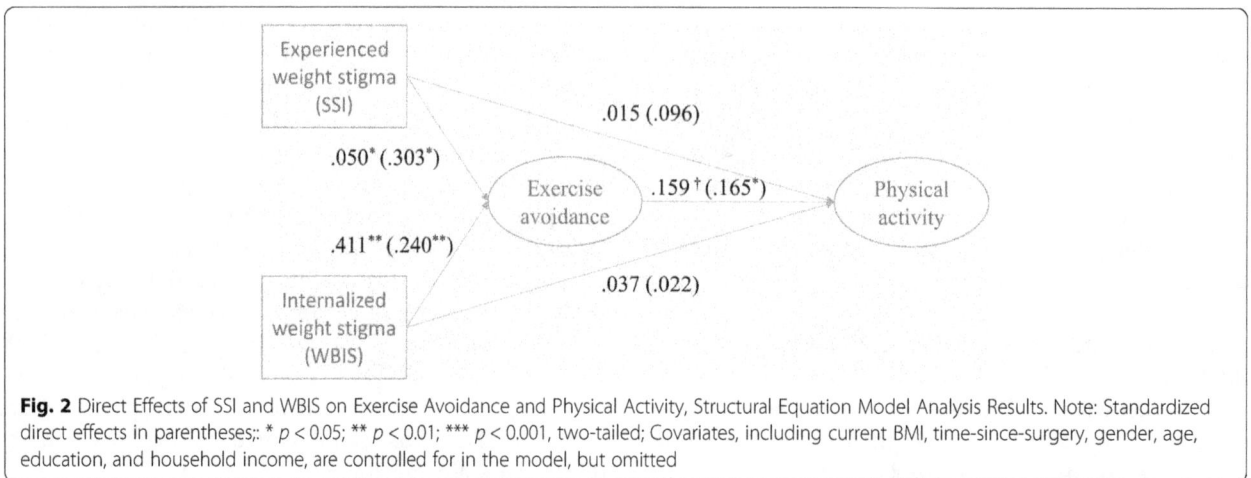

Fig. 2 Direct Effects of SSI and WBIS on Exercise Avoidance and Physical Activity, Structural Equation Model Analysis Results. Note: Standardized direct effects in parentheses;: * p < 0.05; ** p < 0.01; *** p < 0.001, two-tailed; Covariates, including current BMI, time-since-surgery, gender, age, education, and household income, are controlled for in the model, but omitted

Table 2 Indirect, Direct, and Total Effects of Weight Stigma on Physical Activity, Bootstrapping Results

	Coefficient	S.E.	Bias-corrected 99% C.I.
Experienced weight stigma (SSI)			
Indirect effect	**0.008**	0.007	[0.001; 0.030]
Direct effect	0.015	0.016	[−0.011; 0.053]
Total effect	0.023	0.015	[0.000; 0.058]
Internalized weight stigma (WBIS)			
Indirect effect	**0.066**	0.039	[0.013; 0.190]
Direct effect	0.037	0.126	[−0.185; 0.325]
Total effect	0.102	0.122	[−0.091; 0.393]

N = 298 and the number of completed replications = 4856 (out of 5000 requested); **bold** if the result is significant at the p-value 0.05 level; CI stands for confidence intervals, SE stands for standard errors; covariates, such as current BMI, weight loss, time since surgery, gender, age, education, and household income, are controlled for in the model, but omitted; the developers of Mplus recommend reporting non-significance when either the lower bound or the upper bound of the C.I. is reported as 0.000

variable is the same as the scale of the indicator with a factor loading fixed at one, so the scale of the latent variable measuring PA in our model was days per week. In other words, one unit increase in WBIS was, on average, associated with 0.066 days per week (bias-corrected 95% C.I. between 0.013 and 0.190) increase in physical activity. This indirect effect explained 64.7% of the total effect (=0.066/0.102*100). While the magnitude of the effect size may not seem overtly substantive, comparing the lowest and the highest levels of observed WBIS in the data (ranging from 1.2 and 3.5, see Table 1) indicated a clear difference in physical activity of 0.152 days per week. EAM also mediated the association between experienced weight stigma (SSI) and PA. In detail, one unit increase in SSI was, on average, associated with 0. 008 days per week (bias-corrected 95% C.I. between 0. 001 and 0.030) increase in physical activity. This indirect effect explained 35% of the total effect (=0.008/0. 023*100). And the standardized coefficients of two indirect effects indicate that two weight stigma indices have similar impacts on PA through EAM (see Fig. 2).

Discussion

In total, our results indicate that level of physical activity may be influenced by postoperative bariatric patients' internalized and experienced weight-related stigma via exercise avoidance. In other words, the higher the level of weight stigma a patient had when surveyed, the more likely she or he wanted to avoid exercise, and subsequently, the less physically active she or he was. Furthermore, both experienced and internalized weight stigma only indirectly, not directly, affected PA. Studies in non-bariatric populations indicate that weight stigma may significantly lower people's willingness to engage in physical activity [18, 20, 50]. In this sample of

postoperative patients, we identified weight stigma as a factor that may be involved in patient non-compliance with physical activity recommendations, even despite the significant postsurgical weight loss our participants reported. Considering patients and medical providers' concerns with weight recidivism after bariatric surgery, these results indicate stigma interventions may help treatment professionals identify psychosocial barriers to exercise engagement. The enduring influence of internalized weight-related stigma suggests that weight-stigma interventions might help patients meet physical activity goals at any stage after surgery, even years. This study also adds to a small but growing body of research [19, 26] demonstrating that weight stigma has important and direct negative effects on the physical health of people living with obesity, such as exercise aversion.

Our results are consistent with those of previous studies that show for people who consider themselves overweight, higher internalized stigma generates greater sensitivity to the effects of experienced stigma, making them more likely to avoid exercising and/or placing themselves in situations where experienced stigma is more likely (e.g., jogging in public, attending gyms or fitness classes) [18, 51]. In the context of our sample, higher levels of self-stigma cultivated by years spent living with high weight may generate far-reaching psychosocial effects that persist even despite significant weight loss following surgery, and these may manifest as a reluctance to engage in publically visible forms of activity [25, 52]. This is particularly important given research suggesting 200–300 min of weekly physical activity (including exercise) is necessary not only to lose weight, but to maintain weight loss over the long term [53, 54]. This is well over the often recommended 150 min of moderate-intensity physical activity to reduce health risks associated with obesity [55]. There are many known barriers to engagement in physical activity, the most common including lack of time or energy, health-related concerns (e.g., injury/fear of injury, poor health, or physical discomfort), lack of adequate social support (e.g., childcare, regular encouragement), lack of access to resources (e.g., gym, equipment, or training), and low exercise self-efficacy [56–61]. Importantly, several studies have shown a lack of motivation to be among the most prevalent reasons offered by respondents when asked why they did not engage in more physical activity [61, 62].

Our findings suggest that addressing weight stigma may help curtail this barrier. Intervention programs have successfully helped to reduce several such barriers and facilitate weight loss by targeting other psychosocial variables, such as physical activity self-efficacy or behaviors surrounding social support [63, 64]. Similar programs designed to reduce weight stigma may motivate bariatric surgery patients to be more physically active, which would help them achieve the greater overall health benefits to be gained from surgery in combination with regular exercise. As such, medical and healthcare professionals who support bariatric surgery patients may benefit from the development of pre- and post-operative programs designed to help patients cope with the psychological stresses and trauma that arose from negative interactions surrounding body size in tandem with promoting more positive views about the body and higher exercise self-efficacy [22, 64].

These results are also important for health and fitness experts who work in public spaces, particularly nonmedical facilities like gyms and fitness centers which have, in recent decades, increasingly emphasized a holistic focus on health and fitness, of which weight loss is a part [65]. To fully realize these fitness goals, it is necessary for activity centers to provide a welcoming environment that limits stigmatizing situations, ensuring that people of all body types can be motivated to exercise free from both direct and indirect forms of judgement. Habitual inactivity is considered a leading cause of non-communicable disease worldwide, with many such diseases being associated with higher weight (e.g., heart disease, high blood pressure, type two diabetes, or certain types of cancer) [66, 67]. An emphasis on cultivating stigma-free conditions in fitness centers could therefore have beneficial health outcomes for all individuals with relatively larger bodies, not just those who chose bariatric surgery as an option to manage their weight [68]. Such reduced-stigma activity centers may also lower certain barriers to physical activity and incentivize individuals to stick with long-term exercise goals even without active professional guidance.

There are several limitations to this study. First, the level of physical activity was reported in minutes as well as in days, but we could not use data reported in minutes because there were too many missing cases. Further, there remains little consensus on how to measure physical activity based on self-reported data, nor how to construct an index that reflects the combined effects of diverse activity types (e.g., vigorous and moderate physical activity and walking). Instead, a latent variable approach was used to measure physical activity based on three survey items. The World Health Organization (WHO) recommends all adults age between 18 and 65 should do at least 150 min of moderate physical activity, 75 min of vigorous physical activity, or an equivalent combination of moderate and vigorous physical activity on a weekly basis to stay healthy (more details on http://www. who.int/dietphysicalactivity/factsheet_adults/en. However, this validated index could not be used as a variable in the model due to missing cases and their negative effect on statistical power. In addition, over-reporting physical activity is a documented phenomenon especially among obese respondents, meaning the low level of reported moderate and vigorous physical activity may actually have been lower [51]. We are unsure of how systematically it was overestimated nor do we know the implication of this for the analysis. Future research could benefit from more detailed and sophisticated physical activity data collection, perhaps using passive forms of activity documentation (e.g., tracking devices, pedometers, accelerometers) that do not rely solely on self-reported estimates as these tend to be overestimated among bariatric surgery patients [35]. Second, because this project was cross-sectional in design, the findings from these results should be interpreted and discussed in terms of associations, not necessarily causations. A longitudinal study that tracks these variables as individuals move through the treatment program (e.g., pre-surgery to several years afterward) would greatly enhance our understanding of how the relationship between self-stigma, exercise avoidance, and physical activity shifts over time, particularly at the crucial 12–24 month postsurgical window when weight loss often stalls and the 2–5 year window when many patients experience weight regain [69]. This would highlight times at which certain interventions may be most beneficial. Additionally, research that focuses on developing interventions to help ameliorate the psychosocial effects of being/having been overweight would also be a logical extension of this work that may yield promising treatment outcomes for postsurgical patients specifically and weight-loss seeking individuals more generally. Third, BMI was calculated based on patients' self-reported height and weight at the time of survey, not objectively measured height and weight collected by trained researchers. Given consistent evidence that respondents tend to under-report weight and over-report height [70, 71], this is a potential limitation of the study. However, bariatric surgery patients may be more accurate in self-reporting BMI than are other populations [70]. Last, there was a wide range of time between surgery and survey across the study participants. There might be a significant difference in observed patterns of weight stigma, exercise avoidance, and physical activity between patients who recently underwent surgery and those who did so many years ago. Subgroup analysis could not be conducted with the data due to a relatively small sample size limiting statistical power of the analysis.

Conclusion

This study provides additional evidence that weight-related stigma has a likely effect on an individual's capacity to lose and maintain weight via physical activity, even when they are otherwise highly motivated to do so. While more research is needed, our findings suggest that a therapeutic program designed to reduce deeply held feelings of weight-related stigma and working to create judgement-free exercise spaces may indirectly improve weight loss by decreasing an individual's reluctance to engage in physical activity. Stigma-focused programs may therefore be a helpful complement the many nutrition- and exercised-focused programs traditionally offered to bariatric surgery patients.

Abbreviations

BMI: Body mass index; EAM: Exercise avoidance motivation; FIML: Full information maximum likelihood; MVPA: Moderate-to-vigorous physical activity; PA: Physical activity; SEM: Structural equation model; SSI: Stigmatizing situations inventory; WBIS: Weight bias internalization scale

Acknowledgements

We thank the Mayo Clinic Survey Research Center, Sarah Trainer, James Levine, Danielle Raves, Elizabeth Kurtz, Deborah Williams, and Erika Jermé for their various contributions to this study.

Funding

This research was supported by an award to the Obesity Solutions initiative by The Virginia G Piper Charitable Trust.

Authors' contributions

The authors' responsibilities were as follows – AB and AW designed the research study (including tools, sampling, ethics); SH managed the survey data and designed and conducted initial analysis with input from AB; GA assisted with re-analyses. All authors drafted, read, and approved the final manuscript; SH had primary responsibility for final content.

Competing interests

The authors declare that they have no competing interests.

Author details

[1]Mayo Clinic/Arizona State University Obesity Solutions, 1000 Cady Mall Suite 164, Tempe, AZ 85287, USA. [2]School of Human Evolution and Social Change, Arizona State University, 900 Cady Mall, Tempe, AZ 85287, USA.

References

1. Myers A, Rosen JC. Obesity stigmatization and coping: relation to mental health symptoms, body image, and self-esteem. Int J Obes. 1999;23:221–30.

2. Raves DM, Brewis A, Trainer S, Han SY, Wutich A. Bariatric surgery patients' perceptions of weight-related stigma in healthcare settings impair post-surgery dietary adherence. Front Psychol. 2016;7:1–13.

3. Papadopoulos S, Brennan L. Correlates of weight stigma in adults with overweight and obesity: a systematic literature review. Obesity. 2015;23: 1743–60.

4. Puhl RM, Heuer CA. Obesity stigma: important considerations for public health. Am J Public Health. 2010;100:1019–28.

5. Puhl RM, Heuer CA. The stigma of obesity: a review and update. Obesity. 2009;17:941–64.

6. Hatzenbuehler ML, Keyes KM, Hasin DS. Associations between perceived weight discrimination and the prevalence of psychiatric disorders in the general population. Obesity. 2009;17:2033–9.

7. Puhl RM, Brownell KD. Confronting and coping with weight stigma: an investigation of overweight and obese adults. Obesity. 2006;14:1802–15.

8. Haines J, Neumark-Sztainer D, Eisenberg ME, Hannan PJ. Weight teasing and disordered eating behaviors in adolescents: longitudinal findings from project EAT (eating among teens). Pediatrics. 2006;117: e209–15.

9. Hackman J, Maupin J, Brewis A. Weight-related stigma is a significant psychosocial stressor in developing countries: evidence from Guatemala. Soc Sci Med. 2016;161:55–60.

10. Lewis S, Thomas SL, Blood RW, Castle DJ, Hyde J, Komesaroff PA. How do obese individuals perceive and respond to the different types of obesity stigma that they encounter in their daily lives? A qualitative study. Soc Sci Med. 2011;73:1349–56.

11. Li W, Rukavina P. A review on coping mechanisms against obesity bias in physical activity/education settings. Obes Rev. 2009;10:87–95.

12. Corrigan PW, Watson AC. The paradox of self-stigma and mental illness. Clin Psychol. 2002;9(1):35–53.

13. Corrigan PW, Watson AC, Barr L. The self–stigma of mental illness: implications for self–esteem and self–efficacy. J Soc Clin Psychol. 2006; 25(8):875–84.

14. Puhl RM, Moss-Racusin CA, Schwartz MB. Internalization of weight bias: implications for binge eating and emotional well-being. Obesity. 2007; 15(1):19–23.

15. Carels RA, Young KM, Wott CB, Harper J, Gumble A, Oehlof MW, Clayton AM. Weight bias and weight loss treatment outcomes in treatment-seeking adults. Ann Behav Med. 2009;37(3):350–5.

16. Tomiyama AJ. Weight stigma is stressful. A review of evidence for the cyclic obesity/weight-based stigma model. Appetite. 2014;82:8–15.

17. Mensinger JL, Calogero RM, Tylka TL. Internalized weight stigma moderates eating behavior outcomes in women with high BMI participating in a healthy living program. Appetite. 2016;102:32–43.

18. Vartanian LR, Novak SA. Internalized societal attitudes moderate the impact of weight stigma on avoidance of exercise. Obesity. 2011;19:757–62.

19. Brewis AA. Stigma and the perpetuation of obesity. Soc Sci Med. 2014; 118:152–8.

20. Vartanian LR, Shaprow JG. Effects of weight stigma on exercise motivation and behavior a preliminary investigation among college-aged females. J Health Psychol. 2008;13:131–8.

21. Pearl RL, Puhl RM, Dovidio JF. Differential effects of weight bias experiences and internalization on exercise among women with overweight and obesity. J Health Psychol. 2015;20:1626–32.

22. Mensinger JL, Meadows A. Internalized weight stigma mediates and moderates physical activity outcomes during a healthy living program for women with high body mass index. Psychol Sport Exerc. 2017;30: 64–72.

23. Hübner C, Baldofski S, Zenger M, Tigges W, Herbig B, Jurowich C, Kaiser S, Dietrich A, Hilbert A. Influences of general self-efficacy and weight bias internalization on physical activity in bariatric surgery candidates. Surg Obes Relat Dis. 2015;11(6):1371–6.

24. Major B, Eliezer D, Rieck H. The psychological weight of weight stigma. Soc Psychol Personal Sci. 2012;3:651–8.

25. Granberg EM. Now my 'old self' is thin: stigma exits after weight loss. Soc Psychol Q. 2011;74:29–52.

26. Wott CB, Carels RA. Overt weight stigma, psychological distress and weight loss treatment outcomes. J Health Psychol. 2010;15(4):608–14.

27. Corrigan PW, Larson JE, Ruesch N. Self-stigma and the "why try" effect: impact on life goals and evidence-based practices. World Psychiatry. 2009;8(2):75–81.

28. Friedman KE, Ashmore JA, Applegate KL. Recent experiences of weight-based stigmatization in a weight loss surgery population: psychological and behavioral correlates. Obesity. 2008;16:S69–74.

29. Rand CS, Macgregor AM. Morbidly obese patients' perceptions of social discrimination before and after surgery for obesity. South Med J. 1990; 83(12):1390–5.

30. Crocker J, Major B. Social stigma and self-esteem: the self-protective properties of stigma. Psychol Rev. 1989;96(4):608.

31. Pomeranz JL. A historical analysis of public health, the law, and stigmatized social groups: the need for both obesity and weight bias legislation. Obesity. 2008;16(S2):S93–S103.

32. Mechanick JI, Youdim A, Jones DB, Garvey WT, Hurley DL, McMahon MM, et al. Clinical practice guidelines for the perioperative nutritional, metabolic, and nonsurgical support of the bariatric surgery patient—2013 update: cosponsored by American Association of Clinical Endocrinologists, the Obesity Society, and American Society for Metabolic & bariatric surgery. Obesity. 2013;21:S1–27.

33. Egberts K, Brown WA, Brennan L, O'Brien PE. Does exercise improve weight loss after bariatric surgery? A systematic review. Obes Surg. 2012;22:335–41.

34. Haskell WL, Lee IM, Pate RR, Powell KE, Blair SN, Franklin BA, Macera CA, Heath GW, Thompson PD, Bauman A. Physical activity and public health: updated recommendation for adults from the American College of Sports Medicine and the American Heart Association. Circulation. 2007;116:1081–93.

35. Bond DS, Jakicic JM, Unick JL, Vithiananthan S, Pohl D, Roye GD, Ryder BA, Sax HC, Wing RR. Pre-to postoperative physical activity changes in bariatric surgery patients: self report vs. objective measures. Obesity. 2010;18(12):2395–7.

36. Weinsier RL, Hunter GR, Desmond RA, Byrne NM, Zuckerman PA, Darnell BE. Free-living activity energy expenditure in women successful and unsuccessful at maintaining a normal body weight. Am J Clin Nutr. 2002;75:499–504.

37. Wing RR, Hill JO. Successful weight loss maintenance. Annu Rev Nutr. 2001;21:323–41.

38. Klem ML, Wing RR, Lang W, McGuire MT, Hill JO. Does weight loss maintenance become easier over time? Obes Res. 2000;8:438–44.

39. Schoeller DA, Shay K, Kushner RF. How much physical activity is needed to minimize weight gain in previously obese women? Am J Clin Nutr. 1997;66:551–6.

40. Bond DS, Thomas JG, Ryder BA, Vithiananthan S, Pohl D, Wing RR. Ecological momentary assessment of the relationship between intention and physical activity behavior in bariatric surgery patients. Int J Behav Med. 2013;20:82–7.

41. Elkins G, Whitfield P, Marcus J, Symmonds R, Rodriguez J, Cook T. Noncompliance with behavioral recommendations following bariatric surgery. Obes Surg. 2005;15:546–51.

42. Toussi R, Fujioka K, Coleman KJ. Pre-and postsurgery behavioral compliance, patient health, and postbariatric surgical weight loss. Obesity. 2009;17(5):996–1002.

43. Peacock JC, Sloan SS, Cripps B. A qualitative analysis of bariatric patients' post-surgical barriers to exercise. Obes Surg. 2014;24:292–8.

44. Livhits M, Mercado C, Yermilov I, Parikh JA, Dutson E, Mehran A, Ko CY, Gibbons MM. Exercise following bariatric surgery: systematic review. Obes Surg. 2010;20(5):657–65.

45. Wallace AE, Young-Xu Y, Hartley D, Weeks WB. Racial, socioeconomic, and rural–urban disparities in obesity-related bariatric surgery. Obes Surg. 2010;20:1354–60.

46. Allison PD. Missing data techniques for structural equation modeling. J Abnorm Psychol. 2003;112:545–57.

47. Kenny DA. Correlation and causality. New York: Wiley; 1979.

48. Durso LE, Latner JD. Understanding self-directed stigma: development of the weight bias internalization scale. Obesity. 2008;16(S2):S80–6.

49. Hilbert A, Braehler E, Haeuser W, Zenger M. Weight bias internalization, core self-evaluation, and health in overweight and obese persons. Obesity. 2014;22:79–85.

50. Major B, Tomiyama AJ, Hunger, JM. Chapter 27: The Negative and Bi-Directional Effects of Weight Stigma on Health. In: B Major, J Dovidio, B Link (Eds.) Oxford Handbook of Stigma, Discrimination, and Health. 2017.

51. Packer J. The role of stigmatization in fat people's avoidance of physical exercise. Women & Therapy. 1989;8(3):49–63.

52. Brewis A, Trainer S, Han SY, Wutich A. Publically misfitting: extreme weight and the everyday production and reinforcement of felt stigma. Med Anthropol Q. 2016; https://doi.org/10.1111/maq.12309.

53. Jakicic JM. Appropriate intervention strategies for weight loss and prevention of weight regain in adults. American college of sports medicine. Med Sci Sports Exerc. 2001;33:2145–56.

54. Saris WH, Blair SN, Van Baak MA, Eaton SB, Davies PS, Di Pietro L, Fogelholm M, Rissanen A, Schoeller D, Swinburn B, Tremblay A. How much physical activity is enough to prevent unhealthy weight gain? Outcome of the IASO 1st stock conference and consensus statement. Obes Rev. 2003;4(2):101–14.

55. Physical Activity Guidelines Advisory Committee. Physical activity guidelines for Americans. Washington: US Department of Health and Human Services; 2008. Retrieved from https://health.gov/paguidelines/report/

56. Chang MW, Nitzke S, Guilford E, Adair CH, Hazard DL. Motivators and barriers to healthful eating and physical activity among low-income overweight and obese mothers. J Am Diet Assoc. 2008;108(6):1023–8.

57. Hoebeke R. Low-income women's perceived barriers to physical activity: focus group results. Appl Nurs Res. 2008;21(2):60–5.

58. Bauman AE, Reis RS, Sallis JF, Wells JC, Loos RJ, Martin BW, Lancet Physical Activity Series Working Group. Correlates of physical activity: why are some people physically active and others not? Lancet. 2012;380(9838):258–71.

59. Picorelli AM, Pereira LS, Pereira DS, Felício D, Sherrington C. Adherence to exercise programs for older people is influenced by program characteristics and personal factors: a systematic review. J Phys. 2014;60(3):151–6.

60. McGuire A, Seib C, Anderson D. Factors predicting barriers to exercise in midlife Australian women. Maturitas. 2016;87:61–6.

61. Herazo-Beltrán Y, Pinillos Y, Vidarte J, Crissien E, Suarez D, García R. Predictors of perceived barriers to physical activity in the general adult population: a cross-sectional study. Brazilian J Phys Ther. 2017;21(1):44–50.

62. Booth ML, Bauman A, Owen N, Gore CJ. Physical activity preferences, preferred sources of assistance, and perceived barriers to increased activity among physically inactive Australians. Prev Med. 1997;26(1):131–7.

63. Gallagher KI, Jakicic JM, Napolitano MA, Marcus BH. Psychosocial factors related to physical activity and weight loss in overweight women. Med Sci Sports Exerc. 2006;38(5):971–80.

64. Lee LL, Arthur A, Avis M. Using self-efficacy theory to develop interventions that help older people overcome psychological barriers to physical activity: a discussion paper. Int J Nurs Stud. 2008;45(11):1690–9.

65. Andreasson J, Johansson T. The fitness revolution. Historical transformations in the global gym and fitness culture. Sport Sci Rev. 2014;23(3–4):91–111.

66. Booth M. Assessment of physical activity: an international perspective. Res Q Exerc Sport. 2000;71(sup2):114–20.

67. Kohl HW, Craig CL, Lambert EV, Inoue S, Alkandari JR, Leetongin G, Kahlmeier S, Lancet Physical Activity Series Working Group. The pandemic of physical inactivity: global action for public health. Lancet. 2012;380(9838): 294–305.

68. Reiner M, Niermann C, Jekauc D, Woll A. Long-term health benefits of physical activity–a systematic review of longitudinal studies. BMC Public Health. 2013;13(1):813.

69. Magro DO, Geloneze B, Delfini R, Pareja BC, Callejas F, Pareja JC. Long-term weight regain after gastric bypass: a 5-year prospective study. Obes Surg. 2008;18(6):648–51.

70. Christian NJ, King WC, Yanovski SZ, Courcoulas AP, Belle SH. Validity of self-reported weights following bariatric surgery. J Am Med Assoc. 2013;310: 2454–6.

71. Gorber SC, Tremblay M, Moher D, Gorber B. A comparison of direct vs. self-report measures for assessing height, weight, and body mass index: a systematic review. Obes Rev. 2007;8:307–26.

10

Cultural differences in food and shape related attitudes and eating behavior are associated with differences of Body Mass Index in the same food environment: cross-sectional results from the Seafarer Nutrition Study of Kiribati and European seafarers on merchant ships

Joachim Westenhoefer[1]* ⓘ, Robert von Katzler[2], Hans-Joachim Jensen[2], Birgit-Christiane Zyriax[3], Bettina Jagemann[4], Volker Harth[2] and Marcus Oldenburg[2]

Abstract

Background: Overweight and obesity is quite prevalent among seafarers. The present study examined differences in BMI and their association with weight, shape and nutrition related attitudes and perceptions among seafarer from Kiribati, a Pacific Island Group, and European origin.

Methods: The Seafarer Nutrition Study compared 48 Kiribati and 33 European male seafarers from 4 commercial merchant ships. BMI was calculated from measured weight and height. Attitudes to weight, shape and nutrition and disinhibition of control as a characteristic of eating behavior were assessed in a structured interview. Differences between the two groups were examined using t-tests and Chi-square-tests as appropriate. Associations between the variables were examined using Multiple Regression Analysis (MRA) and correlations.

Results: Kiribati seafarer had significantly higher BMI than Europeans (30.3 ± 4.2 vs. 25.6 ± 3.4; $p < 0.001$). However, MRA indicated that Kiribati were choosing thinner shapes as being "most similar" to their appearance than Europeans with the same BMI (B = − 1.14; $p < 0.05$). In addition, Kiribati had significantly higher scores of disinhibition than Europeans (5.6 ± 2.2 vs. 4.3 ± 2.1; $p < 0.01$), and disinhibition correlated with BMI in the Kiribati ($r = 0.39$; $p < 0.01$), but not in the European group ($r = 0.17$; n.s.).

Conclusions: For Kiribati seafarers the nutrition situation on board represents a highly tempting westernized food environment. Their tendency to disinhibited eating facilitates overconsumption and weight gain, and self-evaluation of their shapes as being thinner than comparable Europeans may hamper appropriate weight control behavior.

Keywords: Obesity, Pacific islanders, Body shape, Eating behavior, Disinhibition, Seafarer

* Correspondence: joachim@westenhoefer.de
[1]Competence Center Health, Department Health Sciences, Hamburg University of Applied Science, Ulmenliet 20, 21033 Hamburg, Germany
Full list of author information is available at the end of the article

Background

Several studies have shown that overweight, obesity and cardio-metabolic risk factors are quite prevalent among seafarers [1–5].

The situation on board of commercial merchant ships is characterized by limited individual influence on the quality and variety of the diet, because crew members often stay aboard of the vessels for months, and shore leaves are rare and short. Therefore the possibility to buy food is restricted and the nutrition is largely limited to what is offered on board. Likewise, leisure time physical activity is mainly restricted to voluntary exercise in fitness rooms as recreational walking or cycling for longer distances is not possible on board of a ship.

Nevertheless, there seem to be marked differences in the prevalence of obesity and associated risk factors between crew members with different cultural and/or ethnic background working on the same ships and hence in the same environment. A German shipping company reported that particularly crew members from Kiribati, a Pacific island group, experience significant weight gain and possibly impaired cardio-vascular health (personal communication).

This informal observation is in line with the fact that obesity and associated non-communicable diseases, particularly diabetes, present a prevalent and urgent public health problem in the Pacific Region [6]. On Kiribati, 76.5% of adult men are overweight or obese (BMI ≥ 25), among them 39.3% who are obese (BMI ≥ 30). Among adult women 81.8% are overweight or obese and 55.5% are obese [7]. While genetic factors may play an important role for these high prevalences, also cultural factors might be involved in influencing food choices.

Traditionally, large body sizes were positively valued and encouraged in Pacific Island societies. They were associated with wealth, health and beauty [8, 9]. Cortes et al. [8] for example reported that on the Marshall Islands a common greeting has been: "Oh you look good; you look fatter than you did before". However, these cultural values and perceptions of body size have changed considerably during westernization in the recent decades [9, 10].

A comparison of Samoan and Australian women with similar BMI [11] showed that Samoan woman had similar feelings of fatness as Australian women. However they showed less salience of fatness, felt more attractive and experienced more strength and fitness. While Samoan women had stronger feelings of body disparagement than Australian women, body disparagement was not correlated with BMI in Samoan women whereas is was in Australian women. Brewis et al. [12] reported that Samoan men and women have high levels of obesity, but slim body ideals. However, even when obese they were positive about their body size and weight. A study

in the late 1990s reported that both, men and women from the Marshall Islands feel that healthy bodies are larger bodies, whereas thinner bodies are more attractive [8]. More recently, a study found that ratings of attractiveness of women with different BMIs by British and Samoan male adolescents did not differ [13]. The authors concluded that the traditional veneration of large body sizes is not any longer present in the younger generation of Samoan people.

With regard to eating behavior, research has shown that the "disinhibition of control" [14] is consistently associated with weight gain, higher BMI, less healthful food choices and eating disorders like Bulimia nervosa or Binge Eating Disorder [15]. The disinhibition of control reflects the tendency to overeat in response to environmental stimuli (e.g. sight or smell of food, company of others) or emotional stimuli (e.g. anxiety, feeling blue). Therefor we use "disinhibition" and "tendency to overeat" interchangeably in this paper (see methods section). To the best of our knowledge, it has not been investigated whether this characteristic of eating behavior is associated with the high prevalence of obesity in the pacific region.

Therefore the aim of the present study was to examine potential differences in food and shape related attitudes and differences in eating behavior that might contribute to weight gain and obesity in Kiribati seafarers as opposed to seafarers with European origin. Particularly, we assumed that Europeans and Kiribati differed in the relationship between body mass and attitudes to body shape. In addition, we hypothesized that Kiribati could be characterized by a stronger tendency to overeat. And finally, we assumed that being exposed to a western food environment on board as opposed to the traditional Pacific food habits is a tempting situation and prompts the Kiribati seafarers to eat more than at home.

Methods
Sample

The 81 seafarers participating in this study came from four cargo vessels belonging to a shipping company with a large number of Kiribati crew members. All explored ships were container ships of similar size (mean 99,400 GT) and had a transatlantic route. The participation rate for this study was 90.9%. Five women and four Africans, as well as one person of Asian origin who were on board of the vessels were excluded from the analysis because we felt that five or less subjects per group was not a sufficient sample size to form a meaningful group for the further analyses of group differences. This resulted in two homogeneous male groups: 48 participants with a Kiribati origin and 33 Europeans.

The participation in this study was voluntary and participants gave their written informed consent. The study protocol was approved by the Ethics committee of Medical Association Hamburg.

Measures

All measures and interviews were taken on board of the ships. Weight and height of the participants was measured during harbor stays. The interviews were conducted between the 2nd and the 7th day of a transatlantic sea trip during the leisure time of the seafarers. They took place in a separate room with only the interviewer (RvK) and the interviewee present to assure privacy.

Weight and height was measured using standard procedures. Body Mass Index was calculated as BMI = kg/m^2. A BMI of 25 and more was considered as overweight, a BMI of 30 or more as obese.

Several attitudes regarding weight and shape were assessed in a structured interview with the following questions. Self-evaluation of body weight was assessed with the question "What do you think about your weight? Are you ... much too thin – a little bit too thin – just the right weight – a little bit too fat – much too fat". Answers were scored 1 (much too thin) to 5 (much too fat). Attitudes towards body shape were assessed using a body shape scale [16] which shows 9 different male shapes ranging from thin to obese (see Fig. 1). Subjects were asked to identify the picture that "is most similar to your current shape" (most similar shape), "is most similar to your most desired shape" (most desired shape), "is the most respected shape for a man in your country" (most respected shape), is "the most healthy shape for a man" (most healthy shape). The answers were scored on a rating scale ranging from 1 to 9. If subjects had difficulties to answer the questions on the desired shape and the most respected shape spontaneously, the interviewer explained that "most desired shape" means, what oneself ideally would like to look like oneself, whereas "most respected" refers to what the others in one's country of origin value most.

The tendency to overeat can be reliably measured with the "disinhibition of control" subscale from the Eating Inventory which often is called Three-Factor Eating Questionnaire TFEQ [14]. This subscale comprises 16 items that address the tendency to overeat in response to environmental stimuli (e.g. sight or smell of food, company of others) or emotional stimuli (e.g. anxiety, feeling blue). It has been originally named "disinhibition of control", because people trying to restrict their food intake in order to reduce weight or to maintain their weight, so called restrained eaters, often give up their restricted eating behavior in response to such stimuli. From this scale a score is computed that ranges from 0 to 16 with higher scores representing a stronger tendency to overeat. Results related to this facet of eating behavior will be labeled as "disinhibited eating behavior" within the current paper. In order to avoid overly burden for the subjects we used only the disinhibition subscale and omitted the other two subscales (restrained eating and hunger).

In order to collect information about the different views on the nutrition and food situation, a couple of single choice questions were asked in the interview: "Are you satisfied with the supply of food you have on board?", "Compared to your nutrition at home, do you eat on board ... More/Less/To a similar level?", "Are the foods you receive on board according to your taste?"; "Is the amount of food receiving on your vessel sufficient for you?"; "Does your cook take the preparation of foods for different nationalities into account?" "Is the nutrition on board rich in variety?"

In addition, with regard to the particular food situation on board of the merchant ships, the following open-ended questions were asked in the interview: [1] What do you like most with regard to food and eating on board? [2] Are there things with regard to food and eating that you don't like or find disturbing? [3] If you compare food and eating with the situation at home: what are you missing most? [4] And again, if you compare food and eating with the situation at home: is there

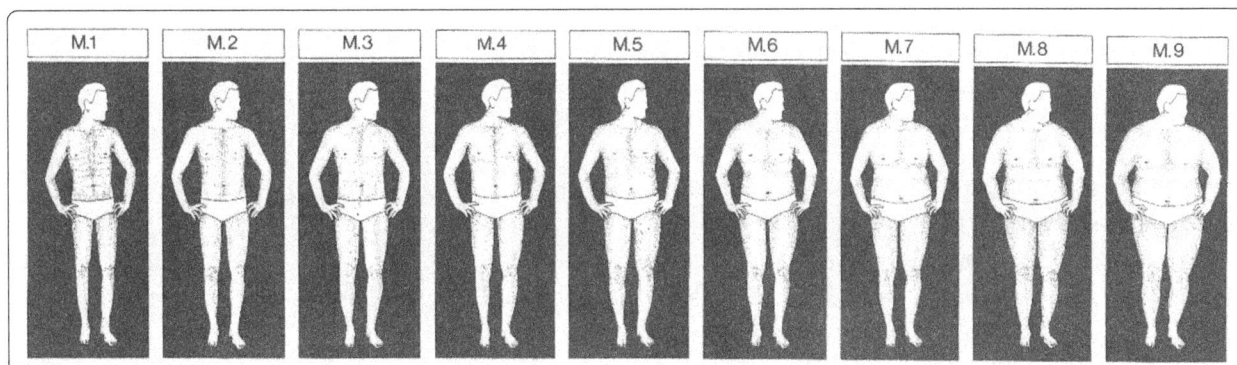

Fig. 1 Body shape picture scale. This figure was reproduced from [16] with permission from Deutsche Gesellschaft für Ernährung e.V

anything that is better on board than at home? The answers to these questions were protocolled verbatim. Using a content analytic approach categories were built by one Author (RvK) [17]: Similar answers were grouped together and a category name was assigned summarizing and abstracting the common content of the answers. The answers were then categorized independently by two raters (RvK and MO). Comparing the results showed an agreement of 95%. Answers without agreement regarding the categorization were excluded from the further analysis.

Statistical analysis

Statistical analyses were computed using IBM SPSS Version 22.0. Descriptive statistics are reported as mean ± standard deviation. Differences between means were tested using the t-test. Differences in frequency distributions of nominal scale variables were examined using the Chi-square test or Fisher's exact test were appropriate. Correlations between two variables were examined using Pearson correlation coefficients. The relationship of one dependent variable to two or more (potential) predictor variables was analyzed using multiple regression analysis with all predictors simultaneously entered. Thus, the relationship of the different shape ratings (dependent variables) to BMI, ethnic group and their interaction (predictors) was analyzed using multiple regression analysis with the predictors centered BMI, dummy coded ethnic group (0 = European, 1 = Kiribati) and the product term of the two for the interaction [18, 19]. We used this type of analysis particularly in order to study whether there was an interaction between ethnicity and BMI in predicting the different shape ratings. This would imply that the slope of the relation of BMI to shape ratings is modified by ethnicity. The significance level for all analyses was set to alpha = 0.05.

Results

The sample consisted of 81 male seafarers, 33 with European and 48 of Kiribati origin. Age did not differ significantly between the European and the Kiribati group (36.8 ± 12.8 resp. 38.9 ± 11.0 years).

Body Mass Index and Attitudes to Weight and Shape.

Kiribati seafarers and European seafarers differed significantly with respect to BMI (see Table 1). Only 8.3% of the Kiribati were normal weight, 39.6% were overweight but not obese, and 52.1% were obese. In contrast, 48.5% of the Europeans were normal weight, 42.4% overweight but not obese, and only 9.1% were obese.

However, both groups did not differ significantly with regard to the self-evaluation of their weight. The mean BMI of the 14 European seafarers who considered themselves as "little bit too fat" or "much too fat" was 28.0 ± 3.3 (range 23.6–35.0), whereas the mean BMI of the 26 Kiribati seafarers who considered themselves as a little or much too fat was 32.5 ± 3.7 (range 25.5–40.5; $p < 0.01$). There was also no significant difference between the two cultural-ethnic groups with regard to the self-evaluation of the "most similar shape" figure. Regression analysis (see Table 1) revealed that the self-evaluation of the "most similar shape" was significantly associated with current BMI. The non-significant interaction indicated that regression slopes in the two cultural-ethnic groups were identical. The significant regression coefficient for the cultural-ethnic group indicated that, on average, Kiribati were choosing the image that was one level smaller than Europeans with the same BMI (see Fig. 2).

The shapes that were selected as the "most healthy" shape were not significantly different between Kiribati and European seafarers, but there were significant differences regarding the "most desirable shape" for oneself and the "most respected shape" in the country of origin. While Kiribati nominated smaller shapes as

Table 1 BMI, self-evaluation of weight and ratings of the most similar shape, the most desirable shape, most respected shape in the country of origin and most healthy shape: Descriptive statistics (Means ± SD and results from t-tests) and regression coefficients from the multiple regression analysis (MRA) of shape ratings (dependent variables) on ethnic-cultural group (0 = European; 1 = Kiribati), centered BMI and interaction term (predictors)

| | Range | Means ± SD | | Raw regression coefficients B from multiple regression analysis | | |
| | | | | Predictors for MRAs | | |
		European	Kiribati	Ethnic Group	BMI	Interaction
BMI		25.6 ± 3,4	30.3 ± 4.2 ***			
Self-evaluation of weight	1–5	3.5 ± 0.8	3.5 ± 0.8			
Dependent variables for MRAs						
Most similar shape	1–9	4.3 ± 1.6	4.7 ± 1.8	− 1.14 *	0.34 *	−0.01
Most desirable shape	1–9	3.6 ± 1.1	2.8 ± 1.3 *	− 1.08 *	0.09	− 0.02
Most respected shape	1–9	4.2 ± 1.3	6.7 ± 2.1 ***	2.85 *	0.04	−0.17
Most healthy shape	1–9	3.2 ± 1.3	2.5 ± 1.6	−0.44	− 0.06	0.04

* $p < 0.05$; *** $p < 0.001$

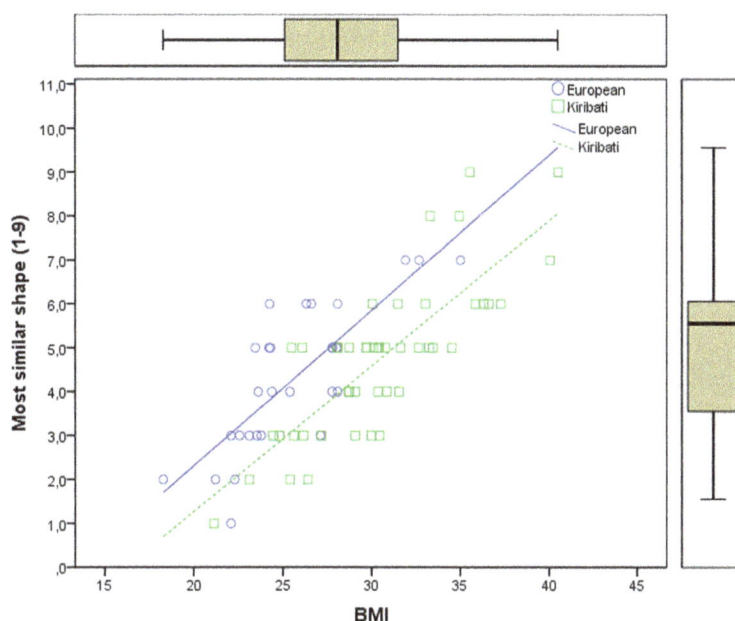

Fig. 2 Scatterplot and regression lines of the ratings of the most similar body shape using the body shape picture scale on Body Mass Index BMI

"most desirable" compared to Europeans, they nominated considerably larger shapes as the "most respected" ones. As a result the difference between the most desirable and the most respected shape was significantly larger (close to three levels) for Kiribati seafarers than for Europeans ($p < 0.001$). Regression analyses showed that the attitudes regarding the most healthy, most desirable and the most respected shapes were not associated with current BMI or with the interaction between BMI and cultural ethnic groups.

Eating Behavior and attitudes to nutrition and food.

Kiribati had significantly higher disinhibition scores than Europeans (5.6 ± 2.2 vs. 4.3 ± 2.1; $p < 0.01$). In addition, BMI was significantly correlated with disinhibition in the Kiribati group ($r = 0.39$; $p < 0.01$), but not in the European group ($r = 0.17$; n.s.) (see Fig. 3).

Kiribati seafarers reported significantly more often than Europeans to be satisfied with the food supply on board and to eat more on board than at home (Fig. 4). However, there were no significant differences between the two groups with regard to the tastiness of the meals ($p = 0.077$) and whether the amount of food is acceptable ($p = 0.65$; data not shown). Furthermore, Kiribati and Europeans differed significantly in their opinion whether the cooks prepare special meals for the different nations on board and in their appraisal of the variety of the food in the meals (Fig. 4). Particularly striking is the high portion of Kiribati who state that they don't know whether meals include a variety of foods.

The relative frequency of the categorized answers to the open questions regarding food and eating on board is shown in Fig. 5. Kiribati mentioned significantly more often than Europeans meat and fish dishes as things they like most. Correspondingly, also one third of the Kiribati, but none of the Europeans mentioned meat dishes as being better on board than at home. In addition, Kiribati mentioned more often meeting with others during meals as something they appreciate. Three quarters of the Kiribati stated that they were missing traditional dishes and fresh products on board, whereas Europeans were missing self-determination and the company of friends and family more often. Last, not least, Europeans appreciated several aspects of convenience of the eating situation considerably more often than Kiribati.

Discussion

Despite living, working and eating in the same food environment for most of the time, namely on commercial merchant ships, there are marked differences in Body Mass Index between Kiribati and European seafarers. The present study examined attitudes and perceptions related to weight, shape, eating and food for differences between the two cultural-ethnic groups and their association to the Body Mass Index.

In summary, the present study found that despite being considerably heavier than Europeans Kiribati perceive their weight and shape as being on the same level as the Europeans. When selecting pictures from the Body Shape Scale representing their appearance, on

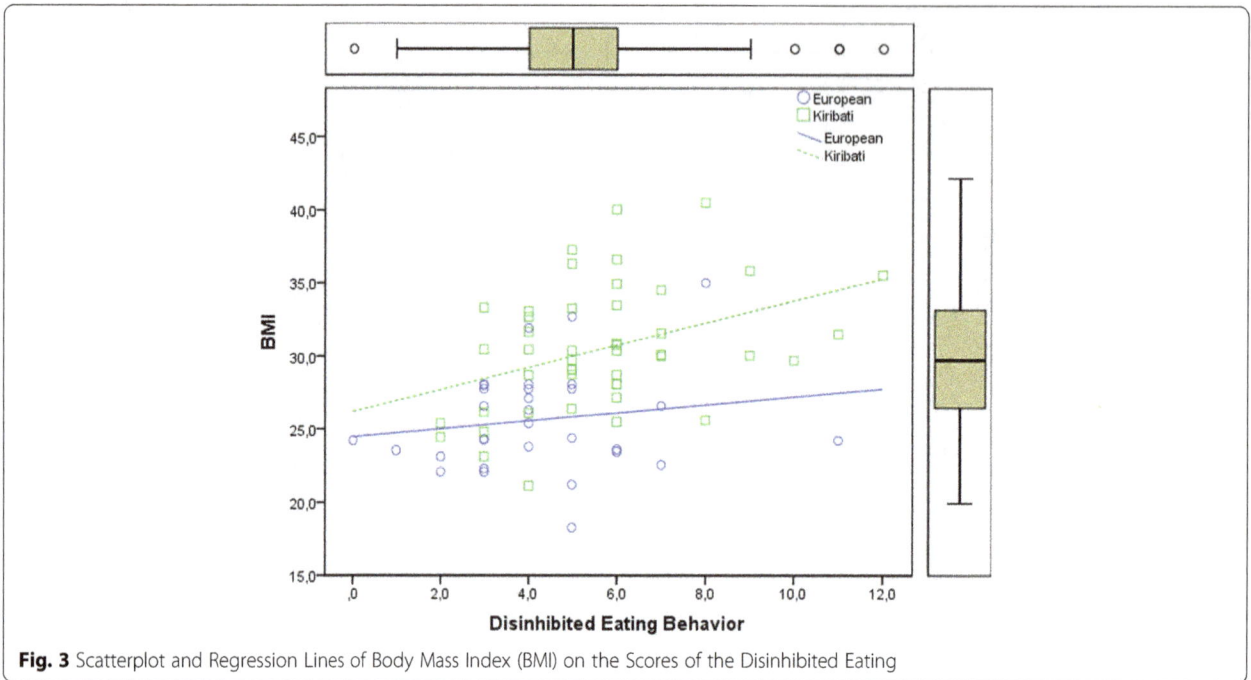

Fig. 3 Scatterplot and Regression Lines of Body Mass Index (BMI) on the Scores of the Disinhibited Eating

average they select thinner shapes than Europeans with the same BMI. Likewise, Europeans considering themselves as being "too fat" have significantly lower BMIs than Kiribati considering themselves as being "too fat". Compared to Europeans, Kiribati nominate thinner body shapes as "most desirable" for a man, but larger shapes as the "most respected" shape in their home country. The question on the "most desired shape" was intended to elicit the view about what the subject himself perceives as an ideal shape for himself, whereas the question of the "most respected shape" was intended to elicit the subjects view about social norms in his country of origin. The difference in the answers to the two questions indicates that the subjects indeed recognized these different perspectives. Thus, the present findings about the "desirable" shape are in line with results from other pacific islands that found that both men and women attributed attractiveness to thinner bodies [8]. The views of Kiribati on the most respected shape reflect the more traditional veneration of large body size in Pacific populations. Such valuation with regard to men seems to persist to a certain degree at least in adult males. This observation questions the idea that such veneration is not any longer present [13].

The higher BMI of Kiribati seafarers corresponds with a significantly higher level of disinhibited eating which reflects the tendency to overeat in response to environmental and emotional stimuli. In addition, the disinhibition of eating behavior correlates with BMI in the Kiribati group, but not in the European group.

The tendency to overeat in response to environmental stimuli could be particularly important, given the finding that the majority of Kiribati reports that they eat more on board than at home, and that they are more satisfied with the nutrition situation on board of the vessels than the Europeans. Particularly, the Kiribati enjoy the availability of meat dishes and fish and they value the social company with others during meals more than the Europeans. Thus, overall it seems that Kiribati experience the food and nutrition environment on board very positive, and this might be potentially stimulating appetite. However, the vast majority of Kiribati is missing traditional dishes and fresh products, and they feel more often than Europeans that food preparation does not take differences between nationalities into account. Hence, Kiribati seem to experience the nutrition situation on board as foreign, but overall quite positive and appetizing for them. This in turn might predispose them to overeating and weight gain.

In addition, differences in the social environment on board from the situation at home could contribute to differences in eating behavior and food intake. Kiribati are considered to be a sociable population group who appreciate meals together with others as an important element of their cultural tradition [20]. The average household has 7 or more members and common meals at home play an essential role in social relationships and familial tradition [21]. In contrast, meals on board are offered in the crew's messroom in immediate vicinity of the working place. Mealtimes are entirely determined by work requirements. Meals are nearly always eaten

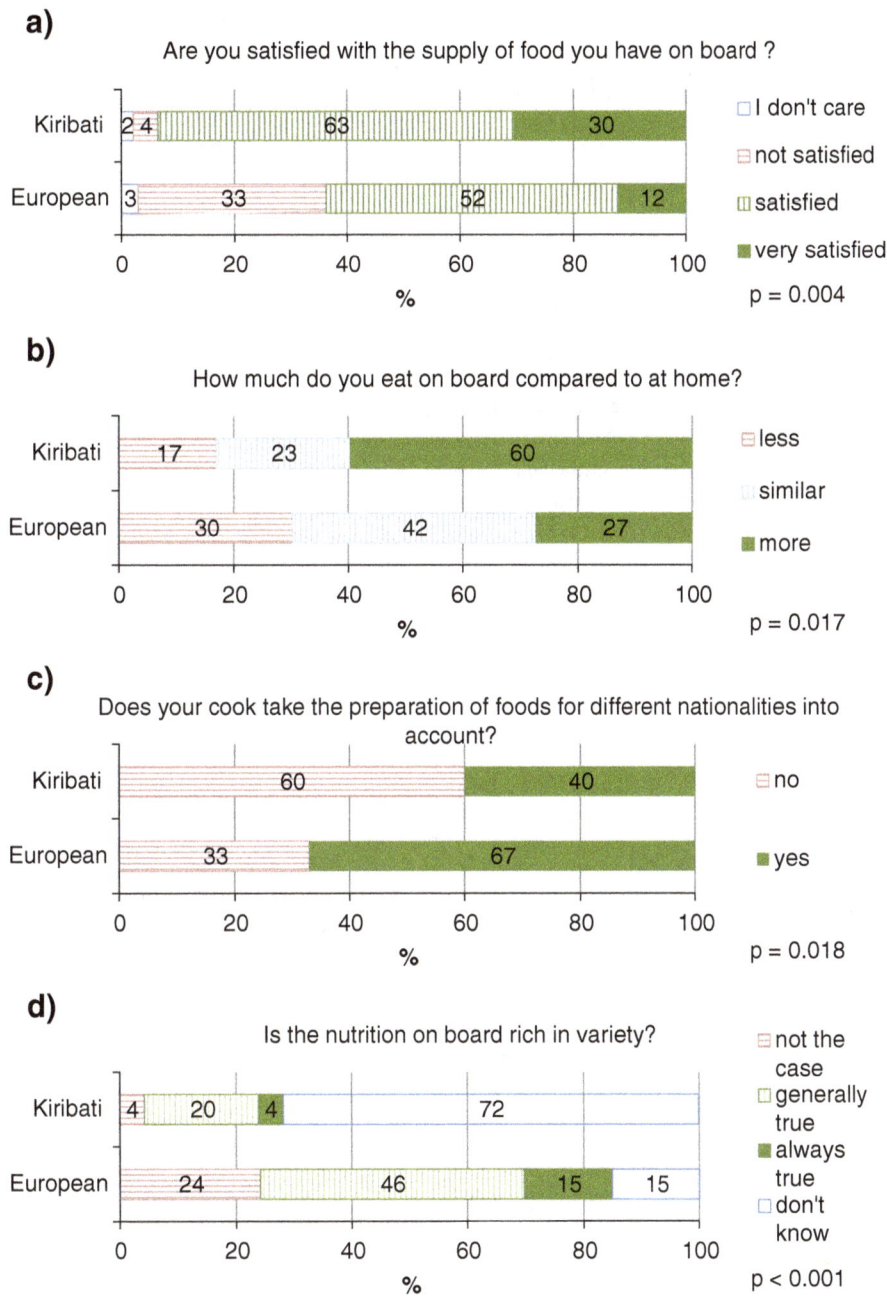

Fig. 4 Evaluation of food and nutrition situation on board of commercial merchant ships by European and Kiribati seafarers. **a** Are you satisfied with the supply of food you have on board? **b** How much do you eat on board compared to at home? **c** Does your cook take the preparation of foods for different nationalities into. **d** Is the nutrition on board rich in variety? account?

together with other crew members who are determined by working conditions, not by familial relations. Preparing own meals is impossible.

In contrast, European seafarers value particularly the convenience aspects of the nutrition situation (being served, no need of cooking, shopping, washing up), but are more unsatisfied with the lack of self-determination regarding food and the restricted choice they have on board. These negative experiences are nearly unmentioned by the Kiribati. Taken together, the findings from the present study suggest that the more western food environment on commercial merchant ships prompts Kiribati seafarers to eat more than at home, enjoying particularly meals with meat. This environment could trigger higher food intakes particularly in view of the higher responsiveness of Kiribati to such environmental stimuli.

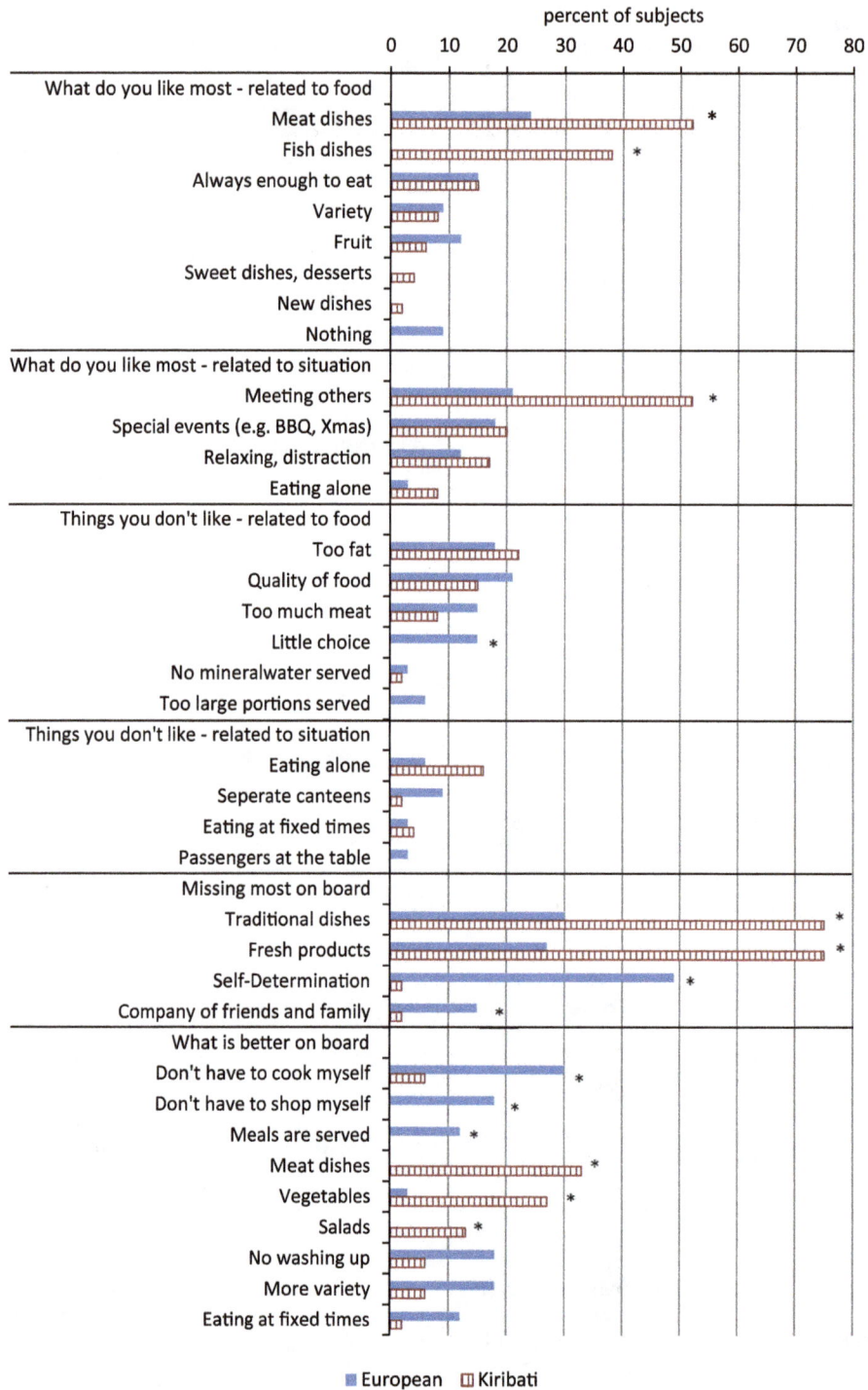

Fig. 5 Percentage of categorized answers to open questions about food and eating on board of commercial merchant ships. Significant differences (p < 0.05) between European and Kiribati seafarers are marked with *

The views of a healthy body shape, and presumably weight, are not much different for Kiribati and Europeans; the desirable shape is even thinner for the Kiribati. However, given the cultural valuation of the larger body shape in Kiribati, they perceive themselves as thinner as Europeans with the same BMI. Such differences in self-evaluation could prevent appropriate adjustment of eating and activity behavior in order to prevent weight gain.

The present study has some underlying limitations which have to be considered when interpreting results and drawing conclusions. First of all, we studied a relatively small sample of 33 European and 48 Kiribati male seafarers. Hence, findings and conclusions have inherent uncertainty. However, this sample represented more than 80% of the total crew of 4 ships and can be considered as highly representative for European and Kiribati crew members. Moreover, our findings are clearly limited to males. However, since most of the research on body image is done in women, the present study adds some insights on the cultural differences between men from European and Oceanian origin. Secondly, the socio-economic position of European and Kiribati crew members is not entirely comparable, because European crew members hold more often higher positions on board. However, this cannot be balanced as it reflects the current reality on board of commercial ships. Third, the present study is cross-sectional and thus precludes any causal interpretations. Forth, our study design does not allow to distinguish between socio-cultural and biological-genetic factors. Thus, we cannot exclude that some differences and associations which we interpreted as cultural differences are at least partially associated with genetic differences.

Conclusions

Having these limitations in mind, our study suggests that men from Kiribati who hire as seamen on commercial merchant ships are more susceptible to overeating in response to environmental stimuli and perceive themselves as thinner than Europeans. For them the nutrition situation on boards represents a highly tempting westernized food environment which facilitates overconsumption and weight gain.

Thus, the present study and its results appear to be small scale model of the much broader problem of the globalization of western influences. On board, food insecurity is no problem: Physical and economic access to food is simply given. Food is provided at little cost, actually for free, in a regular, predictable manner, in amounts that are more than sufficient. Food supply includes foods which are highly valued, particularly meat, and therefore tempting. All of these elements are relatively new for people living in or coming from food environments which have been traditionally characterized by scarcity of food. In parallel, such food scarce environments have traditionally established the ideal of large body sizes [8, 9]. When globalization offers the opportunities to have at little costs and efforts what long has been desired, it is not surprising that people use these opportunities to overeat. Traditional social values may justify to a certain degree weight gain, even though they might be in conflict with individual ideals which in turn are changing to approach the western standard of slenderness. The heightened tendency to overeat has been associated with body mass index of Kiribati in the present study. This is consistent with the body of evidence [15]. However, an interesting question for further research is whether the higher tendency to overeat is a consequence of deprived subjects being exposed to an environment that provides the deprived objects. Experimental research on chocolate "deprivation" suggest that such mechanisms could play a role [22].

Further research should explore the potential of changing some elements of the environment on board to improve food choice and eventually weight development of the seafarers. An obvious option would be the provision of information about healthy food choice directly at the table. However, given the limited influence of nutrition knowledge on eating behavior, this might not be sufficient. A promising option would be to apply the principles of nudging [23], e.g. by offer of fresh fruit and vegetables as first courses of the meals, because research has shown that the order of presentation of food influences food choice and consumption [24]. Additionally, adding more choice options during meals would probably increase satisfaction with the eating situation, particularly the needs of European seafarers for more self-determination.

On board of merchant ships is an interesting research environment, because external influences are rather limited to very short periods of port visits. Thus, ships could represent an ideal "laboratory" environment to study the influence of environmental changes on eating behavior and weight development. Further research should exploit this potential. Particularly, Kiribati seafarers who are susceptible to weight gain, overweight and obesity would directly benefit from the development of environmental measures to encourage adequate energy intakes while maintaining the satisfying features of on board nutrition.

Abbreviations
BMI: Body Mass Index; GT: Gross Tonnage; MRA: Multiple Regression Analysis; n.s.: not significant; resp.: respectively; SD: Standard Deviation; TFEQ: Three factor eating questionnaire; vs.: versus

Acknowledgments
The authors thank the shipping company for their support and all seafarers for participating in this study.

Funding
The study was financially and logistically supported by the shipping company Hamburg Süd 'COLUMBUS' Shipmanagement that made all 4 vessels available for the on-board examination. The company had no role in the design of the study, collection, analysis, and interpretation of data or preparation of the manuscript.

Authors' contributions

JW contributed to the concept of the study, conducted the statistical analysis and wrote the present paper. RvK contributed to the concept of the study, recruited all subjects and collected all data, was involved in drafting the manuscript and made a critical revision of the manuscript. BZ, BJ, HJ and VH contributed to the concept of the study and made a critical revision of the manuscript. MO suggested the study, contributed to the concept of the study, was involved in drafting the manuscript and made a critical revision of the manuscript. All authors read and approved the final manuscript.

Competing interests

The authors declare that they have no competing interests.

Author details

[1]Competence Center Health, Department Health Sciences, Hamburg University of Applied Science, Ulmenliet 20, 21033 Hamburg, Germany. [2]Institute for Occupational and Maritime Medicine (ZfAM) Hamburg, University Medical Center Hamburg-Eppendorf, Hamburg, Germany. [3]Preventive Medicine and Nutrition, Institute for Health Services Research in Dermatology and Nursing (IVDP), University Medical Center Hamburg-Eppendorf, Hamburg, Germany. [4]I. Medical Clinic and Polyclinic, University Medical Center Hamburg-Eppendorf, Hamburg, Germany.

References

1. Baygi F, Jensen OC, Qorbani M, Farshad A, Salehi SA, Mohammadi-Nasrabadi F, et al. Prevalence and associated factors of cardio-metabolic risk factors in Iranian seafarers. Int Marit Health. 2016;67(2):59–65.
2. Hansen HL, Hjarnoe L, Jepsen JR. Obesity continues to be a major health risk for Danish seafarers and fishermen. Int Marit Health. 2011;62(2):98–103.
3. Nas S, Fışkın R. A research on obesity among Turkish seafarers. Int Marit Health. 2014;65(4):187–91.
4. Oldenburg M, Harth V, Jensen H-J. Overview and prospect: food and nutrition of seafarers on merchant ships. Int Marit Health. 2013 Dec 17;64(4): 191–4.
5. Oldenburg M, Jensen H-J, Latza U, Baur X. Coronary risks among seafarers aboard German-flagged ships. Int Arch Occup Environ Health. 2008 May; 81(6):735–41.
6. Hawley NL, ST MG. Obesity and diabetes in Pacific Islanders: the current burden and the need for urgent action. Curr Diab Rep. 2015 May;15(5):29.
7. Ng M, Fleming T, Robinson M, Thomson B, Graetz N, Margono C, et al. Global, regional, and national prevalence of overweight and obesity in children and adults during 1980-2013: a systematic analysis for the global burden of disease study 2013. Lancet. 2014 Aug 30;384(9945):766–81.
8. Cortes LM, Gittelsohn J, Alfred J, Palafox NA. Formative research to inform intervention development for diabetes prevention in the Republic of the Marshall Islands. Health Educ Behav off Publ Soc public Health Educ. 2001 Dec;28(6):696–715.
9. Cultural PNJ. Elaborations of obesity - fattening practices in Pacific societies. Asia Pac J Clin Nutr. 1995;4:357–60.
10. Becker AE. Television, disordered eating, and young women in Fiji: negotiating body image and identity during rapid social change. Cult Med Psychiatry. 2004;28(4):533–59.
11. Wilkinson JY, Ben-Tovim DI, Walker MK. An insight into the personal and cultural significance of weight and shape in large Samoan women. Int J Obes Relat Metab Disord J Int Assoc Study Obes. 1994 Sep;18(9):602–6.
12. Brewis AA, McGarvey ST, Jones J, Swinburn BA. Perceptions of body size in Pacific islanders. Int J Obes Relat Metab Disord J Int Assoc Study Obes. 1998 Feb;22(2):185–9.
13. Swami V, Knight D, Tovée MJ, Davies P, Furnham A. Preferences for female body size in Britain and the South Pacific. Body Image. 2007 Jun;4(2):219–23.
14. Stunkard AJ, Messick S. The three-factor eating questionnaire to measure dietary restraint, disinhibition and hunger. J Psychosom Res. 1985;29(1):71–83.
15. Bryant EJ, King NA, Blundell JE. Disinhibition: its effects on appetite and weight regulation. Obes Rev Off J Int Assoc Study Obes. 2008 Sep;9(5):409–19.
16. Becker K, Pudel V, Westenhöfer J. Ausgewählte sozio-kulturelle Einflüsse auf das Ernährungsverhalten [Some socio-cultural influences on eating behavior]. In: Deutsche Gesellschaft für Ernährung e.V., editor. Ernährungsbericht 1992 [German Nutrition Report 1992]. Frankfurt/Main: Druckerei Henrich; 1992. p. 177–222.
17. Taylor-Powell E, Renner M. Analysing qualitative data [internet]. Wisconsin: University of Wisconsin Extension, Cooperative Extension Madison; 2003 [cited 2017 Jan 4]. Available from: https://learningstore.uwex.edu/assets/pdfs/g3658-12.pdf.
18. Aiken LS, West SG. Multiple regression: testing and interpreting interactions. Newbury Park: Sage; 1991.
19. Cohen J, Cohen P, West SG, Aiken LS. Applied Multiple Regression/Corelation analysis for the behavioral sciences. 3rd edition. Mahwah, London: Lawrence Erlbaum Associates, Inc.; 2003.
20. Coyne T. Lifestyle diseases in Pacific communities. Hughes R, Langi S, editors. Noumea: Secretariat of the Pacific Community; 2000. (Technical Paper, Secretariat of the Pacific Community).
21. Kiribati National Statistics Office, Secretariat of the Pacific Community (SPC). Kiribati Population and Housing Census 2005 [Internet]. [cited 2017 Sep 22]. Available from: http://catalog.ihsn.org/index.php/catalog/4129.
22. Polivy J, Coleman J, Herman CP. The effect of deprivation on food cravings and eating behavior in restrained and unrestrained eaters. Int J Eat Disord. 2005 Dec;38(4):301–9.
23. Thaler RH, Sunstein CR. Nudge: improving decisions about health, wealth and happiness. New internat. Ed. London: Penguin; 2009. 305 p.
24. Wansink B, Hanks AS. Slim by design: serving healthy foods first in buffet lines improves overall meal selection. PLoS One. 2013;8(10):e77055.

11

Prevalence and predictors of overweight and obesity among school-aged children in urban Ghana

Richmond Aryeetey[1*], Anna Lartey[2], Grace S. Marquis[3], Helena Nti[2], Esi Colecraft[2] and Patricia Brown[4]

Abstract

Background: Childhood overnutrition is a serious public health problem, with consequences that extend into adulthood. The aim of this study was to determine the prevalence and determinants of overweight and obesity among school-age children in two urban settings in Ghana.

Methods: This cross-sectional study involved 3089 children (9–15 years) recruited between December 2009 and February 2012 in Accra and Kumasi, Ghana. Socio-demographic, dietary, and physical activity data were collected using pretested questionnaires. BMI-for-age z-scores were used to categorize anthropometric data of the children as thin, normal, or overweight/obese. Determinants of overweight were examined using multiple logistic regressions.

Results: Seventeen percent of children were overweight or obese. Children who reported lower participation (< 3 times/week) in sports activity were 44% more likely to be overweight or obese (AOR = 1.44; 95% CI: 1.07, 1.94). Maternal tertiary education (AOR = 1.91, 95% CI: 1.07, 3.42), higher household socioeconomic status (AOR = 1. 56, 95% CI: 1.18, 2.06), and attending private school (AOR = 1.74, 95% CI: 1.31, 2.32) were also associated with elevated risk of overweight and obesity.

Conclusions: Physical inactivity is a modifiable independent determinant of overweight or obesity among Ghanaian school-aged children. Promoting and supporting a physically active lifestyle in this population is likely to reduce risk of childhood overnutrition.

Keywords: School-age children, Overweight, Obesity, Physical activity, Urban, Ghana

Background

Childhood overweight and obesity is a serious public health challenge affecting both developed and developing countries [1]. The prevalence of overweight and obesity is increasing rapidly in developing countries; in some countries, high rates of childhood overweight (> 15%) have been reported [2]. The current increasing prevalence of overweight has been partly attributed to the nutrition transition which is characterised by systemic societal changes such as increased urbanization, industrialization, trade liberalization, and economic growth. All these changes influence the food system in ways that then fuel behavior changes linked with increased energy-dense food consumption and reduced

physical activity [3, 4]. In particular, living in an urban setting has been linked with increased risk of childhood obesity in developing countries [2, 5].

One suggested pathway through which urbanization influences overnutrition is by reducing opportunities for physical activity [6]. The reported mechanisms of this relationship include increased access to and use of motorized transport [7, 8] as well as computerized devices which displace time which would otherwise be used for activity [9, 10]. Simultaneously, urban-dwelling children do not consume adequate amounts of fruits and vegetables, and also have more access to energy-dense foods high in fat, sugar and salt, including out-of-home, ready-to-eat meals and snacks [11]. In urban Benin, out-of-home prepared foods contributed more than 40% of the daily energy intake of school-going adolescents; those who consumed more than 55% of energy out of home

* Correspondence: raryeetey@ug.edu.gh
[1]School of Public Health, University of Ghana, Box LG 13 Legon, Accra, Ghana
Full list of author information is available at the end of the article

ate more sweetened energy-dense foods, and less fruits and vegetables compared to those who consumed less out of home (< 34% of energy) [12].

Childhood and adolescent overweight and obesity are associated with both short- and long-term adverse effects related to health and development. In the short term, obese young adolescents have an elevated risk of low self-esteem, negative self-image, hyperlipidemia, elevated blood pressure, and hyperinsulinemia compared to non-obese children [13, 14]. In addition, overweight in early childhood is likely to persist into adulthood, and thereby further increase risk of overweight-related chronic disease sequelae in adulthood [15]; this relationship is particularly stronger among older children (>10 years) [16, 17]. Thus, childhood overweight is associated with adverse effects on adult outcomes resulting in an unhealthy workforce, increased cost of health care, and limiting total population productivity. It is therefore important that strategies to address overweight and obesity start among children and adolescents. A critical step towards addressing overweight is a better understanding of the scope of the problem, as well as associated factors.

In Ghana, information on childhood obesity is scarce, particularly for children of school age. The 2007 Global School-based Student Health Survey reported overweight and obesity prevalence of 7% among Ghanaian children 13–15 years [18]. This survey is, however, limited by its use of self-reported anthropometric data among both rural and urban school-going children. There is thus a gap in knowledge on the magnitude and determinants of overweight and obesity among school-going children that is based on a representative sample of the urban population. Identifying risk factors of over-nutrition among children and adolescents will provide the basis for comprehensive interventions to address obesity. Therefore, the main objective of this study was to determine the prevalence and risk factors of overweight and obesity among 9–15 year old school-age children in two urban settings of Accra and Kumasi in Ghana. The study will also explore the key risk factors of overweight and obesity among school-age children in Ghana.

Methods
Study population
This was a cross-sectional survey involving 3089 school-age children between the ages of 9 and 15 years who were recruited from 121 schools located in the two largest urban centres of Ghana: Accra (the capital city of Ghana) and Kumasi (Fig. 1). Children in the 9–15 years age group were recruited from either upper primary level or junior high school level. This age group was selected for two main reasons: 1) under-representation in

nation-wide surveys, and 2) it is a target of on-going school nutrition interventions in the Ghanaian context. The schools included in the study were either exclusively primary, exclusively junior high, or having both primary and junior high level children together in a single school. The study was implemented between December 2009 and February 2012.

The study was approved by the Ethical Review Boards of McGill University (A09-B21-09A), Canada and the Noguchi Memorial Institute for Medical Research (004/09–10), University of Ghana, Legon. Prior to data collection, administrative permissions were also obtained from the national office of the Ghana Education Service as well as from head teachers of all participating schools. Written informed consent was obtained from all parents whose children participated in the study. In addition, each participating child provided signed assent before the questionnaire was administered.

Sampling
Due to expected higher prevalence of overweight and obesity among children attending private schools in Ghana, sample sizes were estimated separately for public and private schools. In public schools, the estimated sample was 954; in private schools, the estimate was 1808. These estimates were based on an overweight prevalence of 10% in private schools and 5% in public schools, a margin of error of 1.5%, and a 95% confidence interval, and allowing for 15% loss due to incomplete data. Using a cluster sampling plan, 57 public schools that had both primary and junior high school (JHS) departments were randomly selected. Assuming 20% parental refusal, a total of 20 pupils (10 males and 10 females) were randomly selected and contacted in each school. Using a similar cluster sampling for the private schools, 64 private primary and junior secondary schools were randomly selected. In each school, 36 pupils (18 females and 18 males) were randomly selected and contacted.

Data collection
Questionnaires were administered to the school children, individually. Data collected with the questionnaire included socio-demographic characteristics, dietary habits, physical activity, and television viewing. Each child and parent had the weight and height measurements taken and recorded by a trained research assistant. The measurements were taken at the school premises.

Socio-demographic data
A structured pre-tested questionnaire was used to collect information on household demographic and socio-economic characteristics including educational, home

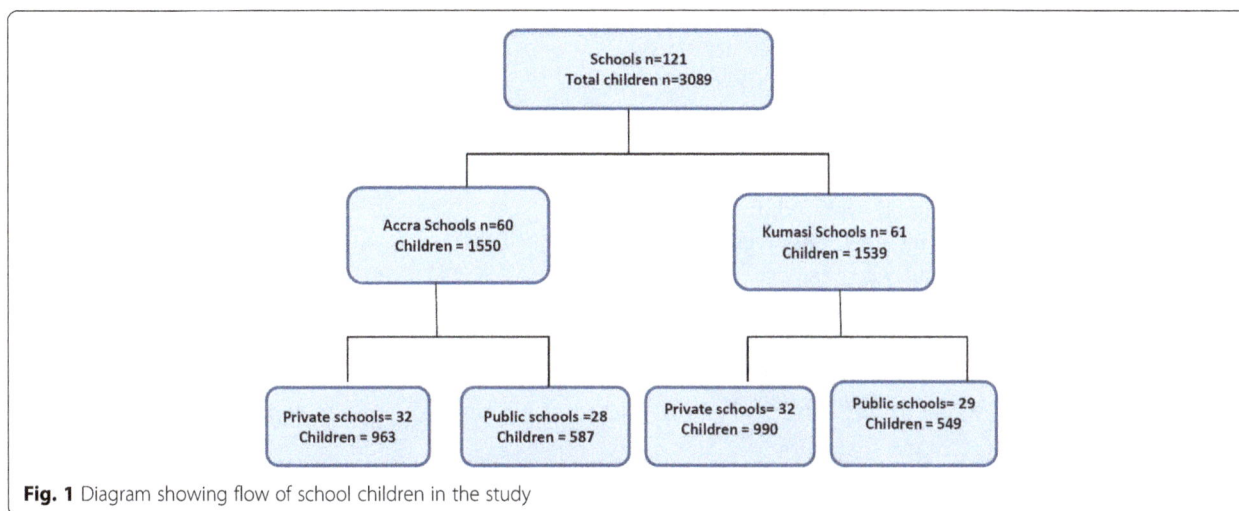

Fig. 1 Diagram showing flow of school children in the study

living arrangements, and occupation of parents. In addition, ownership of household assets, including refrigerator and television, video player, and automobile were documented. This information was obtained from the children with the assistance of parents (where a parent was available).

Dietary and physical activity assessment
Dietary intakes of the school children were assessed using a food frequency questionnaire that had a reference period of one week prior to the survey. The questionnaire consisted of 60 food items and focused on describing patterns of consumption of high fat foods, high sugar foods, sweetened drinks, fruits, and vegetables. The frequencies of intake of the listed foods over time (daily and weekly) by the school children were then determined. The food frequency questionnaire was designed for this study by identifying commonly consumed foods in Ghana under each of 11 food groups. The food groups were sugar-sweetened beverages, milk and dairy products, cereal products (including breads and biscuits), fried foods, animal-source foods, spreads and toppings, fruits, vegetables, soups, sweets and high calorie foods, and other staple foods. An initial list of foods was pre-tested among mothers in Accra, following which additional foods were added. During the survey, opportunity was provided for including additional foods that were reportedly consumed. A pre-tested questionnaire was used to collect information on the level of physical activity and sports participation of study children. The specific questions included the frequency and duration of television viewing, number of days per week child walked to school, and frequency of performing house chores and participation in sporting and other physical activities including football, *ampe* (indigenous Ghanaian jumping game), hockey, table tennis, lawn tennis, rope skipping, volleyball, basketball, swimming and gardening.

Anthropometry
All anthropometric measurements were carried out at the school premises. Participants removed all heavy clothing and accessories (such as shoes or sandals, belts, watches, and sweaters) and emptied their pockets (where necessary), prior to the measurement. Body weight was measured to the nearest 0.1 kg using the Tanita Digital Scale (model BWB-800, Tanita Corporation, USA). Height measurements were taken to the nearest 0.1 cm using the Shorr Board (Shorr Productions, Olney, MD). Parents were invited to the school for weight and height to be taken. All measurements were done and recorded in duplicate. Weight and height measurements were converted to body mass index for age z-scores (BMIZ) based on the WHO Child Growth Standards [19]. Overweight was defined as BMIZ greater than one standard deviation from the median; obesity was determined as BMIZ greater than two standard deviations [20].

Statistical analyses
Two factors were created from a set of seven socio-economic status (SES) variables using factor analysis with varimax rotation as proxy indicators for household socio-economic status. The first factor reflected household items such as television and refrigerator and the second reflected occupation and ownership of items such as home, air conditioner, and vehicle. Tertiles of the factors are reported. Regarding dietary data, proportions were reported for how frequently dietary behaviors and foods with established links to obesity were reported by respondents. Analyses were carried using cases with complete data. The proportion of children who were overweight or obese (BMIZ >1 SD) was computed. Multiple logistic regression procedure was used to examine characteristics that were statistically and independently associated with overweight or obese status. The factors considered were those that were shown to

be either significantly correlated ($p < 0.05$) or tended to be correlated ($p < 0.10$) with overweight and obesity, and included child characteristics (age, sex, dietary habits, physical activity, type of school), maternal characteristics (education, occupation), and household characteristics (household wealth status). The region of residence and correlation within clusters (school) were controlled for in the model. The final model included only factors that were associated with overweight or obesity at $p < 0.05$. We used weights in the analysis to restore the representativeness of the sample. All statistical analyses were conducted using SAS (version 9.2, Cary, NC, USA) and statistical significance in the final model was determined at $p < 0.05$.

Results

The current analysis included 3089 out of the 3444 school children who were sampled (Fig. 1). The majority (90%) of children who were sampled but not included did not show up on the day of data collection; the remainder either refused participation (9%) or were ineligible because of their age (1%). The mean age of children who participated in the study was 12.2 ± 1.7 years and more than half of them were female (Table 1). Most of the children ate breakfast during the school week, with 85% having breakfast more than three days per week (Table 2). Consumption of fruits and vegetables was low. Only 20% and 38% had consumed fruits and vegetables >5 times, respectively, the previous week. About three-quarters of the children (76%) walked to school at least four out of the five school days in a week and more than half (58%) did household chores during the week. However, involvement in sporting activities was low, with less than one-third of the children engaging in a sport at least three times in a week. Television watching was also low among the study sample. Less than 15% watched television at least five times during the week prior to the survey. The overall prevalence of overweight and obesity was 14.7% among the children, with 4.4% being obese (Table 3). A higher proportion of children were overweight (including obese) in the private compared to the public schools (21.4% vs 11.2%, $p < 0.001$).

Risk factors of overweight and obesity

Table 4 shows the factors that were significantly associated with being overweight or obese in the study sample, based on multiple logistic regression. Female children were twice as likely to be overweight or obese compared to male children (AOR = 2.38, 95% CI: 1.79, 3.18). None of the dietary habits that were assessed was significantly associated the risk of overweight or obesity. Physical activity was a determinant of overnutrition among the children. Children who engaged in sports for less than

Table 1 Background characteristics of Ghanaian children 9–15 years

	Total		Private School		Public School	
	n	%	n	%	n	%
Child's sex						
Male	1413	46.6	925	51.1	488	46.7
Female	1617	53.4	1028	48.9	648	53.3
Maternal education						
None	174	56	74	3.8	100	8.8
Primary	1055	34.2	558	28.0	497	43.5
Secondary (JHS/SHS)	637	20.7	458	23.3	179	15.7
Tertiary	357	11.6	287	14.8	70	6.1
Do not know	860	27.9	572	30.1	288	25.9
Maternal occupation						
Artisan	515	16.7	302	15.5	213	18.8
Professional[a]	380	12.3	302	15.5	78	6.7
Office worker[b]	71	2.3	52	2.6	19	1.7
Trading	1884	61.0	1140	58.4	744	65.5
Not employed	195	6.3	126	6.4	69	6.2
Do not know	44	1.4	31	1.6	13	1.1
Household size						
≤ 3	309	10.0	200	10.2	109	9.5
4–6	1785	57.8	1121	57.7	664	58.8
7–9	810	26.2	505	25.7	305	26.6
≥10	185	6.0	127	6.4	58	5.1
Household socioeconomic status factor 1[c]						
Low	1027	33.7	575	30.0	451	40.3
Medium	981	32.2	725	37.7	256	22.6
High	1037	34.1	621	32.3	416	37.1
Household socioeconomic status factor 2[d]						
Low	1199	39.4	603	31.3	596	53.3
Medium	825	27.1	501	26.1	324	28.9
High	1021	33.5	818	42.6	203	17.7

Values presented as number (percentage of private or public)
[a]Includes teachers, lawyers, doctors, and accountants
[b]Includes secretaries and office clerks
[c]Reflects possession of household items such as television, video player, and refrigerator
[d]Reflects occupation and ownership of assets such as home, air conditioner, and vehicle

three times a week were at a 44% higher odds of being overweight or obese when compared to those who were involved in sporting activities at least three times a week. High maternal education and household SES were risk factors for overweight and obesity. Children of mothers who received formal education beyond the secondary level were more likely to be overweight or obese compared to those whose mothers had no education (AOR = 1.91, 95% CI: 1.07, 3.42). However, being educated up to the secondary level was not linked with overweight. Children living in households in the third SES tertile had

Table 2 Dietary and physical activity habits of Ghanaian children 9–15 years

	Total		Private		Public	
	n	%	n	%	n	%
Dietary habits						
Access to soft drinks at home	860	27.8	626	32.1	234	20.3
Breakfast ≤3 days/week	427	13.8	289	14.9	138	12.1
Fried foods ≥5 times/week	1388	44.9	728	37.3	460	40.5
Soft drinks ≥2 bottles previous day	33	1.1	24	1.3	9	0.8
Sweetened drink ≥5 times/week	465	15.1	331	16.9	134	11.8
Cakes, pies, doughnuts ≥3 days/week	1742	56.4	1071	54.5	671	58.6
Fruit consumption (times/week)						
0–5	2464	79.8	1563	80.0	901	79.7
6–10	452	11.7	282	14.4	170	14.6
11–15	138	3.6	89	4.6	49	4.3
> 15	35	0.9	19	1.0	16	1.4
Vegetable consumption (times/week)						
0–5	1899	61.5	1210	62.6	689	60.7
6–10	864	30.0	550	27.7	314	27.6
11–15	236	7.6	138	6.9	98	8.6
> 15	90	2.9	55	2.8	35	3.1
Physical activity						
Transport to school ≥3 days/week	1347	43.6	1034	52.9	313	27.2
Household chores >5 times/week	1795	58.1	1041	53.3	754	65.7
Any sporting activity ≥3 times/week	852	27.6	498	26.2	354	32.0
Playing football/ampe[a] ≥ 3 times/week						
Males	578	18.7	349	9.2	229	21.9
Females	275	8.9	149	7.0	125	10.1
Sedentary behavior						
Watching Television ≥5 times/week	166	5.4	105	13.9	61	13.7
Duration watching TV (hours/week)						
<2	1356	45.1	854	45.1	502	45.2
2–3	1356	45.1	856	45.2	500	45.1
≥4	291	9.8	183	9.7	108	9.7

Values presented as number (percentage of private or public)
[a]A local game involving clapping and jumping

Table 3 Nutritional status of Ghanaian School children ages 9–15 years

Growth status	Total		Private		Public	
	n	%	n	%	n	%
Thin	102	3.3	55	2.9	47	4.4
Normal	2429	78.6	1475	75.7	954	84.3
Overweight	382	12.4	282	14.2	100	8.3
Obese	143	4.6	113	5.8	30	2.5
Severely obese	33	1.1	28	1.4	5	0.4
Stunting	99	3.2	50	2.6	49	4.4

Thin: BAZ < −2SD; Overweight: +1SD < BAZ ≤ +2SD; Obese: +2SD ≤ BAZ ≤ +3SD; Severely Obese: BAZ > +3; Stunting: HAZ < −2SD; (WHO, 2007)

Table 4 Factors associated with overweight and obesity (BMIZ >1 SD) among Ghanaian children 9–15 years

	Adjusted Odds Ratio[b]	95% Confidence Interval	p-value
Child's sex			
Female	2.38	1.79, 3.18	<0.01
Male	1		
Breakfast ≥ 3 days/week			
No	0.76	0.58, 1.00	0.05
Yes	1		
Eats Cakes, pies, doughnuts ≥3 days/week			
Yes	0.83	0.66, 1.04	0.10
No	1		
Fruit consumption (frequency/week)			
> 15	0.41	0.14, 1.17	0.09
11–15	1.13[a]	0.65, 1.93	0.67
6–10	1.07[a]	0.78, 1.46	0.69
0–5	1		
Vegetable consumption (frequency/week)			
> 15	1.27	0.69, 2.32	0.44
11–15	1.48	0.99, 2.23	0.06
6–10	1.16	0.92, 1.46	0.20
0–5	1		
Transported to school (days/week)			
4–5	1.39	1.06, 1.82	0.02
1–3	1.11	0.52, 2.37	0.79
Never	1		
Engaged in any sporting activity ≥ 3 times/week			
No	1.44	1.07, 1.94	0.02
Yes	1		
School type			
Private	1.74	1.31, 2.32	<0.01
Public	1		
Maternal education			
Tertiary	1.91	1.07, 3.42	0.03
Secondary	1.00	0.57, 1.75	0.99
Primary	1.12	0.68, 1.84	0.65
Don't know	1.14	0.69, 1.89	0.61
None	1		
Household socioeconomic status			
High	1.56	1.18, 2.06	<0.01
Medium	1.10	0.81, 1.49	0.54
Low	1		

[a]Borderline significant values (0.05 ≤ P < 0.08)
[b]Other variables controlled in the analysis: age, child engaged in household chores, and frequency of sweetened beverage consumption

56% higher odds of being overweight or obese when compared to those from households in the first tertile (lowest SES). After adjusting for biologic factors, dietary and physical activity habits, and SES, those attending private schools were more likely to be overweight or obese compared those who attended public schools (AOR = 1.74, 95% CI: 1.31, 2.32).

Discussion

Among Ghanaian school children 9–15 years living in Accra and Kumasi, the prevalence of overweight (including obesity) was 15%. Fundamentally, overweight and obesity reflects positive energy balance; physical inactivity and poor dietary habits are two key modifiable factors that can influence this balance in a population. In the current study, low physical activity participation was associated with overweight and obesity among school-going children in urban Ghana, similar to earlier studies in other developing countries [2, 21, 22]. Both low participation in structured (sports) and unstructured forms of physical activity (e.g., walking to school) were related to overweight and obesity, indicating the need to encourage varied opportunities for physical activity among school-aged children.

In line with the WHO global strategy on diet, physical activity, and health, the Ministry of Health in Ghana recommends that children and adolescents have at least one hour of moderate to vigorous physical activity daily, and that physical education (PE) of not less than 2 h per week should be included in the school curriculum [23, 24]. Although PE is part of the basic education curriculum, studies show that the main focus has been on competitive sports [25]. While PE aims to encourage majority of students to participate regularly in physical activities, competitive sports is described as a value-added experience for few students who show the potential for elite performance in specific structured activities. Thus, focusing mainly on competitive sports in school limits opportunity for the majority of children to engage in school-based physical activity.

Parental work habits is known to influence the level of physical activity among children [26]. When parents work mostly away from home, as is commonly observed in urban settings, there is limited time to supervise or engage in recreational activities with their children. Children are thus left on their own to decide the use of the period after school. With the upsurge of video and computer games and television stations, children are likely to engage in sedentary activities that involve spending time in front of a screen, thereby limiting their opportunities for engaging in moderate and vigorous physical activities. An earlier study in the Ga-East district of Ghana reported that obese and overweight school children

(8–18 years) spent more time watching television and playing video games (90 min/day) than engaging in physical activities (50 min/day) [27]. In the current study, more than half of children spent at least two hours/day watching television in the week prior to the survey.

The positive association between SES and overweight (including obesity) observed in this study is similar to studies in other developing countries [2, 21, 28, 29]. The direction of the association between obesity and SES varies from positive in poorer countries to negative among better-off societies [30]. Households with high SES may have more access to and be able to afford processed, fatty, and/or sugary foods and beverages compared to poorer households. Socio-Economic Status may also predict access to technology (e.g., television, cars, computers, and video games). These technology devices are likely to contribute to a more sedentary lifestyle. In our study, however, SES was associated with overweight and obesity independent of physical activity. Thus, there may be other factors that mediate the observed relationship.

Available studies on the relationship between maternal education and overweight/obesity in children and adolescents are mixed. While some studies found a positive association [28, 31], others have reported a negative [32, 33] or no [21] association. In the present study, children whose mothers had received post-secondary education were more likely to be overweight or obese compared to those who had no formal education. High level of maternal education may lead to improved acquisition and use of nutrition knowledge which can translate into good dietary practices [34]. On the other hand, mothers with higher levels of education are likely to earn higher income. The latter has been linked with adverse affects on dietary and/or physical activity habits through the easier accessibility of energy-dense foods and electronic devices that promote sedentary lifestyles. Thus, the relationship between maternal education and overnutrition among children may be modified by other factors and therefore needs further investigations.

Previous studies have established a strong association between diet and risk of overweight in both developed and developing country settings [35–37]. In the current analysis, however, there was no statistically significant association observed between overweight and any of the indicators of dietary behavior. This can be explained by both the inherent imprecision of measuring diet by recall, as well as the detail of dietary analysis reported in the current analysis. It is important, however, that this finding is neither misunderstood nor misrepresented as evidence of the association between overweight and diet. Subsequent analysis of the dietary data will enable better understanding of the links between diet and overweight as well as other biological outcomes examined (including lipid profile).

One of the strengths of this study was the use of the WHO growth reference for school-aged children and adolescents in the determination of overweight and obesity. Compared to the previous NCHS growth curves [38], the WHO reference curves are closely aligned with Child Growth Standards at five years of age as well as the recommended adult cut-offs for overweight and obesity at 19 years, which is the WHO upper age limit for adolescence [20]. It provides, therefore, an appropriate reference for the age group that participated in the current study. Further, the study included more than one hundred schools that were located throughout the two largest cities in Ghana. The use of random sampling to select the children enhanced our sample as representative of the school-going children in urban settings in Ghana.

The findings of the current study should be interpreted bearing in mind its inherent limitations. First, we recognise the inability of this study to establish causality due to its cross-sectional design. Additionally, although parental BMI has been shown to be a risk factor for overweight and obesity among children and adolescents [5, 32, 33, 39], this could not be controlled for in the regression analyses. This was due to the lack of anthropometric data for more than 20% of parents who were interviewed by phone. Finally, and importantly, the dietary information was collected using food frequency questionnaire and thus any interpretations from the diet-related analyses should be viewed with this inherent limitation in mind.

Conclusions

In conclusion, the prevalence of overweight and obesity among school-going children living in urban areas in Ghana was high. This study identified physical activity status, sex of child, maternal education, household SES, and type of school as significant determinants of overweight and obesity in these children. Of these factors, physical activity is the one that can be modified among school-going children. The current physical education curriculum for basic schools in Ghana needs to be reassessed and updated to encourage more children and adolescents to participate regularly in physical activities. Further, there is need to champion the utilization of the PE time for physical activity in schools. This may require placing more emphasis on non-competitive activities. In addition, school children should be encouraged to walk to school as much as possible and this recommendation should be supported by policies that ensure safety on walk routes.

Abbreviations

AOR: Adjusted Odds Ratio; BMI: Body Mass Index; BMIZ: Body Mass Index Z-Score; CI: Confidence Interval; GSHS: School-based Student Health Survey; JHS: Junior High School; PE: Physical education; SD: Standard Deviation; SES: Socio-Economic Status; WHO: World Health Organization

Acknowledgements

The study team appreciates the cooperation and support of teachers, parents and school children for their patience and time spent in participating in the data collection process. We also appreciate the facilitative role of the School officials as well as research assistants (Mawuli Avedzi, Hussein Mohamed, and Deda Ogum). Seth Adu-Afarwuah is acknowledged for support with data analyses.

Funding

This work was carried out with the aid of a grant from the International Development Research Centre, Ottawa, Canada (#104519–017).

Authors' contributions

The study was conceived and designed by AL and GSM. HN supervised data collection. All authors contributed to analyses and interpretation of the data. The manuscript was drafted by RA and AL with substantial contributions by all the other authors (GSM, HN, EC and PB). All authors approved manuscripts, and revisions arising from review process.

Competing interests

The authors declare that they have no competing interests.

Author details

[1]School of Public Health, University of Ghana, Box LG 13 Legon, Accra, Ghana. [2]Department of Nutrition and Food Science, University of Ghana, Box LG 134 Legon, Accra, Ghana. [3]School of Dietetics and Human Nutrition, McGill University, 21,111 Lakeshore Road, Ste-Anne-de-Bellevue, Montreal, QC H9X 3V9, Canada. [4]Department of Biochemistry and Biotechnology, Kwame Nkrumah University of Science and Technology, Kumasi, Ghana.

References

1.　United Nations Childrens Fund (UNICEF), World Health Organization (WHO), (WB) WBG. Levels And Trends In Child Malnutrition: Key findings of the 2016 edition. New York: UNICEF/WHO/WB; 2016.
2.　Gupta N, Goel K, Shah P, Misra A. Childhood obesity in developing Countires: epidemiology, determinants, and prevention. Endocr Rev. 2012;33:48–70.
3.　Popkin BM. The nutrition transition and obesity in the developing world. J Nutr. 2001;131:871S–3S.
4.　Shetty P. Nutrition transition and its health outcomes. Indian J Pediatr. 2013; 80(Suppl 1):S21–7.

5. Kiranmala N, Das M, Arora N. Determinants of childhood obesity: need for a trans-sectoral convergent approach. Indian J Pediatr. 2013;80(Suppl 1):S38–47.

6. Hill J, Peters J. Environmental contributions to the obesity epidemic. Science. 1998;280:1371–4.

7. Lee MC, Orenstein MR, Richardson MJ. Systematic review of active commuting to school and childrens physical activity and weight. J Phys Act Health. 2008; 5(6):930–49.

8. Faulkner GE, Buliung RN, Flora PK, Fusco C. Active school transport, physical activity levels and body weight of children and youth: a systematic review. Prev Med. 2009;48(1):3–8.

9. Boulos R, Vikre EK, Oppenheimer S, Chang H, Kanarek RB. ObesiTV: how television is influencing the obesity epidemic. Physiol Behav. 2012; 107(1):146–53.

10. Reid Chassiakos YL, Radesky J, Christakis D, Moreno MA, Cross C. COUNCIL ON COMMUNICATIONS AND MEDIA. Children and adolescents and digital media. Pediatrics. 2016;138(5).

11. Buscemi S, Barile A, Maniaci V, Batsis JA, Mattina A, Verga S. Characterization of street food consumption in Palermo: possible effects on health. Nutr J. 2011;10:119–27.

12. Chauliac M, Bricas N, Ategbo E, Amoussa W, Zohoun I. Food outside the home of schoolchildren in Cotonou (Benin). Sante. 1998;8(2):101–8.

13. Dietz W. Health consequences of obesity in youth: childhood predictors of adult disease. Pediatrics. 1998;101:518–25.

14. Strauss R. Childhood obesity and self-esteem. Pediatrics. 2000;105:e15–20.

15. Dietz W, Gortmaker S. Preventing obesity in children and adolescents. Annu Rev Public Health. 2001;22:337–53.

16. Rosenbaum M. Special considerations relative to pediatric obesity. In: de Groot LJ, Chrousos G, Dungan K, Feingold KR, Grossman A, Hershman JM, Koch C, Korbonits M, McLachlan R, new M, et al., editors. Endotext. South Dartmouth (MA): MDText.com, Inc.; 2000.

17. Llewellyn A, Simmonds M, Owen CG, Woolacott N. Childhood obesity as a predictor of morbidity in adulthood: a systematic review and meta-analysis. Obes Rev. 2016;17(1):56–67.

18. WHO: Global School-based Student Health Survey: Ghana Fact Sheet. 2007. http://www.who.int/chp/gshs/2007_Ghana_fact_sheet.pdf?ua=1. Accessed 27 Nov 2017.

19. WHO: Software for assessing growth and development of the world's children. In.: Geneva: WHO. 2007. http://www.who.int/childgrowth/software/en/. Accessed 27 Nov 2017.

20. de Onis M, Onyango A, Borghi E, Nishida C, Siekmann J. Development of a WHO growth reference for school-aged children and adolescents. Bull World Health Organ. 2007;85:660–7.

21. Laxmaiah A, Nagalla B, Vijayaraghavan K, Nair M. Factors affecting prevalence of overweight among 12- to 17-year-old urban adolescents in Hyderabad, India. Obesity. 2007;15(6):1384–90.

22. Mushtaq MU, Gull S, Mushtaq K, Shahid U, Shad MA, Akram J. Dietary behaviors, physical activity and sedentary lifestyle associated with overweight and obesity, and their socio-demographic correlates, among Pakistani primary school children. Int J Behav Nutr Phys Act. 2011;8:130–43.

23. Ministry of Health: Dietary and physical activity guidelines for Ghana. In. Accra, Ghana; 2010.

24. WHO: School policy framework: implementation of the WHO global strategy ondiet, physical activity and health. In. Geneva, Switzerland; 2008.

25. Ocansey R, Seidu S, Jatong J. Physical education and after-school sport programs in Ghana: The role of public and private structures. In: Chepyator-Thomson J, Hsu S-H, editors. Global perspectives on physical education and after-school sports. Lanham, MD: University Press of America; 2013. p. 13–35.

26. Kohl IIIH, Hobbs K. Development of physical activity behaviors among children and adolescents. Pediatrics. 1998;101(549–554)

27. Steiner-Asiedu M, Addo P, Bediako-Amoa B, Fiadjoe F, Anderson A. Lifestyle and nutrition profile of overweight and obese school children in the Ga-east district of Ghana. Asian Journal of Medical Sciences. 2012;4(3):99–102.

28. Ullmann H, Buttenheim AM, Goldman N, Pebley AR, Wong R. Socioeconomic differences in obesity among Mexican adolescents. Int J Pediatr Obes. 2011;6: e373–80.

29. Daboné C, Delisle HF, Receveur O. Poor nutritional status of schoolchildren in urban and peri-urban areas of Ouagadougou (Burkina Faso). Nutr J. 2011; 10(34):1–8.

30. Ntandou G, Delisle H, Agueh V, Fayomi B. Physical activity and socioeconomic status explain rural-urban differences in obesity: a cross-sectional study in Benin (West Africa). Ecology of Food and Nutrition. 2008;47:313–37.

31. Mushtaq MU, Gull S, Shahid U, Shafique MM, Abdullah HM, Shad MA, Siddiqui AM. Family-based factors associated with overweight and obesity among Pakistani primary school children. BMC Pediatr. 2011;11:114–22.

32. Keane E, Layte R, Harrington J, Kearney PM, Perry IJ. Measured parental weight status and familial socio-economic status correlates with childhood overweight and obesity at age 9. PLoS One. 2012;7(8)

33. Yi XQ, Yin CY, Chang M, Xiao YF. Prevalence and risk factors of obesity among school-aged children in Xi'an, China. Eur J Pediatr. 2012;171(2):389–94.

34. Armar-Klemesu M, Ruel MT, Maxwell DG, Levin CE, Morris SS: Poor Maternal Schooling is the Main Constraint to Good Child Care Practices in Accra. J Nutr. 2000; 130(6):1597-607.

35. Kuzbicka K, Rachon D. Bad eating habits as the main cause of obesity among children. Pediatric endocrinology, diabetes, and metabolism. 2013;19(3):106–10.

36. Katzmarzyk PT, Broyles ST, Champagne CM, Chaput JP, Fogelholm M, Hu G, Kuriyan R, Kurpad A, Lambert EV, Maia J, et al. Relationship between soft drink consumption and obesity in 9-11 years old children in a multi-National Study. Nutrients. 2016;8(12):E770.

37. Emmett PM, Jones LR. Diet, growth, and obesity development throughout childhood in the Avon longitudinal study of parents and children. Nutr Rev. 2015;73(Suppl 3):175–206.

38. Kuczmarski RJ, Ogden CL, Guo SS, Grummer-Strawn LM, Flegal KM, Mei Z, Wei R, Curtin LR, Roche AF, Johnson CL: 2000 CDC growth charts for the United States: methods and development. In., vol. 11: National Center for Health Statistics; 2002.

39. Moraeus L, Lissner L, Yngve A, Poortvliet E, Al-Ansari U, Sjoberg A. Multi-level influences on childhood obesity in Sweden: societal factors, parental determinants and child's lifestyle. Int J Obes. 2012;36(7):969–76.

12

Exploring the associations between systemic inflammation, obesity and healthy days: a health related quality of life (HRQOL) analysis of NHANES 2005–2008

Jeffrey Wilkins[1†], Palash Ghosh[2†], Juan Vivar[3], Bibhas Chakraborty[2] and Sujoy Ghosh[4*] (iD)

Abstract

Background: Obesity is positively associated with low-level chronic inflammation, and negatively associated with several indices of health-related quality of life (HRQOL). It is however not clear if obesity-associated inflammation is partly responsible for the observed negative associations between obesity and HRQOL, and also whether systemic inflammation independently affects HRQOL. We conducted an exploratory analysis to investigate the relationships between obesity, systemic inflammation and indices of HRQOL, using NHANES survey data.

Methods: Data for the variables of interest were available for 6325 adults (aged 20–75 years, BMI > 18.5 kg/m^2). Demographic, body mass index (BMI), C-reactive protein (CRP), inflammatory disease status, medication use, smoking, and HRQOL data were obtained from NHANES (2005–2008) and analyzed using sampling-weighted generalized linear models. Data was subjected to multiple imputation in order to mitigate information loss from survey non-response. Both main effects and interaction effects were analyzed to evaluate possible mediation or moderation effects. Model robustness was ascertained via sensitivity analysis. Averaged results from the imputed datasets were reported in as odds ratios (OR) and confidence intervals (CI).

Results: Obesity was positively associated with poor physical healthy days (OR: 1.59, 95% CI: 1.15–2.21) in unadjusted models. 'Elevated' and 'clinically raised' levels of the inflammation marker CRP were also positively associated with poor physical healthy days (OR = 1.61, 95% CI: 1.23–2.12, and OR = 2.45, 95% CI: 1.84–3.26, respectively); additionally, 'clinically raised' CRP was positively associated with mental unhealthy days (OR = 1.66, 95% CI: 1.26–2.19). The association between obesity and physical HRQOL was rendered non-significant in models including CRP. Association between 'elevated' and 'clinically raised' CRP and physical unhealthy days remained significant even after adjustment for obesity or inflammation-modulating covariates (OR = 1.36, 95% CI: 1.02–1.82, and OR = 1.75, 95% CI: 1.21–2.54, respectively).

Conclusions: Systemic inflammation appears to mediate the association between obesity and physical unhealthy days. Clinically raised inflammation is an independent determinant of physical and mental unhealthy days. Importantly, elevated (but sub-clinical) inflammation is also negatively associated with physical healthy days, and may warrant more attention from a population health perspective than currently appreciated.

Keywords: Obesity, Inflammation, Healthy days, Health-related quality of life, Mediation

* Correspondence: sujoy.ghosh@duke-nus.edu.sg
†Jeffrey Wilkins and Palash Ghosh contributed equally to this work.
4Program in Cardiovascular & Metabolic Disorders & Centre for Computational Biology, Duke-NUS Medical School, 8 College Road, Singapore 169857, Singapore
Full list of author information is available at the end of the article

Background

Obesity poses one of the most significant public health challenges of the developed and developing nations today. The fundamental process underlying obesity is an energy imbalance between calories consumed and calories expended, resulting in a net positive energy balance. Obesity has accelerated globally due to an increased intake of energy-dense food high in fat and refined carbohydrates, reduced physical activity associated with an increasingly sedentary lifestyle, altered modes of transportation, control of ambient temperature and increasing urbanization [1, 2]. Worldwide obesity rates have nearly tripled between 1975 and 2016, with more than 650 million adults obese worldwide. In addition to weight-related pathologies, obesity is also a gateway to other chronic disorders including type 2 diabetes, cardiovascular disease, musculoskeletal disorders, and specific cancers [3–5]. Regardless of origin, higher levels of obesity are associated with higher relative mortality risk compared to healthy weight [6]. Consequently, obesity and obesity-associated health problems lead to a significant economic impact involving direct and indirect medical costs [7–9].

Obesity is typically associated with a chronic state of systemic low-grade inflammation [10]. Rapid adipose tissue expansion due to overnutrition results in a hypoxic internal core which, along with endoplasmic reticulum and oxidative stress, orchestrates a pro-inflammatory response through the release of various cytokines into systemic circulation [11]. Adipose tissue depots also undergo significant immune cell infiltration further contributing to a sustained inflammatory tone [12, 13]. Although biological studies have strongly implicated a causal role of obesity in promoting inflammation [14–18], Mendelian randomization experiments employing genetic variants in the inflammation biomarker C-reactive protein (CRP) [19] and obesity-associated FTO gene [20–22] have formally established the direction of causality from increased adiposity to elevated systemic inflammation [23]. The same technique has also been recently used to infer a causal role of obesity in promoting inflammatory skin diseases [24]. Obesity-associated chronic inflammation, in turn, has been causally associated with several metabolic complications including insulin resistance, endothelial dysfunction, and type 2 diabetes [5, 25–29].

From a population health perspective, effective interventions and optimized predictions for future health-care costs require a better quantitative understanding of chronic conditions such as inflammation and obesity and their relationship to indices of public health. One index that captures the population level effects of chronic conditions is the health related quality of life (HRQOL) [30]. HRQOL, a self-reported measure of physical and mental functioning and well-being, is increasingly used to assess the effects of chronic illness, treatments, and short- and long-term disabilities.

Previous studies have generally demonstrated a negative correlation between excess adiposity and various dimensions of HRQOL in different populations [31–37]. Much less is known, however, on the effects of chronic inflammation on HRQOL, and whether inflammation mediates some of the association between obesity and HRQOL. Most of the earlier studies investigating inflammation and HRQOL have either focused on small cohorts targeting specific inflammatory disorders [38–40], or interrogated inflammation and HRQOL as separate endpoints. Recently however, the role of systemic inflammation as a co-factor in the disease to HRQOL relationship is beginning to be examined [41, 42]. Systemic inflammation is often measured via the chronic inflammatory biomarker, C-reactive protein (CRP) [43, 44], which is a commonly used predictor in studies of inflammatory disease, and considered an excellent biomarker of baseline and progressive inflammation in chronic conditions [45]. CRP levels in the range consistent with infection or inflammation (> 1 mg/dl) are more common among obese subjects than in non-obese subjects [46]. Additionally, reliable associations between blood levels of the inflammation biomarker CRP and a variety of HRQOL outcomes have also been reported [47, 48].

The temporal precedence of obesity over systemic inflammation, and the reported causal connections between obesity-associated inflammation and secondary disorders [25], raises the question of whether obesity-associated chronic inflammation may also play a similar role in the observed association between obesity and HRQOL. More specifically, such questions may be explored in the mediator-variable framework of Barron and Kenny [49, 50] whereby an antecedent variable (e.g. obesity) may affect a mediating variable (e.g. inflammation), which would then affect an outcome variable (e.g. HRQOL). While acknowledging the potential biases of a cross-sectional mediation analysis, the strong prior biological evidence causally linking obesity to inflammation, and inflammation to obesity-associated disorders led us to explore a similar scenario for obesity and HRQOL. This line of questioning has important implications for prevention and treatment research where interventions may be designed to alter the outcome of interest by controlling the mediating variables, especially where the primary variable is difficult to control. Thus, if chronic inflammation does indeed mediate the association between obesity and poorer HRQOL, then controlling for such inflammation via lifestyle and pharmacologic interventions may provide a path forward for improving the HRQOL index for the obese population. This is particularly relevant, given the current paucity of effective treatments for obesity [51].

Methods
Study design and participants
Study data was downloaded from the National Health and Nutrition Examination Survey (NHANES) collection (years 2005 through 2008, http://www.cdc.gov/nchs/nhanes/nhanes_questionnaires.htm). NHANES is conducted by the Center for Disease Control's National Center for Health Statistics (CDC-NCHS) to assess the health and nutritional status of a representative civilian, non-institutionalized US population using a multistage, stratified, clustered probability design [52]. Data for the variables of interest were available for a total of 6325 adults (aged 20–75 years, BMI > 18.5 kg/m^2) and included missing values. Data for subjects 18–20 years of age were excluded due to the large excess of missing values in this group and to prevent complications from differential growth patterns in childhood and adolescence where the usual BMI categories do not apply [53]. There were no missing values for age, sex and race variables. For the other variables, the extent of missing value ranged from 0.01% (presence of heart disease) to ~ 53% (smoking). BMI and CRP had missing values for ~ 6 and 10% of the observations respectively, whereas both physical and mental healthy days had missing values of ~ 12%. Data collected included demographic information, health-related questionnaire, and laboratory data on C-reactive protein (CRP, a marker of systemic inflammation). Data for confounding factors that can influence inflammation status and HRQOL outcomes such as relevant medical conditions (asthma, arthritis, heart disease, and cancer), anti-inflammatory/analgesic medication, and smoking were also downloaded for statistical modeling. To account for the complexity of survey design including oversampling, survey non-response, or post-stratification issues, NHANES assigns sample 'weights' were also downloaded (additional details available from https://www.cdc.gov/nchs/tutorials/nhanes/SurveyDesign/Weighting/Overview Key.htm, and in Additional file 1: Text 1).

Health related quality of life (HRQOL) measures
Quality of life was assessed by using a subset of the CDC HRQOL-4 questionnaire that was developed to assess physical and mental health in the general U.S population [54, 55]. The HRQOL-4 questionnaire (Additional file 1: Text 2) uses self-reported measures of healthy and unhealthy days as indicators of HRQOL, and have undergone cognitive testing and criterion validity with the Short-Form 36, content and construct validity, predictive validity, internal consistency, test-

retest reliability, and measurement invariance in persons with and without disability [56, 57]. The core Healthy Days consists of four questions focusing on the participant's general health status (Question-1), number of physical unhealthy days in the 30 days preceding the survey (Question-2), number of mental unhealthy days in the 30 days preceding the survey (Question-3), and number of days with activity limitations in the 30 days preceding the survey (Question-4). Question-1 is a predictor of mortality and chronic disease conditions [58], questions – 2 and – 3 assess recent physical symptoms and mental or emotional distress, respectively, and question- 4 measures perceived disability and lost productivity [55]. Only responses to survey Questions-2 and -3 were used in the current study since the focus of the analysis was to determine effects specifically on physical and mental health. Throughout this analysis, an *increase* in the number of physical/mental unhealthy days has been used to indicate poorer health outcomes.

Coding of variables
Participants were divided into 3 categories by age (20–44 yrs., 45–65 yrs., > 65 yrs.) and 5 categories by race/ethnicity as Mexican-American (1), Other Hispanic (2), Non-Hispanic White (3), Non-Hispanic Black (4), and Other (5). Obesity was measured by body mass index (BMI) based on self-reported weight in kilograms divided by measured height in meters-square. Respondents were broadly categorized into 3 BMI groups: normal weight (BMI 18.5–24.9), overweight (BMI 25–29.9), and obese (BMI > 30). Systemic inflammation was measured via blood CRP levels (mg/dl) and grouped into 3 classes according to Visser et al. [44] – non-elevated CRP (< 0.22 mg/dl), elevated CRP (≥0.22 and < 1.0 mg/dl) and clinically raised CRP (≥1.0 mg/dl), respectively. Each medical condition, including asthma (MCQ010), arthritis (MCQ160A), cancer (MCQ220), or any heart disease (a composite variable derived from a positive diagnosis of any one of congestive heart failure (MCQ160B), coronary heart disease (MCQ160C), or heart attack (MCQ160E)) were dichotomized into '0' and '1' categories where '1' indicates a positive response to the question of whether there ever was a diagnosis of the relevant condition by a doctor or healthcare professional. Smoking status was also dichotomized, with '1' assigned to individuals who are current smokers. The use of common analgesic and anti-inflammatory medications (aspirin, acetaminophen, ibuprofen and naproxen) was extracted from the RXDDRUG field of NHANES data, which records the generic name of the drug. Subjects associated with any one of the 4 drugs listed above were marked with '1' and '0'

otherwise. Although acetaminophen is more widely prescribed as an analgesic and antipyretic rather than anti-inflammatory drug, previous studies have reported effectiveness of acetaminophen against lower grade inflammation [59] and acetaminophen overdose has been associated with reductions in circulating CRP levels [60]. Based on these findings, and the close association between inflammation and physical pain, we included the use of acetaminophen in the analysis. For logistic regression analysis each outcome variable (HRQOL measures) was dichotomized into ≤ 15 or > 15 days of poor physical (HSQ470) or mental health (HSQ480), with > 15 unhealthy days denoted by 1, and 0 otherwise. The rationale for dichotomization was based on earlier reports which considered a report of > 14 days of poor physical or mental health as representing a state of 'frequent distress' [61, 62].

Statistical analysis

All statistical analysis was conducted using SAS, version 9.1 (SAS Institute Inc., Cary, NC, USA) or R (version × 64 3.2.3). Data was analyzed using sampling weighted generalized linear models. Both unadjusted and adjusted models linking BMI and CRP to the outcome variables (HSQ470 and HSQ480) were constructed, with adjustments for possible inflammation-regulating medical conditions (asthma, arthritis, heart disease, and cancer), use of over the counter anti-inflammatory/pain medications (acetaminophen, aspirin, ibuprofen and naproxen), and current cigarette smoking status. As several of the surveyed variables contained missing values, any attempt to analyze only complete cases severely reduced the total number of observations, leading to increased risk of biased estimates. To mitigate this problem, we used multiple imputation [63] to estimate probable value ranges for incomplete observations. The original coding for the missing values included bona-fide missing values, plus other types of non-response such as "don't know" (1517 total instances), and "refused to answer" (2 total instances). We converted all missing and non-response cases into missing values, as recommended in the NHANES analytical guidelines [64]. Multiple imputation generates more than one set of replacements for the missing values based on plausible models for data thereby yielding multiple completed datasets for analysis [65]. Five imputed datasets were generated according to multiple imputation procedures described by Rubin [63]. Each of these "completed" datasets were individually analyzed using sampling weighted generalized linear models (GLM), via the *survey* package in R [66]. For each of the imputed datasets, $m = 1...5$, we obtained the estimate of regression coefficient as β_m along with the standard error s_m. The overall estimate was obtained by

averaging the individual estimates from the imputed datasets as

$$\hat{\beta} = \frac{1}{M} \sum_{m=1}^{M} \hat{\beta}_m$$

The estimated variance for $\hat{\beta}$ is given by

$$V(\hat{\beta}) = W + (1 + \frac{1}{M})B,$$

where $W = \frac{1}{M} \sum_{m=1}^{M} s_m^2$, and $B = \frac{1}{M-1} \sum_{m=1}^{M} (\widehat{\beta_m} - \hat{\beta})^2$

Due to the difficulties in combining and interpreting the combined p-values arising from the above analysis, we have chosen to report results in terms of the estimated odds ratio ($e^{\hat{\beta}}$) and their 95% confidence interval for all analysis. The odds ratios (OR) were obtained by exponentiation of the average regression coefficient, $\hat{\beta}$.

The mediation analyses that are presented in Fig. 1, consisted of the following steps, as suggested by MacKinnon et al. [67]. The main association between the independent variable (obesity) and dependent variable (physical unhealthy days) were examined as per Eq. 1 (*c*-coefficient in Fig. 1). Next, we estimated the association of the mediating variable (inflammation, CRP levels) to the dependent variable in the presence of obesity (Eq. 2, *b*-coefficient in Fig. 1). Finally, we investigated the association of the mediating variable to the independent variable (Eq. 3, *a*-coefficient in Fig. 1).

$$Y = i_1 + cX + e_1 \tag{1}$$
$$Y = i_2 + c'X + bM + e_2 \tag{2}$$
$$M = i_3 + aX + e_3 \tag{3}$$

where Y is the number of physical unhealthy days (dependent variable), X is the obesity status (independent variable), M is the inflammation status (mediating variable), c is the coefficient relating X to Y, c' is the coefficient relating X to Y adjusted for M, b is the coefficient relating M to Y adjusted for X, a is the coefficient relating X to M, i_1-i_3 are intercepts and e_1-e_3 are residuals, respectively.

Results
Participants

The general characteristics of the survey respondents are listed in Table 1, with continuous measures reported as the mean (+ standard deviation), and categorical measures expressed as frequencies. The average age of the sampled population was 51.3 years (+ 17.85 years), with

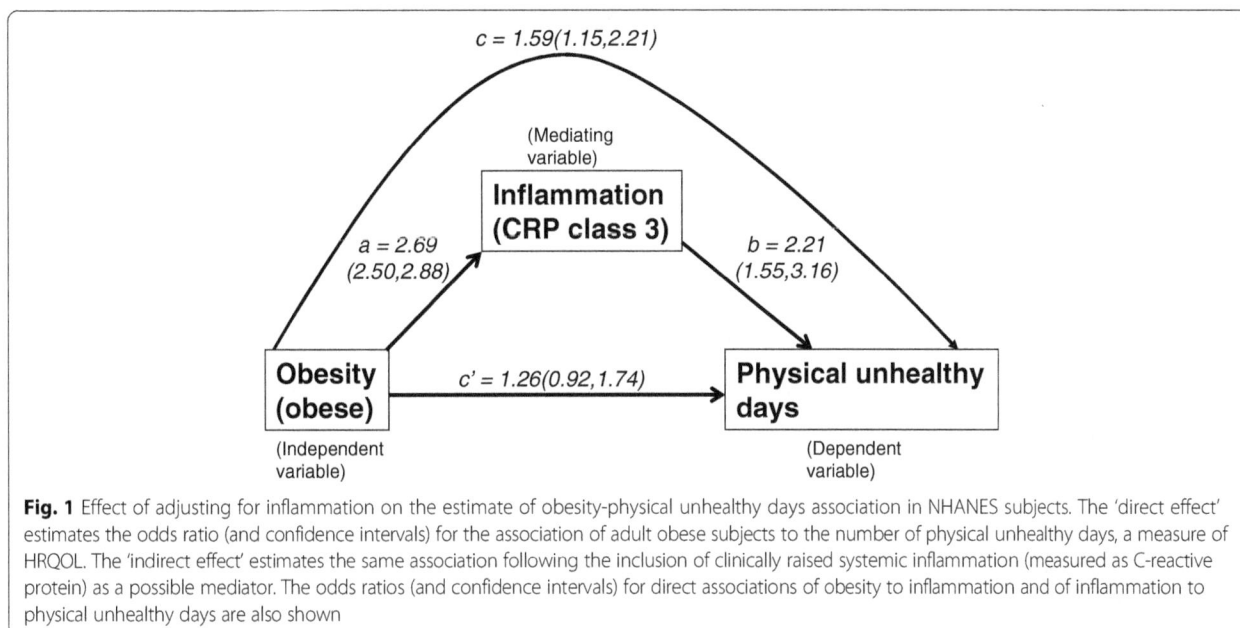

Fig. 1 Effect of adjusting for inflammation on the estimate of obesity-physical unhealthy days association in NHANES subjects. The 'direct effect' estimates the odds ratio (and confidence intervals) for the association of adult obese subjects to the number of physical unhealthy days, a measure of HRQOL. The 'indirect effect' estimates the same association following the inclusion of clinically raised systemic inflammation (measured as C-reactive protein) as a possible mediator. The odds ratios (and confidence intervals) for direct associations of obesity to inflammation and of inflammation to physical unhealthy days are also shown

approximately 49% male subjects. The proportions of normal weight, overweight and obese subjects were 27, 35 and 38%, respectively. CRP levels were in the 'normal' range for 51% of the subjects, 'elevated' in 37%, and 'clinically raised' in 11% of subjects. With the exception of age, sex and race, the data displayed varying levels of missingness for all other variables.

Relationship between body mass index and C-reactive protein

Quantile-quantile plots demonstrated that CRP and BMI values were better approximated to the normal distribution after log transformation (data not shown). We carried out linear regression to determine the association between CRP levels and BMI. Taking log CRP as the dependent variable and log BMI as the predictor variable, the regression coefficient of BMI was 2.69 (95% CI: 2.50, 2.88) (Additional file 1: Table S1, Figure S1, Text 3 and 4), indicating a statistically significant association between BMI and CRP in the study population.

Relationship of body mass index (BMI) and C-reactive protein (CRP) to physical and mental healthy days

Considering physical unhealthy days (HSQ470) as a binary response, we performed logistic regression with BMI groups (normal, overweight and obese) (normal group as reference) (Table 2, model 1). The estimated odds ratio for overweight subjects was 1.06 (95% CI: 0.76, 1.47) and that for obese subjects was 1.59 (95% CI: 1.15, 2.21). Thus, compared to a normal-weight person, an overweight person ($25 \leq BMI \leq 29.9$) was 1.06 times more likely, and an obese person ($BMI \geq 30$) 1.59 times more likely to

experience > 15 physical unhealthy days in a month. Only the estimated OR for the obese, but not overweight, individuals were statistically significant (95% CI excluded 1). In contrast, neither overweight nor obese individuals were significantly associated to mental unhealthy days (95% CI includes 1) (Table 2, model 2).

To further assess the relationship between the obesity class and physical/mental unhealthy days, we focused only on obese subjects ($BMI \geq 30$), divided into 5 subclasses according to increasing values of BMI (Additional file 1: Table S2 and S3). Subjects in the two highest classes of obesity (class IV, BMI 50.0–59.9 and class V, BMI ≥ 60) were found to be significantly associated to physical unhealthy days, compared to baseline (class I obesity, BMI 30.0–34.9). Only class V obesity subgroup was found to be significantly associated to HSQ480, with higher BMI associated with a reduced probability for mental unhealthy days. Although this finding is counterintuitive, we note that the statistical estimates may be unstable due to the very low subject numbers in this group (15 individuals, < 1% of total BMI ≥ 30 population).

Next, we assessed the relationship between plasma CRP levels (with non-elevated CRP class as reference) and the number of physical unhealthy days (Table 2, model 3). The estimated OR of elevated CRP was 1.61 (95% CI: 1.23, 2.12) and that of clinically raised CRP was 2.45 (95% CI: 1.84, 3.26), suggesting statistically significant associations for both CRP categories. The association between elevated CRP to mental unhealthy days (HSQ480) was not significant (OR = 1.05, 95% CI: 0.79, 1.40); however, clinically raised CRP was significantly associated to mental unhealthy days, (OR = 1.66, 95% CI: 1.26, 2.19) (Table 2, model 4).

Table 1 Demographic and Medical Characteristics of Study Subjects

Variable	Mean (SD) or frequency (%)	% missing
Sample size = 6325		
Age (yrs.)	51.30(17.85)	0
Male	48.96%	0
Race		
-Mexican American (1)	17.28%	0
-Other Hispanic (2)	11.38%	0
-Non-Hispanic White (3)	46.75%	0
-Non-Hispanic Black (4)	20.63%	0
-Other Race (Multiracial) (5)	4.03%	0
HSQ470 (days)	4.49(8.71)	11.74
HSQ480 (days)	4.09(8.28)	11.71
BMI (kg/m^2)	29.34(6.77)	5.66
-normal weight(18.5–24.99)	27.1%	
-overweight(25–29.99)	34.8%	
-obese(≥ 30)	38.0%	
CRP(mg/dl)	0.46(0.89)	9.92
-non-elevated (< 0.22)	51.3%	
-elevated (≥ 0.22- < 1.0)	37.4%	
-clinically raised (≥ 1.0)	11.3%	
SMQ040 (=1) [smoking]	21.97%	52.29
MCQ010 (=1) [asthma]	14.01%	0.09
MCQ220 (=1) [cancer]	10.12%	0.17
MCQ160A (=1) [arthritis]	32.21%	0.16
Any heart disease (=1)	9.38%	0.01
Anti-inflammatory drug use	13.72%	38.02

Data is presented as mean(SD) for continuous variables and as frequency(%) for categorical variables. The percent of data missing for each variable is indicated. Inflammation-related variables are coded (as per NHANES 2005–2008) as follows: SMQ040 (current smoking status), MCQ010 (medical diagnosis of asthma), MCQ220 (medical diagnosis of cancer), MCQ160A (medical diagnosis of arthritis), Any heart disease (medical diagnosis of one or more of heart attack, congestive heart failure or coronary heart disease)

Table 2 Relationship of Physical and Mental Healthy Days to BMI and CRP levels

Model	Dependent Variable	Parameter	OR (95% CI)
Model 1	HSQ470 (physical)	(Intercept)	0.06 (0.04,0.09)
		overweight	1.06 (0.76,1.47)
		obese	1.59 (1.15,2.21)
Model 2	HSQ480 (mental)	(Intercept)	0.06 (0.05,0.09)
		overweight	1.20 (0.86,1.68)
		obese	1.25 (0.89,1.75)
Model 3	HSQ470 (physical)	(Intercept)	0.06 (0.04,0.07)
		elevated CRP	1.61 (1.23,2.12)
		clinically raised CRP	2.45 (1.84,3.26)
Model 4	HSQ480 (mental)	(Intercept)	0.07 (0.05,0.09)
		elevated CRP	1.05 (0.79,1.40)
		clinically raised CRP	1.66 (1.26,2.19)
Model 5	HSQ470 (physical)	(Intercept)	0.05 (0.04,0.07)
		overweight	0.98 (0.70,1.35)
		obese	1.26 (0.92,1.74)
		elevated CRP	1.51 (1.14,2.0)
		clinically raised CRP	2.21(1.55,3.16)

Results include estimates of odds ratio (OR) and corresponding 95% confidence intervals under different models indexed by varying dependent variables. The OR is interpreted as the relative changes in odds for physical (HSQ470 > 15 days) or mental (HSQ480 > 15 days) unhealthy days upon changes in the categories of the explanatory variables (BMI and/or CRP) Data was analyzed using sampling weighted generalized linear models (logistic) as described under Methods. Model specifications are as follows: Model 1, HSQ470 vs. BMI; Model 2, HSQ480 vs. BMI; Model 3, HSQ470 vs. CRP; Model 4, HSQ480 vs. CRP; Model 5, HSQ470 vs. BMI and CRP

We next modeled both BMI groups and CRP categories as explanatory variables to ascertain their relative contribution to physical unhealthy days. The estimated odds ratios were 0.98 and 1.26 for overweight and obese BMI groups, respectively, and, 1.51 and 2.21 for elevated CRP and clinically raised CRP, respectively (Table 2, model 5). However, both the 95% CIs corresponding to the overweight (95% CI: 0.70, 1.35) and obese group (95% CI: 0.92, 1.74) now included 1, whereas the corresponding CIs for elevated CRP (95% CI: 1.14, 2.00) and clinically raised CRP (95% CI: 1.55, 3.16) excluded 1. In other words, when both CRP and BMI are included as explanatory variables in the same model, the significant associations observed earlier between BMI level and physical unhealthy days was no longer present. In the context of a mediation-framework according to Eqs. 1–3 listed under Methods, we observed significant relations for the coefficients a, b and c but not for c', suggesting that inflammation may function as a possible mediator of the observed association between obesity and physical unhealthy days (Fig. 1).

Effect modification analysis:

We carried out an effect modification analysis on the relationship of HSQ470 to BMI and CRP by including gender, age-class and race in the models. The interaction effects between 'overweight and gender', 'obese and gender' and 'overweight and Race-5' were significant (Table 3). For example, within the overweight category, a male was 0.42 times less likely to experience > 15 physical unhealthy days compared to a female. All other interactions were non-significant. For HSQ480 (mental unhealthy days), we observed significant interaction effects due to 'obese and gender'; 'clinically raised CRP and gender'; 'overweight and Age (45-65yrs)'; 'obese and Age (45-65yrs)'; 'clinically raised CRP and Age (45-

Table 3 Effect modification for outcome variable HSQ470

	Outcome Variable HSQ470		
	OR (95% CI)		OR (95% CI)
Effect modification due to GENDER			
(Intercept)	0.06 (0.04, 0.09)	(Intercept)	0.06 (0.04, 0.09)
Overweight	1.60 (1.01, 2.54)	elevated CRP	1.72 (1.18, 2.51)
Obese	1.96 (1.24, 3.11)	clinically raised CRP	2.38 (1.61, 3.52)
GENDER1	1.26 (0.80, 1.99)	GENDER1	0.92 (0.63, 1.33)
Overweight:GENDER1	*0.42 (0.26, 0.68)*	elevated CRP: GENDER1	0.83 (0.57, 1.20)
Obese:GENDER1	*0.62 (0.39, 0.99)*	clinically raised CRP: GENDER1	1.03 (0.70, 1.51)
Effect modification due to AGE			
(Intercept)	0.03 (0.02, 0.06)	(Intercept)	0.03 (0.02, 0.05)
Overweight	1.16 (0.64, 2.12)	elevated CRP	1.72 (1.03, 2.89)
Obese	1.64 (0.90, 3.01)	clinically raised CRP	2.16 (1.28, 3.63)
AGE (45-65 yrs)	2.68 (1.47, 4.89)	AGE (45-65 yrs)	2.67 (1.60, 4.45)
AGE (>65 yrs)	3.40 (1.86, 6.21)	AGE (>65 yrs)	2.53 (1.51, 4.24)
Overweight:AGE (45-65 yrs)	0.79 (0.43, 1.45)	elevated CRP: AGE (45-65 yrs)	0.79 (0.47, 1.33)
Obese:AGE (45-65 yrs)	0.89 (0.49, 1.63)	clinically raised CRP: AGE (45-65 yrs)	0.89 (0.53, 1.51)
Overweight:AGE (>65 yrs)	0.78 (0.43, 1.44)	elevated CRP: AGE (>65 yrs)	1.01 (0.60, 1.70)
Obese:AGE (>65 yrs)	0.82 (0.45, 1.50)	clinically raised CRP: AGE (>65 yrs)	1.57 (0.93, 2.66)
Effect modification due to Race			
(Intercept)	0.05 (0.02, 0.11)	(Intercept)	0.05 (0.03, 0.09)
Overweight	1.05 (0.48, 2.30)	elevated CRP	1.22 (0.66, 2.24)
Obese	1.42 (0.65, 3.12)	clinically raised CRP	2.23 (1.23, 4.04)
Race2	1.22 (0.56, 2.67)	Race2	1.40 (0.77, 2.54)
Race3	1.32 (0.60, 2.88)	Race3	1.20 (0.66, 2.17)
Race4	1.05 (0.48, 2.31)	Race4	1.20 (0.66, 2.19)
Race5	0.92 (0.42, 2.02)	Race5	0.63 (0.33, 1.22)
Overweight:Race2	1.53 (0.70, 3.37)	elevated CRP:Race2	1.00 (0.54, 1.85)
Obese:Race2	0.97 (0.44, 2.14)	clinically raised CRP:Race2	1.15 (0.60, 2.21)
Overweight:Race3	1.02 (0.46, 2.24)	elevated CRP:Race3	1.47 (0.79, 2.73)
Obese:Race3	1.17 (0.54, 2.58)	clinically raised CRP:Race3	1.20 (0.65, 2.19)
Overweight:Race4	0.95 (0.43, 2.09)	elevated CRP:Race4	0.96 (0.50, 1.83)
Obese:Race4	1.09 (0.50, 2.40)	clinically raised CRP:Race4	0.63 (0.35, 1.15)
Overweight:Race5	*0.30 (0.14, 0.67)*	elevated CRP:Race5	0.91 (0.33, 2.51)
Obese:Race5	0.58 (0.26, 1.29)	clinically raised CRP:Race5	1.11 (0.37, 3.37)

The modification of the association between physical healthy days (HSQ470) and BMI or CRP was investigated. Data was analyzed using sampling weighted generalized linear models (logistic) as described under Methods.
Significant associations are shown in italics

65yrs)'; 'clinically raised CRP and Age (>65yrs)', and, 'overweight and Race-5' (Additional file 1: Table S4). All other interactions effects were non-significant. These results suggest that the observed association between adiposity or CRP and physical/mental healthy days are modifiable to some extent by age and gender. However, the apparent modification of the association between overweight and HSQ470/ HSQ480 by Race-5 has to be

Table 4 Sensitivity Analysis with respect to different cut-off values of HSQ470 vs BMI and CRP

	OR (95% CI) (outcome variable HSQ470 vs BMI Class)					
Cut-off of HSQ470	12	13	14	16	17	18
Intercept	0.08 (0.06,0.11)	0.08 (0.06,0.11)	0.07 (0.05,0.1)	0.06 (0.04,0.08)	0.06 (0.04,0.08)	0.06 (0.04,0.08)
Overweight	1.21 (0.91,1.59)	1.19 (0.9,1.58)	1.2 (0.89,1.61)	1.03 (0.74,1.43)	1.02 (0.73,1.42)	1.02 (0.73,1.42)
Obese	1.69 (1.27,2.23)	1.7 (1.28,2.25)	1.66 (1.23,2.23)	1.6 (1.15,2.23)	1.58 (1.13,2.2)	1.54 (1.1,2.15)
	OR (95% CI) (outcome variable HSQ470 vs CRP Class)					
Cut-off of HSQ470	12	13	14	16	17	18
Intercept	0.08 (0.06,0.1)	0.08 (0.06,0.1)	0.07 (0.05,0.09)	0.05 (0.04,0.07)	0.05 (0.04,0.07)	0.05 (0.04,0.07)
elevated CRP	1.54 (1.22,1.96)	1.53 (1.2,1.93)	1.55 (1.21,1.98)	1.7 (1.29,2.24)	1.7 (1.28,2.24)	1.73 (1.3,2.28)
clinically raised CRP	2.34 (1.83,2.99)	2.36 (1.84,3.03)	2.46 (1.89,3.2)	2.59 (1.94,3.45)	2.64 (1.97,3.54)	2.7 (2.01,3.62)

The threshold for physical unhealthy days was varied from 12 to 18 days and the effects on the association to BMI or CRP classes was evaluated (upper and lower panels of table, respectively). Data was analyzed by sampling weighted generalized linear models as described under Methods

interpreted with caution due to the very low numbers of subjects belonging to this category (< 5% of the surveyed population, Table 1).

Sensitivity analysis

We performed sensitivity analysis on the relationship of HSQ470 to BMI groups and CRP classes by varying the cut-off value for HSQ470 = 1 from 15 to 12, 13, 14, 16, 17 and 18 days. The obese class was significantly associated to HSQ470 for all the cut-off values tested with stable odds ratio estimates (Table 4). On the other hand, the odds-ratios for overweight were non-significant for all HSQ470 cut-off values tested, consistent with the original findings. Similarly, the odds-ratios corresponding to the different CRP classes (elevated and clinically raised CRP) with different HSQ470 cut-off values were significant, agreeing again with the primary results (HSQ470 cut-off value = 15). These results suggest that the identified associations between BMI or CRP and HRQOL are robust to the threshold used for defining physical unhealthy days.

Relationship of CRP to physical and mental unhealthy days after adjustment for other sources of inflammation

We next investigated whether the effects of CRP classes on physical unhealthy days could be confounded by some of the more common sources of inflammation encountered in the study population (mediator outcome confounding). We carried out multivariable logistic regression analysis by including demographics (age, gender), pro-inflammatory medical conditions, use of common anti-inflammatory/pain medications, and current smoking status, in addition to CRP and BMI categories in the model (Table 5). The CRP.Class variable remained significantly associated to physical unhealthy days, for both the elevated CRP (OR = 1.34, 95% CI: 1.00, 1.79) and clinically raised CRP (OR = 1.71, 95% CI:1.18, 2.48), even after adjustment. A similar analysis against mental unhealthy days showed the association of CRP classes and BMI groups to be non-significant, although significant associations were

observed for presence of asthma, presence of arthritis, current smoking status, occurrence of any heart disease and gender (Additional file 1: Table S5).

Discussion

The present study was undertaken to better define the relationship between obesity, systemic inflammation and measures of HRQOL. We used data from a US population based survey (NHANES 2005–2008) to estimate effects of increasing body mass and increasing inflammation on the number of physical and mental unhealthy days reported by participants. We also tested the impact of common inflammation regulators (inflammatory disease, anti-inflammatory drug use, and smoking) on the association between the inflammation marker CRP, and HRQOL (based

Table 5 Multivariable logistic regression analysis of the association of CRP to physical unhealthy days

Parameter	OR (95% CI)	p-value
(Intercept)	0.04 (0.02, 0.06)	< 0.01
Overweight	0.95 (0.68, 1.33)	0.76
Obese	1.12 (0.79, 1.58)	0.52
CRP.class (2)	1.34 (1.00, 1.79)	0.05
CRP.class (3)	1.71 (1.18, 2.48)	0.01
Anti-inflammatory Drug Use (1)	2.40 (1.74, 3.3)	< 0.01
AGEclass (2)	1.88 (1.35, 2.63)	< 0.01
AGEclass (3)	1.79 (1.2, 2.68)	< 0.01
MCQ010 (1)	1.36 (1.01, 1.83)	0.05
MCQ220 (1)	1.36 (0.96, 1.95)	0.09
MCQ160A (1)	2.32 (1.72, 3.13)	< 0.01
GENDER (1)	0.88 (0.68, 1.15)	0.35
SMQ040 (1)	0.83 (0.69, 1.00)	0.05
Any Heart Disease (1)	1.63 (1.14, 2.32)	0.01

Results include estimates of odds ratio (OR) and corresponding 95% confidence intervals. The OR is interpreted as the increase in odds for physical (HSQ470 > 15 days) unhealthy days upon changes in the categories of the explanatory variables. Data was analyzed using sampling weighted generalized linear models (logistic) as described under Methods

on the CDC HRQOL-4 questionnaire). Compared to the more detailed Medical Outcomes Study Short Form 36 (SF-36), the CDC's "healthy days" serves as a simple proxy measure of HRQOL. It measures perceptions of physical and mental health using one question each, eliminating the need for complex weighting factors to calculate summary scores.

In previous studies, Hassan et al. [32] assessed a US-based sample with the CDC-HRQOL-4 and reported greater likelihood of poor physical and mental quality of life in participants with obesity. Renzaho et al. [34] sampled an Australian population with SF-36 and found that physical, but not mental, HRQOL scores were negatively associated with BMI. Serrano-Aguilar et al. [35] analyzed a European sample using the EuroQol-5d assessment and found that participants with BMI > 40 had lower HRQOL scores than normal weight participants. These findings agree with the positive association between BMI and number of physical unhealthy days observed in the current study in unadjusted models, and also support the general lack of association between BMI and mental unhealthy days [34].

We next conducted an exploratory analysis to examine whether obesity-associated systemic inflammation could potentially mediate some of the observed association between obesity and HRQOL (physical or mental unhealthy days), by employing the well-known causal steps approach to mediation by Barron and Kenny [68, 69]. This approach consists of 4 steps to establish mediation, namely (i) a significant relation of the independent variable (obesity) to the dependent variable (number of physical unhealthy days) (Table 2, model 1); (ii) a significant relation of the independent variable to the hypothesized mediating variable (systemic inflammation) (Additional file 1: Table S1); (iii) a significant relation of the mediating variable to the dependent variable in the presence of independent variable (Table 2, model 5); (iv) a smaller absolute coefficient relating the independent variable to the dependent variable in the presence of the mediating variable (Table 2, model 5). All four conditions were satisfied in the analysis of systemic inflammation as a possible mediator of the relation between obesity and physical healthy days. Notably, the association between BMI and physical HRQOL was non-significant after systemic inflammation (CRP levels) was included in the regression model (Table 2, model 5).

We further investigated whether systemic inflammation was itself a predictor of HRQOL in the NHANES cohort, and whether the association was modified in the presence of other factors such as obesity, common inflammatory disease, anti-inflammatory drug use, etc. We based our analysis on the rationale that chronic inflammation is an important index of population health and provides a unifying pathological mechanism for many seemingly unrelated diseases [70]. Recent research focusing on general associations between specific inflammatory chronic conditions (e.g. asthma, irritable bowel syndrome, Crohn's disease, chronic prostatitis, etc.) and health outcomes have also reported significant associations between symptom severity and HRQOL reductions [71–76]. These reductions are further compounded by psychological distress [77] and allostatic load [78]. Literature on inflammatory disease and HRQOL suggests that these negative associations may be partly mediated by the common medical consequences of chronic illness [79]. For example, pain and disability linked to chronic inflammation has been found to play a small but significant mediating role in the overall HRQOL reduction in older adults [80].

In our analysis, systemic CRP levels were positively and significantly associated with the number of physical and mental unhealthy days, even after adjustments for sex, age, pro-inflammatory co-morbidities, and anti-inflammatory/analgesic drug use. Importantly, the observed association to physical unhealthy days persisted even for levels of inflammation below the clinical threshold. Visser et al. [44] introduced the classification scheme of sub-clinical 'elevated CRP ($\geq$0.22 mg/dl)' and 'clinically raised CRP ($\geq$1.0 mg/dl)' and identified an association of the former with overweight and obesity. In other studies, sub-clinical CRP has been associated with increased risk of cardiovascular disease-related mortality in healthy subjects [81]. Our study now further demonstrates the importance of sub-clinical CRP levels in the domain of HRQOL.

We now discuss some potential limitations of the study and differences from previously published reports. While our study used the number of healthy days as the HRQOL metric, previous studies utilized composite HRQOL measures, based on a summation over several sub-domain scores. Additionally, differences in the sampled populations between the studies could also potentially influence the current findings. Also, since the assessment by CDC HRQOL-4 is based on self-reporting, the study results are also potentially susceptible to the risk of recall error and misreport. In this study, we applied the multiple imputation method to address the missing data, based on the underlying assumption of 'missing at random'(MAR) [82], wherein the systematic differences between the missing and observed values are entirely explicable by other observed variables. Under MAR, the multiple imputation approach maintains the benefits of maximum likelihood estimation, while also allowing for uncertainty due to imputation (infeasible under single imputation) to be included during data analysis. In our study, we have assumed MAR for all the variables, including smoking and anti-inflammatory drug uses that have high proportion of missing values (52 and 38%, respectively). Since the study sample size is reasonably large (6325), we expect the missing values imputation to remain robust, even for variables with a high proportion of missing values. Another possible limitation of the current work is that the mediation analysis has been conducted on a cross-sectional design (the only design available for this type of study at the moment). Although several studies in the mediation literature have employed cross-sectional designs, these designs lack the ability to formally support causal inference and instead must depend on a priori assumptions, based on strong biological rationale, to infer mediation [83]. As explained by Maxwell and Cole [49], cross-sectional approaches to mediation typically generate biased estimates in the absence of true time precedence data [84]. In our case, several biological experiments, including Mendelian randomization studies, strongly implicate the precedence of obesity over chronic inflammation reflected in rising CRP levels [23]. Also as discussed earlier [25–29], other studies have shown obesity-associated inflammation to be causally linked to various biologic endpoints. Finally, the ability of disease-associated inflammation to alter HQOL has also been recently demonstrated for depression and schizophrenia [41, 42]. Given these observations, we think there are reasonable biological grounds for exploring a possible mediation-framework in our study. We would, however, caution about the exploratory nature of the current analysis and emphasize it as only hypothesis-generating at present.

Conclusion

In conclusion, a population-based analysis investigating the roles of obesity and systemic inflammation on indices of health-related quality of life suggests inflammation as a possible mediator of the negative associations between body mass index and the number of reported physical healthy days. Sub-clinical inflammation also appears to be an independent predictor of physical and mental healthy days in the general population. In light of these observations, the relationship of systemic inflammation to quality of life need to be further investigated, and a distinction made between clinically-raised high CRP levels and lower (but possibly chronic) elevations in CRP that can still significantly affect health related quality of life.

Abbreviations

BMI: Body Mass Index; CRP: C-reactive protein; HRQOL: Health Related Quality of Life; HSQ470: Health Status Questionnaire 470; HSQ480: Health Status Questionnaire480; NHANES: National Health and Nutrition Examination Survey

Acknowledgements

The authors thank Drs. Jonathan Livingston, Dwayne Brandon and Sandra Waters from the Department of Psychology, North Carolina Central University, for helpful discussions and suggestions during the design and analysis of the study. The authors also thank Mr. Lavonza Holliman for his assistance with the initial literature review.

Author contributions

JW (acquisition and interpretation of data, writing of manuscript); PG (analysis and interpretation of data, writing of manuscript); JV (analysis of data); BC (interpretation of data, review of statistical analysis); SG (conception and supervision of study, interpretation of data, writing of manuscript). All authors read and approved the final manuscript.

Funding

This work was supported by a NCCU-BBRI fellowship to JW and funding from the National Institutes of Health (HL059868, MD000175 and DK088319), American Heart Association (AHA10SDG4230068) National Medical Research Council, Ministry of Health, Singapore (WBS R913200076263) to SG; funding from the Duke-NUS Medical School, Singapore, to BC.

Competing interests

The authors declare that they have no competing interests.

Author details

[1]Biomedical Biotechnology Research Institute, North Carolina Central University, 1801 Fayetteville Street, Durham, NC 27707, USA. [2]Centre for Quantitative Medicine, Duke-NUS Medical School, 8 College Road, Singapore 169857, Singapore. [3]Center for Tobacco Products, Food and Drug Administration, 10903 New Hampshire Avenue, Silver Spring, MD 20993, USA. [4]Program in Cardiovascular & Metabolic Disorders & Centre for Computational Biology, Duke-NUS Medical School, 8 College Road, Singapore 169857, Singapore.

References

1. Mozaffarian D, Hao T, Rimm EB, Willett WC, Hu FB. Changes in diet and lifestyle and long-term weight gain in women and men. N Engl J Med. 2011;364(25):2392–404.
2. McAllister EJ, Dhurandhar NV, Keith SW, Aronne LJ, Barger J, Baskin M. Ten putative contributors to the obesity epidemic. Crit Rev Food Sci Nutr. 2009;49
3. Bluher M. The distinction of metabolically 'healthy' from 'unhealthy' obese individuals. Curr Opin Lipidol. 2010;21(1):38–43.
4. Kaaks R, Kuhn T. Epidemiology: obesity and cancer-the evidence is fattening up. Nat Rev Endocrinol. 2014;10(11):644–5.
5. Lumeng CN, Saltiel AR. Inflammatory links between obesity and metabolic disease. J Clin Invest. 2011;121(6):2111–7.
6. Flegal KM, Carroll MD, Ogden CL, Curtin LR. Prevalence and trends in obesity among US adults, 1999-2008. JAMA. 2010;303(3):235–41.
7. Wolf AM, Colditz GA. Current estimates of the economic cost of obesity in the United States. Obes Res. 1998;6(2):97–106.
8. Hammond RA, Levine R. The economic impact of obesity in the United States. Diabetes Metab Syndr Obes. 2010;3:285–95.

9. Tsai AG, Williamson DF, Glick HA. Direct medical cost of overweight and obesity in the USA: a quantitative systematic review. Obes Rev. 2011;12(1):50–61.

10. Singer K, Lumeng CN. The initiation of metabolic inflammation in childhood obesity. J Clin Invest. 2017;127(1):65–73.

11. Hotamisligil GS. Endoplasmic reticulum stress and the inflammatory basis of metabolic disease. Cell. 2010;140(6):900–17.

12. Odegaard JI, Chawla A. The immune system as a sensor of the metabolic state. Immunity. 2013;38(4):644–54.

13. Lee YS, Li P, Huh JY, Hwang IJ, Lu M, Kim JI, Ham M, Talukdar S, Chen A, Lu WJ, et al. Inflammation is necessary for long-term but not short-term high-fat diet-induced insulin resistance. Diabetes. 2011;60(10):2474–83.

14. Yang X, Li M, Haghiac M, Catalano PM, O'Tierney-Ginn P, Hauguel-de Mouzon S. Causal relationship between obesity-related traits and TLR4-driven responses at the maternal-fetal interface. Diabetologia. 2016;59(11):2459–66.

15. Emilsson V, Thorleifsson G, Zhang B, Leonardson A, Zink F, Zhu J, Carlson S, Helgason A, Walters G, Gunnarsdottir S, et al. Genetics of gene expression and its effect on disease. Nature. 2008;452(7186):423–8.

16. Chen Y, Zhu J, Lum P, Yang X, Pinto S, MacNeil D, Zhang C, Lamb J, Edwards S, Sieberts S, et al. Variations in DNA elucidate molecular networks that cause disease. Nature. 2008;452(7186):429–35.

17. Hirosumi J, Tuncman G, Chang L, Gorgun CZ, Uysal KT, Maeda K, Karin M, Hotamisligil GS. A central role for JNK in obesity and insulin resistance. Nature. 2002;420(6913):333–6.

18. Weisberg SP, McCann D, Desai M, Rosenbaum M, Leibel RL, Ferrante AW Jr. Obesity is associated with macrophage accumulation in adipose tissue. J Clin Invest. 2003;112(12):1796–808.

19. Yudkin JS, Stehouwer CD, Emeis JJ, Coppack SW. C-reactive protein in healthy subjects: associations with obesity, insulin resistance, and endothelial dysfunction: a potential role for cytokines originating from adipose tissue? Arterioscler Thromb Vasc Biol. 1999;19(4):972–8.

20. Frayling TM, Timpson NJ, Weedon MN, Zeggini E, Freathy RM, Lindgren CM, Perry JR, Elliott KS, Lango H, Rayner NW, et al. A common variant in the FTO gene is associated with body mass index and predisposes to childhood and adult obesity. Science. 2007;316(5826):889–94.

21. Li H, Kilpelainen TO, Liu C, Zhu J, Liu Y, Hu C, Yang Z, Zhang W, Bao W, Cha S, et al. association of genetic variation in FTO with risk of obesity and type 2 diabetes with data from 96,551 east and south Asians. Diabetologia. 2012;55(4):981–95.

22. Tung YC, Yeo GS, O'Rahilly S, Coll AP. Obesity and FTO: changing focus at a complex locus. Cell Metab. 2014;20(5):710–8.

23. Welsh P, Polisecki E, Robertson M, Jahn S, Buckley BM, de Craen AJ, Ford I, Jukema JW, Macfarlane PW, Packard CJ, et al. Unraveling the directional link between adiposity and inflammation: a bidirectional Mendelian randomization approach. J Clin Endocrinol Metab. 2010;95(1):93–9.

24. Budu-Aggrey A, Brumpton B, Tyrrell J, Watkins S, Modalsli EH, Celis-Morales C, Ferguson LD, Vie GÅ, Palmer T, Fritsche LG, et al. Evidence of a common causal relationship between body mass index and inflammatory skin disease: a Mendelian randomization study. In: bioRxiv; 2018.

25. Chmelar J, Chung KJ, Chavakis T. The role of innate immune cells in obese adipose tissue inflammation and development of insulin resistance. Thromb Haemost. 2013;109(3):399–406.

26. Hotamisligil GS. Inflammation and metabolic disorders. Nature. 2006;444(7121):860–7.

27. Shoelson SE, Lee J, Goldfine AB. Inflammation and insulin resistance. J Clin Invest. 2006;116(7):1793–801.

28. Schenk S, Saberi M, Olefsky JM. Insulin sensitivity: modulation by nutrients and inflammation. J Clin Invest. 2008;118(9):2992–3002.

29. Ouchi N, Parker JL, Lugus JJ, Walsh K. Adipokines in inflammation and metabolic disease. Nat Rev Immunol. 2011;11(2):85–97.

30. McHorney CA. Health status assessment methods for adults: past accomplishments and future challenges. Annu Rev Public Health. 1999;20:309–35.

31. Doll HA, Petersen SE, Stewart-Brown SL. Obesity and physical and emotional well-being: associations between body mass index, chronic illness, and the physical and mental components of the SF-36 questionnaire. Obes Res. 2000;8(2):160–70.

32. Hassan MK, Joshi AV, Madhavan SS, Amonkar MM. Obesity and health-related quality of life: a cross-sectional analysis of the US population. International journal of obesity and related metabolic disorders : journal of the International Association for the Study of Obesity. 2003;27(10):1227–32.

33. Jia H, Lubetkin EI. The impact of obesity on health-related quality-of-life in the general adult US population. J Public Health (Oxf). 2005;27(2):156–64.

34. Renzaho A, Wooden M, Houng B. Associations between body mass index and health-related quality of life among Australian adults. Qual Life Res. 2010;19(4):515–20.

35. Serrano-Aguilar P, Munoz-Navarro SR, Ramallo-Farina Y, Trujillo-Martin MM. Obesity and health related quality of life in the general adult population of the Canary Islands. Qual Life Res. 2009;18(2):171–7.

36. Hoare E, Fuller-Tyszkiewicz M, Skouteris H, Millar L, Nichols M, Allender S. Systematic review of mental health and well-being outcomes following community-based obesity prevention interventions among adolescents. BMJ Open. 2015;5(1):e006586.

37. Nemiary D, Shim R, Mattox G, Holden K. The relationship between obesity and depression among adolescents. Psychiatr Ann. 2012;42(8):305–8.

38. Courtney JM, Kelly MG, Watt A, Garske L, Bradley J, Ennis M, Elborn JS. Quality of life and inflammation in exacerbations of bronchiectasis. Chron Respir Dis. 2008;5(3):161–8.

39. Ehrs PO, Sundblad BM, Larsson K. Effect of fluticasone on markers of inflammation and quality of life in steroid-naive patients with mild asthma. Clin Respir J. 2010;4(1):51–8.

40. Farag YM, Keithi-Reddy SR, Mittal BV, Surana SP, Addabbo F, Goligorsky MS, Singh AK. Anemia, inflammation and health-related quality of life in chronic kidney disease patients. Clin Nephrol. 2011;75(6):524–33.

41. Faugere M, Micoulaud-Franchi JA, Alessandrini M, Richieri R, Faget-Agius C, Auquier P, Lancon C, Boyer L. Quality of life is associated with chronic inflammation in schizophrenia: a cross-sectional study. Sci Rep. 2015;5:10793.

42. Faugere M, Micoulaud-Franchi JA, Faget-Agius C, Lancon C, Cermolacce M, Richieri R. Quality of life is associated with chronic inflammation in depression: a cross-sectional study. J Affect Disord. 2018;227:494–7.

43. Greenfield JR, Samaras K, Jenkins AB, Kelly PJ, Spector TD, Gallimore JR, Pepys MB, Campbell LV. Obesity is an important determinant of baseline serum C-reactive protein concentration in monozygotic twins, independent of genetic influences. Circulation. 2004;109(24):3022–8.

44. Visser M, Bouter LM, McQuillan GM, Wener MH, Harris TB. Elevated C-reactive protein levels in overweight and obese adults. JAMA. 1999;282:2131–5.

45. Pepys MB, Hirschfield GM. C-reactive protein: a critical update. J Clin Invest. 2003;111(12):1805–12.

46. Aronson D, Bartha P, Zinder O, Kerner A, Markiewicz W, Avizohar O, Brook GJ, Levy Y. Obesity is the major determinant of elevated C-reactive protein in subjects with the metabolic syndrome. Int J Obes Relat Metab Disord. 2004;28(5):674–9.

47. Nowakowski AC. Chronic inflammation and quality of life in older adults: a cross-sectional study using biomarkers to predict emotional and relational outcomes. Health Qual Life Outcomes. 2014;12:141.

48. Hamer M, Chida Y. Life satisfaction and inflammatory biomarkers: the 2008 Scottish health survey. Jpn Psychol Res. 2011;53(2):133–9.

49. Maxwell SE, Cole DA. Bias in cross-sectional analyses of longitudinal mediation. Psychol Methods. 2007;12(1):23–44.

50. Maxwell SE, Cole DA, Mitchell MA. Bias in cross-sectional analyses of longitudinal mediation: partial and complete mediation under an autoregressive model. Multivariate Behav Res. 2011;46(5):816–41.

51. Khera R, Murad MH, Chandar AK, Dulai PS, Wang Z, Prokop LJ, Loomba R, Camilleri M, Singh S. Association of Pharmacological Treatments for obesity with weight loss and adverse events: a systematic review and meta-analysis. JAMA. 2016;315(22):2424–34.

52. Centers for Disease Control and Prevention (CDC) NCfHS. National Health and nutrition examination survey data. Hyattsville: US Department of Health and Human Services, Centers for Disease Control and Prevention; 2005–2008) (http://www.cdc.gov/nchs/nhanes.htm.

53. Dey M, Gmel G, Mohler-Kuo M. Body mass index and health-related quality of life among young Swiss men. BMC Public Health. 2013;13:1028.

54. Ford ES, Li C. Metabolic syndrome and health-related quality of life among U.S. adults. Ann Epidemiol. 2008;18(3):165–71.

55. Hennessy CH, Moriarty DG, Zack MM, Scherr PA, Brackbill R. Measuring health-related quality of life for public health surveillance. Public Health Rep. 1994;109(5):665–72.

56. Mielenz T, Jackson E, Currey S, DeVellis R, Callahan LF. Psychometric properties of the Centers for Disease Control and Prevention health-related quality of life (CDC HRQOL) items in adults with arthritis. Health Qual Life Outcomes. 2006;4:66.

57. Newschaffer CJ. Validation of behavioral risk factor surveillance system (BRFSS) HRQOL measures in a statewide sample. Atlanta: prevention CfDCa; 1998.

58. Idler EL, Benyamini Y. Self-rated health and mortality: a review of twenty-seven community studies. J Health Soc Behav. 1997;38(1):21–37.

59. Graham GG, Davies MJ, Day RO, Mohamudally A, Scott KF. The modern pharmacology of paracetamol: therapeutic actions, mechanism of action, metabolism, toxicity and recent pharmacological findings. Inflammopharmacology. 2013;21(3):201–32.

60. Craig DG, Lee P, Pryde EA, Walker SW, Beckett GJ, Hayes PC, Simpson KJ. Elevated levels of the long pentraxin 3 in paracetamol-induced human acute liver injury. Eur J Gastroenterol Hepatol. 2013;25(3):359–67.

61. Andresen EM, Catlin TK, Wyrwich KW, Jackson-Thompson J. Retest reliability of surveillance questions on health related quality of life. J Epidemiol Community Health. 2003;57(5):339–43.

62. (CDC) CfDCaP. Self-reported frequent mental distress among adults - United States, 1993-1996. MMWR Morb Mortal Wkly Rep. 1998;47:326–31.

63. Rubin DB. Formalizing subjective notions about the effect of nonrespondents in sample surveys. J Am Stat Assoc. 1977;72:538–43.

64. Johnson CL, Paulose-Ram R, Ogden CL. National Health and Nutrition Examination Survey: Analytic Guidelines, 1999–2010. Vital Health Stat. 2013;2(161):1–24.

65. He Y. Missing data analysis using multiple imputation: getting to the heart of the matter. Circulation Cardiovascular quality and outcomes. 2010;3(1): 98–105.

66. Lumley T. Analysis of complex survey samples. J Stat Softw. 2004;9(8):1–19.

67. MacKinnon DP, Fairchild AJ, Fritz MS. Mediation analysis. Annu Rev Psychol. 2007;58:593–614.

68. Baron RM, Kenny DA. The moderator-mediator variable distinction in social psychological research: conceptual, strategic, and statistical considerations. J Pers Soc Psychol. 1986;51(6):1173–82.

69. Judd CM, Kenny DA. Estimating mediation in treatment Evaluatins. Eval Rev. 1981;5(5):602–9.

70. Ward PA. Cytokines, inflammation, and autoimmune diseases. Hospital practice. 1995;30(5):35–41.

71. Testa MA, Simonson DC. Assessment of quality-of-life outcomes. N Engl J Med. 1996;334(13):835–40.

72. Sprangers MA, de Regt EB, Andries F, van Agt HM, Bijl RV, de Boer JB, Foets M, Hoeymans N, Jacobs AE, Kempen GI, et al. Which chronic conditions are associated with better or poorer quality of life? J Clin Epidemiol. 2000;53(9): 895–907.

73. Schmaling KB, Afari N, Hops H, Barnhart S, Buchwald D. Change in airflow among patients with asthma discussing relationship problems with their partners. J Health Psychol. 2009;14(6):715–20.

74. Drossman DA, Patrick DL, Mitchell CM, Zagami EA, Appelbaum MI. Health-related quality of life in inflammatory bowel disease. Functional status and patient worries and concerns Dig Dis Sci. 1989;34(9):1379–86.

75. Lichtenstein GR, Hanauer SB, Sandborn WJ. Practice Parameters Committee of American College of G: Management of Crohn's disease in adults. The American journal of gastroenterology. 2009;104(2):465–83. quiz 464, 484

76. Nickel JC. Prostatitis: evolving management strategies. Urol Clin North Am. 1999;26(4):737–51.

77. Cummings DM, King DE, Mainous AG 3rd. C-reactive protein, antiinflammatory drugs, and quality of life in diabetes. Ann Pharmacother. 2003;37(11):1593–7.

78. Geronimus AT, Hicken M, Keene D, Bound J. "weathering" and age patterns of allostatic load scores among blacks and whites in the United States. Am J Public Health. 2006;96(5):826–33.

79. McSorley ST, Dolan RD, Roxburgh CSD, McMillan DC, Horgan PG. How and why systemic inflammation worsens quality of life in patients with advanced cancer. Expert Review of Quality of Life in Cancer Care. 2017;2(3): 167–75.

80. Nowakowski AC, Graves KY, Sumerau JE. Mediation analysis of relationships between chronic inflammation and quality of life in older adults. Health Qual Life Outcomes. 2016;14:46.

81. Koenig W, Sund M, Frohlich M, Fischer HG, Lowel H, Doring A, Hutchinson WL, Pepys MB. C-reactive protein, a sensitive marker of inflammation, predicts future risk of coronary heart disease in initially healthy middle-aged men: results from the MONICA (monitoring trends and determinants in cardiovascular disease) Augsburg cohort study, 1984 to 1992. Circulation. 1999;99(2):237–42.

82. Bhaskaran K, Smeeth L. What is the difference between missing completely at random and missing at random? Int J Epidemiol. 2014;43(4):1336–9.

83. Kline RB. The mediation myth. Basic Appl Soc Psychol. 2015;37(4):202–13.

84. Little TD. Longitudinal structural equation modeling. New York: Guilford Press; 2013.

85. US Department of Health and Human Services Code of Federal Regulations, Title 45 (http://www.hhs.gov/ohrp/humansubjects/guidance/45cfr46.html).

13

Informing the development of online weight management interventions: a qualitative investigation of primary care patient perceptions

Samantha B. van Beurden[1*], Sally I. Simmons[1], Jason C. H. Tang[3], Avril J. Mewse[2], Charles Abraham[1] and Colin J. Greaves[1]

Abstract

Background: The internet is a potentially promising medium for delivering weight loss interventions. The current study sought to explore factors that might influence primary care patients' initial uptake and continued use (up to four-weeks) of such programmes to help inform the development of novel, or refinement of existing, weight management interventions.

Methods: Semi-structured interviews were conducted with 20 patients purposively sampled based on age, gender and BMI from a single rural general practice. The interviews were conducted 4 weeks after recruitment at the general practice and focused on experiences with using one of three freely available weight loss websites. Thematic Analysis was used to analyse the data.

Results: Findings suggested that patients were initially motivated to engage with internet-based weight loss programmes by their accessibility and novelty. However, continued use was influenced by substantial facilitators and barriers, such as time and effort involved, reaction to prompts/reminders, and usefulness of information. Facilitation by face-to-face consultations with the GP was reported to be helpful in supporting change.

Conclusions: Although primary care patients may not be ready yet to solely depend on online interventions for weight loss, their willingness to use them shows potential for use alongside face–to-face weight management advice or intervention. Recommendations to minimise barriers to engagement are provided.

Keywords: Weight loss, Obesity, E-health, Internet, Primary care, Qualitative research

Background

Overweight and obesity remain a worldwide problem. Guidelines from the National Institute for Health and Care Excellence (NICE) recommend that GPs monitor patient weight and offer clinical weight management where necessary [1], but the choice of treatments in traditional primary care settings is limited. Currently, patients are offered lifestyle modification, pharmacotherapy (Orlistat), or weight loss surgeries of which the latter two are effective but expensive and often accompanied by negative side effects or complications [2, 3]. Referral to community-based weight loss programmes has been shown to be effective in the short term [4, 5], but resources are limited and face-to-face programmes can be costly to implement [6] and limited access restricts their use in rural areas [7]. Moreover, research suggests that primary care staff feel under-resourced to provide weight loss services [8, 9] and practitioners seldom approach the topic of weight [10–13].

Self-directed interventions delivered via digital platforms (eHealth) are plentiful and could provide a low cost and easily accessible alternative to existing treatment options in primary care [14, 15]. Such interventions can range from educational websites focused on information provision such as NHS Choices, to the more intensive

* Correspondence: s.b.vanbeurden@exeter.ac.uk
[1]University of Exeter Medical School, University of Exeter, Exeter, UK
Full list of author information is available at the end of the article

mobile applications that offer interactive food diary and weight monitoring tools such as MyFitnessPal. With 87.9% of adults in the UK using the internet and the 68.7% increase in prevalence of recent internet use among adults aged 65 to 74 (currently at 74.1%) between 2011 and 2016 [16], these interventions have the potential of reaching a substantial proportion of the UK population. E-Health has been found to be effective for a range of health behaviours including smoking, reducing cholesterol levels, lowering high blood pressure [17, 18], and facilitating weight loss [14, 19]. Technological advances have enabled the delivery of behaviour change techniques that map on to theoretically derived behavioural determinants, which were previously limited to face-to-face delivery such as prompting goal setting, instructing progress monitoring, and providing timely goal-related feedback [20] and are associated with effectiveness in face-to-face weight loss programmes [21]. In addition, service providers are positive about the use of eHealth in terms of its potential to provide continuity of care and opportunities for auditing the provided service [9].

However, not much is known about the experiences of primary care patients with eHealth for weight loss or their willingness to use it when recommended by their GP. This applies particularly to middle-aged and older patients living in rural areas with limited or no access to traditional weight management. Therefore, this study aimed to investigate the experiences of rural primary care patients with GP-facilitated use of such programmes and the factors that may influence their adoption and ongoing use to help inform the development of a novel weight management interventions.

Methods
Study design and setting
A qualitative study was conducted, using face-to-face semi-structured interviews with patients from a single General Practice in rural South West England. Ethical approval was obtained from the East of England Research Ethics Committee (Norfolk) in November 2012. No pre-determined theoretical framework was used to develop the design of the study.

Weight loss websites
Three freely available weight loss websites were selected for use in this study to access a range of experiences to help identify facilitators and barriers to the use of publicly available internet-based weight management programmes. The selection of these websites was based on the additional criteria concerning their compatibility with current US and UK recommendations for healthy eating as checked by a GP (SS):

1. SparkPeople (http://www.sparkpeople.com/) is an online community which requires registration and profile creation. The website provides diet tips & coaching from nutritionists and other experts; healthy recipes; exercise instructions in educational videos; food and weight monitoring tools; visual feedback on progress and goals; access to support via the internal social network such as the forums and blog options as well as the opportunity to link out to personal social media such as Facebook.

2. LiveWell (https://www.nhs.uk/livewell/loseweight/Pages/Loseweighthome.aspx) is part of the NHS Choices website and provides access to a 12-week diet and exercise plan in PDF format that can be printed off and completed by the individual; other information available on the website are healthy recipes; information about BMI and calorie counting; large collection of links out to various related useful information sources and dieting tools.

3. LiveStrong (http://www.livestrong.com/) is an online community which requires registration and profile creation; this website gives access to educational exercise videos; healthy recipes; and information and tools for calorie goals and counting, as well as weight progress monitoring and access to social support via the community forum.

Participants
Participants were identified by a GP (SS) through (a) a single General Practice patient database search and (b) opportunistic recruitment during consultations at that same General Practice situated in rural South West England from which patients are on average older than in the rest of the UK (26.9% aged 65+ vs 17.2%), predominantly Caucasian (99.5%), and living in an area that is among the 40% least deprived (IMD 12.8) [16, 20]. Searches were conducted using the inclusion criteria in Table 1. Of the 649 eligible participants, 64 were invited

Table 1 Inclusion and exclusion criteria

Inclusion criteria:

(1) desire to lose weight

(2) aged 35–60

(3) BMI of 30 to 45 kg/m^2

(4) able to access to the internet via a computer or other device.

Exclusion criteria:

(1) medical-conditions, such as coronary artery disease, type I diabetes or insulin-treated type 2 diabetes, stroke or cognitive impairment, terminal illness

(2) unable to read, write, or understand English

(3) learning difficulties

(4) taking medication that could affect weight.

using a purposive sampling framework [22] to select for diversity in terms of gender and BMI.

A total of 24 participants agreed to take part. Participant identification, recruitment and follow-up can be found in Fig. 1.

Materials and procedures

Eligible participants attended a 20-min recruitment meeting at the surgery with the GP (SS). The study was discussed, written informed consent was requested and participants were asked to complete a questionnaire providing baseline information on BMI and age. Participants were then provided with the three web-addresses (as above), asked to explore each and select their preferred choice for the following 4 weeks. The meeting ended with a 30-min semi-structured lifestyle consultation (see Additional file 1 for consultation guide).

After 4 weeks semi-structured face-to-face interviews were conducted by two female researchers (SS the GP and SvB an MSc student at the time; both attended a University of Exeter Qualitative Interviewing and NVivo course) at the General Practice Surgery, using a topic guide (see Additional file 1) which was adapted after the first few interviews. Interviews lasted approximately 30 to 50 min. Participant checking was conducted during the interview to ensure understanding of the data. The topic guide was adapted from the one used by Tang and colleagues [23] that helped explore the views of young adults (19-33 yrs) on similar websites. The interviews were audio-recorded and transcribed verbatim.

Data analysis

Two researchers (SS & SvB) conducted inductive thematic analysis as described by Braun and Clarke [24] of the transcripts, to identify overarching themes and create hierarchies of thematic categories and presenting a realist account of the data. Using constant comparison techniques, themes were updated iteratively as new data came in. Coding continued until data saturation was reached (i.e., last 5 transcripts did not add substantially to the thematic framework). We constructed explanations of the data both within-cases (representing the patient's journey through the intervention process) and between-cases (to identify themes that were common or divergent between people preferring different websites). We used NVivo 8 to organise the data. Thematic analysis is widely used in similar exploratory studies [25, 26].

After initial independent reading and coding of a sample of the data (10 transcripts) the two researchers noted and discussed preliminary themes in a draft coding framework. Coding of the remainder of the data continued independently. Any new emerging themes on the remainder of the transcripts were captured in an "other" node which were discussed by four members of the research team along with the existing themes in subsequent meetings (SS, SvB, AM, and CG).

Results

Of the 24 participants recruited in the initial meeting, 20 (70% female) took part in the follow-up interview (See Fig. 1. above for participant flow). Participant characteristics and website choices are shown in Table 2.

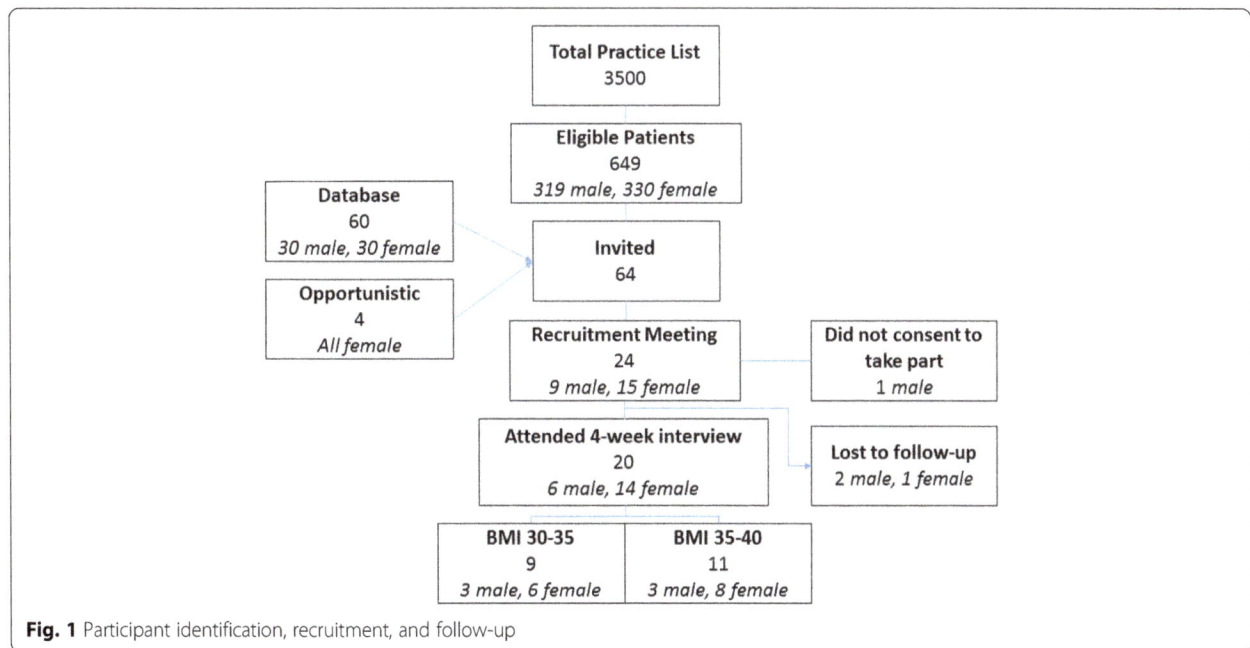

Fig. 1 Participant identification, recruitment, and follow-up

Table 2 Participant characteristics and website choice

	Men	Women	All
Age	35–57	40–57	35–57
	(M = 47.3)	(M = 51.4)	(M = 49.5)
BMI	32–44.8	30.4–43.4	30–47.8
	(M = 36.2)	(M = 35.7)	(M = 35.9)
Website Choice			
Livestrong	2	1	3
LiveWell	2	6	8
SparkPeople	2	7	9

All participants were familiar with the use of the internet and selected their preferred website to continue with. Only seven participants indicated they were either still using their chosen website or aimed to continue using it at the four-week interview. However, some of those who were no longer using their website reported they would be interested in using a different website providing it encompassed some of the suggestions they provided (as below).

The key stages of our participant journey in engaging with weight management websites form the four overarching themes (Table 3) and provide the framework for structuring our analysis and subsequent results section. Each of these overarching themes comprises several subthemes and these are described and evidenced in detail. Organising the results in this order will allow exploration of facilitators and barriers at each stage which may help inform ways of minimising programme drop-out and nonadherence to optimise potential effectiveness. Some similar subthemes weave across various stages, these are highlighted as facilitators and barriers in Table 4 with reference to the respective stages.

Stage 1: Initial interest and website choice
Motivation
Participants were motivated to lose weight to improve physical appearance, self-confidence and health consequences, and due to feelings of obligation to others. For example:

> "I have a BMI of 41, I have to find a way of conquering that. My daughter is graduating in September and I'd love to be a stone and a half lighter, y'know I have got goals." (Participant 1, F, 57)

Table 3 Key stages of patient journey

(1) initial interest and website choice

(2) engagement with and use of the website

(3) implementation of changes

(4) continued use of the website and behaviour change. Within these stages a number of themes were identified.

Table 4 Main facilitators and barriers identified across the key stages

Facilitator/Barrier to website use	Influencing factor
Facilitators	(1) Motivation (Stage 1–4); from Tracking features and Email reminders.
	(2) Personal preferences (Stage 1&2); Appeal of website; Email reminders
Barriers	(1) Effort (Stage 2–4); Time and commitment (Stage 3)
	(2) Lack of novel or useful information (Stage 4)
	(3) Accessibility and disposability; (Stage 4)
	(4) Email Reminders (Stage 2)
	(5) Perceived target group (Stage 4); Appeal of website (Stage 1)

> "I wouldn't say life expectancy is an issue that drives me erm I will live however long I live … however I think the key things are how I feel and how I look. They're the motivation factors." (Participant 17, M, 48)

It is important to note that some participants credited the initial GP recruitment meeting for motivating them to try out the websites for weight loss.

Internet as a source of information
Participants described regularly using the internet to look up topics of interest and this may have facilitated their willingness to try online weight loss programmes. Few participants had prior experiences with eHealth and none had heard of the three websites offered in the study. Their choice of website was influenced by the website's ability to satisfy their information needs about weight loss and its potential health consequences. For example:

> "That's the one that seemed to have got more of the information that I was looking for really... I like the fact they send you, you have lots of recipes y'know so it's sort of easy then to buy ingredients and to put together meals er it just, it just seemed to me to be the one that best suited me really." (Participant 20, F, 47 years)

Appeal of the website
Participants wanted the amount of information provided to be satisfactory and relevant but not overwhelming or bombarding as this could result in difficulties with navigating the website itself.

> "Just a lot of information to go through I didn't find them, any of them actually particularly easy to move through." (Participant 20, F, 47 years)

Only three participants chose the LiveStrong website and said that this was to try something new. The other participants felt that LiveStrong was not aimed at them and chose either SparkPeople or LiveWell.

"I'm an overweight, middle-aged woman and it seemed to me that this was geared up to young, fit people who wanted to exchange views about being even younger and fitter." (Participant 9, F,49)

The features that were appealing to those choosing one of the latter two websites, seemed to be the exact features that led to dismissal of that particular website for the others.

"...if you can imagine a glossy magazine that you buy... it was very much like that, but on the website [SparkPeople] instead of a magazine. So I felt involved, I felt invited and I wanted to interact more with it." (Participant 17, M, 48 years)

"Well the American websites [SparkPeople and LiveStrong] just seemed a bit blotchy... it's like when you watch shopping channels it was like trying to sell you something and I didn't like it..." (Participant 18, M, 35 years)

Although personal preferences influenced the initial choice of a website, the overall appeal of weight loss websites seemed to be increased by having a clear structure, ease of navigation, and being relevant to the target audience.

Stage 2: Engagement with and use of the website
Tracking features
Most participants appreciated and enjoyed using the self-monitoring features such as food and activity trackers.

"...they track you... I also find that doing that made you want to eat more healthily, because you want to come in under... it's probably a human nature competitive y'know... I can beat this." (Participant 12, M, 50 years)

Participants using these tools seemed to gain motivation from the continuous reflection involved in monitoring their goals and lifestyle changes. The tools highlighted the discrepancy between current behaviour and their goals, showing what changes worked for them and which did not.

"it is like a sort of working document that you can update regularly and just having something like that is in itself a motivation because you're reminding yourself of something you wanted to do, you know,

maybe I set a target a month ago and as I'm getting older my memory's not so good anyway, I can't remember what I've done, but I can look back, oh yes that's what I said I'd do then, review it now, review it again in a month's time, change it, adapt it and keep it moving on so it's the sort of continuous reflection and making yourself decide what your priorities are and where you want to be in three, six months' time" (Participant 05, F, 54 years).

Although most participants thought it was easy to use the tools, by the end of the 4 weeks all participants reported that it had become too much of an effort. This was especially true for food trackers which required accurate logging of ingredients and quantities.

"But you put in something like potatoes or something, mash potato and then they'd come up with a whole great long list of mash potato,... then it gave you how many ounces or whatever like that, so you had to be really thinking all the time." (Participant 15, F, 57 years)

Some mentioned that they would have liked some sort of useful feedback on or reward for their progress and this was suggested as a possible way of minimizing the perceived effort. With regards to the food tracking features, some participants showed an aversion to the *"old message of calorie counting"* as *"I know it doesn't work for me"* (Participant 3, F, 56). In some cases a boomerang effect of calorie counting was also referred to. When the food tracker showed the intake to be below the daily target, this prompted some to eat more to make up the missing calories. This was also mentioned in relation to using calories burned through exercise as an excuse to allow increased eating.

"...oh I'm doing all this exercise; I can eat all this food." (Participant 23, F, 40 years)

Email reminders
Both SparkPeople and LiveStrong send out regular emails including weekly newsletters, health tips, and tracking (self-monitoring) prompts. In some cases the abundance of emails led participants to avoid the website. For example:

"I see Sparkpeople Sparkpeople... Sparkpeople, and I think OH, and walk away." (Participant 11, F, 56 years)

However, other participants enjoyed reading these emails and accredited their ongoing use of the website to them.

"They actually sort of instigated my use of their website by these emails, ok? and I find that kept

me going back, I mean, other than that, I probably wouldn't have gone there so often." (Participant 12, M, 50 years)

This variability in responses to emails shows the strong influence of personal preferences on engagement with online weight loss interventions. This is a common subtheme that cuts through various stages, and was previously encountered in Stage 1 where personal preferences influenced initial use and website choice (See also Table 2). Importantly, even those who did not like the emails mentioned they did not wish to entirely cut them.

"I wouldn't want more than an email every couple of weeks really, I find it really off putting that they just email and email and email, but the occasional email, yes, if it's got some pertinent information on it." (Participant 09, F, 49 years)

Social networking in relation to weight loss

All three websites provide access to a social support system in the form of internal online forums, linking to existing forums, or linking to the user's Facebook account allowing progress to be posted onto their personal profile. Although participants thought these forums were helpful for gathering information, they showed an aversion to engaging interactively. None of our participants actively posted in the available forums or uploaded their progress to Facebook.

"You can read all these other people's comments which are quite helpful but I certainly wasn't gonna put anything about myself on there..." (Participant 10, F, 54 years)

Stage 3: Implementation of changes
Time and commitment

The time taken to fully engage with the websites' features and implement the encouraged lifestyle changes was a substantial barrier.

"I s'pose you have to do it like that to be accurate but I haven't got enough hours in the day I'm afraid to weigh my mash out." (Participant 15, F, 57 years)

Some participants mentioned that to commit to the lifestyle changes and the time needed to fully use the website, these changes would ideally need to feel effortless or they need to be more convinced that making these changes would guarantee weight loss. .

"I'd like just something with simple recipes on it, and a choice of recipes for like, for a whole week, with simple ingredients that you know, you could, you would know, that if you followed this, this plan for a week, erm, bit like Weight Watchers but, if you, if you followed this plan for a week, you would definitely lose weight and if you did exercise as well." (Participant 11, F, 56).

Translating motivation into action

Most participants reported being able to successfully integrate small changes into their lives, such as walking to work instead of driving and joining -grandchildren, partner, clients, or dog- for walks' and changing snacking habits. Some of these changes were attributed to the information provided on the websites or community forums, for example:

"...the good thing from it is I've changed a lot of habits... I really have changed... It's just about thinking before you put it in your mouth sort of thing you know. I've not, this is a shocker, I've not touched a soft drink since looking, I just drink sparkling water now. Probably 4 or 5 pints a day which is a shock for me. So yeah it's sort of changed me a little bit as well cos when I first looked at it me and my wife, cos it's telling you about sugars." (Participant 18, M, 35)

In some cases successful implementation of changes was facilitated by other behaviour change techniques such as the need to record behaviour.

"I've been more conscious of what I've been eating and again a sense of guilt because if you have to record it." (Participant 5, F, 54 years)

Making small and manageable changes also seemed to be associated with a higher chance of success. For example:

"I've been eating a bit less but I haven't changed what I eat, I've just been eating a little bit less and it hasn't taken me an awful lot of effort and I think I have lost some weight according to my own scales and that's fine, I'm quite happy with that." (Participant 16, M, 55)

The same was found for changes in physical activity. In contrast, the promotion of intense physical activity was reported to be off-putting.

"The two things that I've tapped into are the walking one because that's what I can, I like to walk, I've always liked to walk, I also walk for a purpose cos I gotta take my dog places. I can even measure the

distance I have to walk from the house to the bus stop so that was very practical." (Participant 19, M, 50)

Although participants credited their initial motivation to GP (Stage 1), they also wanted further facilitated support alongside internet-based weight loss programmes used in primary care settings in the form of face-to-face meetings with a health professional, as this would give them an extra push to make lifestyle changes.

"...to be totally honest, the whole thing, just the talking with you [the GP: SS] was just amazing, but that really, and as I now hate groups, it's actually nice talking to a real person, than it is to looking at a website. I think you'd have to have a combination of the two." (Participant 10, F, 54 years)

Stage 4: Continued use
Lack of novel or useful information
The participants reported going back to the website as long as the information was still considered to be new and helpful. However, most participants mentioned that they felt the information was often just the same as everywhere else.

"Maybe I'm too simplistic, but it all basically comes down to eating less and exercising more and there's only so many people that you can listen to telling you that..." (Participant 24, F, 52 years)

They mentioned that instead of being told what to eat or not eat (which they already knew), they needed help with, or strategies for dealing with temptations or the pressure to revert to old habits to eat unhealthily in various situations such as when under time pressure, in social situations, or when confronted with tempting foods.

"you can be motivated but in all the different points during the day where there is the option to, every time again you have to make the choice, shall I or shan't I?... So you're constantly confronted with it as well." (Participant 24, F, 52)

"I'm trying to feed the family with things that they normally like and they're very entrenched in set behaviours and my husband does the shopping and it's quite difficult to get him to buy different things." (Participant 5, F, 54)

Effort
Another reason people gave for not maintaining changes was that the intervention methods promoting them were considered to be arduous and too much of a hassle for continued use. This was particularly true when monitoring efforts involved weighing of food, converting measurements, logging of eating and exercise behaviours, and reading emails. Some participants remarked that integrating the websites with a smartphone app might be a way to minimise the effort involved in engaging with certain behaviour change techniques.

"... if you wanted to make a food diary then you've got to keep logging back in and it would be much easier to have something maybe by your side, that you could use almost, on your phone or something like an app." (Participant 20, F, 47 years)

Accessibility and disposability
Continued use of the websites was also influenced by the way participants accessed the internet in day-to-day life. Although all participants were confident computer users, some reported a lack of interest in using them in their leisure time. They considered these programmes to be more beneficial for those who 'love being on the computer' (Participant 11, F, 56). Some also hinted at the disposability of weight loss websites - they are easily closed and soon lose their novelty value.

"No staying power... I just get bored of this all eventually, move on to the next exciting thing..." (Participant 17, M, 48 years)

Smartphone apps were mentioned again as a way to improve accessibility.

"If you had a smartphone and you used one and it was beside you when you were cooking or something, it might be more intuitive to do it that way because it's with you all the time." (Participant 15, F, 57)

Continued motivation
Although the participants were recruited based on their desire to lose weight, their comments suggested a loss of motivation over time. A greater emphasis on health risk information was suggested as a means of increasing motivation. For example:

"I don't want them saying to me, you should eat less fat and you should eat more of this and less of that because I already know that. What I think they should be doing is saying, if you're more than 10% overweight or whatever it is then you're putting yourself at quite a big risk of diabetes, this is what happens to you if you get diabetes, and that was sort of missing I felt." (Participant 16, M, 55)

However, for some, information on long-term health consequences did not feel like an imminent threat. Those who perceived the problem to be more urgent reported being more vigilant in terms of adhering to the lifestyle changes.

"Somehow even threats of diabetes and goodness knows what...it's perhaps not immediate enough." (Participant 24, F, 52 years)

"some days I have said no to eating something 'cause I do know that this is the long haul so I'm quite excited that I'm just going to keep going... I just know I've got to, I can't give up now 'cause of my health so I've just got to keep going." (Participant 10, F, 54)

Perceived target group

Finally, the matching of the website content to individual preferences is not only important to initial uptake, but also crucial to continued use. Although all three websites were aimed at people who wanted to lose weight through diet and exercise, some participants still felt the websites were *'too young'* and *'too modern' (Participant 11, F, 56)* or that the website wasn't quite aimed at them which particularly hindered continued use. For example:

"...It [LiveStrong] was certainly more for a sort of like bodybuilder, and I wasn't going to do bodybuilding... that was the impression that I got, and that was why I didn't really use it, because it just didn't feel like it was pertinent to me and what I wanted." (Participant 12, M, 50 years)

Discussion
Summary

This study explored primary care patients' experiences of using weight loss websites facilitated by a single brief contact with a GP. A number of facilitators and barriers to website use were identified (See also Table 4). Website components that were considered facilitative by some participants were seen as barriers by others (e.g., multiple email reminders). In addition, features that facilitate initial engagement may discourage continued use over time (e.g., food logs). These individual differences in the appraisal of components highlight the need for personal tailoring in online weight loss websites. The data driven recommendations for eHealth selection and development for use in primary care settings are summarized in Table 5 which have helped inform the development of a novel smartphone app-based weight management

Table 5 Recommendations for future development and refinement of internet-based weight loss interventions

1. Future internet-based interventions that are designed to facilitate weight loss consultations given in primary care settings should be personally tailored where possible, to allow for choice of style (e.g. technical, health-focused) and delivery formats (e.g. internet, smartphone), and ideally allowing users to adjust the number of reminders to prevent users from feeling harassed.

2. To maintain interest, content and features need to be novel (e.g., temptation resistance strategies) and updated, yet require very little effort from the user to find and use (i.e. good organisation of detailed information allowing users to find what they want easily).

3. Tracking features should be appealing and require less effort from the user than current methods (e.g., use of smartphone barcode scanners, auto tracking of activity using devices, tracking weight or success with planned changes, rather than total calories consumed).

4. Lifestyle changes should be presented in a manner that reduces the perceived effort and time to implement such changes (i.e., reduce portion size vs weighing and logging every ingredient).

5. The intervention may need to address issues of motivation and prioritisation to support more resource-intensive changes.

6. Particular care is needed to ensure that social support elements of interventions provide a safe environment in which to disclose sensitive information.

7. The use of face-to-face support alongside web-based support may be advantageous when implementing internet-based interventions in primary care settings.

intervention focused on the modification and management of nonconscious processes to facilitate dietary change.

Strengths and limitations

To our knowledge, this is the first qualitative investigation of middle-aged adults' use of eHealth for weight loss in the context of primary care service delivery. The study's strengths include use of a real-world health care context where participants were offered weight management treatment by a GP as part of their clinical care and the rigorous application of qualitative research methods. However, some limitations need to be acknowledged. Some participants acknowledged that involvement in a research study had motivated their use of the website, so the findings may not translate to a non-research context. In addition, the study used self-reported accounts of engagement with the websites and of lifestyle changes. Further research could incorporate actual website usage data and objective measures of behaviour change such as accelerometry and weight. The gender distribution (70% female) is a further limitation, restricting the range of views and experiences captured in this study. Unfortunately, the gender distribution in this study is seen in other internet-based intervention studies [14, 27] which highlights the need for further investigation of strategies to improve male engagement with, and adherence to, weight management interventions. Due to this distribution, as well as the sample size we did not explore gender (or age) differences in depth. However, no potential differences were noted during analysis. Our sample was drawn from a rural population in South West England. The findings may not transfer well to the wider rural primary care population in the UK.

Comparison with existing literature
Previous research has shown that monitoring features are positively perceived in behaviour change interventions [28] and techniques such as self-monitoring, and goal setting are associated with effectiveness in facilitating weight loss [21, 29], although the evidence linking these change techniques to effectiveness in eHealth interventions is limited [30]. Our research shows that, although such features are often useful they may result in disengagement from the intervention if they are time-consuming.

Our participants disliked interactive use of social support tools which required disclosure of intentions and/or progress, yet evidence suggests that social support is positively associated with weight loss both in eHealth [31] and other weight management programmes [32]. Therefore, it is important to investigate strategies to enhance engagement with social support tools. However, public online platforms can be perceived as untrustworthy [23]. This suggests that additional forms of support may be required such as encouraging the (offline or online) involvement of an existing relation or friend. Age may be a factor affecting the use of these social support tools. Tang and colleagues [23] identified that young adults (age range 19–33) who are familiar with internet applications value attractive user interface, structure, ease of use, personalisation and accessibility when using eHealth for weight management. Social support tools were motivating for some, but not all. This contrasts with our findings where none actively engaged, or were interested in actively using, social networks for weight loss support. Intervention developers also need to consider the age of their target group when developing their materials. LiveStrong was particularly off-putting to our sample due to the images of young and healthy active people and therefore confusing the target population. Additional file 1: Table S1 compares the findings of Tang and colleagues [23] with the findings of the current study. This table highlights differences in views about social networking, as well as similarities in factors affecting the appeal of, and initial engagement with, weight loss websites.

Finally, personal-tailoring has been suggested to be of importance for adherence to eHealth [23, 32, 33]. The current study supports this idea, suggesting that personal-tailoring should involve allowing participants to set preferences for feedback and email frequency as well as units of measure. Tailoring content to individual motivations

and barriers to change (which can be assessed by questionnaire) might also help to engage people more strongly.

Conclusion
Although primary care patients are willing to use and engage with eHealth, they expressed a strong preference for additional support or facilitation. There is therefore potential for the use of such interventions in primary care settings alongside standard weight loss advice. This study has helped inform the development of a smartphone app-based intervention that provides strategies and in-the-moment support to help individuals resist food-related temptations in order to facilitate weight loss. It is crucial to identify or develop weight management eHealth options that enhance the facilitative features and minimize barriers identified in this study. Although this does not guarantee treatment effectiveness, ignoring such changes may result in non-use and therefore ineffectiveness.

Abbreviations
eHealth : Electronic Health; GP: General Practitioner; NICE : National Institute for Health and Care Excellence

Acknowledgements
The listed order of the authors represents extent of contribution. The authors would like to thank the Wyndham House Surgery for its help in identifying suitable patients.

Funding
Sally Simmons, Jason Tang, Charles Abraham and Colin Greaves' input was supported by the UK National Institute for Health Research (NIHR) through an Academic Clinical Fellowship, the Collaboration for Leadership in Applied Health Research and Care in the South West Peninsula (PenCLAHRC) and a Career Development Fellowship (CDF-2012-05-259) respectively. The views expressed in this publication are those of the authors and not necessarily those of the NHS, the National Institute for Health Research or the UK Department of Health. The funders have not contributed to the research design or text of the article.

Authors' contributions
SS, SvB, AM, and CG designed the study, building on a pre-existing protocol and topic guide written by JT, CA and CG. SS, SvB, AM, and CG were involved in the analysis and all authors contributed to writing the manuscript. All authors read and approved the final manuscript."

Competing interests
The authors declare that they have no competing interests.

Author details
[1]University of Exeter Medical School, University of Exeter, Exeter, UK.
[2]Psychology, University of Exeter, Exeter, UK. [3]School of Medicine, University of Dundee, Dundee, UK.

References
1. National Institute for Health and Care Excellence. Obesity. CG43. London: National Institute for Health and Care Excellence; 2006.
2. Chaudhari D, Crisostomo C, Ganote C, Youngberg G. Acute oxalate nephropathy associated with orlistat: a case report with a review of the literature. Case Rep Nephrol. 2013;2013:124604.
3. Chang S, Stoll CT, Song J, Varela J, Eagon CJ, Colditz GA. The effectiveness and risks of bariatric surgery: an updated systematic review and meta-analysis, 2003-2012. JAMA Surg. 2014;149(3):275–87.
4. Jebb SA, Ahern AL, Olson AD, Aston LM, Holzapfel C, Stoll J, et al. Primary care referral to a commercial provider for weight loss treatment versus standard care: a randomised controlled trial. Lancet. 2011;378(9801):1485–92.
5. Jolly K, Lewis A, Beach J, Denley J, Adab P, Deeks JJ, et al. Comparison of range of commercial or primary care led weight reduction programmes with minimal intervention control for weight loss in obesity: lighten up randomised controlled trial. BMJ. 2011;343:d6500.
6. Muñoz RF, Mendelson T. Toward evidence-based interventions for diverse populations: the San Francisco general hospital prevention and treatment manuals. J Consult Clin Psychol. 2005;73(5):790–9.
7. Weinstein PK. A review of weight loss programs delivered via the internet. J Cardiovasc Nurs. 2006;21(4):251–8.
8. Huang J, Yu H, Marin E, Brock S, Carden D, Davis T. Physicians' weight loss counseling in two public hospital primary care clinics. Acad Med. 2004;79(2):156–61.
9. Ware LJ, Williams S, Bradbury K, Brant C, Little P, Hobbs FR, et al. Exploring weight loss services in primary care and staff views on using a web-based programme. Inform Prim Care. 2012;20(4):283–8.
10. Kraschnewski JL, Sciamanna CN, Stuckey HL, Chuang CH, Lehman EB, Hwang KO, et al. A silent response to the obesity epidemic: decline in US physician weight counseling. Med Care. 2013;51(2):186–92.
11. Tham M, Young D. The role of the general practitioner in weight management in primary care – a cross sectional study in general practice. BMC Fam Pract. 2008;9:66.
12. Booth HP, Prevost AT, Gulliford MC. Access to weight reduction interventions for overweight and obese patients in UK primary care: population-based cohort study. BMJ Open. 2015;5(1):e006642.
13. Potter MB, Vu JD, Croughan-Minihane M. Weight management: what patients want from their primary care physicians. J Fam Pract. 2001;50(6):513.
14. Tang J, Abraham C, Greaves C, Yates T. Self-directed interventions to promote weight loss: a systematic review of reviews. J Med Internet Res. 2014;16(2):e58.
15. Manzoni GM, Pagnini F, Corti S, Molinari E, Castelnuovo G. Internet-based behavioral interventions for obesity: an updated systematic review. Clin Pract Epidemiol Ment Health. 2011;7:19–28.
16. Office for National Statistics. Internet users in the UK - Office for National Statistics. London: Office for National Statistics; 2016.
17. Free C, Knight R, Robertson S, Whittaker R, Edwards P, Zhou W, et al. Smoking cessation support delivered via mobile phone text messaging (txt2stop): a single-blind, randomised trial. Lancet. 2011;378(9785):49–55.
18. Neuhauser L, Kreps GL. Rethinking communication in the E-health era. J Health Psychol. 2003;8(1):7–23.
19. Wieland LS, Falzon L, Sciamanna CN, Trudeau KJ, Folse SB, Schwartz JE, et al. Interactive computer-based interventions for weight loss or weight maintenance in overweight or obese people. Cochrane Database Syst Rev. 2012;8:CD007675.
20. McEwan D, Harden SM, Zumbo BD, Sylvester BD, Kaulius M, Ruissen GR, et al. The effectiveness of multi-component goal setting interventions for changing physical activity behaviour: a systematic review and meta-analysis. Health Psychol Rev. 2016;10(1):67–88.
21. Greaves CJ, Sheppard KE, Abraham C, Hardeman W, Roden M, Evans PH, et al. Systematic review of reviews of intervention components associated with increased effectiveness in dietary and physical activity interventions. BMC Public Health. 2011;11:119.
22. Marshall MN. Sampling for qualitative research. Fam Pract. 1996;13(6):522–5.
23. Tang J, Abraham C, Stamp E, Greaves C. How can weight-loss app designers' best engage and support users? A qualitative investigation. Br J Health Psychol. 2015;20(1):151–71.
24. Braun V, Clarke V. Using thematic analysis in psychology. Qual Res Psychol. 2006;3(2):77–101.
25. Dennison L, Morrison L, Conway G, Yardley L. Opportunities and challenges for Smartphone applications in supporting health behavior change: qualitative study. J Med Internet Res. 2013;15(4):e86.
26. Urowitz S, Wiljer D, Dupak K, Kuehner Z, Leonard K, Lovrics E, et al. Improving diabetes management with a patient portal: a qualitative study of diabetes self-management portal. J Med Internet Res. 2012;14(6):e158.
27. Pagota SL, Schneider KL, Oleski JL, Luciani JM, Bodenlos JS, Whited MC. Male inclusion in randomized controlled trials of lifestyle weight loss interventions. Obesity. 2012;20(6):1234–9.
28. Carter MC, Burley VJ, Nykjaer C, Cade JE. Adherence to a Smartphone application for weight loss compared to website and paper diary: pilot randomized controlled trial. J Med Internet Res. 2013;15(4):e32.
29. Michie S, Abraham C, Whittington C, McAteer J, Gupta S. Effective techniques in healthy eating and physical activity interventions: a meta-regression. Health Psychol. 2009;28(6):690–701.
30. Tang JCH, Abraham C, Greaves CJ, Nikolaou V. Self-directed interventions to promote weight loss: a systematic review and meta-analysis. Health Psychol Rev. 2016;10(3):358–72.
31. Hwang KO, Ning J, Trickey AW, Sciamanna CN. Website usage and weight loss in a free commercial online weight loss program: retrospective cohort study. J Med Internet Res. 2013;15(1):e11.
32. Hankonen N, et al. Which behavior change techniques are associated with changes in physical activity, diet and body mass index in people with recently diagnosed diabetes? Ann Behav Med. 2015;49(1):7–17.
33. Saperstein SL, Atkinson NL, Gold RS. The impact of internet use for weight loss. Obes Rev. 2007;8(5):459–65.

14

Intake of non-nutritive sweeteners is associated with an unhealthy lifestyle: a cross-sectional study in subjects with morbid obesity

Robert Winther[1,2], Martin Aasbrenn[3,4] and Per G. Farup[1,4*] (iD)

Abstract

Background: Subjects with morbid obesity commonly use Non-Nutritive Sweeteners (NNS), but the health-related effects of NNS have been questioned. The objectives of this study were to explore the associations between the use of NNS and the health and lifestyle in subjects with morbid obesity.

Methods: This cross-sectional study included subjects with morbid obesity (BMI $\geq$ 40 kg/m^2 or $\geq$35 kg/m^2 with obesity-related comorbidity). Information about demographics, physical and mental health, and dietary habits was collected, and a blood screen was taken. One unit of NNS was defined as 100 ml beverages with NNS or 2 tablets/units of NNS for coffee or tea. The associations between the intake of NNS and the health-related variables were analyzed with ordinal regression analyses adjusted for age, gender and BMI.

Results: One hundred subjects (women/men 83/17; mean age 44.3 years (SD 8.5)) were included. Median intake of NNS was 3.3 units (range 0 – 43). Intake of NNS was not associated with BMI ($p = 0.64$). The intake of NNS was associated with reduced heavy physical activity ($p = 0.011$), fatigue ($p < 0.001$), diarrhea ($p = 0.009$) and reduced well-being ($p = 0.046$); with increased intake of total energy ($p = 0.003$), fat ($p = 0.013$), carbohydrates ($p = 0.002$), sugar ($p = 0.003$) and salt ($p = 0.001$); and with reduced intake of the vitamins A ($p = 0.001$), C ($p = 0.002$) and D ($p = 0.016$).

Conclusions: The use of NNS-containing beverages was associated with an unhealthy lifestyle, reduced physical and mental health and unfavourable dietary habits with increased energy intake including sugar, and reduced intake of some vitamins.

Keywords: Diet, General health, Life style, Non-nutritive sweeteners, Obesity

Background

In adults, the global prevalence rates of overweight and obesity, defined as Body Mass Index (BMI) above 25 and 30 kg/m^2, were in 2014 39% and 13% respectively [1]. The prevalence rates have more than doubled since 1980 and the disorders have been mentioned as one of the largest public health concerns worldwide because of the increased

risk of serious non-communicable diseases such as cancer, cardiovascular diseases, and diabetes [1–3]. In Norway, 1 in 4 middle-aged men and 1 in 5 women have a BMI above 30 kg/m^2 [4].

The "obesity epidemic" (the rapidly increasing prevalence) is caused by environmental and societal changes with increased intake of energy-dense food and increased physical inactivity [1]. Interventions at the societal level should facilitate regular physical activity and make healthier dietary choices available [1]. At the individual level, it is recommended to limit the energy intake from fat and sugar, to increase the intake of fruits,

* Correspondence: per.farup@ntnu.no
[1]Department of Research, Innlandet Hospital Trust, PB 104, N-2381 Brumunddal, Norway
[4]Unit for Applied Clinical Research, Department of Clinical and Molecular Medicine, Faculty of Medicine and Health Sciences, Norwegian University of Science and Technology, N-7491 Trondheim, Norway
Full list of author information is available at the end of the article

vegetables, legumes, whole grains and nuts, and to increase the regular physical activity [1].

To maintain the pleasure of the sweet taste and at the same time reduce the energy intake, subjects with obesity commonly replace sugar by non-nutritive sweeteners (NNS). The reasoning is logical and the producers of NNS have promoted the use and raised the global market to $ 5.5 billion in 2014 [5]. The effect of NNS on weight prevention and reduction is controversial, and serious safety concerns have been raised [6–11]. The controversies are in part related to the study design. Observational studies indicate weight gain and interventional studies the opposite [12]. Both designs are prone to bias. Bias is also introduced by the industry; the relative risk to have favourable results in industry-sponsored reviews was 17.25 (95%CI 2.34 to 127.29) times that of industry independent ones [2]. Most studies have focused on the effect on body weight, whereas associations with lifestyle and general health have been less studied.

The aims of this study in subjects with morbid obesity were to assess associations between the use of NNS and demographics, lifestyle, physical and mental health, dietary habits, comorbidity and a blood screen.

Methods

Study design

This cross-sectional study was performed at the unit for morbid obesity at Innlandet Hospital Trust, Gjøvik, Norway. Consecutive subjects were included from December 2012 through September 2014. A medical history was taken, a physical examination was performed, and a blood sample was collected for further analyses. The patients filled in paper-based questionnaires. A trained study nurse was responsible for the care of the patients and the practical work.

Subjects

Consecutive subjects aged 18 – 65 years old with a BMI ≥ 40 kg/m^2 or ≥35 kg/m^2 with obesity-related complications referred for evaluation of bariatric surgery or conservative treatment were included in a comprehensive study. Subjects with serious somatic and psychiatric disorders judged as unrelated to obesity and subjects with previous major surgery including bariatric surgery were excluded. Only subjects with satisfactorily filled in food frequency questionnaires (FFQ) were included in this study.

Variables

Demographics: Gender; age (years); body weight (kg), height (meter), body mass index (BMI, kg/m^2); cohabitant (yes/no); working (no / part-time / full-time); smoking (never / previously / daily); and overall physical activity (score 0 – 8) and heavy physical activity (hours per week: no / <1 / 1-2 / >2).

Diseases, disorders and well-being: Perceived state of health (poor / not quite good / good / very good); present or previous somatic disorders including hypertension, diabetes, and fibromyalgia (yes / no); muscle-skeletal pain score (score 0-12); WHO-5 well-being index (score 0-100; score ≤ 28 = likely depression; score ≤ 50 = low mood); Hopkins Symptom Checklist –10 (HSCL-10) for measurement of mental distress (score 1-4; mental distress ≥1,85); Fatigue severity scale (FSS; score 9-63, score ≥ 36 = fatigue) [13–15]. The functional gastrointestinal disorders Irritable bowel Syndrome (IBS), functional constipation, functional diarrhea, and functional bloating were diagnosed with a validated Norwegian translation of the Rome III criteria; and the degree of gastrointestinal complaints with Gastrointestinal Symptom Rating Scale – IBS (GSRS-IBS) with subscales for GSRS-diarrhea, –constipation and -bloating (scores 1-7) [16, 17].

The dietary intake of nutrients, energy, and NNS was assessed with an FFQ prepared and validated by the Department of Nutrition at the University of Oslo, Norway who also analyzed the FFQs with their in-house calculation program (KBS, version 7.3, food database AE-14) based on the official Norwegian food composition table from 2016 (http://www.matvaretabellen.no). The frequency was reported as less than once/week; 1-2 times/week; 3-4 times/week; 5-6 times/week; once daily; 2 times/day; 3 times/day; ≥ 4 times/day. The portion size was reported in liter (1/5, 1/3: 1/2, 1) and/or glasses and the amounts converted into gram/day. As the FFQ did not capture the type or amount of NNS used in beverages or NNS tablets, the calculation of the NNS intake was performed pragmatically. One unit of NNS was defined as 100 ml NNS-containing beverage (divided into carbonated and non-carbonated beverage). This was considered as the amount of NNS that would equal the sweetening of regular sugar containing beverages with 10% of sugar (10 g/100 ml). One tablet of NNS was approximately equal to 1 teaspoon of sugar (5 g). Thus, 2 NNS tablets/units for use in tea or coffee were judged as equally amount of 100 ml NNS in beverages. 100 ml was chosen as the unit because the subjects reported the intake in liter and/or glasses and the unit is easy to understand. Intakes of NNS from other sources than beverages and tablets used in beverages were not included in the FFQ. Sugar alcohols and naturally-derived sweeteners not defined as NNS were not included. A range of hematological and biochemical blood tests including vitamins and minerals were analyzed.

Statistics

The results have been reported as mean (SD), median (range), and number (proportion in percentage). Because the intake of NNS varied markedly and was clustered in groups, the intake was ordered in groups with roughly uniform intake and analyzed with ordinal regression analyses. Associations between NNS and the subjects' characteristics and blood tests were analyzed with ordinal logistic regression analyses adjusted for age, gender and BMI and reported as B- and *p*-values. The associations between NNS and dietary intake were not linear and were analyzed with Spearman's correlation test reported as rho, and the p-values were calculated with ordinal logistic fractional polynomial regression adjusted for gender, age and BMI. The analyses were performed with IBM SPSS Statistics for Windows, Version 24.0. Armonk, NY: IBM Corp, and the fractional polynomial regression analyses with STATA v14, StatCorp LLC, Texas, USA. *P*-values <0.05 were judged as statistically significant.

Ethics
The study was approved by the Norwegian Regional Committees for Medical and Health Research Ethics, PB 1130, Blindern, 0318 Oslo, Norway (reference number 2012/966) and performed in accordance with the Declaration of Helsinki. Written informed consent to participate was given by all participants before inclusion.

Results
Out of 350 consecutive subjects visiting the obesity unit, 100 (83 women and 17 men with a mean age of 44.3 years (SD 8.5)) were included in the study. The reasons for the exclusion of 250 subjects are given in Fig. 1. Table 1 gives the participants' characteristics in detail and the results of the blood tests. Table 2 gives the daily dietary intake of energy, energy-yielding nutrients, NNS, vitamins, and salt. The total intake of NNS varied from

zero to 43 units per day. High intake of NNS was associated with diabetes, reduced physical activity, fatigue, reduced well-being, and diarrhea (Table 3). Table 4 gives all the associations between intake of NNS and the dietary intake of energy, energy-yielding nutrients, vitamins, and salt. Intake of NNS was associated with increased intake of energy and salt, and reduced intake of vitamins. The positive associations between the intake of NNS and energy and salt were most pronounced for the use of NNS in carbonated beverages and are presented in Fig. 2.

Discussion
The study confirms the findings from studies in the general population that the use of NNS is high in overweight and obese adults [18–21]. Half of the subjects used more than 3.3 units of NNS per day, which corresponds to 330 ml beverages with NNS. An intake of 2 – 4 l was not uncommon.

The main finding was the associations between NNS and an unhealthy lifestyle. In literature, less is known about these clinically relevant outcomes than about the weight. In this study, NNS was associated with a less healthy diet, reduced physical activity, low well-being and fatigue, which indicate an unhealthy lifestyle. The results indicate that the intake of NNS-containing beverages was approximately 100 ml higher in subjects with diabetes than in those without, and the same difference was seen between those with strong physical activity less than 1 hour/week compared to those with more than 2 h, and in subjects with low mood. The clinical significance of these effects are uncertain, but is indicative of an unhealthy lifestyle associated with the use of NNS.

A high intake of NNS was associated with increased intake of fat, proteins, carbohydrates including sugar,

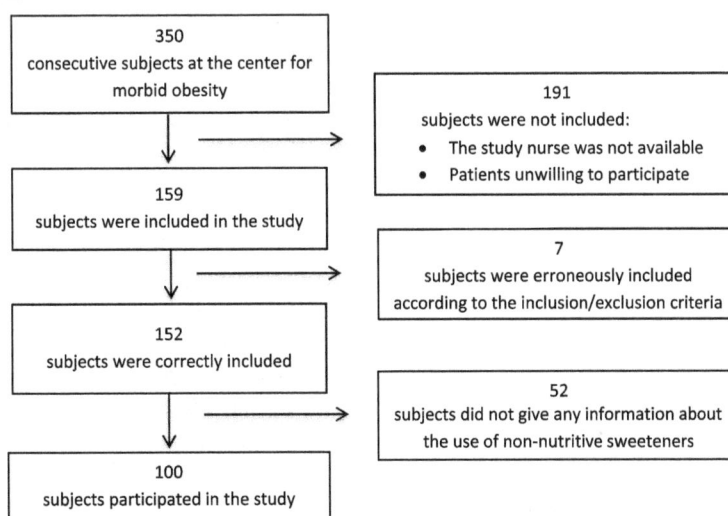

Fig. 1 A flow chart of the subjects in the study

Table 1 The characteristics of the participants in the study

Participants' characteristics (if less than 100, the number is given in brackets)	Mean Median Number	SD Range Proportion (%)
Gender (female/male)	83 / 17	83% / 17%
Age (years)	44.3	8.5
Body weight (kg)	121.8	16.2
BMI (kg/m2)	41.9	3.5
Living with someone (99)	84	85%
Working (no / part time / full-time) (98)	23 / 32 / 43	23%/33%/44%
Smoking (never/previously/daily)	43 /44 / 13	43%/44%/13%
Total physical activity (score 0-8)	4.6	2.2
Heavy physical activity (hrs. Per week: no / <1 / 1-2 / >2)	28/29/32/ 11	28%/29%/32%/ 11%
State of health (98) (Poor/Not quite good/ Good/ Very good)	10/54/30/ 4	10%/55%/31%/ 4%
Fibromyalgia	19	19%
Muscle-skeletal pain score (range 0-12)	4.0	0 – 12
Hypertension (96)	57	59%
Diabetes	20	20%
HSCL10 > 1.85 (mental distress)	27	27%
WHO-5 (low mood) (cut-off <50)	30	30%
Fatigue (cut-of >36) (99)	48	48%
Irritable bowel syndrome (97)	27	28%
Functional bloating (96)	14	15%
Functional diarrhea (97)	2	2%
GSRS-diarrhea (score 1 - 7) (80)	1.5	1.0 – 4.8
GSRS-bloating (score 1 - 7) (80)	2.3	1.0 – 6.0
Blood tests		
Haemoglobin (F: 11-15; M: 13-17 g/dl) (98)	14.4	1.1
Serum iron (9-34 µmol/L) (98)	15.0	5.5
Transferrin saturation (0.10-0.57) (97)	0.23	0.09
Ferritin (10-380 µg/dL) (98)	96	7 - 584
CRP (<5 mg/L) (98)	5	0 - 28
s-Glucose (4.2-6.3 mmol/L) (98)	5.7	4.0 – 23.2
HbA1C (4.3-5.6%) (98)	5.4	4.6 – 11.5
C-peptide (0.3-2.4 nmol/L) (98)	1.47	0.53 – 4.31
Cholesterol (3-7 mmol/L) (98)	5.0	1.0
HDL (F: 1.0-2.7; M: 0.8-2.1 mmol/L) (98)	1.2	0.3
LDL (1-5 mmol/L) (98)	3.3	0.9
Vitamin A (1.2-3.4 µmol/L) (91)	2.0	0.4
Vitamin B1 (122-223 nmol/l) (97)	158	27
Vitamin B6 (27-273 nmol/l) (96)	23	6 - 209
Vitamin B12 (141-700 pmol/L) (98)	338	173 - 1401
Vitamin D (45-161 nmol/L) (98)	58	23
Folic acid (9-36 nmol/l)	17	7 – 46

HSCL10 Hopkins Symptom Checklist 10, *WHO-5* WHO-5 Well-Being Index, *GSRS* Gastrointestinal Symptom Rating Scale, *HDL* High Density Lipoprotein, *LDL* Low Density Lipoprotein

Table 2 Daily intake of total energy, energy-yielding nutrients, non-nutritive sweeteners, vitamins and salt

Daily dietary intake	Median	Range
Energy		
Total energy (kJ)	9737	2648 - 21,816
Protein (g)	109	40 - 212
Fat (g)	90	21 - 283
Carbohydrates (g)	251	65 - 903
Sugar (g)	26	1 - 632
Non-nutritive sweeteners (NNS) (unit[a])		
NNS total	3.3	0.0 – 43.0
NNS carbonated beverages	0.4	0.0 – 40.0
NNS non-carbonated beverages	0.1	0.0 – 32.0
NNS sweeteners in coffee and tea	0.0	0.0 – 27.0
Vitamins and salt		
Vitamin A (µg)	1341	352 - 4460
Vitamin B1 (mg)	2.6	0.8 – 7.8
Vitamin B2 (mg)	3.0	1.1 – 8.8
Vitamin B6 (mg)	2.7	0.9 – 10.0
Vitamin B12 (µg)	9.3	3.0 – 33.7
Vitamin C (mg)	170	11 - 623
Vitamin D (µg)	12.5	2.2 – 44.6
Folic acid (µg)	391	131 – 1077
β-carotene (µg)	4947	340 – 24,306
Salt (g)	7.5	2.4 – 18.8

[a] *NNS* One unit = 100 ml beverages with NNS or 2 units of NNS for coffee/ tea

and salt; and reduced intake of some vitamins. The high intake of energy is harmful to obese subjects. The association with the intake of sugar could support the hypothesis that NNS encourage sugar craving and dependence by an altered metabolism and processing of sweet taste in the brain [22, 23]. Most of the unfavorable associations were related to the use of NNS in carbonated beverages, probably because the highest intake of NNS was from carbonated beverages. The stongest correlations were between intake of NNS containing beverages and salt. It is likely that these users combine the beverages with intake of salted food and snacks, which has also been shown by others [18]. Most of the associations between intake of NNS and energy and nutrients were weak (rho <0.2) and NNS explain only a minor part of the variation. The negative associations between intake of NNS and c-peptid, HbA1c and perhaps also Hb might have been confounded by diabetes. To adjust the analyses for all comorbidity including diabetes, in addition to age, gender and BMI was judged as inappropriate. The users of NNS in non-carbonated beverages, tea, and coffee seem to have a more conscious and correct use of NNS with a slightly reduced intake of total energy,

Table 3 Associations between non-nutritive sweeteners (dependent variable) and subjects' characteristics

Patient characteristics	NNS total		NNS carb. beverages		NNS non-carb. beverages		NNS sweeteners	
	B	p-value	B	p-value	B	p-value	B	p-value
Gender (female/male)	−0.10	0.838	0.519	0.285	−0.049	0.924	−2.896	**0.005**
Age (years)	−0.04	0.073	−0.014	0.544	−0.045	0.063	0.002	0.951
BMI (kg/m2)	−0.025	0.640	−0.007	0.902	−0.032	0.582	0.040	0.510
Living with someone	−0.728	0.151	−0.030	0.953	−0.981	0.060	−0.011	0.985
Working	−0.124	0.594	0.383	0.114	−0.379	0.126	−0.047	0.858
Smoking	0.194	0.485	0.196	0.492	−0.043	0.884	−0.110	0.715
Perceived general health	0.011	0.965	0.070	0.793	0.098	0.722	0.083	0.771
Total physical activity	−0.184	**0.029**	−0.086	0.308	−0.030	0.732	0.014	0.883
Heavy physical activity	−0.477	**0.011**	−0.368	0.052	−0.212	0.278	0.116	0.576
Hypertension	0.201	0.607	0.261	0.518	−0.128	0.759	−0.340	0.442
Diabetes	0.971	**0.039**	0.639	0.174	1.227	**0.012**	0.171	0.748
Fibromyalgia	0.696	0.131	0.202	0.664	0.718	0.132	0.568	0.249
Muscle-skeletal pain score (range 0-12)	−0.004	0.952	0.001	0.987	−0.097	0.149	0.058	0.397
HSCL10 > 1.85	0.073	0.855	−0.194	0.639	−0.664	0.137	−0.028	0.951
WHO-5 (poor wellbeing)	0.452	0.249	0.805	**0.046**	−0.135	0.746	−0.297	0.509
Fatigue	1.232	**0.001**	0.490	0.184	0.316	0.408	0.575	0.159
IBS	0.317	0.444	−0.193	0.651	0.207	0.633	−0.047	0.915
Functional bloating	−0.379	0.486	0.600	0.280	−0.714	0.258	−1.365	0.067
Functional diarrhea	NA	NA	NA	NA	NA	NA	NA	NA
GSRS-diarrhea (score)	0.625	**0.009**	0.178	0.447	0.176	0.467	0.626	**0.012**
GSRS-bloating (score)	−0.112	0.509	−0.033	0.849	−0.324	0.084	−0.184	0.320
Blood tests								
Haemoglobin (g/dl)	−0.299	0.149	−0.063	0.765	−0.625	**0.007**	−0.534	**0.022**
Serum iron (µmol/L	−0.015	0.648	−0.042	0.237	−0.011	0.768	−0.049	0.205
Transferrin saturation	−0.875	0.673	−0.025	0.255	−0.011	0.631	−0.033	0.167
Ferritin (µg/dL)	0.002	0.311	−0.001	0.450	0.000	0.909	−0.001	0.615
CRP (mg/L)	0.040	0.226	0.029	0.393	0.081	**0.020**	0.042	0.228
s-Glucose (mmol/L)	0.110	0.082	0.122	0.055	0.044	0.492	0.005	0.944
HbA1C (%)	0.294	0.052	0.235	0.117	0.367	**0.018**	0.076	0.644
c-peptide (nmol/L)	0.662	**0.005**	0.410	0.077	0.279	0.244	0.509	0.052
Cholesterol (mmol/L)	0.116	0.542	0.188	0.339	−0.043	0.830	−0.096	0.661
HDL (mmol/L)	−0.612	0.291	−0.164	0.782	−1.017	0.115	0.541	0.394
LDL (mmol/L)	0.164	0.427	0.164	0.438	−0.026	0.907	−0.179	0.457
Vitamin A (µmol/L)	0.291	0.536	−0.725	0.136	−0.232	0.644	0.050	0.921
Vitamin B1 (nmol/L)	0.008	0.243	0.006	0.356	0.001	0.876	0.007	0.363
Vitamin B6 (nmol/L)	0.004	0.479	0.005	0.407	−0.011	0.178	−0.002	0.759
Vitamin B12 (pmol/L)	−0.001	0.384	0.000	0.727	0.000	0.940	−0.001	0.503
Vitamin D (nmol/L)	0.006	0.458	0.012	0.166	0.001	0.952	0.000	0.966
Folic acid (nmol/L)	−0.024	0.269	−0.007	0.759	−0.021	0.362	−0.018	0.433

HSCL10 Hopkins Symptom Checklist 10, *WHO-5* WHO-5 Well-Being Index, *IBS* Irritable bowel syndrome, *GSRS* Gastrointestinal Symptom Rating Scale, *HDL* High Density Lipoprotein, *LDL* Low Density Lipoprotein

The analyses have been performed with ordinal logistic regression analyses adjusted for gender, age and BMI)

Table 4 Associations between the intake of NNS and intake of energy, energy-yielding nutrients, vitamins and salt

Diet	NNS Total		NNS Carbonated		NNS Non-carb		NNS Sweeteners	
	rho	p-value	rho	p-value	rho	p-value	rho	p-value
Total energy (kcal)	0.138	**0.003**	0.235	**0.004**	- 0.101	**0.0329**	0.014	0.080
Protein (g)	0.081	0.106	0.198	**0.012**	- 0.066	0.551	- 0.007	**0.028**
Fat (g)	0.172	**0.013**	0.273	**0.005**	- 0.053	**0.043**	0.083	0.094
Carbohydrates (g)	0.145	**0.002**	0.221	**0.014**	- 0.097	**0.031**	- 0.048	**0.031**
Sugar (g)	0.204	**0.003**	0.257	**0.003**	- 0.037	0.091	- 0.111	**0.012**
Vitamin A (µg)	- 0.242	**0.001**	- 0.092	0.077	- 0.185	**0.014**	- 0.016	0.659
Vitamin B1 (mg)	- 0.076	0.062	- 0.017	0.121	- 0.171	0.088	0.025	0.595
Vitamin B2 (mg)	- 0.092	0.060	- 0.016	0.088	- 0.190	0.053	0.026	0.054
Vitamin B6 (mg)	- 0.033	0.238	- 0.005	0.111	- 0.091	0.558	0.060	0.611
Vitamin B12 (µg)	0.027	0.804	0.103	0.584	- 0.017	0.622	0.066	0.595
Folic acid (mg)	- 0.028	0.074	0.043	**0.036**	- 0.150	0.160	0.065	0.730
β-Carotene (µg)	- 0.154	0.091	- 0.084	0.145	- 0.175	**0.033**	0.107	0.428
Vitamin C (mg)	- 0.194	**0.002**	- 0.050	0.051	- 0.172	**0.026**	0.084	0.083
Vitamin D (µg)	- 0.198	**0.016**	- 0.146	**0.033**	- 0.217	0.079	- 0.052	0.069
Salt (g)	0.261	**0.001**	0.321	**<0.001**	0.051	**0.001**	0.070	**0.028**

NNS Non-Nutritive Sweeteneres
The correlations have been calculated with Spearmans' rho, and the p-values with ordinal logistic fractional polynomial regression adjusted for gender, age and BMI

carbohydrates, and sugar. They also reduced the intake of β-Carotene and vitamin C, indicating that they reduced all kinds of food including the healthy fruits and vegetables. Opposed to the findings in this study, population-based studies in the UK, US and Canada suggest a higher dietary quality in NNS consumers than in nonconsumers [19, 20]. The way NNS are used and the physiological and psychological effect of NNS might differ between subjects randomly selected from the population and subjects referred for treatment of morbid obesity at a spesialised hospital unit. Although NNS have been accused of a diabetogenic effect, the associations between NNS and diabetes and c-peptide in this study are probably explained by the higher use of NNS by subjects with diabetes [24, 25].

Reduced physical and mental health was also associated with NNS. The users of NNS had a feeling of poor well-being and more fatigue, and were less physically

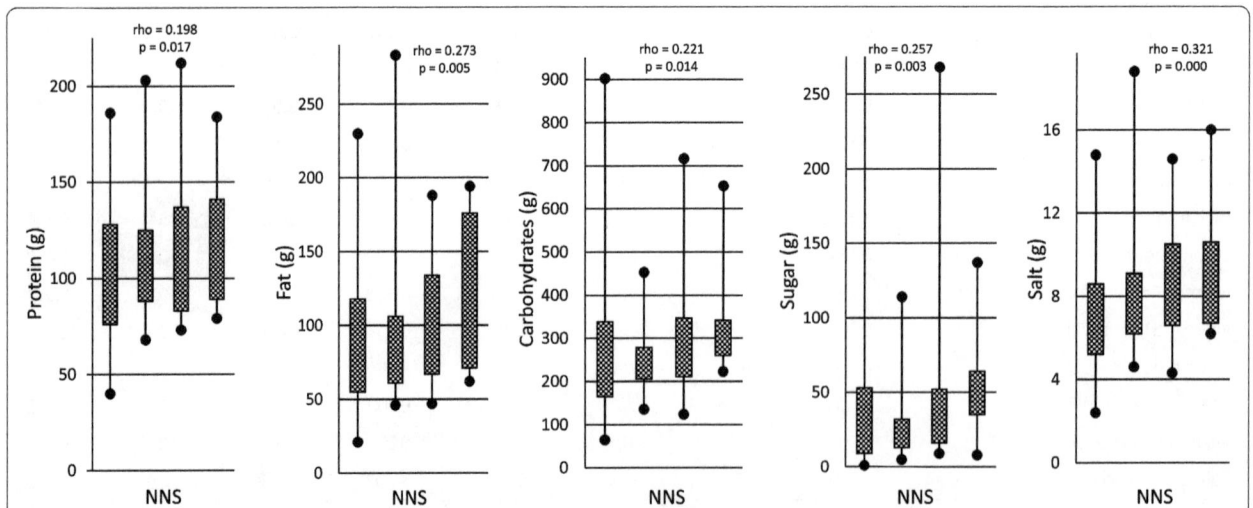

Fig. 2 Associations between the intake of NNS in carbonated beverages and intake of nutrients and salt. NNS: Non-Nutritive Sweeteners. The box-and-whisker plots indicate no (0 unit) /low (0.1 – 2.0 units) / medium (2.1 – 9.0 units) / high (9.0 – 40.0 units) intake of non-nutritive sweeteners in carbonated beverages. One unit = 100 ml NNS-beverage/day. The correlations have been calculated with Spearmans' rho, and the p-values with ordinal logistic fractional polynomial regression.

active. These aspects have not been focused on in literature as far as we know. Caffeine- and NNS-containing beverages might have been used to counteract fatigue and as an excuse for less physical activity. Diarrhea associated with NNS for use in coffee and tea might have been an adverse event related to some of the NNS.

The association between the use of NNS and BMI is not clear [8, 26]. The lack of associations between the use of NNS and BMI in this study was likely because all subjects were morbidly obese, but could indicate a lack of weight-reducing effect of NNS. In population-based observational studies, the use of NNS is higher in overweight and obese subjects than in healthy-weight subjects [18–20]. The findings could indicate that NNS induce weight gain, but it more likely reflects the use of NNS for weight reduction by overweight and obese subjects.

Numerous studies from agriculture, in the laboratory and in humans indicate a counterintuitive effect of NNS with increased food intake and body weight, accumulation of fat, weaker caloric compensation, metabolic syndrome and cardiovascular diseases [27–29]. Animal studies have shown weight gain and metabolic dysregulation after intake of NNS [29, 30]. NNS are not inert substances, and physiological effects on metabolism and energy balance have been proposed to explain an unexpected weight-inducing effect in long-term follow-up studies in children and adults [7, 31–33]. NNS affect the glucose metabolism and have been associated with type 2 diabetes [24, 34–36]. Concerns have also been raised about effects on appetite, eating behaviour, satiation, satiety, craving, reward, addiction, cognitive functions, neurophysiology, and brain function [22, 23, 37–40].

More recently, the effect of NNS on the gut microbiome has achieved considerable attention. The disturbed gut-brain interaction caused by the NNS-induced dysbiosis might in part explain the effects associated with obesity such as weight gain, metabolic changes including glucose intolerance, neurophysiological and psychological changes [41–43].

Except for a slightly favourable effect in the subgroup of subjects using NNS-containing non-carbonated beverages, the overall findings were discouraging. It was anticipated that subjects who were referred for obesity and therefore motivated for weight-reducing interventions, had a conscious relation to the use of NNS as a way to reduce energy intake. Most of them had bariatric surgery later on.

Despite numerous concerns and an extensive literature, the correct use of NNS is unknown [25]. The actual knowledge has been summarized by the U.S. Department of Health and Human Services and U.S. Department of Agriculture in "Dietary Guidelines for Americans 2015-2020": *".... replacing added sugar with*

high-intensity sweeteners may reduce calorie intake in the short-term, yet questions remain about their effectiveness as a long-term weight management strategy", and *"Based on available scientific evidence, these high-intensity sweeteners have been determined to be safe for the general population"* [44]. Shankar et al. gave an intelligent advice *"...for optimal health it is recommended that only minimal amounts of both sugar and NNS be consumed"* [45].

Strengths and limitations

The focus on an unselected group of consecutive subjects with morbid obesity from a general hospital and their health and lifestyle, and not on overweight and obesity in general and body weight only, was a strength. This study from a general hospital is likely to be representative of unselected consecutive subjects referred to a specialized unit for morbid obesity. The validity of the results for all subjects with overweight and obesity is unknown. The lack of information about the use of NNS in other products than beverages and the different types of NNS was a limitation. The FFQ only asked for the use of NNS-containing carbonated beverages, non-carbonated beverages and units of NNS in tea and coffee and not the specific products. Information about NNS in packets added to other beverages or food was not asked for. The limited sample size reduces the ability to control for confounders. No correction was performed for the numerous correlations, which increased the risk of type I errors.

Conclusions

The use of NNS-containing beverages in subjects with morbid obesity was associated with an unhealthy lifestyle, reduced physical and mental health, and unfavourable dietary habits. Lifestyle and dietary advice are therefore particularly important to subjects with morbid obesity using NNS-containing beverages. There were no significant associations between the use of NNS-containing beverages and BMI. The study gave no support for the recommendation of NNS-containing beverages to subjects with morbid obesity.

Abbreviations
BMI: Body Mass Index; CI: Confidence interval; FFQ: Food Frequency Questionnaire; GSRS: Gastrointestinal Symptom Rating Scale; HDL: High-Density Lipoprotein; HSCL-10: Hopkins Symptoms Checklist 10; IBS: Irritable Bowel Syndrome; LDL: Low-Density Lipoprotein; NNS: Non-Nutritive Sweeteners; SD: Standard Deviation; WHO: World Health Organization

Acknowledgements
The authors want to thank Anne Stine Kvehaugen for the collection and scoring of the dietary data, Anja Byfuglien for conscientious help with the practical work and Innlandet Hospital Trust for the funding.

Authors' contribution

RW prepared the data file for the statistical analyses, performed parts of the statistical analyses and drafted the manuscript. MAa was responsible for the collection of the clinical data and prepared the data file for the statistical analyses together with RW. PGF is the guarantor of the project. He designed the main study, was responsible for the practical implementation, performed the statistical analyses, finalized the manuscript and is responsible for the integrity of the work. All authors have given valuable comments on the manuscript and approved the last version.

Funding

The work was supported by a grant from Innlandet Hospital Trust, Brumunddal, Norway.
Availability of data and materials.
Case report forms (CRFs) on paper were used for collection of the clinical data, and all the CRFs are safely stored. The data were transferred manually to SPSS for statistical analyses. The data files are stored by Innlandet Hospital Trust, Brumunddal, Norway, on a server dedicated to research and with security according to the rules given by The Norwegian Data Protection Authority, P.O. Box 8177 Dep. NO-0034 Oslo, Norway. The data are available on request to the authors.

Competing interests

The authors declare that there are no conflicts of interest.

Author details

[1]Department of Research, Innlandet Hospital Trust, PB 104, N-2381 Brumunddal, Norway. [2]Faculty of Medicine, University of Aalborg, DK-9100 Aalborg, Denmark. [3]Department of Surgery, Innlandet Hospital Trust, N-2819 Gjøvik, Norway. [4]Unit for Applied Clinical Research, Department of Clinical and Molecular Medicine, Faculty of Medicine and Health Sciences, Norwegian University of Science and Technology, N-7491 Trondheim, Norway.

References

1. WHO Fact sheet N 311, Obesity and overweight. Updated June 2016. http://www.who.int/mediacentre/factsheets/fs311/en/. Accessed 17 Nov 2017.
2. Mandrioli D, Kearns CE, Bero LA. Relationship between research outcomes and risk of bias, study sponsorship, and author financial conflicts of interest in reviews of the effects of artificially sweetened beverages on weight outcomes: a systematic review of reviews. PLoS One. 2016;11:e0162198.
3. Mitchell NS, Catenacci VA, Wyatt HR, Hill JO. Obesity: overview of an epidemic. Psychiatr Clin North Am. 2011;34:717–32.
4. Overweight and obesity in Norway. Norwegian Institute of Public Health. https://www.fhi.no/en/op/public-health-report-2014/risk%2D-protective-factors/overweight-and-obesity-in-norway-%2D-/. Accessed 18 Nov 2017.
5. Kumar A. Global Markets for non-Sugar Sweeteners. BCC Research LLC. https://www.bccresearch.com/market-research/food-and-beverage/non-sugar-sweeteners-global-markets-report-fod044b.html. Accessed 17 Nov 2017
6. Fowler SP. Low-calorie sweetener use and energy balance: results from experimental studies in animals, and large-scale prospective studies in humans. Physiol Behav. 2016;164:517–23.
7. Chia CW, Shardell M, Tanaka T, Liu DD, Gravenstein KS, Simonsick EM, et al. Chronic low-calorie sweetener use and risk of abdominal obesity among older adults: a cohort study. PLoS One. 2016;11:e0167241.
8. Rogers PJ, Hogenkamp PS, de Graaf C, Higgs S, Lluch A, Ness AR, et al. Does low-energy sweetener consumption affect energy intake and body weight? A systematic review, including meta-analyses, of the evidence from human and animal studies. Int J Obes. 2016;40:381–94.
9. Peters JC, Beck J. Low calorie sweetener (LCS) use and energy balance. Physiol Behav. 2016;164:524–8.
10. Soffritti M, Padovani M, Tibaldi E, Falcioni L, Manservisi F, Belpoggi F. The carcinogenic effects of aspartame: the urgent need for regulatory re-evaluation. Am J Ind Med. 2014;57:383–97.
11. Schernhammer ES, Bertrand KA, Birmann BM, Sampson L, Willett WC, Feskanich D. Consumption of artificial sweetener- and sugar-containing soda and risk of lymphoma and leukemia in men and women. Am J Clin Nutr. 2012;96:1419–28.
12. Roberts JR. The paradox of artificial sweeteners in managing obesity. Curr Gastroenterol Rep. 2015;17:423.
13. Strand BH, Dalgard OS, Tambs K, Rognerud M. Measuring the mental health status of the Norwegian population: a comparison of the instruments SCL-25, SCL-10, SCL-5 and MHI-5 (SF-36). Nord J Psychiatry. 2003;57:113–8.
14. Topp CW, Ostergaard SD, Sondergaard S, Bech P. The WHO-5 well-being index: a systematic review of the literature. Psychother Psychosom. 2015;84: 167–76.
15. Whitehead L. The measurement of fatigue in chronic illness: a systematic review of unidimensional and multidimensional fatigue measures. J Pain Symptom Manag. 2009;37:107–28.
16. Longstreth GF, Thompson WG, Chey WD, Houghton LA, Mearin F, Spiller RC. Functional bowel disorders. Gastroenterology. 2006;130:1480–91.
17. Wiklund IK, Fullerton S, Hawkey CJ, Jones RH, Longstreth GF, Mayer EA, et al. An irritable bowel syndrome-specific symptom questionnaire: development and validation. Scand J Gastroenterol. 2003;38:947–54.
18. Bleich SN, Wolfson JA, Vine S, Wang YC. Diet-beverage consumption and caloric intake among US adults, overall and by body weight. Am J Public Health. 2014;104:e72–8.
19. Drewnowski A, Rehm CD. Consumption of low-calorie sweeteners among U.S. adults is associated with higher healthy eating index (HEI 2005) scores and more physical activity. Nutrients. 2014;6:4389–403.
20. Gibson SA, Horgan GW, Francis LE, Gibson AA, Stephen AM. Low calorie beverage consumption is associated with energy and nutrient intakes and diet quality in British adults. Nutrients. 2016;8(1):9.
21. Bouchard DR, Ross R, Janssen I. Coffee, tea and their additives: association with BMI and waist circumference. Obes Facts. 2010;3:345–52.
22. Yang Q. Gain weight by "going diet?" artificial sweeteners and the neurobiology of sugar cravings: neuroscience 2010. Yale J Biol Med. 2010;83:101–8.
23. Green E, Murphy C. Altered processing of sweet taste in the brain of diet soda drinkers. Physiol Behav. 2012;107:560–7.
24. Imamura F, O'Connor L, Ye Z, Mursu J, Hayashino Y, Bhupathiraju SN, et al. Consumption of sugar sweetened beverages, artificially sweetened beverages, and fruit juice and incidence of type 2 diabetes: systematic review, meta-analysis, and estimation of population attributable fraction. Br J Sports Med. 2016;50:496–504.
25. Romo-Romo A, Aguilar-Salinas CA, Brito-Cordova GX, Gomez Diaz RA, Vilchis Valentin D, Almeda-Valdes P. Effects of the non-nutritive sweeteners on glucose metabolism and appetite regulating hormones: systematic review of observational prospective studies and clinical trials. PLoS One. 2016;11: e0161264.
26. Peters JC, Wyatt HR, Foster GD, Pan Z, Wojtanowski AC, Vander Veur SS, et al. The effects of water and non-nutritive sweetened beverages on weight loss during a 12-week weight loss treatment program. Obesity (Silver Spring). 2014;22:1415–21.
27. Swithers SE, Martin AA, Davidson TL. High-intensity sweeteners and energy balance. Physiol Behav. 2010;100:55–62.
28. Swithers SE. Artificial sweeteners produce the counterintuitive effect of inducing metabolic derangements. Trends Endocrinol Metab. 2013;24:431–41.
29. Shearer J, Swithers SE. Artificial sweeteners and metabolic dysregulation: lessons learned from agriculture and the laboratory. Rev Endocr Metab Disord. 2016;17:179–86.
30. Swithers SE, Martin AA, Clark KM, Laboy AF, Davidson TL. Body weight gain in rats consuming sweetened liquids. Effects of caffeine and diet composition. Appetite. 2010;55:528–33.
31. Burke MV, Small DM. Physiological mechanisms by which non-nutritive sweeteners may impact body weight and metabolism. Physiol Behav. 2015; 152:381–8.

32. Pepino MY. Metabolic effects of non-nutritive sweeteners. Physiol Behav. 2015;152:450–5.
33. Laverty AA, Magee L, Monteiro CA, Saxena S, Millett C. Sugar and artificially sweetened beverage consumption and adiposity changes: national longitudinal study. Int J Behav Nutr Phys Act. 2015;12:137.
34. Kuk JL, Brown RE. Aspartame intake is associated with greater glucose intolerance in individuals with obesity. Appl Physiol Nutr Metab. 2016;41:795–8.
35. Gul SS, Hamilton AR, Munoz AR, Phupitakphol T, Liu W, Hyoju SK, et al. Inhibition of the gut enzyme intestinal alkaline phosphatase may explain how aspartame promotes glucose intolerance and obesity in mice. Appl Physiol Nutr Metab. 2017;12:77–83.
36. Sylvetsky AC, Brown RJ, Blau JE, Walter M, Rother KI. Hormonal responses to non-nutritive sweeteners in water and diet soda. Nutr Metab (Lond). 2016;13:71.
37. Hill SE, Prokosch ML, Morin A, Rodeheffer CD. The effect of non-caloric sweeteners on cognition, choice, and post-consumption satisfaction. Appetite. 2014;83:82–8.
38. Choudhary AK, Lee YY. Neurophysiological symptoms and aspartame: what is the connection? Nutr Neurosci. 2017;2017:1–11.
39. Rudenga KJ, Small DM. Amygdala response to sucrose consumption is inversely related to artificial sweetener use. Appetite. 2012;58:504–7.
40. Low YQ, Lacy K, Keast R. The role of sweet taste in satiation and satiety. Nutrients. 2014;6:3431–50.
41. Nettleton JE, Reimer RA, Shearer J. Reshaping the gut microbiota: impact of low calorie sweeteners and the link to insulin resistance? Physiol Behav. 2016;164:488–93.
42. Suez J, Korem T, Zilberman-Schapira G, Segal E, Elinav E. Non-caloric artificial sweeteners and the microbiome: findings and challenges. Gut Microbes. 2015;6:149–55.
43. Suez J, Korem T, Zeevi D, Zilberman-Schapira G, Thaiss CA, Maza O, et al. Artificial sweeteners induce glucose intolerance by altering the gut microbiota. Nature. 2014;514:181–6.
44. U.S. Dept of Health and Human Services and U.S. Dept of Agriculture. 2015 – 2020 Dietary Guidelines for Americans. 8th Edition.. https://health.gov/dietaryguidelines/2015/guidelines/.Accessed 18 Nov 2017.
45. Shankar P, Ahuja S, Sriram K. Non-nutritive sweeteners: review and update. Nutrition. 2013;29:1293–9.

15

Measurement equivalence of child feeding and eating measures across gender, ethnicity, and household food security

Marisol Perez[1*], Tara K. Ohrt[1], Amanda B. Bruening[1], Aaron B. Taylor[4], Jeffrey Liew[2], Ashley M. W. Kroon Van Diest[3] and Tatianna Ungredda[4]

Abstract

Background: Although there have been extensive studies that make group comparisons on child eating and feeding practices, few studies have examined measurement equivalence to ensure that measures used to make such group comparisons are equivalent across important group characteristics related to childhood obesity.

Methods: Using a sample of 243 caregivers with children between the ages of 4 to 6 years, we conducted a measurement equivalence analysis across gender, ethnicity (Latino versus non-Latino White), and household food security. The subscales of the Child Feeding Questionnaire (CFQ) and the Child Eating Behaviour Questionnaire (CEBQ) were examined separately using a one factor multi-group confirmatory factor analysis.

Results: For the CFQ, Concern about Child Weight and Parental Responsibility subscales were consistent across all groups examined. In contrast, Pressure to Eat, Restriction, and Perceived Parent Weight subscales varied or fit poorly across the groups. For the CEBQ, Emotional Overeating, Enjoyment of Food, and Satiety Responsiveness performed consistently across the groups. On the other hand, Food Fussiness, Desire to Drink, Slowness in Eating, and Emotional Undereating subscales varied or fit poorly across the groups.

Conclusions: Findings from this study suggest both of these measures need continued psychometric work, and group comparisons using some subscales should be interpreted cautiously. Some subscales such as Food Responsiveness and Parental Restriction may be assessing behaviors that occur in food secure households and are less applicable to food insecure environments.

Keywords: Child feeding questionnaire, Child eating behaviour questionnaire, Child feeding, Eating behaviors, Latino, Hispanic, Food security, Gender, Measurement invariance

Background

Research has demonstrated that contextual factors such as gender, food security (e.g., limited or uncertain availability of nutritionally appropriate foods), and ethnicity play a role in the development of pediatric obesity [1–3]. For example, research has found that when compared to boys, girls have more fat mass with a different fat distribution pattern, are less sensitive to insulin across childhood, and are more susceptible to family and environmental risk factors that contribute to pediatric

obesity [4]. Boys, in turn, are more physically active throughout childhood and adolescence, receive more benefits from physical activity, and tend to have lower leptin levels when compared to girls [4]. This suggests there may be differential risk factors and susceptibility across groups such as sex. Research on ethnicity has demonstrated that Latino children and adolescents have higher rates of overweight and pediatric obesity than their non-Latino White counterparts [3]. Similarly, there is an association with food insecurity and higher rates of overweight and obesity in children [2, 5–7]. Despite studies demonstrating the influence of these contextual factors on pediatric obesity, limited research has been conducted to ensure that questionnaires on key risk

* Correspondence: Marisol.Perez@asu.edu
[1]Department of Psychology, Arizona State University, 950 S McAllister Avenue, Tempe, AZ 85287-1104, USA
Full list of author information is available at the end of the article

factors for pediatric obesity are invariant across gender, ethnicity, and food security. Measurement invariance is important, because construct validity is threatened when items of a scale function inconsistently across groups.

Existing cross-sectional and longitudinal research suggests that parental beliefs and feeding practices contribute to pediatric obesity [8–12]. Two commonly used measures to assess parental beliefs and feeding practices are the Child Feeding Questionnaire [9] and Child Eating Behaviour Questionnaire [13]. Both questionnaires have been used to make group comparisons despite limited psychometric research examining the appropriateness of these measures across key contextual factors related to pediatric obesity.

The Child Feeding Questionnaire (CFQ), one of the most widely used scales in the child feeding literatures, assesses parent's concern about a child's weight, responsibility for feeding a child, and the extent a parent pressures a child to eat or restricts a child's food intake [9]. The CFQ was initially developed with a 7-factor model and validated among an ethnically diverse sample of mothers and fathers with children ranging from 2- to 11-years of age [9]. However, a replication study of low-income Latino and African American families with boys and girls failed to replicate the original factor structure and proposed an alternate model [14]. This same study also found cross-cultural conceptual problems resulting in the authors dropping the perceived weight subscales, as well as a number of items in each of the remaining subscales in order to achieve cross-cultural equivalence [14]. Despite these issues, the CFQ has been used to make group comparisons across a number of different groups, such as parents with boys versus girls [15], Latino versus European Americans [11, 16], food secure and food insecure households [5, 17] and among low-income families without an assessment of food security [18, 19].

The Children's Eating Behavior Questionnaire (CEBQ) is a parent-report questionnaire that assesses individual eating styles of children that have been found to relate to pediatric obesity [12, 13]. The CEBQ was initially developed with an 8 factor model and validated among mothers and fathers with children between the ages of 3- to 8-years old in the United Kingdom [13]. Additional studies have validated the original factor structure among children, with only a slight variation where food responsiveness and emotional overeating at times load onto the same factor [20, 21]. Within the United States, one study replicated the original factor structure among low income families with pre-school aged children and found measurement equivalence across White and Black participants [22]. Yet, another study of low-income Hispanic and African American families failed to replicate the original factor structure [23]. An additional study of minority low-income families has suggested there may be conceptual issues with some of the scales in the CEBQ [24]. Despite these concerns, the CEBQ has been used to make group comparisons across gender [21, 25], and ethnicity [22, 23, 25]. In addition, the CEBQ has been used across socioeconomic status [25, 26]. If there are problems with measurement invariance, validity of the inferences and interpretations of the results associated with the measure may be threatened.

Research has suggested there may be cross-cultural conceptual problems with the CFQ and CEBQ, and highlighted the need to examine measurement equivalence of these widely used scales, particularly among low-income minority groups [24]. The goal of the current study was to examine measurement equivalence of the CFQ and CEBQ across key contextual factors that influence pediatric obesity (gender, ethnicity, food security). To facilitate across study comparisons of both measures, the current study targeted caregivers with children between the ages of 4- to 6-years old. Both measures have psychometric studies that recruited families from preschool centers, thereby increasing our ability to compare our findings to the extant literature [14, 22–24, 27].

Method

Participants and procedures

This study includes 243 caregivers (169 maternal caregivers) with children between the ages of 4- to 6-years old who resided in the home with the children the majority of the time. Table 1 displays the sample characteristics. Approximately 51% of the children were male, and 33.6% were Latino. The majority of caregivers (51.5%) reported a monthly household income of $3000 or below. There were 72 children whose caregiver reported household food insecurity. The number of persons per household ranged from 2 to 10 ($M = 4.27$, $SD = 1.14$). Child body mass index (BMI) was calculated as BMI-for-age (age- and sex-specific) using experimenter-measured child weight and height with Centers for Disease Control and Prevention (CDC) growth charts [28]. Among the children, 66.7% had a BMI percentile score below the 85th percentile and considered of healthy weight, while 23.8% of the sample had a BMI percentile score between 85th and 95th and considered overweight, and 9.5% of the children were considered obese with a 95th or greater BMI percentile score.

Using flyers, participants were recruited from waiting rooms of pediatricians' offices, daycare centers, preschools, and local stores or businesses that were frequented by families. Families called if they were interested in participating in the study and were screened by phone. Caregivers were excluded if (1) they were unable to use English fluently, (2) had a significant

Table 1 Means, standard deviation, and sample characteristics

Characteristic/Scale	Total (N = 243)	Males (n = 125)	Females (n = 116)	Latino (n = 81)	Non-Latino (n = 160)	Insecure (n = 72)	Secure (n = 167)
Age	4.80(0.85)						
Income							
0 - $2000	36.4%						
$2001-$3000	15.1%						
$3001-$5000	15.5%						
$5001-$7000	9.2%						
$7001 – more	23.8%						
Child BMI							
Healthy	66.7%						
Overweight	23.8%						
Obese	9.5%						
Caregiver BMI							
Healthy	36.8%						
Overweight	27.1%						
Obese	36.1%						
Child feeding questionnaire							
Perceived Parent Weight	12.81(1.83)	12.75(1.64)	12.86(2.02)	12.85(1.70)	12.78(1.90)	13.29(1.81)	12.60(1.82)
Concern Child Weight	6.67(3.86)	6.53(3.86)	6.83(3.88)	7.59(4.14)	6.21(3.64)	6.97(3.99)	6.53(3.83)
Parental Responsibility	13.26(2.18)	13.12(2.36)	13.41(1.96)	13.51(2.65)	13.14(1.90)	13.71(1.96)	13.06(2.25)
Restriction	27.28(7.82)	27.59(7.91)	26.94(7.73)	27.09(9.05)	27.37(7.14)	28.18(7.99)	26.85(7.77)
Pressure to Eat	10.52(4.44)	10.99(4.47)	10.04(4.38)	10.86(4.14)	10.35(4.59)	11.33(4.72)	10.21(4.30)
Child eating behaviour questionnaire							
Food Responsiveness	11.56(4.03)	11.64(4.07)	11.47(4.00)	11.38(4.87)	11.64(3.54)	12.17(4.96)	11.24(3.44)
Emotional Overeating	6.83(2.93)	6.78(2.87)	6.89(2.99)	6.95(3.41)	6.78(2.66)	7.24(3.44)	6.67(2.68)
Enjoyment of Food	14.09(2.98)	14.07(2.99)	14.11(2.97)	14.09(3.05)	14.09(2.95)	14.21(3.28)	14.01(2.83)
Desire to Drink	9.83(3.21)	10.31(3.19)	9.30(3.15)	10.26(3.29)	9.61(3.15)	10.69(3.32)	9.39(3.05)
Satiety Responsive	15.29(3.29)	15.19(3.33)	15.39(3.28)	14.69(3.59)	15.59(3.10)	14.88(3.52)	15.46(3.14)
Slowness in Eating	11.75(3.12)	11.68(2.93)	11.82(3.32)	11.36(3.46)	11.94(2.93)	11.61(3.20)	11.82(3.05)
Emotional Undereat	10.79(3.21)	10.70(3.18)	10.88(3.24)	10.39(3.13)	10.99(3.24)	10.50(3.34)	10.88(3.15)
Food Fussiness	14.64(5.34)	18.20(5.30)	17.04(5.33)	16.79(4.86)	18.08(5.53)	17.69(5.33)	17.70(5.33)

Note: Total = total sample; Insecure = food insecurity; Secure = food security; Income is monthly household income. Child BMI percentile score below the 85th percentile is healthy weight, percentile score between 85th -95th is considered overweight, and 95th percentile score or greater is considered obese. Caregiver BMI was calculated using experimenter-measured weight and height. Data reported as Means (SD)

disability that would prevent them from completing the tasks in this proposal, such as blindness, or (3) did not have a child between the ages of 4- to 6-years old. Parents completed online questionnaires on their behavior patterns and those of their children, and were paid for their participation.

Measures
Child Feeding Questionnaire (CFQ)
The CFQ is a 28 item measure given to parents that assesses parent's perceived responsibility for feeding, perceived parent weight across development, concern about child weight and risk for being overweight, food

restriction, and pressure to eat [12, 13]. Items are rated on a scale from 1 to 5. Scores on the subscales range from 4 to 20 for Perceived Parent Weight, 3 to 15 for Concern about Child Weight, 3 to 15 for Parental Responsibility, 8 to 40 for Restriction, and 4 to 20 for Pressure to Eat. Confirmatory factor analyses have tested the factor structure of this measure across Caucasian and Latino samples [14]. Among Caucasian and Latino samples, internal reliability coefficients range from .70 to .92 [14]. In the current study, internal reliability coefficients are: .64 Parent Perceived Weight, .85 Concern about Child weight, .88 Parental Responsibility, .81 Restriction, and .75 Pressure to Eat.

Children's Eating Behaviour Questionnaire (CEBQ)

The Children's Eating Behaviour Questionnaire is a 35 item measure that assesses parents' perceptions on child's eating behaviors with items rated on a scale from 1 to 5. The subscales include child's responsiveness to food (scores range 5–25), enjoyment of food (scores range 4–20), satiety responsiveness (scores range 5–25), slowness in eating (scores range 4–20), food fussiness (scores range 6–30), emotional overeating (scores range 4–20), emotional undereating (scores range 4–20), and desire for drinks (scores range 3–15) [13]. Past research reports internal reliability coefficients ranging from .74 to .91 [13]. In the current study, internal reliability coefficients are: .79 Food Responsiveness, .86 Emotional Overeating, .82 Enjoyment of Food, .87 Desire to Drink, .71 Satiety Responsiveness, .74 Slowness in Eating, .73 Emotional Undereating, and .88 Food Fussiness.

Food security

The United States Department of Agriculture Household Food Security questionnaire was used to assess food security [29, 30]. This is an 18 item questionnaire that categorizes families into high food security (score of 0), marginal food (scores of 1–2) security, low food security (scores 3–7) and very low food security (scores of 8 or more). This measure has been used with different ethnic groups [31]. For this study, individuals with scores of 2 or less were considered food secure, and individuals with a score of 3 or more were considered food insecure. However, among those with a score of 1 or 2, if caregivers reported skipping meals or not eating so that their children may eat, they were classified as food insecure.

Data analytic approach

Descriptive analyses were conducted using SPSS software. Descriptive statistics were calculated by gender, ethnicity, and household food security via independent sample t tests. Internal consistency was calculated and reported across all of the groups.

Power analyses

Research has determined that no general rule of thumb will suffice when determining the needed sample size for CFA [32, 33]. Research has found that communality of indicators (i.e., reliability of the indicators), and factor overdetermination (i.e., number of factors/number of indicators) are important when determining sample size requirements for CFAs [33, 34]. MacCallum et al. suggested communalities of .6 or greater, and a minimum of 3 indicators per factor [34]. Using Monte Carlo data simulation techniques, Wolf and colleagues [32] found that for CFAs with one factor loading of .50 and with 3 or 4 indicators required a sample size of 190 or a sample size of 90 if the indicators increased to 6 or 8. Given the

findings from Wolf and colleagues [32], our sample size should be sufficient. To further ensure sufficient power, retrospectively the RMSEA analyses were all entered into the Preacher and Coffman online software and yielded power of .80 through .98 [35].

Measurement invariance

To conduct the measurement equivalence analyses, confirmatory factor analyses (CFAs) in Mplus [36] were conducted following the procedures recommended by Mulaik and Millsap [37]. For all analyses, we used full information maximum likelihood to handle missing data as this method produces more unbiased results [38]. Little MCAR tests with expectation-maximization methods were performed to evaluate if data was missing at random. For the CFQ, missing data for all the items ranged from 1.2 to 3.2%, and analyses indicate the data is indeed missing at random, χ^2 (247) = 225.451, p = .83. For the CEBQ, missing data for all items ranges from 1.6 to 2.8% and analyses indicate the data is missing at random, χ^2 (101) = 116.648, p = .14. We evaluated model fit using various fit statistics, including the chi-square significance test [39], the root-mean-square error of approximation (RMSEA) [40], and the comparative fit index (CFI) [41]. The Akaike Information Criterion (AIC) was used to compare different models with the lowest AIC value relative to another model is the optimal model [41]. Adequate fit was considered to be a lack of significance on chi-square difference test, a RMSEA <.08, and CFI > .90 [41, 42]. To examine measurement invariance across groups (males vs. females, Latino vs. non-Latino Whites, food secure vs. food insecure) we used a step-wise approach (instead of constraining all the parameters) to identify at which point invariance is no longer achieved between the two groups [43]. The first step entails examining single group solutions of each subscale of the CFQ and CEBQ for each subgroup. For example, we examined Pressure to Eat subscale of CFQ among males and females, separately. If model fit was adequate for each of these samples, then we proceeded to the next step; otherwise, we stopped. The second step involved examining configural invariance, which assesses if the number of factors and pattern of indicator-factor loadings fit both groups equally well. Both the factor loadings and item thresholds were allowed to be freely estimated in each group. If model fit was adequate, then we proceeded to the next step; otherwise, we stopped. The third step examined loading invariance, which constrained loadings to be equal across both groups. Differences in factor loadings would suggest that items were not assessing the same construct across groups. For example, this test would examine if the items in the Pressure to Eat subscale of the CFQ were associated with comparable relationships to the latent construct (parents pressuring their children to eat) across the gender groups in this sample. If model fit was adequate, then we proceeded to the next step; otherwise, we stopped. The fourth step examined item intercept invariance, which constrained loadings and intercepts to be equal across both groups. Lack of invariance would suggest that the groups had different thresholds for endorsing a particular item, such that one group endorsed the item at higher severity despite having similar levels of the latent construct. For example, Latino parents may produce different raw scores on the items that comprise the Pressure to Eat subscale than non-Latino parents despite having similar global Pressure to Eat subscale scores.

Results

Means and standard deviations on all subscales across all groups are reported in Table 1.

Invariance across male and female samples
CFQ
Independent CFAs indicated poor fit of the single latent factor for either females or males on Perceived Parent Weight, Restriction, and Pressure to Eat subscales. Throughout gender invariance examination, males were used as the reference group. Results support configural, loading, and intercept invariance for the Concern about Child Weight and Parental Responsibility subscales. This indicates these subscales appear to be assessing the same underlying constructs across males and females, and the groups are endorsing items at similar thresholds. Comparatively, the AIC values indicate that the intercept invariance model appears to be the optimal model for both subscales (Table 2).

CEBQ
Independent CFAs indicated poor fit of the single latent factor for either females or males on Emotional Overeating, Slowness in Eating, Emotional Undereating and Food Fussiness. Results support configural, loading, and intercept invariance for the Food Responsiveness, Enjoyment of Food, and Satiety Responsiveness subscales indicating these subscales appear to be assessing the same underlying constructs across males and females. In addition, males and

Table 2 Independent and multi-group CFAs for parent feeding in males and females

Subscale	Overall fit indices			Comparative fit
	χ^2 (df)	CFI	RMSEA (90% CI)	AIC
Child feeding questionnaire				
Perceived parent weight				
Female	4.063(2), p = .13	.960	.091 (.000 - .220)	–
Male	37.804(2), p < .01	.687	.395 (.291 - .509)	–
Concern child weight				
Female	0.000(0)	1.000	.000	–
Male	0.000(0)	1.000	.000	–
Configural Invariance	0.000(0)	1.000	.000	36.000
Loading Invariance	1.851(2), p = .40	1.000	.000 (.000 - .125)	33.851
Intercept Invariance	4.212(5), p = .52	1.000	.000 (.000 - .082)	30.212
Parental responsibility				
Female	0.000(0)	1.000	.000	–
Male	0.000(0)	1.000	.000	–
Configural Invariance	0.000(0)	1.000	.000	36.000
Loading Invariance	1.844(2), p = .40	1.000	.000 (.000 - .075)	34.756
Intercept Invariance	6.854(5), p = .23	.996	.039 (.000 - .104)	32.854
Restriction				
Female	127.385(20), p < .01	.711	.208 (.174 - .243)	
Male	200.813(20), p < .01	.599	.280 (.246 - .316)	
Pressure to eat				
Female	5.092(2), p = .08	.975	.112 (.000 - .237)	
Male	4.140(2), p = .13	.981	.096 (.000 - .230)	

Note. Italicized analyses represent independent CFAs examining each subscale as a latent single factor. Perceived Parent Weight has 4 indicators, Concern about Child Weight has 3 indicators, Parental Responsibility has 3 indicators, Restriction has 8 indicators and Pressure to Eat has 4 indicators. AIC is a comparative fit index for two or more groups

females appear to be endorsing items at similar thresholds. The AIC values indicated the intercept invariance model to be the optimal model for all of these subscales. However, Desire to Drink only achieved configural and loading, with the model poorly fitting for intercept invariance. The AIC value further confirms the configural invariance model to be the optimal model for Desire to Drink Table 3.

Table 3 Independent and multi-group CFAs for child eating in males and females

Subscale	Overall fit indices			Comparative fit
	χ^2 (df)	CFI	RMSEA (90% CI)	AIC
Child eating behaviour questionnaire				
Food responsiveness				
Female	6.485(5), p = .26	.991	.049 (.000 - .141)	–
Male	6.844(5), p = .23	.991	.057 (.000 - .150)	–
Configural Invariance	13.329(10), p = .21	.991	.037 (.000-.084)	73.329
Loading Invariance	14.308(14), p = .43	.999	.010 (.000-.064)	66.308
Intercept Invariance	14.661(19), p = .74	1.000	.000 (.000-.041)	56.661
Emotional overeating				
Female	2.280(2), p = .32	.999	.034 (.000 - .185)	–
Male	8.973(2), p = .01	.977	.174 (.070 - .297)	–
Enjoyment of food				
Female	0.462(2), p = .79	1.000	.000 (.000 - .113)	–
Male	1.041(2), p = .59	1.000	.000 (.000 - .153)	–
Configural Invariance	1.504(4), p = .83	1.000	.000 (.000 - .058)	49.504
Loading Invariance	3.590(7), p = .83	1.000	.000 (.000 - .048)	45.590
Intercept Invariance	3.988(11), p = .97	1.000	.000 (.000 - .000)	37.988
Desire to drink				
Female	0.000(0)	1.000	.000	–
Male	0.000(0)	1.000	.000	–
Configural Invariance	0.000(0)	1.000	.000	36.000
Loading Invariance	6.196(2), p = .05	.991	.094 (.012 - .182)	38.196
Intercept Invariance	14.395(5), p = .01	.979	.089 (.037 - .144)	40.395
Satiety responsiveness				
Female	2.429(5), p = .79	1.000	.000 (.000 - .082)	–
Male	2.271(5), p = .81	1.000	.000 (.000 - .080)	–
Configural Invariance	4.700(10), p = .91	1.000	.000 (.000 - .028)	64.700
Loading Invariance	9.674(14), p = .79	1.000	.000 (.000 - .042)	61.674
Intercept Invariance	12.222(19), p = .88	1.000	.000 (.000 - .029)	54.222
Slowness in eating				
Female	6.864(2), p = .03	.932	.140 (.035 - .261)	–
Male	18.374(2), p < .01	.909	.267 (.164 - .384)	–
Emotional undereating				
Female	6.013(2), p = .05	.961	.127 (.005 - .250)	–
Males	6.481(2), p = .04	.967	.140 (.027 - .266)	–
Food fussiness				
Female	55.537(9), p < .01	.880	.204 (.155 - .257)	–
Male	35.779(9), p < .01	.932	.161 (.108 - .218)	–

Note. Italicized analyses represent independent CFAs examining each subscale as a single latent factor. Food Responsiveness has 5 indicators, Emotional Overeating has 4 indicators, Enjoyment of Food has 4 indicators, Desire to Drink has 3 indicators, Satiety Responsiveness has 5 indicators, Slowness in Eating has 4 indicators, Emotional Undereating has 4 indicators, and Food Fussiness has 6 indicators. AIC is a comparative fit index for two or more groups

Invariance across Latino and non-Latino samples
CFQ

Independent CFAs indicated poor fit of the single latent factor for either Latinos or Non-Latinos on Perceived Parent Weight, Restriction, and Pressure to Eat subscales. Results support configural, loading, and intercept invariance for Concern about Child Weight subscale. This subscale appears to be assessing the same underlying construct across ethnic groups, and the groups appear to be endorsing items at similar thresholds. Comparatively, the loading invariance model appears to be the optimal model for this subscale. Parental Responsibility achieved configural invariance but not loading invariance (Table 4).

CEBQ

Independent CFAs indicated poor fit of the single latent factor for either Latinos or Non-Latinos on Slowness in Eating, Emotional Undereating, and Food Fussiness. Results support configural, loading, and intercept invariance for all other scales. For Food Responsiveness, the best fitting model was the loading invariance model when compared to the other models. For Emotional

Overeating, the configural invariance model was the best fitting of the three invariance models. For Enjoyment of food, Desire to Drink, and Satiety Responsiveness the intercept model was the optimal model with the lowest AIC values (Table 5).

Invariance across food secure and insecure households
CFQ

Independent CFAs indicated poor fit of the single latent factor for either food secure or insecure households on Perceived Parent Weight, Restriction, and Pressure to Eat. Results support configural, loading and intercept invariance for Concern about Child Weight, with the intercept invariance model being the best fitting based on AIC values. For the Parental Responsibility subscale, only configural invariance was achieved, with loading invariance model fitting poorly (Table 6).

CEBQ

Independent CFAs indicated poor fit of the single latent factor for either food secure or insecure households on Food Responsiveness, Emotional Overeating, Slowness in Eating, Emotional Undereating, and Food Fussiness.

Table 4 Independent and multi-group CFAs for parent feeding in non-Latino and Latino samples

Subscale	Overall fit indices			Comparative fit
	χ^2 (df)	CFI	RMSEA (90% CI)	AIC
Child feeding questionnaire				
Perceived parent weight				
Non-Latino	38.046(2), p < .01	.734	.337 (.248 - .434)	–
Latino	2.509(2), p = .29	.986	.056 (.000 - .237)	–
Concern child weight				
Non-Latino	0.000(0)	1.000	.000	–
Latino	0.000(0)	1.000	.000	–
Configural Invariance	0.000(0)	1.000	.000	36.000
Loading Invariance	0.152(2), p = .93	1.000	.000 (.000 - .041)	32.152
Intercept Invariance	9.751(5), p = .08	.984	.063 (.000 - .122)	35.751
Parental responsibility				
Non-Latino	0.000(0)	1.000	.000	–
Latino	0.000(0)	1.000	.000	–
Configural Invariance	0.000(0)	1.000	.000	36.000
Loading Invariance	10.143(2), p < .01	.981	.131 (.059 - .215)	42.143
Restriction				
Non-Latino	221.360(20), p < .01	.547	.252 (.222 - .282)	–
Latino	147.769(20), p < .01	.680	.283 (.241 - .326)	–
Pressure to eat				
Non-Latino	3.787(2), p = .15	.990	.075 (.000 - .190)	–
Latino	5.446(2), p = .07	.939	.147 (.000 - .301)	–

Note. Italicized analyses represent independent CFAs examining each subscale as a single factor. Perceived Parent Weight has 4 indicators, Concern about Child Weight has 3 indicators, Parental Responsibility has 3 indicators, Restriction has 8 indicators and Pressure to Eat has 4 indicators. AIC is a comparative fit index for two or more groups

Table 5 Independent and multi-group CFAs for child eating in Non-Latino and Latinos

Subscale	Overall fit indices			Comparative fit
	χ^2 (df)	CFI	RMSEA (90% CI)	AIC
Child eating behaviour questionnaire				
Food responsiveness				
Non-Latino	*6.408(5), p = .27*	.992	*.042 (.000 - .124)*	–
Latino	*4.478(5), p = .48*	1.000	*.000 (.000 - .147)*	–
Configural Invariance	10.892(10), p = .37	.998	.019 (.000 - .074)	70.892
Loading Invariance	12.700(14), p = .55	1.000	.000 (.000 - .057)	64.700
Intercept Invariance	28.388(19), p = .08	.974	.045 (.000 - .078)	70.388
Emotional overeating				
Non-Latino	*2.467(2), p = .29*	.999	*.038 (.000 -.167)*	–
Latino	*0.339(2), p = .84*	1.000	*.000 (.000 -.124)*	–
Configural Invariance	2.803(4), p = .59	1.000	.000 (.000 -.083)	50.803
Loading Invariance	12.486(7), p = .09	.990	.057 (.000 - .108)	54.486
Intercept Invariance	22.522(11), p = .02	.980	.066 (.025 - .105)	56.522
Enjoyment of food				
Non-Latino	*1.600(2), p = .45*	1.000	*.000 (.000 - .147)*	–
Latino	*0.539(2), p = .76*	1.000	*.000 (.000 - .149)*	–
Configural Invariance	2.139(4), p = .71	1.000	.000 (.000 -.072)	50.139
Loading Invariance	4.800(7), p = .68	1.000	.000 (.000 - .062)	46.800
Intercept Invariance	9.141(11), p = .61	1.000	.000 (.000 - .059)	43.141
Desire to drink				
Non-Latino	*0.000(0)*	1.000	*.000*	–
Latino	*0.000(0)*	1.000	*.000*	–
Configural Invariance	0.000(0)	1.000	.000	36.000
Loading Invariance	0.344(2), p = .84	1.000	.000 (.000 - .072)	32.344
Intercept Invariance	3.740(5), p = .59	1.000	.000 (.000 - .077)	29.740
Satiety responsiveness				
Non-Latino	*1.689(5), p = .89*	1.000	*.000 (.000 - .050)*	–
Latino	*4.471(5), p = .45*	1.000	*.000 (.000 - .151)*	–
Configural Invariance	6.420(10), p = .78	1.000	.000 (.000 - .048)	66.420
Loading Invariance	13.890(14), p = 46	1.000	.000 (.000 - .062)	65.890
Intercept Invariance	22.116(19), p = .28	.988	.026 (.000 - .065)	64.116
Slowness in eating				
Non-Latino	*21.501(2), p < .01*	.861	*.248 (.160 - .347)*	–
Latino	*3.795(2), p = .15*	.980	*.106 (.000 -.268)*	–
Emotional undereating				
Non-Latino	*11.464(2), p < .01*	.951	*.173 (.085 - .275)*	–
Latino	*2.221(2), p = .33*	.995	*.037 (.000 - .228)*	–
Food fussiness				
Non-Latino	*57.979(9), p < .01*	.916	*.185 (.141 - .232)*	–
Latino	*22.373(9), p < .01*	.928	*.136 (.066 - .208)*	–

Note. Italicized analyses represent independent CFAs examining each subscale as a single latent factor. Food Responsiveness has 5 indicators, Emotional Overeating has 4 indicators, Enjoyment of Food has 4 indicators, Desire to Drink has 3 indicators, Satiety Responsiveness has 5 indicators, Slowness in Eating has 4 indicators, Emotional Undereating has 4 indicators, and Food Fussiness has 6 indicators. AIC is a comparative fit index for two or more groups

Table 6 Independent and multi-group CFAs for parent feeding in food secure and insecure households

Subscale	Overall fit indices			Comparative fit
	χ^2 (df)	CFI	RMSEA (90% CI)	AIC
Child feeding questionnaire				
Perceived parent weight				
Food Secure	*36.347(2), p < .01*	*.724*	*.322 (.235 - .417)*	–
Food Insecure	*2.912(2), p = .23*	*.973*	*.080 (.000 - .263)*	–
Concern child weight				
Food Secure	*0.000(0)*	*1.000*	*.000*	–
Food Insecure	*0.000(0)*	*1.000*	*.000*	–
Configural Invariance	0.000(0)	1.000	.000	36.000
Loading Invariance	3.195(2), p = .20	.996	.050 (.000 - .148)	35.195
Intercept Invariance	6.362(5), p = .27	.996	.034 (.000 - .101)	32.362
Parental responsibility				
Food Secure	*0.000(0)*	*1.000*	*.000*	–
Food Insecure	*0.000(0)*	*1.000*	*.000*	–
Configural Invariance	0.000)0)	1.000	.000	36.000
Loading Invariance	8.605(2), p = .01	.986	.118 (.046 - .204)	40.605
Restriction				
Food Secure	*207.007 (20), p < .01*	*.651*	*.237 (.209 - .267)*	–
Food Insecure	*92.144 (20), p < .01*	*.706*	*.225 (.180 - .273)*	–
Pressure to eat				
Food Secure	*1.848(2), p = .40*	*1.000*	*.000 (.000 - .150)*	–
Food Insecure	*9.570(2), p < .01*	*.911*	*.231 (.099 - .386)*	–

Note. Italicized analyses represent independent CFAs examining each subscale as a single factor. Perceived Parent Weight has 4 indicators, Concern about Child Weight has 3 indicators, Parental Responsibility has 3 indicators, Restriction has 8 indicators and Pressure to Eat has 4 indicators. AIC is a comparative fit index for two or more groups

The models for Enjoyment of Food, Desire to Drink, and Satiety Responsiveness all supported the configural, loading and intercept invariance. Thus, these subscales appear to be assessing the same underlying constructs and samples are endorsing items at similar threshold levels. Based on the AIC index, the intercept invariance model for Enjoyment of Food, the loading invariance model for Desire to Drink, and configural invariance model for Satiety Responsiveness are the optimal models (Table 7).

Discussion

Although there have been extensive studies that make group comparisons on child eating and feeding practices, few studies have examined measures to ensure group comparisons are equivalent across important group characteristics related to childhood obesity. Of note, there have been association studies relating minority groups' responses and scores on child eating and feeding practices measures to childhood obesity with limited research examining the appropriateness of these measures among minority groups. To further strengthen the research base for assessing child feeding practices and eating behaviors, we sought to evaluate the factor

structure and measurement invariance of the CFQ and CEBQ across gender and ethnicity. A unique contribution of our study was the examination of household food security. It is important to ensure that child eating and feeding practices measures perform consistently across diverse environments.

Overall, results regarding the factor structure yielded mixed results for each measure and highlight some important issues to consider in assessing child eating and feeding practices. For the CFQ, the factor structures did not differ across any of the groups for the subscales Concern about Child Weight and Parental Responsibility. Our study is consistent with and adds to the existing psychometric literature. Cumulatively, Concern about Child Weight and Parent Responsibility, are invariant across Latinos (current study, [14]), African Americans [14], preschool-aged boys and girls (current study, [14, 27]) and diverse food secure environments [current study]. Most notably, the factor structures for Restriction, and Pressure to Eat from the CFQ varied across the ethnic and food security groups in the current study. It is important to note our findings add to the existing literature. There have been cross-cultural conceptual issues for the Restriction

Table 7 Independent and multi-group CFAs for child eating in food secure and insecure households

Subscale	Overall fit indices			Comparative fit
	χ^2 (df)	CFI	RMSEA (90% CI)	AIC
Child eating behaviour questionnaire				
Food responsiveness				
Food Secure	*7.902(5), p = .16*	*.985*	*.059 (.000 - .133)*	–
Food Insecure	*14.460(5), p = .01*	*.939*	*.163 (.068 - .265)*	–
Emotional overeating				
Food Secure	*9.252(2), p = .01*	*.982*	*.148 (.062 - .250)*	–
Food Insecure	*3.071(2), p = .22*	*.994*	*.087 (.000 - .267)*	–
Enjoyment of food				
Food Secure	*0.919(2), p = .63*	*1.000*	*.000 (.000 - .122)*	–
Food Insecure	*1.103(2), p = .58*	*1.000*	*.000 (.000 - .198)*	–
Configural Invariance	2.026(4), p = .73	1.000	.000 (.000 - .071)	50.026
Loading Invariance	2.618(7), p = .92	1.000	.000 (.000 - .029)	44.618
Intercept Invariance	5.375(11), p = .91	1.000	.000 (.000 - .026)	39.375
Desire to drink				
Food Secure	*0.000(0)*	*1.000*	*.000*	–
Food Insecure	*0.000(0)*	*1.000*	*.000*	–
Configural Invariance	0.000(0)	1.000	.000	36.000
Loading Invariance	0.038(2), p = .98	1.000	.000 (.000 - .000)	32.038
Intercept Invariance	11.416(5), p = .04	.985	.074 (.012 - .131)	37.416
Satiety responsiveness				
Food Secure	*2.167(5), p = .83*	*1.000*	*.000 (.000 - .064)*	–
Food Insecure	*4.392(5), p = .49*	*1.000*	*.000 (.000 - .154)*	–
Configural Invariance	6.579(10), p = .77	1.000	.000 (.000 - .049)	66.579
Loading Invariance	20.049(14), p = .13	.976	.043 (.000 - .082)	72.049
Intercept Invariance	25.077(19), p = .16	.976	.037 (.000 - .072)	67.077
Slowness in eating				
Food Secure	*17.342(2), p < .01*	*.904*	*.215 (.129 - .313)*	–
Food Insecure	*2.063(2), p = .36*	*.999*	*.021 (.000 - .237)*	–
Emotional undereating				
Food Secure	*2.852(2), p = .24*	*.996*	*.051 (.000 - .171)*	–
Food Insecure	*10.301(2), p < .01*	*.843*	*.242 (.111 - .397)*	–
Food fussiness				
Food Secure	*27.170(9), p < .01*	*.969*	*.110 (.064 - .159)*	–
Food Insecure	*48.759(9), p < .01*	*.797*	*.249 (.183 - .320)*	–

Note. Italicized analyses represent independent CFAs examining each subscale as a single latent factor. Food Responsiveness has 5 indicators, Emotional Overeating has 4 indicators, Enjoyment of Food has 4 indicators, Desire to Drink has 3 indicators, Satiety Responsiveness has 5 indicators, Slowness in Eating has 4 indicators, Emotional Undereating has 4 indicators, and Food Fussiness has 6 indicators. AIC is a comparative fit index for two or more groups

subscale among samples of Latinos (current study, [14]), African American [14, 40] and an Australian sample [27], and diverse food secure groups [current study]. It is important to note, that all of these studies, including the current study, assessed parents of preschool age children. For Pressure to Eat subscale, cross-cultural issues were found in the current study and Boles and colleagues [44], but Anderson and colleagues [14] found this scale to be invariant. In our study, the Perceived Parent Weight factor fit poorly across all the groups. Consistent with our findings, Anderson et al. [14] found issues with this factor and subsequently dropped it altogether. Given all of these findings, caution should be given to conclusions derived from studies that used these subscales across food secure samples [17, 18]. Similarly, the lack of measurement invariance on Pressure to Eat and Restriction suggests findings from published studies demonstrating higher rates among Latinos compared to other ethnic and racial groups (i.e., [11, 16]) should be interpreted with caution. Overall, results of the current study suggest that research should continue to validate the CFQ.

Results on the CEBQ revealed that three of the eight factors (Enjoyment of Food, Desire to Drink, and Satiety Responsiveness) performed well and did not vary across any of the groups. However, the intercepts did vary for Food Responsiveness where Latinos report lower thresholds for endorsing these items. In contrast, the intercepts varied for Emotional Overeating as well, but Latinos reported higher thresholds for endorsing these items when compared to non-Latino Whites. Importantly, the Food Fussiness factor showed poor fit across all of the groups. Other factors (i.e., Desire to Drink, Slowness in Eating, and Emotional Undereating) varied across the groups, suggesting the items in these subscales do not assess the same underlying construct across groups.

Cumulatively, the findings from the psychometric research on the CEBQ are mixed. Domoff et al. [22] conducted a validation study of the CEBQ among an ethnically diverse sample of low-income parents of preschool age children within the United States and replicated the original factor structure. A second study conducted on predominantly Hispanic and Black parents of preschool age children within the United States failed to replicate the original factor structure of the CEBQ and proposed three new factors [23]. Consistent with Domoff et al. [22], our study found that three of the food approach subscales (Food Responsiveness, Emotional Overeating, Enjoyment of Food) and one food avoidance subscale (Satiety Responsiveness) performed well across gender and ethnicity. But, consistent with Sparks & Radnitz [23], Food Fussiness, Slowness in Eating, and Emotional Undereating had cross-cultural conceptual problems. It is important to note that all studies used parents of preschool age children, but differed in mode of administration. The current study along with Sparks & Radnitz [23] administered self-report questionnaires while Domoff and colleagues [22] administered the questionnaire orally. At best, the collective research within the United States is inconclusive with regards to the construct validity of the CEBQ and highlights the need for further research.

A unique contribution of this study was an examination of measurement invariance across food secure and insecure households. For the CEBQ, Food responsiveness, which assesses external eating (e.g., responsiveness to sight, smell, and taste of palatable foods), and Food Fussiness, which assesses picky eating, failed to fit the data adequately. A closer examination of participants from food insecure households and their responses to

food responsiveness and food fussiness items revealed higher rates of "untrue" endorsements. In addition, some parents wrote comments on these items stating those behaviors or situations did not occur. This might suggest that within food insecure environments, items from these subscales do not apply or fail to capture the living context of these families. In other words, the behaviors assessed in these items might be specific to households with consistent and stable food availability. Similarly, parental food restriction also may be only applicable in food secure environments given that within food insecure households the family economics and resources are placing food restrictions on the family. It is important to highlight that household food security is associated with income, however, food insecurity in children can still be quite high at incomes that are two or three times the poverty level [2]. Similarly, caregiver disability can influence the risk of food insecurity in children, but high rates can still be evident among households with employed caregivers [2]. Recent research has found that numerous factors aside from income and employment can influence household food insecurity including caregiver incarceration, immigration status, and caregiver's mental and physical health ([2] for a review). Since these analyses are unique to our study, replication is needed. Further research is need to explore how the presence of poor caregiver mental health or disability influences parent-report of child eating behaviors, if at all.

The results of this study should be interpreted in light of several limitations. First, the findings are limited to White and Latino samples fluent in English who are parents of preschool aged children. Second, the data are parent-report and may be influenced by context-specific eating behaviors and/or the desire to respond with socially expected answers. The very low food insecure and low food insecure were combined into one food insecure group due to sample size. Future research should consider separating this group as the very low food insecure group may differ significantly in feeding practices than the other groups. A larger sample size would have allowed for examining the entire factor structure of the scales within one CFA analysis. Relatedly, the number of analyses conducted increase the chance of family-wise error rate and the probability of making a type I error. This signifies that some of the p-values were significant simply by chance. Furthermore, this study was cross-sectional in nature and cannot address longitudinal measurement invariance or distinguish between important differences among individuals that exist within specific racial groups, genders, or food security groups (i.e., genetics or individual experiences). Future research should consider conducting longitudinal measurement invariance with these variables, as this can address if changes on measurement over time reflect individual change or change in the properties of the measurement instrument.

Conclusions

In summary, continued psychometric research and scale refinement is needed on the CFQ and CEBQ. For the CFQ, Concern about Child Weight and Parental Responsibility subscales perform consistently across gender, ethnicity, and food secure environments. For the CEBQ, Enjoyment of Food, Desire to Drink, and Satiety Responsiveness subscales were invariant across all the contextual factors. Given that pediatric obesity is influenced by contextual factors such as gender, food security, and ethnicity, it is imperative that assessments perform consistently across these factors. The ability to assess risk factors for pediatric obesity, or to detect change across time in treatment studies or longitudinal studies, is compromised if the measures used are influenced by contextual factors.

Abbreviations
BMI: Body mass index; CEBQ: Children's Eating Behaviour Questionnaire; CFA: Confirmatory factor analysis; CFI: Comparative fit index; CFQ: Child Feeding Questionnaire; RMSEA: Root mean square error of approximation

Acknowledgements
The authors express gratitude for the families that participated in this research, and all the research assistants who helped and contributed to the efforts of Project ABC-EAT and the lab.

Funding
The project described was supported by Award Number R03HD058734 from the Eunice Kennedy Shriver National Institute of Child Health & Human Development. The content is solely the responsibility of the authors and does not necessarily represent the official views of the Eunice Kennedy Shriver National Institute of Child Health & Human Development or the National Institutes of Health.

Authors' contributions
MP and JL are the principal investigators on the grant and thus designed the study, operationalized study variables, and oversaw all aspects of the current study. MP, TO, AB conducted literature reviews, and drafted the manuscript. AT conducted analyses and drafted results. JL, AKVD and TU gave critical revision of the manuscript. MP finalized the manuscript. All authors read and approved the final manuscript.

Competing interests
The authors declare that they have no competing interests.

Author details
[1]Department of Psychology, Arizona State University, 950 S McAllister Avenue, Tempe, AZ 85287-1104, USA. [2]Department of Educational Psychology, Texas A&M University, College Station, TX 77843-4225, USA. [3]Nationwide Children's Hospital Department of Pediatric Psychology and Neuropsychology, The Ohio State University Department of Pediatrics, Cleveland, OH 44195, USA. [4]Department of Psychology, Texas A&M University, College Station, TX 77843-4235, USA.

References
1. Bhargava A, Jolliffe D, Howard LL. Socio-economic, behavioural and environmental factors predicted body weights and household food insecurity scores in the early childhood longitudinal study-kindergarten. Brit J Nutr. 2008;100:438–44.
2. Gundersen C, Ziliak JP. Childhood food insecurity in the U.S.: trends, causes, and policy options. The future of children, fall 2014.
3. Ogden CL, Carroll MD, Kit BK, Flegal KM. Prevalence of childhood and adult obesity in the United States, 2011-2012. JAMA. 2014;311:806–14.
4. Wisniewski AB, Chernausek SD. Gender in childhood obesity: family, environment, hormones, and genes. Gender Med. 2009;6(Suppl 1):76–85.
5. Gross RS, Mendelsohn AL, Fierman AH, Racine AD, Messito MJ. Food insecurity and obesogenic maternal infant feeding styles and practices in low-income families. Pediatrics. 2012;130:254–61.
6. Martin KS, Ferris AM. Food insecurity and gender are risk factors for obesity. J Nutr Educ Behav. 2007;39:31–6.
7. Metallinos-Katsaras E, Sherry B, Kalio J. Food insecurity is associated with overweight children in younger than 5 years of age. J Am Diet Assoc. 2009; 109:1790–4.
8. Ashcroft J, Semmier C, Carnell S, van Jaarsveld CHM, Wardle J. Continuity and stability of eating behavior traits in children. Euro J Clin Nutr. 2008;62:985–90.
9. Birch LL, Fisher JO, Grimm-Thomas K, Markey CN, Sawyer R, Johnson SL. Confirmatory factor analysis of the child feeding questionnaire: a measure of parental attitudes, beliefs and practices about child feeding and obesity proneness. Appetite. 2001;36:201–10.
10. Hughes SO, Anderson CB, Power TG, Micheli N, Jaramillo S, Nicklas TA. Measuring feeding in low-income African-American and Hispanic parents. Appetite. 2006;46:215–23.
11. Taveras EM, Gillman MW, Kleinman K, Rich-Edwards JW, Rifas-Shiman SL. Racial/ethnic differences in early-life risk factors for childhood obesity. Pediatrics. 2010;125:686–95.
12. Wardle J, Guthrie C, Sanderson S, Birch L, Plomin R. Food and activity preferences in children of lean and obese parents. Int J Obesity. 2001;25:971–7.
13. Wardle J, Guthrie CA, Sanderson S, Rapoport L. Development of the Children's eating behaviour questionnaire. J Child Psychol Psyc. 2001;42:963–70.
14. Anderson CB, Hughes SO, Fisher JO, Nicklas TA. Cross-cultural equivalence of feeding beliefs and practices: the psychometric properties of the child feeding questionnaire among blacks and Hispanics. Prev Med. 2005;41:521–31.
15. Blissett J, Meyer C, Haycraft E. Maternal and paternal controlling feeding practices with male and female children. Appetite. 2006;47:212–9.
16. Cardel M, Willig AL, Dulin-Keita K, Casazza K, Beasley M, Fernandez JR. Parental feeding practices and socioeconomic status are associated with child adiposity in a multi-ethnic sample of children. Appetite. 2012;58:347–53.
17. Matheson DM, Robinson TN, Varady A, Killen JD. Do Mexican-American mothers' food-related parenting practices influence their children's weight and dietary intake? J Am Diet Assoc. 2006;106:1861–5.
18. Gross RS, Velazco NK, Briggs RD, Racine AD. Maternal depressive symptoms and child obesity in low-income urban families. Acad Pediatrics. 2013;13:356–63.
19. Wehrly SE, Bonilla C, Perez M, Liew J. Controlling parental feeding practices and child body composition in ethnically and economically diverse preschool children. Appetite. 2014;73:163–71.
20. Mallan KM, Liu W, Mehta RJ, Daniels LA, Magarey A, Battistutta D. Maternal reports of young children's eating styles. Validation of the Children's eating behaviour questionnaire in three ethnically diverse Australian samples. Appetite. 2013;64:48–55.
21. Svensson V, Lundborg L, Cao Y, Nowicka P, Marcus C, Sobko T. Obesity related eating behaviour patterns in Swedish preschool children and association with age, gender, relative weight and parental weight-factorial validation of the Children's eating behaviour questionnaire. Int J Behav Nutr Phy. 2011;8:134.

22. Domoff SE, Miller AL, Kaciroti N, Lumeng JC. Validation of the Children's eating behaviour questionnaire in a low-income preschool-aged sample in the United States. Appetite. 2015;95:415–20.

23. Sparks MA, Radnitz CL. Confirmatory factor analysis of the Children's eating behaviour questionnaire in a low-income sample. Eat Behav. 2012;13:267–70.

24. Cross MB, Hallett AM, Ledoux TA, O'Connor DP, Hughes SO. Effects of children's self-regulation of eating on parental feeding practices and child weight. Appetite. 2014;81:76–83.

25. Webber L, Hill C, Saxton J, van Jaarsveld CHM, Wardle J. Eating behaviour and weight in children. Int J Obesity. 2009;33:21–8.

26. Spence JC, Carson V, Casey L, Boule N. Examining behavioural susceptibility to obesity among Canadian pre-school children: the role of eating behaviours. Pediatric Obesity. 2011;6:e501–7.

27. Corsini N, Danthiir V, Kettler L, Wilson C. Factor structure and psychometric properties of the child feeding questionnaire in Australian preschool children. Appetite. 2008;51:474–81.

28. Kuczmarski RJ, Ogden CL, Grummer-Strawn LM, Flegal KM, Guo SS, Wei R, et al. CDC growth charts: United States. Adv Data. 2000;314:1–27.

29. Bickel G, Nord M, Price C, Hamilton W, Cook J. Guide to measuring household food security. Department of Agriculture Food and Nutrition Service. 2000.

30. Nord M, Andrews M, Winicki J. Frequency and duration of food insecurity and hunger in US households. J Nutr Educ Behav. 2002;34:194–200.

31. Rose D, Bodor JN. Household food insecurity and overweight status in young school children: results from the early childhood longitudinal study. Pediatrics. 2006;117:464–70.

32. Wolf EJ, Harrington KM, Clark SL, Miller MA. Sample size requirements for structural equation models: an evaluation of power, bias, and solution propriety. Educ Psychol Meas. 2013;76:913–34.

33. Meade AW, Bauer DJ. Power and precision in confirmatory factor analytic tests of measurement invariance. Struct Equ Modeling. 2007;14:611–35.

34. MacCallum RC, Widaman KF, Zhang S, Hong S. Sample size in factor analysis. Psychol Methods. 1999;4:84–99.

35. Preacher KJ, Coffman DL. Computing power and minimum sample size for RMSEA [computer software] 2006. Available from: http://quantpsy.org.

36. Muthén B, Muthén L. Mplus [computer software]. Los Angeles: Muthén & Muthén; 1998.

37. Mulaik SA, Millsap RE. Doing the four-step right. Struct Equ Model. 2000;7:36–73.

38. Enders CK, Bandalos DL. The relative performance of full information máximum likelihood estimation for missing data in structural equation models. Struct Equ Model. 2001;8:430–57.

39. Bollen KA. Structural equations with latent variables. New York City: Wiley; 1989.

40. Steiger JH. Structural model evaluation and modification: an interval estimation approach. Multivar Behav Res. 1990;25:173–80.

41. Bentler PM. Comparative fit indices in structural models. Psychol Bull. 1990; 107:238–46.

42. Browne MW, Cudeck R. Alternative ways of assessing model fit. In: Bollen KA, Long JS, editors. Testing structural equation models. Newbury Park: Sage; 1993. p. 136–62.

43. Brown T. Confirmatory factor analysis for applied research. New York: Guilford Press; 2006.

44. Boles RE, Nelson TD, Chamberlin LA, Valenzuela JM, Sherman SN, Johnson SL, Powers SW. Confirmatory factor analysis of the child feeding questionnaire among low-income African American families of preschool children. Appetite. 2010;54:402–5.

16

The negative impact of sugar-sweetened beverages on children's health: an update of the literature

Sara N. Bleich[1*] and Kelsey A. Vercammen[2]

Abstract

While sugar sweetened beverage (SSB) consumption has declined in the last 15 years, consumption of SSBs is still high among children and adolescents. This research synthesis updates a prior review on this topic and examines the evidence regarding the various health impacts of SSBs on children's health (overweight/obesity, insulin resistance, dental caries, and caffeine-related effects). We searched PubMed, CAB Abstracts and PAIS International to identify cross-sectional, longitudinal and intervention studies examining the health impacts of SSBs in children published after January 1, 2007. We also searched reference lists of relevant articles. Overall, most studies found consistent evidence for the negative impact of SSBs on children's health, with the strongest support for overweight/obesity risk and dental caries, and emerging evidence for insulin resistance and caffeine-related effects. The majority of evidence was cross-sectional highlighting the need for more longitudinal and intervention studies to address this research question. There is substantial evidence that SSBs increase the risk of overweight/obesity and dental caries and developing evidence for the negative impact of SSBs on insulin resistance and caffeine-related effects. The vast majority of literature supports the idea that a reduction in SSB consumption would improve children's health.

Keywords: Sugar-sweetened beverages, Children's health

Background

Sugar sweetened beverages (SSB) – which include drinks with added sugar such as soda, fruit drinks and energy drinks – are frequently consumed by children and adolescents in the United States (U.S.) [1]. There is evidence that consumption of SSBs has recently begun to decline in the U.S., with this decrease largely driven by fewer children consuming these beverages [2, 3]. From 2003 to 2014, the percentage of children in the U.S. consuming at least one sugar-sweetened beverage on a typical day declined significantly from 80% to 61% [3]. Much of this decline was driven by a decrease in the percentage of young children ages 2 to 5 consuming SSBs, although the decline was significant for all age groups. Over the same period, consumption from caloric beverages (SSBs, milk and 100% juice) declined from 463 to 296 daily calories, and the fraction of all beverage calories from

SSBs decreased from 49% to 45% [3]. Within SSBs, the number of calories from soda and fruit drinks consumed per day declined from 116 kcal to 49 kcal and 70 kcal to 31 kcal, respectively [3]. Despite these important declines, consumption of SSBs by children and adolescents in the U.S. still remains high. In 2013–2014, 46.5% of children aged 2–5, 63.5% of children aged 6–11 and 65.4% of adolescents aged 12–19 reported consuming at least one SSB on a given day [3]. Additionally, high levels of SSB consumption persist among low-income and racial and ethnic minorities.

In light of the frequent consumption of SSBs among children and adolescents in the U.S., there has been an interest in critically examining associated health consequences. As a result, there has been a substantial rise in the number of studies investigating the health effects of SSBs over the past decade. Evidence has emerged linking SSB consumption to a number of health consequences among adults including weight gain [4, 5], cardiovascular risk factors (e.g., dyslipidemia) [6], insulin resistance and type 2 diabetes [7, 8] and non-alcoholic fatty liver

* Correspondence: sbleich@hsph.harvard.edu
[1]Department of Health Policy and Management, Harvard T.H. Chan School of Public Health, Boston, MA, USA
Full list of author information is available at the end of the article

disease [9]. Studies among children are more limited and have generally focused on weight gain [4] and dental caries [10], as well as insulin resistance to a lesser extent [11, 12]. An emerging body of research has also examined the association between caffeinated SSBs (e.g., energy drinks or colas) and caffeine-related health consequences including reduced sleep quality and headaches [13]. Given the growing number of studies assessing SSB-related health consequences, concise summaries of the evidence base are needed in order to inform policy and advocacy efforts focused on reducing SSB consumption.

This review aims to synthesize the existing evidence regarding the impact of SSB consumption on children's health. Unlike previous reviews which have been limited in scope (e.g., focusing on a single outcome such as weight gain) [14, 15], this review summarizes evidence from cross-sectional, longitudinal and intervention studies on a broad range of health outcomes relevant to children including: obesity, insulin resistance, dental caries, and caffeine-related effects. A previous review published in 2009 summarized many early studies on SSBs and children's health [16]. Using a narrative review approach, we update the literature by reviewing more recent studies published up until 2017.

Search selection
For each of the health impacts (obesity, insulin resistance, dental caries and caffeine-related effects), separate searches were conducted of PubMed, Web of Science and PAIS International. For all searches, a search hedge was created in three parts: 1) terms relevant to SSBs including "beverage" and "sodas", 2) terms restricting to children and adolescents including "pediatric" and "teens" and 3) terms specific to the outcome being examined such as "body mass index" and "body weight" for the search on overweight and obesity risk (see Additional file 1: Appendix for full list of search terms). These search terms were chosen to retrieve the most relevant results using an iterative process in consultation with a medical librarian. For searches of PubMed, MeSH subject headings were used. In addition to database searches, reference lists of SSB reviews and articles were searched. Following the removal of duplicate studies, one author (K.V.) screened titles, abstracts and full-texts and another author (S.B.) confirmed the inclusion of these studies. Included studies had to be peer-reviewed articles examining the effects of SSBs on a specific health outcome, be limited to children and adolescents, and be published after January 1, 2007. We selected 2007 as the start date because the most recent relevant review [16] included studies published prior to this. Studies were excluded if they were not published in English, were not conducted in high-income countries (defined as membership in Organisation for Economic

Co-operation and Development) or were grey literature. We limited our scope to high-income countries to promote generalizability of results.

Effects of SSBs on health outcomes in children
Overweight and obesity risk
A large number of studies have reported on the association between SSB consumption and overweight/obesity risk, with the majority of a cross-sectional [17–35] or longitudinal design [36–54] and only a few intervention studies (Table 1).

Cross sectional studies
Most cross-sectional studies found significant positive associations between SSB intake and obesity risk among children and adolescents [17–19, 21–25, 27, 29–32, 34, 35, 55]. For example, among 12 to 19 year olds in the 1999–2004 National Health and Nutritional Examination Survey (NHANES), each additional SSB serving (250 g) consumed per day was associated with a 0.93-percentile increase in Body Mass Index (BMI) z-score [34]. These positive findings were well-replicated across a range of OECD countries, including Canada, Spain, Greece and in Australia where those who consumed more than one SSB servings (≥250 g) per day were 26% more likely to be overweight or obese compared to those who consumed less than one serving per day [27]. They are also consistent with results focused on specific subgroups such as among Mexican-American children aged 8–10 years where each additional SSB serving (240 mL) per week was associated with a 1.29 greater odds of obesity [17] and among toddlers living in low-income families where no SSB intake was associated with a 31% lower obesity prevalence compared to households where toddlers consumed two or more SSB servings (serving = 12 fluid ounces) per day [23].

Some of the cross-sectional studies found positive associations only within subsets of the sample [18, 19, 21, 29, 32, 35, 55], including: boys [32, 35], boys aged 6 to 11 [21], children aged 9 to 11 [29], and among Mexican-American and non-Hispanic White adolescents only [18].

A small number of cross-sectional studies reported null findings [20, 26, 33], and one study conducted in Korea among 9 to 14 year olds reported an inverse association among males [28].

Longitudinal studies
Like the cross-sectional data, longitudinal studies generally demonstrated that increased SSB consumption was associated with weight-related outcomes among children and adolescents [38, 39, 47–49, 51, 53, 56]. For example, among a nationally representative survey of 2 to 5 year olds in the U.S., children who consumed more than one

Table 1 Studies on the the overweight/obesity risk associated with SSB consumption

Author, Year	Setting	Sample Size	Sample Age	Method of Diet Assessment	SSB Unit of Analysis	Primary Outcome	Direction of Association	Findings
Cross-Sectional Studies								
Beck, 2013	Mexican American children recruited from enrollees of Kaiser Permanente Health Plan of Northern California	319	8-10 years	Youth/ Adolescent FFQ	Increment of a serving/day of soda (1 serving = 240ml)	Odds of obesity	Positive	OR = 1.29 [95%CI: 1.13, 1.47]*
Bremer, 2010A	Nationally representative sample of U.S. adolescents, NHANES, 1988-1994, 1999-2004	1988-1994: 3234 1999-2004: 6967	12-19 years	Single 24-hour dietary recall interview	Increment of a serving/day of SSB (1 serving =250g)	Change in BMI percentile for age-sex	Mixed Null for one follow-up Positive for one follow-up	1988-1994 $\beta = 0.38$ [SE: 0.45] 1999-2004 $\beta = 0.93$ [SE: 0.18]*
Bremer, 2010B	Nationally representative sample of U.S. adolescents, NHANES, 1999-2004	6967	12-19 years	Single 24-hour dietary recall interview	Increment of a serving/day of SSB (1 serving =250g)	Change in BMI percentile for age-sex	Mixed Positive in two sub-groups Null in one sub-group	Non-Hispanic White: $\beta = 1.08$ [SE: 0.21]* Mexican-American: $\beta = 0.59$ [SE: 0.29]* Non-Hispanic Black: $\beta = 0.37$ [SE: 0.26]
Clifton, 2011	Australian children as part of Australian National Children's Nutrition and Physical Activity Survey	4400	2-16 years	Single 24-hour dietary recall interview	Consumed any amount of SSB in last 24 hours	Proportion of overweight or obese children who consumed SSBs vs. proportion of non-overweight children Proportion of obese children who consumed SSBs compared to proportion of non-overweight children	Mixed Null for one comparison Positive for one comparison	Overweight and Obese vs. Normal Weight 50% vs. 47% No measure of variation reported Obese vs. Normal Weight 59% vs. 47%* No measure of variation reported
Coppinger, 2011	British schoolchildren in south-west London, UK	248	9-13 years	Three day diary (Friday-Sunday)	mL/day of SSB	Correlation with BMI or BMI z-score	Null	No significant correlation [$r=$ 0.05 for soft drinks and BMI, $r=0.10$ for fruit beverages]
Danyliw, 2012	Representative survey of Canadian children and adolescents	10,038	2-18 years	Single 24-hour dietary recall interview	Soft drink beverage cluster vs. moderate beverage pattern (mean beverage consumption in each cluster differed by gender and age group)	Odds of overweight-obesity	Mixed Positive in one sub-group Null in other sub-groups	Males, 6-11 years old OR= 2.3 [95%CI: 1.2, 4.1] * Females, 6-11 years old OR = 0.8 [95%CI: 0.4, 1.7] Males, 12-18 years old OR = 0.7 [95%CI: 0.4-1.2] Females 12-18 years old OR: 1.1 [0.6, 1.9]
Davis, 2012	Low-income Hispanic toddlers from Los Angeles WIC program, 2008 data	1483	2-4 years	Interview about early-life feeding practices and nutritional intake	No SSB vs. High SSB (≥2 SSBs/day) (1 serving = 12 ounces)	Odds of obesity	Positive	OR= 0.69 [95%CI: 0.47, 1.00]*
Davis, 2014		2295	2-4 years			Odds of obesity	Positive	AOR = 0.72 [95%CI: 0.5, 1.0]*

Table 1 Studies on the the overweight/obesity risk associated with SSB consumption *(Continued)*

Author, Year	Setting	Sample Size	Sample Age	Method of Diet Assessment	SSB Unit of Analysis	Primary Outcome	Direction of Association	Findings
	Low-income Hispanic toddlers from Los Angeles WIC program, 2011 data			Interview about early-life feeding practices and nutritional intake	No SSB vs. High SSB (≥2 SSBs/day) (1 serving = 12 ounces)			
Denova-Gutiérrez, 2009	Adolescent children of workers at two institutes and one university in Mexico	1055	10-19 years	Semi-quantitative FFQ	Increment of a serving/day of sweetened beverage (1 serving = 240mL)	Change in BMI Odds of obesity	Positive	β =0.33 95%CI: 0.2, 0.5]* OR=1.55 [95%CI: 1.32, 1.80]*
Gibson, 2007	Children in the UK part of the UK National Dietary and Nutritional Survey of Young People	1294	7-18 years	Seven day weighed food records	Top tertile of caloric soft drink intake (>396kJ/day)) vs. bottom tertile (<163kJ/day)	Odds of overweight	Weakly Positive	OR=1.39 [95%CI: 0.96, 2.0]
Grimes, 2013	Nationally representative sample of Australian children	4283	2-16 years	Two 24-hour dietary recalls	More than one serving/day vs. less than one serving/day (1 serving = 250g)	Odds of overweight-obese	Positive	OR=1.26 [95%CI: 1.03, 1.53]*
Gómez-Martinez, 2009	Representative sample of urban Spanish adolescents	1523	13-18 years	Single 24-hour dietary recall	Non-consumers vs. moderate consumption (<336g/day) vs. high consumption (>336g/day) of sweetened soft drinks	Mean BMI	Null	No significant differences in BMI across SSB consumption groups
Ha, 2016	Combination of 5 studies conducted on Korean children between 2002 and 2011	2599	9-14 years	Three day dietary records	More than one serving/day vs. no SSB (1 serving = 200mL)	Odds of obesity	Mixed Negative in one sub-group Null in one sub-group	Males OR: 0.52 [95%CI: 0.26, 1.05]* Females OR: 1.36 [95%CI: 0.62, 2.97]
Jiménez-Aguilar, 2009	Representative sample of Mexican adolescents who participated in Mexican National Health and Nutrition Survey	10,689	10-19 years	Semi-quantitative FFQ	Increment of a serving/day of soda (1 serving = 240ml)	Change in BMI	Mixed Positive in one sub-group Null in one sub-group	Males β =0.17 [95%CI: 0.02, 0.32]* Females β =-0.07 [95%CI: -0.23, 0.10] Note: these results are for soda. See full paper for fruit drinks, sugar beverages and SSBs.
Kosova, 2013	Nationally representative sample of U.S. children from NHANES, 1994-2004	4880	3-11 years	Single 24-hour dietary recall interview	Increment of a serving/day of SSB (1serving = 250g)	Change in BMI percentile	Mixed Null overall and in some sub-groups Positive in one sub-group	Overall β =0.71 [SE=0.38] 3-5 year olds β =0.46 [SE=0.68] 6-8 year olds β =0.19 [SE=0.65] 9-11 year olds β =1.42 [SE=0.46]*

Table 1 Studies on the the overweight/obesity risk associated with SSB consumption (*Continued*)

Author, Year	Setting	Sample Size	Sample Age	Method of Diet Assessment	SSB Unit of Analysis	Primary Outcome	Direction of Association	Findings
Linardakis, 2008	Children in public kindergartens in a single county in Greece	856	4-7 years	Three day weighed dietary records	High consumers (>250g/day) vs. non/low consumers of sugar-added beverage	Odds of obesity	Positive	OR= 2.35* No measure of variation reported
Papandreou, 2013	Greek children in Thessaloniki	607	7-15 years	Three 24-hour dietary recalls	High consumers (>360mL/day) vs. low (<180mL/day) of SSBs	Odds of obesity	Positive	OR = 2.57 [95%CI: 1.06, 3.38]*
Schröder, 2014	Representative sample of Spanish adolescents	1149	10-18 years	Single 24-hour dietary recall	Soft drink beverage cluster (mean= 553g) vs. whole milk cluster	One-unit increase in BMI z-score	Positive	Males OR = 1.29 [95%CI: 1.01, 1.65]* Note: No soft drink cluster was identified for females
Valente, 2010	Elementary school children in Portugal	1675	5-10 years	Semi-quantitative FFQ	>2 servings/day (330mL) vs. less than 1 serving/day	Odds of overweight	Null	Males OR: 0.64 [95%CI: 0.33, 1.52] Females OR: 0.63 [95%CI: 0.33, 1.22]
Longitudinal Studies								
Ambrosini, 2013	Adolescent offspring from Australian Pregnancy Cohort (Raine) Study	1433	14 years old, followed-up at 17 years old	FFQ, at baseline and follow-up	Movement into top tertile of SSB consumption (>1.3 servings/day) at follow-up vs. remaining in lower SSB tertile	Odds of overweight-obesity at follow-up	Mixed Null in one sub-group Positive in one sub-group	Males: OR: 1.2 [95%CI: 0.6, 2.7] Females OR: 4.8 [95%CI: 2.1, 11.4] *
Chaidez, 2013	Convenience sample of Latino mother and toddler pairs	67 mothers	1-2 years, followed-up for 6 months	Four 24-hour dietary recall (2 at baseline, 2 at follow-up)	High SSB consumption (higher than median) vs. low SSB consumption (lower than median)	BMI z-score, weight for height z-score, and weight for age z-score at follow-up	Mixed Positive for one measure. Null for other measures.	*Weight for height z-score* β =0.46* *BMI z-score* β =0.47 *Weight for age z-score* β =0.13 *No measure of variation reported*
DeBoer, 2013	Nationally representative sample of toddlers in the U.S.	9600	9 months, 2, 4 and 5 years (followed-up at each age)	Computer-assisted interview with questions about beverage consumption, at each follow-u	≥1 serving/day vs. <1 serving/day of SSB (1 serving = 8 ounces)	BMI z-score at follow-up (between 2 and 4 years and between 4 and 5 years)	Mixed	Measure of association not reported. Positive for change between 2 and 4 years, null for change between 4 and 5 years.
Dubois, 2007	Representative sample of children in Quebec, Canada	1944	2.5, 3.5, 4.5 years (followed-up at each age)	Single 24-hour dietary recall and FFQ at each follow-up	Regular consumers (4-6 servings/week between meals) between ages 2.5 and 4.5 years vs. non-consumers of SSBs	Odds of being overweight at follow-up	Positive	OR: 2.36 [OR: 1.10, 5.05]*
Field, 2014	Children of participants in the	7559		Youth/ Adolescent FFQ, at baseline and follow-up	Increment of baseline and change in sports drink	BMI score at follow-up	Mixed	Results differed depending on type of SSB and whether

Table 1 Studies on the the overweight/obesity risk associated with SSB consumption (Continued)

Author, Year	Setting	Sample Size	Sample Age	Method of Diet Assessment	SSB Unit of Analysis	Primary Outcome	Direction of Association	Findings
	Nurses' Health Study 2 in the U.S.		9-16 years, followed-up for 7 years		serving/day (serving =1 can)			predictor was baseline intake or change in intake. Results below are for sports drink intake. Females Baseline: β =0.29 [95%CI: 0.03, 0.54]* Change: β =0.05 [95%CI: =-0.19, 0.29] Males: Baseline: β =0.33 [95%CI: 0.09, 0.58]* Change: β =0.43 [95%CI: 0.19, 0.66]*
Fiorito, 2009	Non-Hispanic white girls in the U.S.	170	5 years, assessed biennially until 15 years	Three 24-hour dietary recalls at each follow-up	≥2 servings of SSB/day vs. < 1 serving of SSB/day at age 5, (1 serving = 8 ounces)	Percentage overweight in each SSB consumption group at each follow-up	Positive	5 years old ≥2: 38.5% <1: 16.1% 7 years old ≥2: 46.2% <1: 15.1 % 9 years old ≥2: 46.2% <1: 24.2% 11 years old ≥2: 53.9% <1: 21.7% 13 years old ≥2: 46.2% <1: 22.2 15 years old ≥2: 32.0 <1: 18.5 *Significant main effect
Jensen, 2013A	Danish children entering school in Copenhagen participating in intervention study	366	6, 9, 13 years (followed-up at each age)	7 day dietary record at 6 and 9 years	Increment of a serving/day of SSBs at 6 or 9 years, (1 serving = 100g)	Change in BMI from 6 to 9 years, 6 to 13 years or 9 to 13 years	Null	Intake at age 6, change from 6 to 9 years β =-0.005 [95%CI: -0.059, 0.0489] Intake at age 6, change from 6 to 13 years β =-0.059 [95%CI: -0.145, 0.027] Intake at age 9, change from 9 to 13 years β =-0.008 [95%CI: -0.098, 0.113] Note: these results are for SSBs. See full paper for sweet

Table 1 Studies on the the overweight/obesity risk associated with SSB consumption (*Continued*)

Author, Year	Setting	Sample Size	Sample Age	Method of Diet Assessment	SSB Unit of Analysis	Primary Outcome	Direction of Association	Findings
								drinks and soft drinks separately.
Jensen, 2013B	Comparison groups of two quasi-experimental intervention studies in Australia (BAEW, IYM)	1465	4-18 years, followed-up approximately 2 years later	Asked participants how much SSB consumed yesterday or last school day	Increment of a serving/day of sweet drink at baseline, (1 serving = 100mL)	BMI z-score at follow-up	Null	BAEW study: B=0.005 [95%CI: -0.03, 0.012] IYM study: β =0.004 [95%CI: -0.002, 0.01]
Kral, 2008	Cohort of white children in U.S. born at different risks for obesity (based on maternal pre-pregnancy BMI)	49	3-6 years, followed-up at ages 3, 4, 5 and 6 years	Three day weighed food record	Change in calories from SSB from ages 3-5	Change in BMI z-score over follow-up	Null	Measure of association not reported
Laska, 2012	Adolescents enrolled in two longitudinal cohort studies in the U.S. (IDEA, ECHO)	693	6th to 11th grade, followed-up 2 years later	Three telephone-administered 24-hour dietary recalls	Increment of a serving/day (1 serving = not reported)	BMI at follow-up	Mixed Positive in one sub-group Null in one sub-group	Males β =0.25 [SE: 0.10]* Females β =-0.09 [SE: 0.16] Note: Above association was no longer significant when correcting for multiple testing
Laurson, 2008	Cohort of children in three rural U.S. states	268	10 years, followed-up for 18 months	Questionnaire asking about SSB consumption	SSB consumption (1 serving = not reported)	Spearman correlation with BMI at baseline or follow-up or change in BMI	Null	Males Baseline r= 0.009 Follow-up r= 0.033 Change r=0.041 Females Baseline 0.073 Follow-up 0.077 Change -0.033
Lee, 2015	Non-Hispanic Caucasian and African-American girls in the U.S.	2021	9-10 years, followed-up for 1 year	Three day food records	Increment of one teaspoon of added sugar (liquid form)	Change in BMI z-score at follow-up	Positive	β = 0.002 [95%CI: 0.001, 0.003]*
Leermakers, 2015	Dutch children in population-based prospective cohort study	2371	13 months, followed-up at ages 2, 3, 4 and 6	Semi-quantitative FFQ, validation against 24-hour recalls	High intake (15 servings/week) vs. low intake (3 servings/week) of sugar-containing beverages at 13 months, (1 serving = 150ml)	Change in BMI z-score at different follow-up ages	Mixed Null in some sub-groups	Males 2 year olds β =-C.01 [95%CI: -0.15, 0.12] 3 year olds β = -0.01 [95%CI: -0.15, 0.12] 4 year olds

Table 1 Studies on the the overweight/obesity risk associated with SSB consumption (*Continued*)

Author, Year	Setting	Sample Size	Sample Age	Method of Diet Assessment	SSB Unit of Analysis	Primary Outcome	Direction of Association	Findings
							Positive in other sub-groups	β =0.01 [95%CI: -0.12, 0.09] 6 year olds β =0.05 [95%CI: -0.08, 0.18] Females 2 year olds β =0.15 [95%CI: 0.01, 0.30]* 3 year olds β =0.14 [95%CI: 0.01, 0.27]* 4 year olds β =0.13 [95%CI: 0.01, 0.25]* 6 year olds β =0.11 [0.00, 0.23]*
Libuda, 2008	German adolescents participating in longitudinal study (DONALD)	244	9-18 years, followed-up for 5-years	Three day weighed dietary records	Baseline and change in regular soft drink consumption	BMI z-score at follow-up	Null	Males *Baseline soft drink consumption* β =0.046 *Change in baseline soft drink consumption* β =0.009 Females *Baseline soft drink consumption* β =-0.291 *Change in baseline soft drink consumption* β =0.055 *Measures of variation not reported*
Lim, 2009	Low-income African-American children	365	3-5 years, followed-up for 2 years	Block Kids FFQ	Increment of an ounce/day of SSB at baseline	Odds of incidence of overweight at 2-year follow-up	Positive	OR=1.04 [95%CI: 1.01, 1.07]*
Millar, 2014	Nationally representative cohort of Australian children	4164	4-10 years, followed-up for 6 years	Parental interview asked about SSB consumption in past 24 hours	Increment of a serving/day (serving = not reported)	Change in BMI z-score at follow-up	Positive	β =0.015 [95%CI: 0.004, 0.025]*
Pan, 2014	Children in Infant Feeding Practices Cohort Study in U.S.	1189	10-12 months, followed-up at 6 years	Survey including questions about SSB consumption	Ever consumed SSBs vs. never consumed during infancy High intake of SSBs (≥3 times/week) vs. no intake of SSBs during infancy	Odds of obesity at 6 years	Positive	*Ever Consumed vs. Never consumed:* OR: 1.71 [95%CI: 1.09, 2.68]* *High vs. No SSBs* OR: 2.00 [95%CI: 1.02, 3.90]*
Vanselow, 2009	U.S. Adolescents from various socioeconomic and ethnic background in	2294	Adolescents, followed-up for 5 years	Youth/ Adolescent FFQ	Stratified by different number of soft drinks serving/week (0, 0.5-6, ≥6)	Change in BMI over 5-year follow-up	Null	0 servings β =1.74 [SEM= 0.18] 0.5-6 servings β =1.92 [SEM=0.10] ≥7 servings

Table 1 Studies on the the overweight/obesity risk associated with SSB consumption (Continued)

Author, Year	Setting	Sample Size	Sample Age	Method of Diet Assessment	SSB Unit of Analysis	Primary Outcome	Direction of Association	Findings
	Minneapolis/St Paul metropolitan area							1.80 [SEM=0.15] No significant differences across groups Note: these results are for soft drinks. See full paper for punch, low-calorie soft drinks, etc.
Weijs, 2011	Dutch children	120	4-13 months, followed-up 8 years later	Two day dietary record	Beverage sugar intake per one percent of energy intake	Odds of overweight	Positive	OR: 1.13 [95%CI: 1.03, 1.24]*
Zheng, 2014	Danish children part of European Youth Study	283	9 years, followed-at ages 15 and 21	24-hour dietary recall, supplemented by qualitative food record from same day, conducted at baseline and first follow-up	≥1 serving (12 ounces) vs. none at 9 years or 15 years Increase in SSB serving from 9 to 15 years vs. no change	Change in BMI from 9 to 21 years or from 15 to 21 years	Mixed	Change in BMI from 9 to 21 years, using 9 years SSB as predictor 1.42 [SE: 0.68] Change in BMI from 15 to 21 years, using 15 years SSB as predictor 0.92 [SE: 0.54]* Change in BMI from 15 to 21 years, using change in SSB from 9 to 15 years as predictor 0.91 [SE: 0.57]

Intervention Studies

Author, Year	Setting	Sample Size	Sample Age	Intervention	Control	Primary Outcome	Direction of Association	Findings
de Ruyter, 2012	Normal weight Dutch children	641	4-11 years	250mL sugar-free, artificially sweetened beverage	Similar sugar-containing beverage (104 calories)	Difference in change of BMI z-score from baseline at 18-month follow-up	Positive	-0.13 [95%CI: -0.21, -0.05]*
Ebbeling, 2012	Overweight and obese adolescents in U.S. who reported consuming at least 12oz of SSB/day	224	Grade 9 or 10	1-year intervention designed to decrease SSB consumption	No beverage (given supermarket gift cards as retention strategy)	Difference in change of BMI z-score from baseline to 1 year and from 1 year to 2 years (Change in experimental group minus change in control group)	Mixed	1-year follow-up -0.57 [SE: 0.28]* 2-year follow-up -0.3 [SE: 0.40]
James, 2007	Longitudinal follow-up of children involved in intervention in United Kingdom	434	7-11 years	Discouraged children from consuming SSBs and provided one hour of additional health education during each of four school terms	No beverage	Odds of overweight at 1 year and 3-years after baseline intervention (intervention ended at 1 year)	Mixed	1-year follow-up OR=0.58 [95%CI: 0.37, 0.89]* 3-year follow-up OR=0.79 [95%CI: 0.52, 1.21]

Note: *indicates statistical significance (p<0.05) as reported by each study

SSB serving (serving = 8 fluid ounces) per day at 2 years old had a significantly greater increase in BMI z-score over the next 2 years compared to infrequent/non SSB drinkers [38]. Two of the positive studies examined longitudinal associations between SSB consumption and obesity risk among minority populations, with one finding that high SSB intake (defined as greater than median intake in study population) among Latino toddlers was associated with a 0.46 unit increase in weight for height z-score at 6-month follow-up [37] and the other finding that SSBs were positively associated with 2-year overweight risk among African-American preschool children [47].

Some studies found mixed results [36–38, 40, 44, 45, 52], with two reporting the positive association between SSB intake and increased weight was only significant among girls [36, 45]. The first study found high SSB intake (≥15 servings/week) at 13 months old was significantly associated with an increased BMI among girls at ages 2, 3, 4, and 6 years old [45]. Another study found that girls who moved to the top tertile of SSB consumption (>335 g/day) between 14 and 17 years of age had increased BMI and nearly a five-fold greater odds of overweight or obesity risk compared to girls who remained in the lowest tertile of SSB consumption [36]. One study found a positive association when using SSB consumption at 15 years to predict change in BMI from ages 15–21 and found null results when using SSB consumption at 9 years as a predictor [52].

Some of the longitudinal studies found no association between SSBs and BMI or BMI z-scores [41–44, 46, 50, 54, 57].

Intervention studies

A small number of intervention studies have examined SSB consumption and overweight and obesity risk among children [58–60]. Three recent randomized controlled trials found a reduction in BMI or obesity risk in the intervention group compared to the control. De Ruyter and colleagues conducted a double-blinded placebo-controlled trial wherein 641 normal weight Dutch children were randomized to receive either a 250 mL of an SSB or a sugar-free beverage each day for 18 months [58]. At the end of the trial, the difference in BMI z-score was significantly different between the two groups, with the SSB group increasing on average by 0.15 units (compared to 0.02 units in the sugar-free group). The second study randomized 224 overweight and obese American adolescents who regularly consumed SSBs to either participate in a program to reduce SSB consumption or receive no intervention [59]. At the end of the 1-year intervention, those in the intervention group had beneficial changes in BMI and weight compared to those who did not receive the intervention, but these differences were no longer significant when participants were followed-up for an additional year after

the end of the intervention. However, in a pre-planned subgroup analysis of Hispanic participants, there were significant differences in BMI between groups at both follow-up periods. The third study was a cluster randomized trial in which schools in the United Kingdom were randomized to either an intervention discouraging consumption of SSBs or no intervention for one year [61]. A significant difference in BMI z-score and overweight/obesity risk between groups was observed at the end of the first year, supporting a positive association between SSBs and obesity risk [61]. Two years after the intervention had been discontinued, the researchers completed a follow-up assessment and reported the differences between the groups were no longer significant [60].

Insulin resistance

A modest number of studies reported a positive association between SSB consumption and insulin resistance risk among children and adolescents, with the majority conducted cross-sectionally [62–65], one conducted longitudinally [66] and no intervention studies conducted (Table 2).

Cross sectional studies

A number of cross-sectional studies found a positive association in the whole or a subset of their study population [62–65]. For example, among 12–19 year olds in NHANES, each additional SSB serving (250 g) consumed per day was associated with a 5% increase in HOMA-IR (a marker of insulin resistance which is calculated using fasting glucose and insulin levels) [55]. One study reported associations by race, with positive associations found among White and African Americans, but null associations among Mexican Americans [18]. Another study reported a stronger association between SSB consumption and higher HOMA-IR among overweight/obese participants compared to normal weight participants [64].

Longitudinal studies

Only one longitudinal study was conducted to examine this association, reporting that an additional 10 g/day of added sugar from liquid sources was associated with a 0.04 mmol/L higher fasting glucose, 2.3 pmol/L higher fasting insulin and a 0.01 unit increase in HOMA-IR over two year follow-up [66].

Dental caries

A growing number of studies have examined the relationship between SSB consumption and dental caries (cavities or tooth decay) among children and adolescents, with almost all evidence pointing towards a strong positive association (Table 3). While the majority of

Table 2 Studies on the insulin resistance risk associated with SSB consumption

Author, Year	Setting	Sample Size	Sample Age	Method of Diet Assessment	SSB Unit of Analysis	Primary Outcome	Direction of Association	Findings
Cross-Sectional Studies								
Bremer, 2009	Nationally representative sample of U.S. adolescents, NHANES, 1994-2004	6967	12-19 years	Single 24-hour dietary recall interview	Increment of a serving/day (serving = 250g)	Change in HOMA-IR	Positive	β = 0.05 [SE= 0.02]*
Bremer, 2010	Nationally representative sample of U.S. adolescents, NHANES, 1999-2004	6967	12-19 years	Single 24-hour dietary recall interview	Increment of a serving/day (serving = 250g)	Change in HOMA-IR	Mixed	Non-Hispanic White: β= 0.06 [SE=0.02]* Non-Hispanic Black: β=0.12 [SE=0.05]* Mexican Americans: β=0.04 [SE=0.04]
Kondaki, 2012	Adolescents in large multicenter European study	546	12-17 years	Mini FFQ from Health Behavior in School-Aged Children study	≥1 time/day vs. <1 time/week 5-6 times/week vs. <1 time/week 2-4 times/week vs. <1 time/week (serving = not reported)	Change in HOMA-IR	Positive	≥1 time/day vs. ≤ 1 time/week β = 0.19 [95%CI: 0.003, 0.38]* 5-6 times/week vs. ≤1 time/week β = 0.28 [95%CI: 0.07, 0.49]* 2-4 times/week vs. ≤ 1 time/week β =-0.080 [95%CI: -0.084, 0.245]
Santiago-Torres, 2016	Hispanic children attending inner-city school in Milwaukee	187	10-14 years	Block for kid's FFQ with Hispanic foods	SSB consumption, (serving = not reported)	Change in HOMA-IR	Positive	β =0.104* No measure of variation reported
Wang, 2012	Caucasian children recruited from primary schools in Canada	632	8-10 years	Three 24-hour dietary recalls	Increment of a serving/day (serving = 100ml)	Change in HOMA-IR	Mixed Null overall Positive in one sub-group Null in one sub-group	Among all children: β =0.024 > 85th BMI percentile β = 0.097* <85th BMI percentile β =-0.027 No measure of variation reported
Longitudinal Studies								
Wang, 2014	Caucasian Canadian children with at least one obese parent	564	8-10 years	Three 24-hour dietary recalls	Increment of 10g/day of added sugar from liquid sources	HOMA-IR	Positive	Among all children: 0.091 [95%CI: 0.034, 0.149] * Overweight/ obese: 0.121 [95%CI: 0.013, 0.247] * Normal weight: 0.046 [95%CI: -0.003, 0.096]

Note: *indicates statistical significance (p<0.05) as reported by each study

Table 3 Studies on the dental caries risk associated with SSB consumption

Author, Year	Setting	Sample Size	Sample Age	Method of Diet Assessment	SSB Unit of Analysis	Primary Outcome	Direction of Association	Findings
Cross-Sectional Studies								
Armfield, 2013	Australian children enrolled in school dental services	16,508	5-16 years	Questionnaire given to parents asked about SSB consumption	≥3/day, 1-2/day vs. 0/day, (1 serving = "1 medium glass")	Decayed, missing and filled deciduous teeth (for ages 5-10) Decayed, missing and filled permanent teeth (for ages 11-16)	Positive	5-10 years old ≥3 vs. 0 servings/day β = 0.46 [95%CI: 0.29, 0.64]* 1-2 vs. 0 servings/day β = 0.34 [95%CI: 0.23, 0.45]* 11-16 years old ≥3 vs. 0 servings/day β = 0.27 [95%CI: 0.13, 0.41]* 1-2 vs. 0 servings/day β = 0.16 [95%CI: 0.06, 0.26]*
Chi, 2015	Convenience sample of Alaska Native Yup'ik children	51	6-17 years	Verbally administered survey, including questions on beverage consumption adapted from Beverage and Snack Questionnaire	40 grams/day of added sugar (i.e. amount of sugar in 12-ounce soda) measured using hair biomarker and self-report. Note: Biomarker would include all sources of added sugar, not just liquid.	Proportion of carious tooth surfaces	Mixed	Biomarker: 6.4% [95%CI: 1.2, 11.6%]* Self-Report: Null. No measure of association reported.
Declerck, 2008	Preschool children in four distinct geographical areas of Belgium	2533	3 and 5 year olds	Questionnaire given to parents with structured open-ended questions about dietary habits	Daily or more consumption of SSBs at night vs. none Daily consumption of SSBs between meals vs. none	Odds of caries experience (using criteria from British Association for the Study of Community Dentistry)	Positive	SSB consumption at night 3 year-olds OR= 7.96 [95%CI: 1.57, 40.51] * 5 year-olds OR = 1.64 [95%CI: 0.18, 14.63] SSB consumption between meals 3 year-olds OR=1.47 [95%CI: 0.36, 6.04] 5-year olds OR= 2.60 [95%CI: 1.16, 5.84] *
Evans, 2013	Low-income children recruited from pediatric dental	883	2-6 years	Parent-completed 24-hour recall and interviewer-administered FFQ	Using 24-hour recall 1.7 to 14 servings SSB/day vs. 0 servings/day	Odds of severe early childhood caries	Positive	Using 24-hour recall OR = 2.02 [95%CI: 1.33, 3.06]*

Table 3 Studies on the dental caries risk associated with SSB consumption (*Continued*)

Author, Year	Setting	Sample Size	Sample Age	Method of Diet Assessment	SSB Unit of Analysis	Primary Outcome	Direction of Association	Findings
	clinics in D.C. and Ohio				Using FFQ 0.63 to 7 servings SSB/day vs. <0.16 servings/day (1 serving = 8 ounces)			Using FFQ OR = 4.63 [95%CI: 2.86, 7.49]*
Guido, 2011	Children from small rural villages in Mexico	162	2-13 years	Questionnaire with questions about beverage consumption specific to ones sold in local stores	Drinking soda at least onece/day	Decayed, missing and filled deciduous teeth Decayed, missing and filled permanent teeth	Positive	No measures of association reported p=0.71 p=0.04*
Hoffmeister, 2015	Random sample of children in southern Chile from a daycare center register	2987	2 and 4 years	Survey filled out by parents with questions about sugary drink frequency	>3 servings of sugary drinks/week at bedtime vs. ≤ 3 servings of sugar drinks/week at bedtime (1 serving = not reported)	Prevalence ratio of decayed, missing and filled deciduous teeth	Positive	2 year olds PR = 1.43 [95%CI: 0.97, 2.10] * 4 year olds PR = 1.30 [95%CI: 1.06, 1.59] *
Jerkovic, 2009	Children recruited from primary schools in northern region of the Netherlands, including low and high SES schools	301	6 and 10 years	Questionnaire filled out by parents including information on nutritional care	≥5 glasses of fruit juice/soft drinks vs. ≤4 glasses of fruit juice/soft drinks	Prevalence of caries	Positive	Measures of association not reported. p<0.001 *
Jurzak, 2015	Pediatric patients from university dental clinic in Poland	686	1-6 years	Questionnaire including questions about SSB consumption	Frequent consumption of fruit juices and carbonated drinks vs. Infrequent consumption (1 serving = not reported)	Odds of decayed, missing and filled teeth	Mixed, depending on age	1-2 years old 2.60 [95%CI: 0.77, 8.74] 3-4 years old 2.23 [95%CI: 1.25, 3.96] * 5 years old OR=2.134 [95%CI: 0.84, 5.44] 6 years old OR= 2.25 [95%CI: 1.03, 4.92]*
Kolker, 2007	African American children with household incomes below 250% of the 2000 federal poverty level	436	3-5 years	Block Kids FFQ	Consumption of soda (1 serving = not reported)	Odds of higher score of decayed, missing and filled deciduous teeth	Null	OR = 1.00 [95%CI: 1.0, 1.1] Note: this result is for soda. See full paper for powdered drinks, sports drinks, fruit drinks, etc.
Lee, 2010	Convenience sample of healthy primary	266	4-12 years	Prat Questionnaire asked about consumption of sweet drinks	Sweet drinks consumed in the evening/night vs.	Caries experience in past 12 months	Positive	18% vs. 29% p=0.004*

Table 3 Studies on the dental caries risk associated with SSB consumption *(Continued)*

Author, Year	Setting	Sample Size	Sample Age	Method of Diet Assessment	SSB Unit of Analysis	Primary Outcome	Direction of Association	Findings
	school children in Australia				no sweet drinks consumed			Measure of association not reported.
Majorana, 2014	Italian toddlers born to mothers attending two obstetric wards	2395	24-30 months	Self-administered questionnaire for mothers with questions about SSB consumption	≥2 servings day vs. ≤1 servings of SSBs, (1 serving = 250mL)	Odds of higher International Caries Detection and Assessment System score	Positive	OR = 1.18 [95%CI: 0.99-1.40]*
Mello, 2008	Sample of schoolchildren in Portugal	700	13 years	Semi-quantitative FFQ	≥2 servings/week vs. ≤2 servings/week of soft drinks derived from cola, other soft drinks and any soft drinks (1 serving = not reported)	Odds of ≥4 decayed, missing and filled teeth	Positive	Soft drinks from cola OR = 2.23 [95%CI: 1.50, 3.31]* Other soft drinks OR = 1.54 [95%CI: 1.05, 2.26]* Any soft drinks OR = 1.88 [95%CI: 1.07, 3.29]*
Nakayama, 2015	Japanese infants	1675	18-23 months	Questionnaire for parents or guardian with questions about SSB consumption	Drinking soda ≥4 times/week vs. <4 times/week (1 serving = not reported)	Odds of early childhood caries	Positive	OR = 3.70 [95%CI: 1.07, 12.81] *
Pacey, 2010	Inuit preschool-aged children in Nunavut, Canada	388	3-5 years	Past-month qualitative FFQ, 24-hour dietary recall (with repeat 24-hour recalls on 20% of sub-sample)	Mean SSB consumption compared between groups of Reported Caries Experience	Reported Caries Experience (RCE)	Positive	Mean SSB consumption /day among those with RCE 0.8 [SE=0.1] Mean SSB consumption /day among those without RCE 0.5 [SE=0.1] *Significant difference between groups.
Skinner, 2015	Random sample of adolescents in Australia	1187	14 to 15 years	Questionnaire including questions about SSB consumption	0 cup of soft drinks or cordial vs. 1-2 cups per day vs. 3+ cups per day	Mean decayed, missing and filled permanent teeth	Positive	0 cups per day Male: 1.14 Female: 0.81 1-2 cups per day Male: 1.12 Female: 1.47 3+ cups per day Male: 1.69 Female: 1.39 *Significant difference between groups.

Table 3 Studies on the dental caries risk associated with SSB consumption (*Continued*)

Author, Year	Setting	Sample Size	Sample Age	Method of Diet Assessment	SSB Unit of Analysis	Primary Outcome	Direction of Association	Findings
								Measure of variation not reported Note: this result is for soft drinks or cordial. See full paper for sweetened fruit juice, diet soft drinks and sports drinks.
Wilder, 2016	School-based sample of third grade students in Georgia, U.S.	2944	8 and 9 years	Supplemental survey including questions about SSB consumption	Increment of a serving/ day of SSB, (1 serving = not reported)	Prevalence ratio of caries experience	Positive	PR: 1.22 [95%CI: 1.13, 1.32]*
Longitudinal Studies								
Lim, 2008	Low-income African American children in Detroit	369	3-5 years, followed-up 2 years later	Block Kids FFQ	Change from low SSB consumption cluster to high SSB consumption cluster vs. low consumers at both time periods	Incident decayed, missing and filled deciduous teeth and incident filled surfaces at follow-up	Positive	New d_2mfs: IRR=1.75 [95%CI: 1.16, 2.64]* New filled surface: IRR=2.67 [95%CI: 1.36, 5.23]*
Park, 2015	U.S. children in Infant Feeding Practices Study II and Follow-up Study	1274	10-12 months, followed-up at 6 years of age	10 postpartum surveys through infancy, which asked about intake of SSBs during past 7 days	Any SSBs vs. no SSBs during infancy SSB introduction at or after 6 months, SSB introduction before 6 months vs. Never consumed SSBs during infancy SSB consumption < 1 time/week, 1-3 times/week, ≥3 times/week vs. No SSBs	Dental caries in child's lifetime at follow-up	Mixed	Any vs. No intake during infancy OR = 1.14 [95%CI: 0.82, 1.57] SSB intro at or after 6 months vs. no SSB OR = 1.07 [95%CI: 0.76, 1.52] SSB intro before 6 months vs. no SSB OR = 1.29 [95%CI: 0.77, 2.17] Consumed <1 time/week vs. No SSBs during infancy OR = 1.15 [95%CI: 0.61, 2.18] Consumed 1-3 times/week vs. No SSBs during infancy OR = 0.85 [95%CI: 0.48, 1.49] Consumed ≥3 times/week vs. No SSBs during infancy

Table 3 Studies on the dental caries risk associated with SSB consumption (Continued)

Author, Year	Setting	Sample Size	Method of Diet Assessment	Sample Age	SSB Unit of Analysis	Primary Outcome	Direction of Association	Findings
								OR = 1.83 [95%CI: 1.14, 2.92]*
Warren, 2009	Children in rural community in Iowa enrolled in WIC program	212	Questionnaire asking about SSB consumption at each follow-up	6-24 months, followed-up 9 and 18 months later	SSB consumption vs. no SSB consumption at baseline	Odds of caries at 18-month follow-up	Positive	OR = 3.0 [95%CI: 1.1, 8.6]*
Warren, 2016	American Indian infants from Northern Plains Tribal community	232	Validated beverage frequency questionnaire for parents adapted from Iowa Fluoride study, a 24-h dietary recall tool and food habit questionnaire	Infants followed-up at 4, 8, 12, 16, 22, 28 and 36 months	Added-sugar beverage intake as proportion of total	Odds of caries experience at follow-up	Positive	OR = 1.02 [95%CI: 1.00, 1.04]*
Watanabe, 2014	Japanese infants recruited from Kobe City Public Health Center	31,202	Questionnaire for parents asking about SSB consumption and frequency	1.5 years, followed-up 21 months later (at ~3 years old)	Daily SSB consumption vs. no SSB consumption, at baseline	Odds of dental caries at 3-years	Positive	OR = 1.56 [95%CI: 1.46, 1.65]*
Wigen, 2015	Children in the Norwegian Mother and Child Cohort Study	1095	Questionnaire for parents asking about SSB consumption	1.5 years, followed-up at 5 years old	SSBs offered at least once a week vs. less than once a week, at 1.5 years	Odds of decayed, missing and filled deciducus teeth	Positive	OR = 1.8 [95%CI: 1.1, 2.9]*

Intervention Studies

Author, Year	Setting	Sample Size	Intervention	Sample Age	Control	Primary Outcome	Direction of Association	Findings
Maupomé, 2010	American Indian toddlers in U.S.	Four geographically separate tribal groups (3 intervention groups, 1 control group); Group A = 63 enrolled, 53 completed. Group B = 62 enrolled, 56 completed; Group C = 80 enrolled, 69 completed. Group D = NR.	3-pronged approach: 1) increase breastfeeding, 2) limit SSB consumption, 3) promote consumption of water for thirst. Each intervention group measured at pre and post; also compared to control group to account for secular trends	18-30 months,	No intervention received.	Post-pre difference in fraction of affected mouths by incident caries (d1t and d2t)	Positive	$d1t$ Group A: -0.574 [SDE: 0.159]* Group B: -0.300 [SDE: 0.140]* Group C: -0.631 [0.157]* $d2t$ Group A: -0.449 [SDE: 0.180]* Group B: -0.430 [SDE: 0.153]* Group C: -0.342 [SDE: 0.181]

Note: * indicates statistical significance ($p<0.05$) as reported by each study

studies examining SSB intake and dental caries are cross-sectional [67–82], there have been several longitudinal studies [83–88] and one intervention study [89].

Cross sectional studies

The vast majority of cross-sectional studies found evidence for a positive association between SSB consumption and dental caries [67, 69–82]. For example, one study reported that the prevalence of caries was 22% higher for each additional SSB serving consumed by children per day [81]. Several studies replicated this positive association among low-income children [70, 73, 75], with one study reporting that high SSB consumption (≥5 oz/day) was associated with a 4.6 greater odds of dental caries compared to those with lower SSB consumption [70]. Some studies examined how specific timing of SSB consumption affects dental caries, with one study [72] finding an association with dental caries and SSBs consumed at bedtime and another [69] finding an association with dental caries and SSBs consumed at nighttime among 3 year-olds and for SSBs consumed between meals among 5-year olds.

One cross-sectional study reported null results, finding no association between self-reported SSB consumption and dental caries among Alaska Natives – a result which may have been related to the small sample size ($N = 51$) [68].

Longitudinal studies

All longitudinal studies included in this review found a positive or mixed association between SSB consumption and dental caries in at least part of the study population [83–88]. One study reported that a high consumption of SSBs (≥3 servings per week) among infants 10 to 12 months old was associated with a 1.83 greater odds of dental caries at age 6, compared with infants who did not consume SSBs during infancy [84]. Some studies reported these positive findings among specific subgroups including: low-income [86], African American [83] and American Indian children [85]. For example, Lim et al. conducted a cluster analysis and reported that African American children who changed from being low consumers of SSBs at baseline (mean consumption = 567.4 mL/day) to high consumers of SSBs at 2-year follow-up (mean consumption = 1032.4 mL/day) had a 1.75 times higher mean number of new dental caries compared with high consumers of milk-juice at both baseline and 2-year follow-up [83].

Intervention studies

Only one intervention study has been conducted to assess SSB consumption and dental caries [89]. Maupomé et al. conducted community-wide interventions to reduce SSB consumption, improve breastfeeding practices, and promote consumption of water for thirst among American Indian toddlers. While the intervention communities demonstrated improvements in the number of dental caries, it is not possible to attribute this specifically to reduction in SSB consumption as the intervention was a multi-pronged approach.

Caffeine-related effects

A growing number of studies reported on the caffeine-related effects associated with SSB consumption with studies almost exclusively cross-sectional (Table 4).

Cross sectional studies

A number of cross-sectional studies examined the effects of energy drink consumption among children and adolescents [90–97], with each study often reporting on multiple outcomes. Some studies found evidence for an association between energy drink consumption and sleep-related issues such as sleep dissatisfaction, tiredness/fatigue and late bedtime [92, 93, 95], and others reported an association between energy drink intake and increased headaches [91–93]. One study reported an association between energy drink consumption and risk-taking behaviors such as cigarette, marijuana and drug use [90], and two studies found an association between energy drink consumption and stress, depressive symptoms, and suicidal ideation, plan or attempt [90, 95]. Other outcomes examined in these cross-sectional studies reported include irritation [92], stomach ache and low appetite [93].

Some of the cross-sectional studies examined caffeine-related effects of cola drinks [93, 96, 97]. One found that both low and high consumption of cola were associated with lower stress and found null associations with anxiety and depression [96]. Another examined both cola and energy drinks and found that higher consumption of both beverages was associated with headaches, stomach-aches, sleeping problems and low appetite [93]. More specifically, among males, drinking more than one cola per day was associated with a 1.34 greater odds of sleeping problems and among females drinking more than one cola per day was associated with a 1.55 greater odds of sleeping problems.

Longitudinal studies

One longitudinal study was conducted and it found evidence that increased energy drink consumption was associated with attention deficit/hyperactivity disorder inattention and hyperactivity at 16-month follow-up, but did not find evidence for associations with depression, panic and anxiety [94].

Table 4 Studies on caffeine-related effects associated with SSB consumption

Author, Year	Setting	Sample Size	Sample Age	Method of Diet Assessment	SSB Unit of Analysis	Primary Outcome	Direction of Association	Findings
Cross-Sectional Studies								
Azagba, 2014	Adolescents attending public schools in Atlantic Canada	8210	Grades 7, 9, 10 and 12	Self-reported survey with question asking about consumption of caffeinated energy drinks in past year	Energy drink more than once a month vs. one to two times	Odds of depression, sensation seeking, substance use	Positive	*Sensation Seeking* OR = 1.17 [95%CI: 1.11, 1.22]* *Depressive symptoms, very elevated* OR = 1.95 [95%CI: 1.36, 2.79]* *Depressive symptoms, somewhat elevated* OR = 1.08 [95%CI: 0.80, 1.47] *Cigarette use* OR = 2.58 [95%CI: 1.71, 3.89]* *Marijuana use* OR = 1.87 [95%CI: 1.37, 2.56]* *Alcohol use* OR = 2.48 [95%CI: 1.83, 3.36]* *Other drug use* OR = 1.80 [95%CI: 1.26, 2.57]*
Bashir, 2016	Convenience sample of patients in waiting areas of emergency department in U.S.	612	12-18 years	Questionnaire asking about frequency of energy drink consumption	Frequent (at least once a month) vs. Infrequent (less than once a month) consumers of energy drinks	Proportion of frequent vs. infrequent consumers experience of headache, anger and increased urination	Positive	*Headache* 76% [95%CI: 69-81] vs. 60% [95%CI: 55-64]* *Anger* 47% [95%CI: 40-54] vs. 32% [95%CI: 27-36]* *Increased urination* 24 [95%CI: 18-30] vs. 13 [95%CI: 10-16]* Study provides a number of outcomes. See paper for full results.
Koivusilta, 2016	Classroom survey of 7th grade students in Finland	9446	13 years	Self-reported online survey asking about frequency of energy drink consumption	Several times a day vs. not at all	Odds of headache, sleeping problems, irritation, tiredness/fatigue, late bedtime	Positive	*Headache* OR = 4.6 [95%CI: 2.8, 7.7] *Sleeping problems* OR = 3.6 [95%CI: 2.2, 5.8] *Irritation*

Table 4 Studies on caffeine-related effects associated with SSB consumption (*Continued*)

Author, Year	Setting	Sample Size	Sample Age	Method of Diet Assessment	SSB Unit of Analysis	Primary Outcome	Direction of Association	Findings
								OR= 4.1 [95%CI: 2.7, 6.1] *Tiredness/ fatigue* OR=3.7 [95%CI: 2.4, 5.7] *Late bedtime* OR = 7.9 [95%CI: 5.7, 10.9]
Kristjansson, 2013	School survey of children in Iceland	11,267	10-12 years	Questions on population-based survey asking about frequency of energy drink and cola consumption	≥1 cola/day vs. none ≥1 energy drink/ day vs. none	Odds of headaches, stomachaches, sleeping problems, low appetite	Positive	Colas *Headaches* Females: OR = 1.13 [95%CI: 0.87, 1.47] Males: OR = 1.29 [95%CI: 1.03, 1.62]* *Stomachaches* Females: OR = 1.40 [95%CI: 1.08, 1.80]* Males: OR = 1.31 [95%CI: 1.03, 1.67]* *Sleeping problems* Females: OR = 1.55 [95%CI: 1.21, 1.98]* Males: OR = 1.34 [95%CI: 1.09, 1.66]* *Low appetite* Females OR = 1.37 [95%CI: 1.03, 1.83]* Males OR = 1.44 [95%CI: 1.12, 1.86]* Energy Drinks *Headaches* Females: OR = 1.68 [95%CI: 1.17, 2.41]* Males: OR = 1.87 [95%CI: 1.43, 2.46]*

Table 4 Studies on caffeine-related effects associated with SSB consumption (*Continued*)

Author, Year	Setting	Sample Size	Sample Age	Method of Diet Assessment	SSB Unit of Analysis	Primary Outcome	Direction of Association	Findings
								Stomachaches Females: OR = 1.76 [95%CI: 1.21, 2.54]* Males: OR = 2.45 [95%CI: 1.86, 3.23]* *Sleeping problems* Females: OR = 1.56 [95%CI: 1.07, 2.25]* Males: OR = 1.63 [95%CI: 1.25, 2.12]* *Low appetite* Females OR = 2.31 [95%CI: 1.58, 3.39]* Males OR = 1.30 [95%CI: 0.95, 1.78]
Park, 2016	Nationally representative cohort of Korean adolescents	68,043	12-18 years	Web-based survey with questions on energy drink consumption	Highly frequent energy drink consumer (≥5 times/week) vs. infrequent energy drink consumer (<1 time/week) Moderate frequent energy drink consumer (1-4 times/week) vs. infrequent energy drink consumer	Odds of sleep dissatisfaction, perceived stress, persistent depressive mood, suicidal ideation, suicide plan, suicide attempt	Positive	Highly frequent energy drink consumer vs. infrequent energy drink consumer *Sleep dissatisfaction* OR = 1.64 [95%CI 1.61, 1.67]* *Perceived stress* OR = 2.23 [95%CI: 2.19, 2.27]* *Depressive mood* 2.59 [95%CI: 2.54, 2.65]* *Suicidal ideation* 3.14 [95%CI: 3.07, 3.21]* *Suicidal plan* 4.65 [95%CI: 4.53, 4.78]* *Suicide attempt* 6.79 [95%CI: 6.59, 7.00]* Moderate frequent energy drink consumer vs.

Table 4 Studies on caffeine-related effects associated with SSB consumption *(Continued)*

Author, Year	Setting	Sample Size	Sample Age	Method of Diet Assessment	SSB Unit of Analysis	Primary Outcome	Direction of Association	Findings
								infrequent energy drink consumer *Sleep dissatisfaction* OR = 1.25 [95%CI: 1.25, 1.26]* *Perceived stress* OR = 1.38 [95%CI: 1.37, 1.39]* *Depressive mood* OR=1.51 [95%CI: 1.49, 1.52]* *Suicidal ideation* OR=1.43 [95%CI: 1.42, 1.45]* *Suicidal plan* OR=1.78 [95%CI: 1.75, 1.81]* *Suicide attempt* OR=1.91 [95%CI: 1.87, 1.95]*
Richards, 2015	Adolescents from three secondary schools in the South West of England	2307	11-17 years	DABS survey (assesses intake of common dietary variables), including questions on energy drink and cola consumption	High consumption (≥1 can of energy drink or cola) vs. no consumption Low consumption (<1 can of energy drink or cola) vs. no consumption	Odds of stress, anxiety and depression	Mixed	High consumption vs. no consumption Energy Drinks *Stress* OR = 1.10 [95%CI: 0.80, 1.50] *Anxiety* OR = 1.05 [95%CI: 0.77, 1.43] *Depression* OR = 1.11 [95%CI: 0.81, 1.52] Cola *Stress* OR = 0.68 [95%CI: 0.52, 0.90]* *Anxiety* 0.83 [95%CI: 0.64, 1.09] *Depression* 1.23 [95%CI: 0.93, 1.62] Low consumption vs. no consumption Energy Drinks *Stress*

Table 4 Studies on caffeine-related effects associated with SSB consumption (*Continued*)

Author, Year	Setting	Sample Size	Sample Age	Method of Diet Assessment	SSB Unit of Analysis	Primary Outcome	Direction of Association	Findings
								1.38 [95%CI: 1.05, 1.80]* *Anxiety* 1.26 [95%CI: 0.97, 1.64] *Depression* 0.99 [95%CI: 0.76, 1.31] Cola Stress 0.72 [95%CI: 0.56, 0.94]* *Anxiety* 0.86 [95%CI: 0.67, 1.10] *Depression* 1.18 [95%CI: 0.91, 1.54]
Longitudinal Studies								
Marmorstein, 2016	Cohort of middle-school students in the U.S.	144	10-14 years, followed-up 16 months later	Self-reported questionnaire with questions on energy drink consumption	Energy drink consumption at baseline	Change in ADHD inattention, ADHD hyperactive, conduct disorder, depression, panic, anxiety at follow-up (controlling for coffee)	Mixed	*ADHD inattention* β = 0.20* *ADHD hyperactive* β = 0.20* *Conduct disorder* β = 0.18 *Depression* β = 0.08 *Panic* β = 0.17 *Generalized anxiety* β = 0.09 *Social Anxiety* β = -0.02

Note: * indicates statistical significance (*p*<0.05) as reported by each study

Summary of evidence

Since the most recent relevant review was published on this topic in 2009 [16], there has been a substantial increase in research examining the health consequences of SSB consumption among children and adolescents. For example, 227 studies indexed in PubMed were published on SSBs in 2017 compared to 16 studies published in 2007.[1] Many more studies are now conducted exclusively on children and adolescents, while previous evidence was based on results found among adults. While the majority of this research is still cross-sectional (limiting the ability to make inferences about causality), the past decade has seen a growing number of longitudinal studies being implemented, as well as an increasing amount of intervention trials.

The majority of this research on SSBs over the past decade has centered on the relationship with weight gain. The findings of this review confirm that there is clear and consistent evidence that the consumption of SSBs heightens obesity risk among children and adolescents. Although a formal quality assessment or strength of evidence evaluation was not conducted, the vast majority of cross-sectional, longitudinal and intervention studies find strong evidence for a positive relationship in all or part of their study population. The exact mechanism through which SSBs impact childhood obesity is not entirely understood. Generally, the research points to the low satiety of SSBs and incomplete compensation [98, 99]. In other words, drinking calories in liquid form does not decrease hunger in the same way as solid food. Additionally, people do not sufficiently reduce their total energy intake to make up for the excess calories obtained from SSBs. There is also a lively debate about whether the effect of calories from SSBs on body weight is worse than some other foods or nutrients [100, 101].

The association between SSB consumption and weight gain is paramount, given that childhood obesity affects roughly one in six (13 million) children in the U.S., disproportionately impacting children who are low-income and racial and ethnic minorities [102]. From 1976 to 2016, the prevalence of childhood obesity in the U.S. more than doubled in children ages 2 to 5 (from 5% to 13.9%), nearly tripled in children aged 6 to 11 (from 6.5% to 18.4%) and quadrupled in adolescents' ages 12 to 19 (from 5% to 20.6%) [103–105]. While there is some indication that childhood obesity rates may leveling in the U.S. [104], the overall prevalence of obesity among children in 2016–2016 was estimated at 18.5% [105], meaning it is still considerably higher than the Healthy People 2020 goal of 14.5% [4]. Given that children who are overweight and obese youth are likely to remain so as adults [106], obesity and its adverse health consequences create a serious threat to children's current and future health [107]. Hence, reducing SSB consumption is an important intervention point to reduce the burden of childhood obesity in the U.S.

This review also finds strong and consistent evidence that consumption of SSBs is associated with dental caries among children and adolescents. The mechanism for the association between SSB consumption and dental caries is well understood: dental caries are caused by acids produced by bacteria metabolizing sugar in the mouth. Increased sugar from SSBs intensifies the acid production and causes further decay of teeth [108]. The majority of studies examining this relationship are cross-sectional, but a modest number of longitudinal studies as well as one intervention study also support the association.

While evidence has shown a positive relationship between SSB consumption and type 2 diabetes among adults [5, 12, 109], the available literature among child and adolescents is limited. The majority of studies among children and adolescents do not directly examine the link between SSB consumption and type 2 diabetes and instead measure insulin resistance, a biomarker of increased cardio-metabolic risk and type 2 diabetes. It is hypothesized that the high content of sucrose and high-fructose corn syrup present in SSBs may increase dietary glycemic load leading to insulin resistance and inflammation [7]. While not as strong and consistent as the relationships between SSB consumption and weight gain or dental caries, most studies in this review generally support an association between SSB consumption and insulin resistance among children and adolescents. However, this is limited by a small number of studies and the predominance of a cross-sectional study design.

The findings of this review also point to an association between caffeinated SSBs and a wide range of health issues including poor quality or reduced sleep, headaches, risk-seeking behavior and depressive symptoms. The presence of caffeine in energy drinks and other caffeinated SSBs (e.g., cola), in conjunction with the large volumes consumed, can lead to neurological and psychological effects associated with high caffeine consumption. The majority of studies examining the caffeine-related effects of SSBs focus on energy drinks, with very few analyzing the effects of other caffeinated SSBs such as colas. One reason for this may be the considerably higher level of caffeine content in energy drinks: a 250 mL energy drink has an average of 80 mg of caffeine (range: 27-87 mg), compared to 40 g of caffeine (range: 30-60 mg) in a 330 mL cola drink [110]. Additionally, studies examining caffeine-related effects have almost exclusively been cross-sectional, limiting the strength of inferences that can be made and bringing forth issues of reverse causation.

While there is a large and growing body of research examining the impact of SSBs on children's health, important gaps remain. First, researchers should utilize more rigorous study designs (intervention trials and longitudinal studies) and move away from a reliance on cross-sectional studies. This will strengthen the evidence base and allow firmer conclusions to be made regarding the causal relationships between SSB consumption and negative health consequences. Second, more consistency is needed in the definition of SSBs (e.g., specifying which beverages are included and what is a typical serving size) and measurement strategy (e.g., FFQ vs. 24-h recall). Similarly, more uniformity is needed in assessing outcomes, particularly in the risk of overweight/obesity where studies vary considerably in the outcomes measured (e.g., BMI, BMI z-score, BMI percentile, overweight/obese status). Third, researchers should more rigorously examine differences in health risks by subpopulations (e.g., race/ethnicity, socioeconomic status, age and gender) to determine if the intake of SSBs in particularly harmful in certain population subsets. While it is established that low-income and racial and ethnic minorities consume more SSBs, it is unclear the extent to which health consequences are magnified among these groups. This is important particularly for targeting interventions and policy approaches to reduce children's SSB consumption. Better insights in these areas have the potential to inform real-world policies and recommendations that may greatly benefit children's health. Finally, additional research is needed about caffeinated SSBs and their impact on children's health. Energy and sport drink consumption is rising rapidly in the U.S. [13] and so studies examining the negative health effects of caffeinated SSBs are needed to inform future efforts to reduce consumption.

This review has several limitations. First, it only focuses on four main health effects associated with SSB consumption and does not address other potential consequences which have been documented among consumers of SSBs (e.g., hyperlipidemia, non-alcoholic fatty liver disease). Second, our conclusions for a particular health consequence did not include a quality assessment and was limited to an informal evaluation of consistency and lack of conflicting studies. Third, article screening was not done in duplicate, although all included articles were confirmed by a second reviewer.

Conclusion

This review provides clear and consistent evidence that consumption of SSBs increases obesity risk and dental caries among children and adolescents, with emerging evidence supporting an association with insulin resistance and caffeine-related effects. In general, the strength of evidence for all four health consequences could be improved through the implementation of more longitudinal and intervention studies. Additionally, more consistency is needed from studies in the measurement of exposures

(e.g., standardized measurement and definition of SSBs) and outcomes (e.g., assessment of weight-related outcomes) to create a stronger evidence base. Future research should compare low-income and racial/ethnic minority subgroups in order to determine if differences in health risks associated with SSBs exist. Although SSB consumption has declined in the last 15 years, consumption still remains high (61% of children consume at least one SSB per day). The vast majority of the available literature suggests that reducing SSB consumption would improve children's health.

Abbreviations
BMI: Body mass index; NHANES: National Health and Nutritional Examination Survey; OECD: Organisation for Economic Co-operation and Development; SSB: Sugar-sweetened beverage

Acknowledgements
Not applicable

Funding
This work was funded by the Robert Wood Johnson Foundation Healthy Eating Research Program.

Authors' contributions
SNB designed the research. KAV conducted the review. SNB and KAV drafted and revised the paper for intellectual content. SNB had primary responsibility for final content. Both authors read and approved the final manuscript.

Competing interests
The authors declare that they have no competing interests.

Author details
[1]Department of Health Policy and Management, Harvard T.H. Chan School of Public Health, Boston, MA, USA. [2]Department of Epidemiology, Harvard T.H. Chan School of Public Health, Boston, USA.

References

1. US Department of Health and Human Services USDoA. 2015–2020 Dietary guidelines for Americans. 8th ed.. Washington (DC): USDA. 2015.

2. Bleich SN, Wolfson JA. Trends in SSBs and snack consumption among children by age, body weight, and race/ethnicity. Obesity. 2015;23(5):1039–46.

3. Bleich SN, Vercammen KA, Kom JW, Zhonghe L. Trends in beverage consumption among children and adults, 2003-2014. Obesity. 2017;

4. Malik VS, Pan A, Willett WC, Hu FB. Sugar-sweetened beverages and weight gain in children and adults: a systematic review and meta-analysis. Am J Clin Nutr. 2013;98(4):1084–102.

5. Resolved HFB. There is sufficient scientific evidence that decreasing sugar-sweetened beverage consumption will reduce the prevalence of obesity and obesity-related diseases. Obesity reviews : an official journal of the International Association for the Study of Obesity. 2013;14(8):606–19. https://doi.org/10.1111/obr.12040.

6. Malik VS, Popkin BM, Bray GA, Després J-P, Hu FB. Sugar-sweetened beverages, obesity, type 2 diabetes mellitus, and cardiovascular disease risk. Circulation. 2010;121(11):1356–64.

7. Malik VS, Popkin BM, Bray GA, Després J-P, Willett WC, Hu FB. Sugar-sweetened beverages and risk of metabolic syndrome and type 2 diabetes. Diabetes Care. 2010;33(11):2477–83.

8. Schulze MB, Manson JE, Ludwig DS, Colditz GA, Stampfer MJ, Willett WC, et al. Sugar-sweetened beverages, weight gain, and incidence of type 2 diabetes in young and middle-aged women. JAMA. 2004;292(8):927–34.

9. Nseir W, Nassar F, Assy N. Soft drinks consumption and nonalcoholic fatty liver disease. World J Gastroenterol: WJG. 2010;16(21):2579.

10. Tahmassebi J, Duggal M, Malik-Kotru G, Curzon M. Soft drinks and dental health: a review of the current literature. J Dent. 2006;34(1):2–11.

11. Davis JN, Ventura EE, Weigensberg MJ, Ball GD, Cruz ML, Shaibi GQ, et al. The relation of sugar intake to β cell function in overweight Latino children. Am J Clin Nutr. 2005;82(5):1004–10.

12. Hu FB, Malik VS. Sugar-sweetened beverages and risk of obesity and type 2 diabetes: epidemiologic evidence. Physiol Behav. 2010;100(1):47–54. https://doi.org/10.1016/j.physbeh.2010.01.036.

13. Al-Shaar L, Vercammen K, Lu C, Richardson S, Tamez M, Mattei J. Health effects and public health concerns of energy drink consumption in the United States: a mini-review. Front Public Health. 2017;5:225.

14. Forshee RA, Anderson PA, Storey ML. Sugar-sweetened beverages and body mass index in children and adolescents: a meta-analysis. Am J Clin Nutr. 2008;87(6):1662–71.

15. Harrington S. The role of sugar-sweetened beverage consumption in adolescent obesity: a review of the literature. J Sch Nurs. 2008;24(1):3–12.

16. Gortmaker S, Long M, Wang YC. The negative impact of sugar-sweetened beverages on Children's health: a research synthesis. Robert Wood Johnson Foundation; 2009.

17. Beck AL, Tschann J, Butte NF, Penilla C, Greenspan LC. Association of beverage consumption with obesity in Mexican American children. Public Health Nutr. 2014;17(2):338–44. https://doi.org/10.1017/s1368980012005514.

18. Bremer AA, Byrd RS, Auinger P. Differences in male and female adolescents from various racial groups in the relationship between insulin resistance-associated parameters with sugar-sweetened beverage intake and physical activity levels. Clin Pediatr. 2010;49(12):1134–42. https://doi.org/10.1177/0009922810379043.

19. Clifton PM, Chan L, Moss CL, Miller MD, Cobiac L. Beverage intake and obesity in Australian children. Nutrition & metabolism. 2011;8:87. https://doi.org/10.1186/1743-7075-8-87.

20. Coppinger T, Jeanes Y, Mitchell M, Reeves S. Beverage consumption and BMI of British schoolchildren aged 9-13 years. Public Health Nutr. 2013;16(7):1244–9. https://doi.org/10.1017/s1368980011002795.

21. Danyliw AD, Vatanparast H, Nikpartow N, Whiting SJ. Beverage patterns among Canadian children and relationship to overweight and obesity. Applied physiology, nutrition, and metabolism = Physiologie appliquee, nutrition et metabolisme. 2012;37(5):900–6. https://doi.org/10.1139/h2012-074.

22. Davis JN, Koleilat M, Shearrer GE, Whaley SE. Association of infant feeding and dietary intake on obesity prevalence in low-income toddlers. Obesity (Silver Spring, Md). 2014;22(4):1103–11. https://doi.org/10.1002/oby.20644.

23. Davis JN, Whaley SE, Goran MI. Effects of breastfeeding and low sugar-sweetened beverage intake on obesity prevalence in Hispanic toddlers. Am J Clin Nutr. 2012;95(1):3–8. https://doi.org/10.3945/ajcn.111.019372.

24. Denova-Gutierrez E, Jimenez-Aguilar A, Halley-Castillo E, Huitron-Bravo G, Talavera JO, Pineda-Perez D, et al. Association between sweetened beverage consumption and body mass index, proportion of body fat and body fat distribution in Mexican adolescents. Annals of nutrition & metabolism. 2008;53(3–4):245–51. https://doi.org/10.1159/000189127.

25. Gibson S, Neate D. Sugar intake, soft drink consumption and body weight among British children: further analysis of National Diet and nutrition survey data with adjustment for under-reporting and physical activity. Int J Food Sci Nutr. 2007;58(6):445–60. https://doi.org/10.1080/09637480701288363.

26. Gómez-Martínez S, Martín A, Romeo Marín J, Castillo Garzón MJ, Mesena M, Baraza J et al. Is soft drink consumption associated with body composition? A cross-sectional study in Spanish adolescents. 2009.

27. Grimes CA, Riddell LJ, Campbell KJ, Nowson CA. Dietary salt intake, sugar-sweetened beverage consumption, and obesity risk. Pediatrics. 2013;131(1):14–21. https://doi.org/10.1542/peds.2012-1628.

28. Ha K, Chung S, Lee H, Kim C, Joung H, Paik H, et al. Association of dietary sugars and sugar-sweetened beverage intake with obesity in Korean children and adolescents. Nutrients. 2016;8(1):31.

29. Kosova EC, Auinger P, Bremer AA. The relationships between sugar-sweetened beverage intake and cardiometabolic markers in young children. J Acad Nutr Diet. 2013;113(2):219–27. https://doi.org/10.1016/j.jand.2012.10.020.

30. Linardakis M, Sarri K, Pateraki MS, Sbokos M, Kafatos A. Sugar-added beverages consumption among kindergarten children of Crete: effects on nutritional status and risk of obesity. BMC Public Health. 2008;8:279. https://doi.org/10.1186/1471-2458-8-279.

31. Papandreou D, Andreou E, Heraclides A, Rousso II. Beverage intake related to overweight and obesity in school children? Hippokratia. 2013;17(1):42–6.

32. Schroder H, Mendez MA, Ribas L, Funtikova AN, Gomez SF, Fito M, et al. Caloric beverage drinking patterns are differentially associated with diet quality and adiposity among Spanish girls and boys. Eur J Pediatr. 2014; 173(9):1169–77. https://doi.org/10.1007/s00431-014-2302-x.

33. Valente H, Teixeira V, Padrao P, Bessa M, Cordeiro T, Moreira A, et al. Sugar-sweetened beverage intake and overweight in children from a Mediterranean country. Public Health Nutr. 2011;14(1):127–32. https://doi.org/10.1017/s1368980010002533.

34. Bremer AA, Auinger P, Byrd RS. Sugar-sweetened beverage intake trends in US adolescents and their association with insulin resistance-related parameters. Journal of nutrition and metabolism. 2010;2010 https://doi.org/10.1155/2010/196476.

35. Jiménez-Aguilar A, Flores M, Shamah-Levy T. Sugar-sweetened beverages consumption and BMI in Mexican adolescents: Mexican National Health and nutrition survey 2006. Salud Publica Mex. 2009;51:S604–S12.

36. Ambrosini GL, Oddy WH, Huang RC, Mori TA, Beilin LJ, Jebb SA. Prospective associations between sugar-sweetened beverage intakes and cardiometabolic risk factors in adolescents. Am J Clin Nutr. 2013;98(2):327–34. https://doi.org/10.3945/ajcn.112.051383.

37. Chaidez V, McNiven S, Vosti SA, Kaiser LL. Sweetened food purchases and indulgent feeding are associated with increased toddler anthropometry. J Nutr Educ Behav. 2014;46(4):293–8. https://doi.org/10.1016/j.jneb.2013.05.011.

38. DeBoer MD, Scharf RJ, Demmer RT. Sugar-sweetened beverages and weight gain in 2- to 5-year-old children. Pediatrics. 2013;132(3):413–20. https://doi.org/10.1542/peds.2013-0570.

39. Dubois L, Farmer A, Girard M, Peterson K. Regular sugar-sweetened beverage consumption between meals increases risk of overweight among preschool-aged children. J Am Diet Assoc. 2007;107(6):924–934; discussion 34-5. https://doi.org/10.1016/j.jada.2007.03.004.

40. Field AE, Sonneville KR, Falbe J, Flint A, Haines J, Rosner B, et al. Association of sports drinks with weight gain among adolescents and young adults. Obesity (Silver Spring, Md). 2014;22(10):2238–43. https://doi.org/10.1002/oby.20845.

41. Jensen BW, Nichols M, Allender S, de Silva-Sanigorski A, Millar L, Kremer P, et al. Inconsistent associations between sweet drink intake and 2-year change in BMI among Victorian children and adolescents. Pediatric obesity. 2013;8(4):271–83. https://doi.org/10.1111/j.2047-6310.2013.00174.x.

42. Jensen BW, Nielsen BM, Husby I, Bugge A, El-Naaman B, Andersen LB, et al. Association between sweet drink intake and adiposity in Danish children participating in a long-term intervention study. Pediatric obesity. 2013;8(4):259–70. https://doi.org/10.1111/j.2047-6310.2013.00170.x.

43. Kral TVE, Stunkard AJ, Berkowitz RI, Stallings VA, Moore RH, Faith MS. Beverage consumption patterns of children born at different risk of obesity. Obesity. 2008;16(8):1802–8. https://doi.org/10.1038/oby.2008.287.

44. Laska MN, Murray DM, Lytle LA, Harnack LJ. Longitudinal associations between key dietary behaviors and weight gain over time: transitions through the adolescent years. Obesity (Silver Spring, Md). 2012;20(1):118–25. https://doi.org/10.1038/oby.2011.179.

45. Leermakers ET, Felix JF, Erler NS, Cerimagic A, Wijtzes AI, Hofman A, et al. Sugar-containing beverage intake in toddlers and body composition up to age 6 years: the generation R study. Eur J Clin Nutr. 2015;69(3):314–21. https://doi.org/10.1038/ejcn.2015.2.

46. Libuda L, Alexy U, Sichert-Hellert W, Stehle P, Karaolis-Danckert N, Buyken AE, et al. Pattern of beverage consumption and long-term association with body-weight status in German adolescents–results from the DONALD study. Br J Nutr. 2008;99(6):1370–9. https://doi.org/10.1017/s0007114507862362.

47. Lim S, Zoellner JM, Lee JM, Burt BA, Sandretto AM, Sohn W, et al. Obesity and sugar-sweetened beverages in African-American preschool children: a longitudinal study. Obesity (Silver Spring, Md). 2009;17(6):1262–8. https://doi.org/10.1038/oby.2008.656.

48. Millar L, Rowland B, Nichols M, Swinburn B, Bennett C, Skouteris H, et al. Relationship between raised BMI and sugar sweetened beverage and high fat food consumption among children. Obesity (Silver Spring, Md). 2014; 22(5):E96–103. https://doi.org/10.1002/oby.20665.

49. Pan L, Li R, Park S, Galuska DA, Sherry B, Freedman DS. A longitudinal analysis of sugar-sweetened beverage intake in infancy and obesity at 6 years. Pediatrics. 2014;134(Suppl 1):S29–35. https://doi.org/10.1542/peds. 2014-0646F.

50. Vanselow MS, Pereira MA, Neumark-Sztainer D, Raatz SK. Adolescent beverage habits and changes in weight over time: findings from project EAT. Am J Clin Nutr. 2009;90(6):1489–95. https://doi.org/10.3945/ajcn.2009.27573.

51. Weijs PJ, Kool LM, van Baar NM, van der Zee SC. High beverage sugar as well as high animal protein intake at infancy may increase overweight risk at 8 years: a prospective longitudinal pilot study. Nutr J. 2011;10:95. https://doi.org/10.1186/1475-2891-10-95.

52. Zheng M, Rangan A, Olsen NJ, Andersen LB, Wedderkopp N, Kristensen P, et al. Sugar-sweetened beverages consumption in relation to changes in body fatness over 6 and 12 years among 9-year-old children: the European youth heart study. Eur J Clin Nutr. 2014;68(1):77–83. https://doi.org/10.1038/ejcn.2013.243.

53. Fiorito LM, Marini M, Francis LA, Smiciklas-Wright H, Birch LL. Beverage intake of girls at age 5 y predicts adiposity and weight status in childhood and adolescence. Am J Clin Nutr. 2009;90(4):935–42.

54. Laurson K, Eisenmann JC, Moore S. Lack of association between television viewing, soft drinks, physical activity and body mass index in children. Acta Paediatr. 2008;97(6):795–800.

55. Bremer AA, Auinger P, Byrd RS. Sugar-sweetened beverage intake trends in US adolescents and their association with insulin resistance-related parameters. Journal of nutrition and metabolism. 2009;2010

56. Lee A, Chowdhury R, Welsh J. Sugars and adiposity: the long-term effects of consuming added and naturally occurring sugars in foods and in beverages. Obesity science & practice. 2015;1(1):41–9.

57. Stoof SP, Twisk JWR, Olthof MR. Is the intake of sugar-containing beverages during adolescence related to adult weight status? Public Health Nutr. 2013; 16(7):1257–62. https://doi.org/10.1017/s1368980011002783.

58. de Ruyter JC, Olthof MR, Seidell JC, Katan MBA. Trial of sugar-free or sugar-sweetened beverages and body weight in children. N Engl J Med. 2012; 367(15):1397–406.

59. Ebbeling CB, Feldman HA, Chomitz VR, Antonelli TA, Gortmaker SL, Osganian SK, et al. A randomized trial of sugar-sweetened beverages and adolescent body weight. N Engl J Med. 2012;367(15):1407–16.

60. James J, Thomas P, Kerr D. Preventing childhood obesity: two year follow-up results from the Christchurch obesity prevention programme in schools (CHOPPS). BMJ. 2007;335(7623):762.

61. James J, Thomas P, Cavan D, Kerr D. Preventing childhood obesity by reducing consumption of carbonated drinks: cluster randomised controlled trial. BMJ. 2004;328(7450):1237.

62. Kondaki K, Grammatikaki E, Jiménez-Pavón D, De Henauw S, Gonzalez-Gross M, Sjöstrom M, et al. Daily sugar-sweetened beverage consumption and insulin resistance in European adolescents: the HELENA (healthy lifestyle in Europe by nutrition in adolescence) study. Public Health Nutr. 2013;16(03): 479–86.

63. Santiago-Torres M, Cui Y, Adams AK, Allen DB, Carrel AL, Guo JY, et al. Familial and individual predictors of obesity and insulin resistance in urban Hispanic children. Pediatric obesity. 2016;11(1):54–60.

64. Wang J, Mark S, Henderson M, O'loughlin J, Tremblay A, Wortman J, et al. Adiposity and glucose intolerance exacerbate components of metabolic syndrome in children consuming sugar-sweetened beverages: QUALITY cohort study. Pediatric obesity. 2013;8(4):284–93.

65. Bremer AA, Auinger P, Byrd RS. Relationship between insulin resistance–associated metabolic parameters and anthropometric measurements with sugar-sweetened beverage intake and physical activity levels in US adolescents: findings from the 1999-2004 National Health and nutrition examination survey. Archives of pediatrics & adolescent medicine. 2009;163(4):328–35.

66. Wang J, Light K, Henderson M, O'loughlin J, Mathieu M-E, Paradis G, et al. Consumption of added sugars from liquid but not solid sources predicts impaired glucose homeostasis and insulin resistance among youth at risk of obesity. J Nutr. 2014;144(1):81–6.

67. Armfield JM, Spencer AJ, Roberts-Thomson KF, Plastow K. Water fluoridation and the association of sugar-sweetened beverage consumption and dental caries in Australian children. Am J Public Health. 2013;103(3):494–500.

68. Chi DL, Hopkins S, O'Brien D, Mancl L, Orr E, Lenaker D. Association between added sugar intake and dental caries in Yup'ik children using a novel hair biomarker. BMC oral health. 2015;15(1):121.

69. Declerck D, Leroy R, Martens L, Lesaffre E, Garcia-Zattera MJ, Broucke SV, et al. Factors associated with prevalence and severity of caries experience in preschool children. Community Dent Oral Epidemiol. 2008;36(2):168–78.

70. Evans EW, Hayes C, Palmer CA, Bermudez OI, Cohen SA. Must a. Dietary intake and severe early childhood caries in low-income, young children. J Acad Nutr Diet. 2013;113(8):1057–61.

71. Guido JA, EA MM, Soto A, Eggertsson H, Sanders BJ, Jones JE, et al. Caries prevalence and its association with brushing habits, water availability, and the intake of sugared beverages. Int J Paediatr Dent. 2011;21(6):432–40.

72. Hoffmeister L, Moya P, Vidal C, Benadof D. Factors associated with early childhood caries in Chile. Gac Sanit. 2016;30(1):59–62.

73. Jerkovic K, Binnekade J, Van der Kruk J, Van d, Most J, Talsma A, van der Schans C. Differences in oral health behaviour between children from high and children from low SES schools in the Netherlands. Community Dent Health. 2009;26(2):110.

74. Jurczak A, Kościelniak D, Gregorczyk-Maga I, Kołodziej I, Ciepły J, Olczak-Kowalczyk D, et al. Influence of socioeconomic and nutritional factors on the development of early childhood caries in children aged 1-6 years. Nowa Stomatologia. 2015;

75. Kolker JL, Yuan Y, Burt BA, Sandretto AM, Sohn W, Lang SW, et al. Dental caries and dietary patterns in low-income African American children. Pediatr Dent. 2007;29(6):457–64.

76. Lee J, Messer EPL. Intake of sweet drinks and sweet treats versus reported and observed caries experience. european archives of Paediatric Dentistry. 2010;11(1):5–17.

77. Majorana A, Cagetti MG, Bardellini E, Amadori F, Conti G, Strohmenger L, et al. Feeding and smoking habits as cumulative risk factors for early childhood caries in toddlers, after adjustment for several behavioral determinants: a retrospective study. BMC Pediatr. 2014;14(1):45.

78. Mello T, Antunes I, Waldman E, Ramos E, Relvas M, Barros H. Prevalence and severity of dental caries in schoolchildren of Porto, Portugal. Community Dent Health. 2008;25(2):119–25.

79. Pacey A, Nancarrow T, Egeland G. Prevalence and risk factors for parental-reported oral health of Inuit preschoolers: Nunavut Inuit child health survey, 2007–2008. Rural Remote Health. 2010;10(2):1368.

80. Skinner J, Byun R, Blinkhorn A, Johnson G. Sugary drink consumption and dental caries in new South Wales teenagers. Aust Dent J. 2015;60(2):169–75.

81. Wilder JR, Kaste LM, Handler A, McGruder T C, Rankin KM. The association between sugar-sweetened beverages and dental caries among third-grade students in Georgia. J Public Health Dent. 2015;

82. Nakayama Y, Mori M. Association between nocturnal breastfeeding and snacking habits and the risk of early childhood caries in 18-to 23-month-old Japanese children. Journal of Epidemiology. 2015;25(2):142–7.

83. Lim S, Sohn W, Burt BA, Sandretto AM, Kolker JL, Marshall TA, et al. Cariogenicity of soft drinks, milk and fruit juice in low-income african-american children: a longitudinal study. J Am Dent Assoc. 2008;139(7):959–67.

84. Park S, Lin M, Onufrak S, Li R. Association of sugar-sweetened beverage intake during infancy with dental caries in 6-year-olds. Clinical nutrition research. 2015;4(1):9–17.

85. Warren JJ, Blanchette D, Dawson DV, Marshall TA, Phipps KR, Starr D, et al. Factors associated with dental caries in a group of American Indian children at age 36 months. Community Dent Oral Epidemiol. 2016;44(2):154–61.

86. Warren JJ, Weber-Gasparoni K, Marshall TA, Drake DR, Dehkordi-Vakil F, Dawson DV, et al. A longitudinal study of dental caries risk among very young low SES children. Community Dent Oral Epidemiol. 2009;37(2):116–22.

87. Watanabe M, Wang D-H, Ijichi A, Shirai C, Zou Y, Kubo M, et al. The influence of lifestyle on the incidence of dental caries among 3-year-old Japanese children. Int J Environ Res Public Health. 2014;11(12):12611–22.

88. Wigen TI, Wang NJ. Does early establishment of favorable oral health behavior influence caries experience at age 5 years? Acta Odontol Scand. 2015;73(3):182–7.

89. Maupomé G, Karanja N, Ritenbaugh C, Lutz T, Aickin M, Becker T. Dental caries in American Indian toddlers after a community-based beverage intervention. Ethnicity & disease. 2010;20(4):444.

90. Azagba S, Langille D, Asbridge M. An emerging adolescent health risk: caffeinated energy drink consumption patterns among high school students. Prev Med. 2014;62:54–9.

91. Bashir D, Reed-Schrader E, Olympia RP, Brady J, Rivera R, Serra T, et al. Clinical symptoms and adverse effects associated with energy drink consumption in adolescents. Pediatr Emerg Care. 2016;32(11):751–5.

92. Koivusilta L, Kuoppamäki H, Rimpelä A. Energy drink consumption, health complaints and late bedtime among young adolescents. International journal of public health. 2016;61(3):299–306.

93. Kristjansson AL, Sigfusdottir ID, Mann MJ, James JE. Caffeinated sugar-sweetened beverages and common physical complaints in Icelandic children aged 10–12years. Prev Med. 2014;58:40–4.

94. Marmorstein NR. Energy drink and coffee consumption and psychopathology symptoms among early adolescents: cross-sectional and longitudinal associations. Journal of caffeine research. 2016;6(2):64–72.

95. Park S, Lee Y, Lee JH. Association between energy drink intake, sleep, stress, and suicidality in Korean adolescents: energy drink use in isolation or in combination with junk food consumption. Nutr J. 2016;15(1):87.

96. Richards G, Smith A. Caffeine consumption and self-assessed stress, anxiety, and depression in secondary school children. J Psychopharmacol. 2015: 0269881115612404.

97. Franckle RL, Falbe J, Gortmaker S, Ganter C, Taveras EM, Land T, et al. Insufficient sleep among elementary and middle school students is linked with elevated soda consumption and other unhealthy dietary behaviors. Prev Med. 2015;74:36–41.

98. DiMeglio DP, Mattes RD. Liquid versus solid carbohydrate: effects on food intake and body weight. Int J Obes. 2000;24(6):794.

99. Malik VS, Schulze MB, Intake HFB. Of sugar-sweetened beverages and weight gain: a systematic review. Am J Clin Nutr. 2006;84(2):274–88.

100. Ludwig DS. Lifespan weighed down by diet. JAMA. 2016;315(21):2269–70.

101. Slavin J. Beverages and body weight: challenges in the evidence-based review process of the carbohydrate subcommittee from the 2010 dietary guidelines advisory committee. Nutr Rev. 2012;70(suppl 2):S111–S20.

102. Wang Y. Disparities in pediatric obesity in the United States. Advances in nutrition: an international review. Journal. 2011;2(1):23–31.

103. Ogden C, Carroll M. Prevalence of obesity among children and adolescents: United States, trends 1963-1965 through 2007-2008. Centers for Disease Control and Prevention. June 2010. 2013.

104. Ogden CL, Carroll MD, Lawman HG, Fryar CD, Kruszon-Moran D, Kit BK, et al. Trends in obesity prevalence among children and adolescents in the United States, 1988-1994 through 2013-2014. JAMA. 2016;315(21):2292–9.

105. Hales C, Carroll M, Fryar C, Ogden C. Prevalence of obesity among adults and youth: United States, 2015–2016. NCHS data brief. Number 288. National Center for Health Statistics. 2017;

106. Wang LY, Chyen D, Lee S, Lowry R. The association between body mass index in adolescence and obesity in adulthood. J Adolesc Health. 2008;42(5):512–8.

107. Dietz WH. Health consequences of obesity in youth: childhood predictors of adult disease. Pediatrics. 1998;101(Supplement 2):518–25.

108. Touger-Decker R, Van Loveren C. Sugars and dental caries. Am J Clin Nutr. 2003;78(4):881S–92S.

109. Malik VS, Hu FB. Fructose and Cardiometabolic health: what the evidence from sugar-sweetened beverages tells us. J Am Coll Cardiol. 2015;66(14): 1615–24. https://doi.org/10.1016/j.jacc.2015.08.025.

110. Ruxton C. The suitability of caffeinated drinks for children: a systematic review of randomised controlled trials, observational studies and expert panel guidelines. J Hum Nutr Diet. 2014;27(4):342–57.

17

Capsaicinoids supplementation decreases percent body fat and fat mass: adjustment using covariates in a post hoc analysis

James Rogers[1], Stacie L. Urbina[2], Lem W. Taylor[2], Colin D. Wilborn[2], Martin Purpura[3], Ralf Jäger[3] and Vijaya Juturu[4*]

Abstract

Background: Capsaicinoids (CAPs) found in chili peppers and pepper extracts, are responsible for enhanced metabolism. The objective of the study was to evaluate the effects of CAPs on body fat and fat mass while considering interactions with body habitus, diet and metabolic propensity.

Methods: Seventy-five ($N = 75$) volunteer (male and female, age: 18 and 56 years) healthy subjects were recruited. This is a parallel group, randomized, double-blind, placebo controlled exploratory study. Subjects were randomly assigned to receive either placebo, 2 mg CAPs or 4 mg CAPs dosing for 12 weeks. After initial screening, subjects were evaluated with respect to fat mass and percent body fat at baseline and immediately following a 12-week treatment period. The current study evaluates two measures of fat loss while considering six baseline variables related to fat loss. Baseline measurements of importance in this paper are those used to evaluate body habitus, diet, and metabolic propensity. Lean mass and fat mass (body habitus); protein intake, fat intake and carbohydrate intake; and total serum cholesterol level (metabolic propensity) were assessed. Body fat and fat mass were respectively re-expressed as percent change in body fat and change in fat mass by application of formula outcome = (12-week value – baseline value) / baseline value) × 100. Thus, percent change in body fat and change in fat mass served as dependent variables in the evaluation of CAPs. Inferential statistical tests were derived from the model to compare low dose CAPs to placebo and high dose CAPs to placebo.

Results: Percent change in body fat after 12 weeks of treatment was 5.91 percentage units lower in CAPs 4 mg subjects than placebo subjects after adjustment for covariates ($p = 0.0402$). Percent change in fat mass after 12 weeks of treatment was 6.68 percentage units lower in Caps 4 mg subjects than placebo subjects after adjustment for covariates ($p = 0.0487$).

Conclusion: These results suggest potential benefits of Capsaicinoids (CAPs) on body fat and fat mass in post hoc analysis. Further studies are required to explore pharmacological, physiological, and metabolic benefits of both chronic and acute Capsaicinoids consumption.

Keywords: Capsicum, Capsaicinoids, Statistical modelling, Body fat, Fat mass

* Correspondence: v.juturu@omniactives.com
Presented at The World Congress on Insulin Resistance, Diabetes & Cardiovascular Disease, Dec 1–3, 2016; Abstract published in ENDOCRINE PRACTICE 2017; 23 (1): 44.
[4]OmniActive Health Technologies Inc., 67 East Park Place, Suite 500, Morristown, NJ 07950, USA
Full list of author information is available at the end of the article

Background

Since approximately 7500 BC, chili peppers belonging to the species *Capsicum annuum* have been a part of the human diet in South, Middle, and North America. The plants were domesticated between 5200 and 3400 BC in U.S. and used as a food preserving substance in Mexico [1]. In U.S. consumption of all peppers has increased, rising from an average of 15.3 pounds per person in 2005 to 19.1 pounds per person in 2012 and consumption of bell peppers grew from 9.2 pounds to 11.7 pounds, while chili pepper consumption grew from 6.1 pounds to 7.4 pounds [2]. Red/Chili Peppers are widely cultivated in South America, Asia, Africa, and Mediterranean countries [3]. Pure Capsaicin measures 16,000,000 Scoville heat units (SHU). The spicy varieties of Capsicum are commonly called chili peppers, or simply "chilies".

Capsicum (*Capsicum annuum* L. or *Capsicum frutescens* L.) and paprika (*Capsicum annuum* L.) are among the spices and other natural seasonings and flavorings that are generally recognized as safe (GRAS) for their intended use in food [4]. Capsicum and paprika are also listed among the essential oils, oleoresins (solvent-free), and natural extractives (including distillates) that are GRAS for their intended use in food [5, 6]. Capsaicinoids are mainly ingested as naturally occurring pungency-producing components of capsicum spices (chili, cayenne pepper, red pepper). The bell pepper is the only member of the *Capsicum* genus that does not produce capsaicin, a lipophilic chemical that can cause a strong burning sensation when it comes in contact with mucous membranes. The lack of capsaicin in bell peppers is due to a recessive form of a gene that eliminates capsaicin and, consequently, the "hot" taste usually associated with the rest of the *Capsicum* genus.

Parrish [7] reported that CAPs typically range from 0.10 mg/g in chili pepper to 2.50 mg/g in red pepper and 60 mg/g in red pepper oleoresin. In another study, Thomas et al. [8] reported that Capsicum varieties contain 0.22–20 mg total CAPs/g of dry weight. The amount of chili pepper used varies from country-to-country. For example, it was reported that the mean daily consumption of chili peppers in Mexico, Korea, Thailand, India and the United States are 15, 8, 5, 2.5, and 0.05–0.50 g/person/day, respectively [9]. Assuming that 1 g of chili contains 3 mg CAPs, the intake of CAPs in Mexico, Korea, Thailand, India and the United States will be approximately 45, 24, 15, 7.5, and 0.15–1.5 mg/person/day, respectively. The 2012 data from US indicate chili pepper consumption to be 9 g/person (CAPs consumption will be approximately 27.00 mg/person/day).

Capsaicinoids (CAPs, Fig. 1) are the major pungent, naturally occurring active compounds in chilli peppers [10, 11]. The available information indicates that CAPs possess a wide variety of biological and physiological activities, including neuropathic pain, inflammation, [12], reducing oxidative stress [13], antilithogenic effect, diabetic neuropathy, psoriasis, cardio protective, arthritis, and cancer [14]. Whiting et al. [15] indicated that CAPs play a beneficial role, as part of a weight management program. Capsaicinoids may have potential benefits on weight loss, lipolysis and stimulates thermogenesis and energy burning by activating receptors. These receptors include white and brown fat cells. The weight loss benefits of capsaicinoids are at the transient receptor potential cation channel subfamily V member 1, which is also known as vanilloid 1 or TRPV1. Whiting [15] met analysis showed that CAPs ingestion prior to a meal reduced ad libitum energy intake by 309.9 kJ (74.0 kcal) $p < 0.001$ during the meal. These results should be viewed as heterogeneity was high (I (2) =75.7%). Study findings suggest a minimum dose of 2 mg of CAPs may contribute to reductions in ad libitum energy intake. The molecular metabolic signaling mechanisms are by influencing metabolic rate, findings demonstrate CAPs appear to regulate hunger and satiety, blood metabolites, and catecholamine release [11, 15].

Weight management strategies consist of therapeutic lifestyle changes including increased physical activity and reduced caloric intake; however, some of these cases fail and/or significant weight loss is maintained only in the short term because of lack of compliance and potential weight recycling. Natural weight management ingredients aid weight reduction and compliance due to faster weight loss and increasing compliance. Weight management is known to be a complex function of genetic, metabolic, and behavioral components. It was theorized that in the absence of extremely large sample sizes, models taking these factors and the interactions between them into account would be needed to properly evaluate the impact of CAPs from Capsicum extract. Three background factors were thought to be of prima facie merit, namely, baseline body habitus, baseline diet and baseline metabolic propensity. The causes of the obesity epidemic are undoubtedly multifactorial [16, 17]. Recent research suggest body composition variables by covariate factors revealed 35, 28 and 21% of percentage of body fat (PBF), fat mass index (FMI), and fat free mass index (FFMI), respectively [18] and weight gain [19]. Baseline covariates include food intake, physical activity, alterations in sleep patterns, and the stresses impact the outcome in many clinical trials. Conducting exploratory analyses including such variables when large baseline imbalances are observed might be helpful to assess the robustness of the primary analysis.

This study investigates the impact on fat loss of CAPs, a nutraceutical specifically designed to facilitate the loss of fat. However, this is accomplished through the lens of a statistical model designed to control three prima facie background dimension of known relevance to fat loss. It

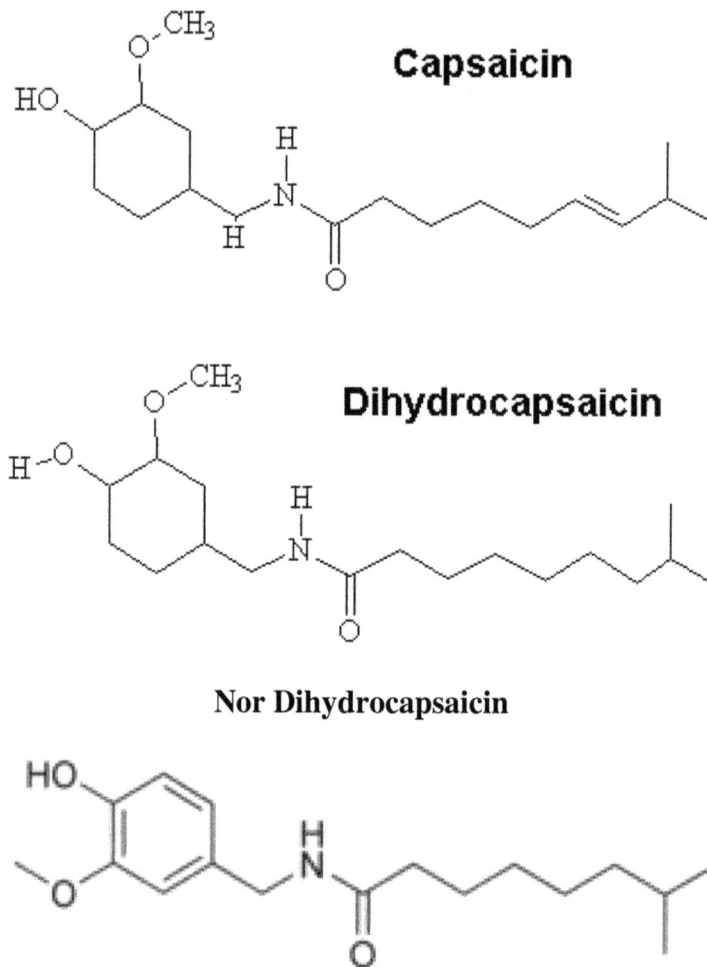

Fig. 1 Components of Capsaicinoids from Capsicum extract

was felt that this exploratory study, without facilitation using such a model, might from the beginning be doomed to failure due to lack of statistical power. By modeling the data, a type II error (i.e., the false denial of a supportive treatment outcome) is lessened.

Methods

This is a parallel group, randomized, double-blind, placebo controlled study conducted at University of Mary Hardin-Baylor, TX, USA. Subjects included 54 Caucasians (34 female/20 male), 13 Hispanics (8 female/5 male), 8 African American (4 female/4 male) and 2 Asians (1 female/1 male). Subjects were evaluated with respect to percent fat mass and body fat at baseline and immediately following a 12-week treatment period. Subjects were randomly assigned to receive either placebo (Corn starch,), 2 mg CAPs dosing [100 mg Capsimax providing 2 mg capsaicinoids] or 4 mg CAPs dosing (100 mg × 2 Capsimax providing 4 mg capsaicinoids). Thus, this study employed a pretest – posttest design with three between

subject conditions created by random assignment. Baseline measurements were prior to dosing and therefore qualify as covariates free of conflation with treatment. All experimental protocols were approved by the University of Mary Hardin-Baylor Institutional Review Board prior to initiation of research activities (ISRCTN registry #10458693).

Subjects

The subjects were recruited based on paper advertisements, via flyers, telephone (verbal guide), email, social media, and internet targeting research participants to determine their eligibility and interest. Subjects were recruited who exhibited the following study inclusion characteristics: 1) male or female volunteers ranging between 18 and 56 years of age; 2) healthy; 3) no ergogenic supplement ingestion in the last 6 months; 4) able to comply with required study activities; 5) expressing agreement to avoid strenuous activity 24–48 h prior to study visits; 6) expressing agreement to avoid smoking, caffeine use and tobacco use for 12-h prior to study visits; 6) exhibiting a BMI between of

24.5–29.5 kg/m^2; and 7) able to provide a written and dated informed consent for study participation.

Subjects were excluded from the study on the basis of the following characteristics: 1) consumption of ergogenic levels of nutritional supplements that may affect muscle mass or aerobic capacity (e.g., creatine, HMB, etc) or anabolic/catabolic hormones (e.g., androstenedione, DHEA, etc.) within 6 months of study start; 2) presence of any absolute or relative contraindication regarding exercise testing or study prescription as outlined by the ACSM; 3) reporting of any unusual adverse events associated with the study that in consultation with the supervising physician would results in recommended study removal; 4) presence of strong history of food or drug allergy of any kind; 5) ingestion of any dietary supplement (excluding multivitamins) within 1 month of study start; 6) existence of any chronic disease and or condition(s) that the principal investigator believes may jeopardize the study; or 7) existing pregnancy prior to or during the study.

There were 28 placebo subjects, 27 subjects in CAPs 2 mg (low dose) treatment and 22 subjects in CAPs 4 mg (high dose) treatment group completed the study. Seventy five subjects completed the treatments. Inclusion and exclusion criteria were used to screen patients for study entrance but were not used for treatment assignment which was random.

Variables

Multiple study parameters were collected over various time points during the study. These variables included a diet log, laboratory values, cardio-metabolic parameters, body composition and anthropometric measurements, adverse events, and QoL (quality of life) indices.

In this study, dietary supplementation of Capsicum for 12 weeks has shown to promote appetite suppression, which translated to reduced self-reported caloric intake after 12 weeks of supplementation. While Capsicum administration resulted in improved body circumferences in a main effects analysis, it did not apparently affect DEXA fat mass or fat-free mass in a statistically significant way [20]. The current study evaluates two measures of fat loss while considering six baseline variables related to fat loss. Baseline measurements of importance in this paper are those used to evaluate body habitus, diet and metabolic propensity. The following parameters *at baseline* were respectively used for these variable types: lean mass and fat mass (body habitus); protein intake, fat intake and carbohydrate intake (diet); and total serum cholesterol level (metabolic propensity).

It was determined that in the statistical modeling for fat loss in this study, body habitus would be captured as baseline lean mass and baseline fat mass; diet would be captured in three variables, namely, baseline protein intake, fat intake, and carbohydrate intake assessed through food frequency questionnaires; and metabolic tendency would be capture as baseline total serum cholesterol level. The author reasoned that if fat loss could be modeled using these variables along with treatment assignment, the model predicted outcome of weight loss as a function of treatment, while controlling for these background factors, would afford an assessment of the impact of CAPs on fat loss. Without taking background factors into account, evaluation of CAPs would be carried out under suboptimal conditions relative to the available sample size. This paper has both an empirical and a methodologic intent. Studies of economically feasible sizes with the goal of screening a panel of outcome variables for treatment signals are important venues of discovery. These formative studies narrow future investigative windows and generate data based hypotheses. As such, they are an important contribution to the scientific literature. When such studies address complex outcome variables (which often are the variables of greatest interest) such as fat loss, too often they are analyzed with statistical models best suited for large summative trials (e.g., Phase III trials). This paper illustrates the utility of a model based approach to discovery in studies of a moderate size. The value of statistical modeling that accounts for important concomitant factors in fat loss is illustrated in this paper by evaluating fat loss using a simple analysis of variance model without covariates or interactions and a generalized linear model that includes both of these features.

Investigational product

Capsicum extract is a Capsaicinoids enriched standardized product obtained from dried red fruits of *Capsicum annuum* L. The Capsicum extract is standardized into bead lets form (Capsimax) with food grade carbohydrates that is useful for food applications. Capsimax is a faint pinkish white colored free flowing uniform spheroidal bead lets with spicy odor, characteristics of dried ripe fruits of Capsicum. The product contains a minimum of 2% Capsaicinoids. The product is standardized to 2% Capsaicinoids, of which 1.2–1.35% is Capsaicin, 0.6–0.8% is dihydrocapsaicin, and 0.1–0.2% is nordihydrocapsaicin. The final product contains 15–25% extract from capsicum, 45–55% sucrose and 30–35% cellulose gum coatings.

Body composition and blood chemistries

Participants received a whole-body dual x-ray absorptiometry (DEXA) scan for body composition assessment at baseline and 12 weeks (Hologic Wi; Hologic Inc., Bedford, MA). Prior to their study evaluations, subjects fasted overnight. Participants had a venous blood drawn from their arm via standard phlebotomy techniques at baseline visit and 12 weeks. A panel of blood health markers (lipid profile, metabolic health markers and complete blood counts) was assessed by sending samples to a commercial laboratory (Quest Diagnostics, Irving, TX).

A power analysis was done on 25 subjects and 21 subjects per group yield a power of 0.85 and 0.81 in terms of body composition changes.

Statistical modeling

Prior to implementation of a statistical model to evaluate fat loss it was conceptualized that subject variation on three background dimension should be addressed during the evaluation process. These were baseline body habitus, baseline diet and baseline metabolic propensity. The objective was to parsimoniously capture these dimensions in as few variables as possible. Baseline lean mass and fat mass were used to capture body habitus; baseline carbohydrate intake, fat intake and protein intake were used to capture baseline diet; and baseline total cholesterol level was used to capture baseline metabolic propensity. Once selected, these baseline variables were used as independent variables in the statistical model used to evaluate fat loss. Percent body fat and fat mass were respectively re-expressed as percent change in body fat and change in fat mass by application of formula outcome = (12-week value − baseline value) / baseline value) × 100. Thus, percent change in body fat and fat mass served as dependent variables in the evaluation of CAPs.

After considering potential interactions among the baseline covariates and treatment, a comprehensive evaluation model was defined that expressed percent change in body fat (or fat mass) as a function of the baseline covariates noted previously, the treatment main effect and interactions between treatment and covariates. Interactions were a key component of the model as these were thought to capture the complex interplay between background factors and weight loss. We determined that the baseline variables and interactions could reasonably be expected to impact fat loss. Taking them into account during the evaluation of a nutraceutical designed to facilitate fat loss therefore seemed sensible.

In summary, two identical statistical models were used to respectively assess percent change in body fat and fat mass. Each model contained 1) the treatment effect (placebo, low dose and high dose); 2) six baseline covariates (carbohydrate intake, fat intake, protein intake, fat mass, lean mass and total cholesterol value); and 3) the interaction of each of the six covariates with treatment.

The above generalized linear model was used to estimate mean values and standard errors for percent change in body fat and fat mass. Inferential statistical tests were derived from the model to compare low dose CAPs to placebo and high dose CAPs to placebo. Covariate adjustment was Type III (each effect adjusted for all others); the model was obtained using Restricted Maximum Likelihood Estimation; and the model solution was accomplished using

Newton-Raphson iterations [21–23]. Individual models were fit to percent change in percent body fat and to percent change in fat mass. Normal model convergence was observed. Missing values were accommodated in a manner that is typical for the generalized linear model. If a covariate value was missing at baseline, the subject was not evaluated in the model. No attempt was made to estimate the missing baseline value. As noted above, there were 77 total subjects in the study. Missing baseline values were concentrated in two subjects. Therefore, the net effect of missing baseline values was that 75 of the 77 total patients were available to each of the two models used to evaluate fat loss. Twenty-six rather than 27 patients were available from the Capsimax 2 mg treatment; all 22 patients were available from the Capsimax 4 mg treatment; and 27 of the 28 patients were available from the placebo group. Otherwise, as is an advantage of the generalized linear model, any missing values in the dependent variable were accommodated by the variance-covariance matrix to obtain model predicted means (i.e., Least Squares (LS) Means) and associated standard errors.

Tables present basic comparisons between treatment groups for the baseline variables serving as covariates. Tables also show the predicted means and standard errors as well as the significance levels for each treatment vs. control contrast obtained from the generalized linear model used to adjust for background factors. Finally, a one-way Analysis of Variance model was used to evaluate three treatments "without" covariate adjustment. These results were used to provide a base of comparison that modeled the data without accounting for the background factors of known importance to fat loss that were included as covariates in the generalized linear model described above.

This paper provides a comparison between the results obtained when important background factors are and are not included in the modeling of outcome data that concern complex physiological response variables such as fat loss. To do this, adjustments for multiplicity of comparisons must be avoided. Then, the unaltered p-values from the model with and the model without covariate adjustment will be available for "direct" comparison. If the more comprehensive model has increased statistical power, the contrast p-value for the comprehensive model should be lower than for the model that eliminates covariates and their interactions with treatment.

Baseline variables

Age, height, weight, BMI, waist circumference, hip circumference and waist to hip ratio were compared to show that the treatment groups were similar with respect to variables of obvious relevance to fat loss; systolic blood pressure, diastolic blood pressure, and calorie intake were compared as these variables, too, are often associated with a history of resistance to fat loss. Descriptive statistics across the treatment groups are presented in Table 1. Additionally, analyses were conducted to compare the three treatment groups on all baseline variables simultaneously (i.e., a multivariate analysis was conducted) as well as individually (i.e., a univariate analysis of variance was conducted on each baseline variable).

Results

Results for comparisons at baseline are first presented. Thereafter results for percent change in body fat and fat mass are presented.

Baseline characteristics and baseline covariates

Table 1 presents descriptive statistics across the three treatment groups. The three groups are quite similar on baseline variable values as well as baseline covariate values. Both multivariate and univariate analyses carried out on baseline variables and baseline covariates resulted in unremarkable statistical significance levels ($p > 0.05$ in all instances).

Body fat anf fat mass
Percent change in percent body fat

To provide a baseline against which the modeled data analysis can be compared, Table 2 presents the findings of a both a one-way ANOVA without control for background variables and the full generalized linear model that accommodates covariates and treatment by covariate interactions. Without consideration of baseline characteristics there is little difference between low dose CAPs 2 mg and placebo (difference = 0.20, $p = 0.99$) and no significant difference was observed. On the other hand, high dose CAPs 4 mg subjects evidence an improvement in percent change in percent body fat (– 0.70) while the placebo group exhibited a deterioration in percent change in percent body fat (2.70). However, the difference between these (– 3.39) was not statistically significant. P-values respectively for the CAPs 2 mg vs. placebo contrast and the CAPs 4 mg vs. placebo contrast are $p = 0.99$ (extreme non- significance) and $p = 0.20$ (not significant).

The basic directional findings are very similar in the modeled data found in the Table 2 "With Baseline Covariates" analysis but the guiding p-values from the model suggest that the intuitive interpretation given above for the analysis lacking control for baseline factors meets the traditional 0.05 significance level for the high dose CAPS 4 mg vs. placebo contrast. Table 2 presents the model predicted means and treatment vs. placebo contrasts. Due to the considerable reduction in the model generated standard errors for the means (i.e., due to attribution of error variance to the covariates used as control variables) and

Table 1 Descriptive statistics at baseline by treatment group

	Capsimax 2 mg		Capsimax 4 mg		Placebo	
Baseline variables						
	N	Mean ± SD	N	Mean ± SD	N	Mean ± SD
Age	27	31.07 ± 12.02	22	28.86 ± 11.58	28	28.71 ± 10.57
Height	27	170.13 ± 9.49	22	170.17 ± 8.58	28	173.05 ± 11.11
Weight	27	79.02 ± 20.12	22	80.16 ± 16.80	28	83.51 ± 19.67
SBP	27	115.04 ± 14.75	22	117.95 ± 10.28	28	118.89 ± 10.02
DBP	27	70.22 ± 10.18	22	73.18 ± 8.02	28	72.89 ± 9.64
BMI	27	27.02 ± 5.88	22	27.42 ± 4.15	28	27.80 ± 6.01
Waist	25	86.84 ± 17.38	22	89.90 ± 12.44	25	94.58 ± 17.87
Hip	25	102.44 ± 17.35	22	106.83 ± 10.27	25	107.36 ± 12.85
WHR	25	0.85 ± 0.06	22	0.84 ± 0.08	25	0.88 ± 0.09
Covariates						
Lean Mass	27	50,234.82 ± 14,130.64	22	52,153.33 ± 12,140.28	28	53,581.51 ± 14,316.47
Fat Mass	27	20,570.47 ± 11,206.61	22	19,903.67 ± 9337.78	28	20,960.33 ± 11,799.70
Protein Intake	26	82.52 ± 38.95	22	100.32 ± 68.52	27	88.66 ± 39.97
Carbohydrate Intake	26	239.61 ± 287.44	22	186.27 ± 70.64	27	188.05 ± 80.82
Fat Intake	26	66.67 ± 24.71	22	76.99 ± 34.58	27	77.75 ± 45.28
Serum Total-C	27	173.33 ± 27.97	22	168.36 ± 37.87	28	178.93 ± 42.75

Total-C Total cholesterol; *BMI* Body mass index; *SBP* Systolic blood pressure; *DBP* Diastolic Blood Pressure; *WHR* Waist Hip Ratio
1) Main Effect Multivariate p (Wilks' Lambda) = 0.7073 for Baseline Variables. Univariate Main Effect p-values in all instances were $p > 0.05$ and ranged from $p = 0.3047$ to $p = 0.8695$. 2) Main Effect Multivariate p (Wilks' Lambda) = 0.0.8562 for Baseline Covariates. Univariate Main Effect p-values in all instances were $p > 0.05$ and ranged from $p = 0.3540$ to $p = 0.9438$. 3) Baseline covariates explained extraneous variance and increased statistical power. Covariates did not dramatically change mean outcomes. There were no baseline differences. 3) *N* Number of subjects

Table 2 Percent change in percent body fat compared between active and placebo groups using model generated means (LS Means)

Contrast	Treatment	N	LS Mean (SE)	LS Mean Difference (SE)	P Value
Without Baseline Covariates					
Capsimax 2 mg vs Placebo	Capsimax 2 mg	27	2.68 (1.78)	0.20	0.9939
	Placebo	28	2.70 (1.75)		
Capsimax 4 mg vs Placebo	Capsimax 4 mg	22	− 0.70 (1.97)	3.39	0.2014
	Placebo	28	2.70 (1.75)		
With Baseline Covariates					
Capsimax 2 mg vs Placebo	Capsimax 2 mg	26	3.51 (2.09)	−1.47	0.6030
	Placebo	27	4.99 (2.28)		
Capsimax 4 mg vs Placebo	Capsimax 4 mg	22	− 0.92 (2.06)	− 5.91	0.0402
	Placebo	27	4.99 (2.28)		

Analysis "Without Baseline Covariates" was a One-way ANOVA model. Analysis "With Baseline Covariates" was a generalized linear model containing treatment, variates and treatment x covariate interactions. Two subjects were lost to the "With Baseline Covariates" analysis due to missing values at baseline

the modeled equalization of covariates at baseline, the significance levels are greatly improved (i.e., statistical power is improved). For example, the model adjusted difference between CAPs 4 mg and placebo is − 5.91 percentage units ($p = 0.0402$). If the two analyses in Table 2 exhibited markedly different pattern of mean differences, one might doubt the validity of the model. In this case, the intuitive approach using basic unadjusted ANOVA and the generalized linear model approach that captures baseline factors of known a priori importance to fat loss, provide the same substantive message, albeit the latter with markedly improved statistical power and statistical significance for the high dose vs. placebo contrast.

Percent change in fat mass
As would be expected, the results for percent change in fat mass parallel those for percent change in percent body fat. Table 3 shows the presence of a favorable difference between high dose 4 mg CAPs and placebo of about 4 percentage points but this difference fails to

obtain statistical significance (difference = − 4.07, $p = 0.20$). A small directional difference exists between low dose CAPs and placebo but this difference is distantly non-significant (− 0.82, $p = 0.79$). When adjustment for covariates is carried out through the model, Table 3 reveals the same general pattern of outcome (little difference between low dose CAPs 2 mg and placebo but a substantial difference between CAPs 4 mg and placebo), but after adjustment for baseline factors, the high dose CAPs 4 mg vs. placebo contrasts is statistically significant (difference = − 6.68, $p = 0.05$).

Discussion
The simpler analysis without adjustment for covariance points to the same substantive understanding of the impact of CAPs on fat loss as the results derived from the generalized linear model that adjusts for covariates. The difference is a substantial increase in statistical power using the model. If the results were distinctly different between the basic analysis and those found after complex

Table 3 Percent change in fat mass compared between active and placebo groups using model generated means (LS Means)

Contrast	Treatment	N	LS Mean (SE)	LS Mean Difference (SE)	P Value
Without Baseline Covariates					
Capsimax 2 mg vs Placebo	Capsimax 2 mg	27	2.44 (2.14)	−0.82	0.7860
	Placebo	28	3.26 (2.10)		
Capsimax 4 mg vs Placebo	Capsimax 4 mg	22	−0.81 (2.37)	−4.07	0.2037
	Placebo	28	3.26 (2.10)		
With Baseline Covariates					
Capsimax 2 mg vs Placebo	Capsimax 2 mg	26	3.45 (2.79)	−2.43	0.5044
	Placebo	27	5.88 (2.76)		
Capsimax 4 mg vs Placebo	Capsimax 4 mg	22	−0.80 (2.37)	−6.68	0.0487
	Placebo	27	5.88 (2.76)		

Analysis "Without Baseline Covariates" was a One-way ANOVA model. Analysis "With Baseline Covariates" was a generalized linear model containing treatment, covariates and treatment x covariate interactions. Two subjects were lost to the "With Baseline Covariates" analysis due to missing values at baseline

adjustment, it would be necessary to carefully unravel the reasons for such a difference. A decision would need to be made concerning whether the model, in fact represented a plausible outcome or presented an artefactual finding. In this case, however, the same general finding is present by both methods of analysis, the difference being that adjustment for background factors has markedly increased statistical power. The reasonable conclusion is CAPs at the high dose reduces percent body fat and fat mass.

A second supportive feature of the analysis is the presence of a dose response. However, in both analyses, there is a small directional finding favoring CAPs 2 mg over placebo, but the difference fails to reach statistical significance, markedly so in the basic analysis with an improved level of significance in the adjusted analysis that nevertheless is still clearly greater than the 0.05 benchmark. Overall, however, the results are consistent and plausible. The worst outcome was evidenced by placebo.

Capsicum has been shown to help improve metabolism and hormone function [24], diabetes [25], and reduce insulin and leptin resistance [26]. Capsicum and CAPs have also been linked to cardiovascular health, endothelial function [27], LDL-cholesterol oxidation [28], stimulate energy expenditure [11, 29–31]. This thermogenic effect has been exploited for purposes of weight management. Capsaicinoids have been reported to reduce appetite [32–34], increase thermogenesis [25, 35–38], and increase lipolysis [25, 35, 36, 39], or changes in serum glycerol and free fatty acids [10, 11]. The thermogenic effect of Capsaicinoids is mediated, at least in part, by a Capsaicinoid sensitive structure located in the rostral ventrolateral medulla [40]. Capsaicinoids treatment may also stimulate vasodilation [27], which may indirectly impact thermogenesis, as any resultant loss of heat may necessitate an increase in metabolism.

Ludy et al. [41] reported effects of red pepper on energy balance from a combination of metabolic and sensory inputs. It was also suggested that individuals may become desensitized to red pepper. Capsaicin's effect on appetite suppression, analgesia and lipolysis are mediated in part by expression of multiple genes involved in the lipid catabolic pathway, including those involved in thermogenesis [i.e., UCP2] and may be due to vanilloid receptor subtype 1 (VR1) binding capsaicin [42–45].

The following section explores potential biological pathways for the study findings on fat loss and influence of diet and body habitus. The methodological lesson from the current study is that in complex processes involving behavior, social and physiological components, such as fat loss, it is very important to control for at least some of the important subject background factors that might contribute to the directionality of the outcome parameter. In this instance, it was reasoned prior to final analysis that diet, body habitus and metabolic

tendency would be important considerations when assessing fat loss. The data base contained three variables directly related to diet (baseline protein, fat and carbohydrate intake), two factors directly related to baseline body habitus (lean mass and fat mass), and a single encompassing variable that at least in part should capture metabolic tendency, namely, total cholesterol. Upon controlling for these factors, the statistical power of the inferential testing procedure was greatly increased. It was shown that higher dose 4 mg CAPs positively influenced fat loss, and after adjustment for background factors of obvious importance to fat loss, a resulting favorable CAPs vs. placebo difference existed with a probability of a type I error (i.e., a false positive conclusion) of less than 0.05.

In our first analysis for the study of CAPs effect on body composition, repeated measures without baseline covariate adjustments did not provided statistical significance for body fat and fat mass [46]. In the current analysis, baseline covariate adjustment resulted in statistical significance for body fat and fat mass in 4 mg CAPs treatment. This outcome *fact* suggests that baseline covariate analysis should have been considered at the point of protocol development. However, that it was not in the current instance does not eliminate the importance of fitting an appropriate model after the fact, particularly in light of the *known* relationship of the covariates selected here to fat loss. Models leading to insight at any point are contributory. A case might be made that it should be common practice in studies involving complex outcomes with suspected interactions with predisposing factors, that methodologies that anticipate the need for modeling be described a priori. For example, it is possible to include meaningful covariates in the data capture process at the beginning of a study and to outline methods of model development that will use those covariates, even if the precise model ultimately used is not described in advance. The limitations of the study are the L-CAP and H-CAP groups were supplemented with 2 mg/d and 4 mg/d of capsaicinoids, and other studies have supplemented participants with much higher doses (i.e., 135 mg/d [6]). In addition, our participants were healthy and were mildly overweight but not obese. Thus, if capsaicinoid supplementation is indeed effective at improving body composition, then more double blind clinical studies need to be performed in participants with greater BMIs.

Whitting et al. [15] observed an increase in energy expenditure (50 kcal/day) with capsaicinoid consumption, and that this would produce clinically significant levels of weight loss in 1–2 years. It was also observed that regular consumption significantly reduced abdominal adipose tissue levels and reduced appetite and energy intake [15]. In a met analysis, it was observed that CAPs increased lipid oxidation (recorded by measuring respiratory gases) or a decrease in fat stores. Further clarification is needed in terms of the specific 'doses' needed to reduction in abdominal body fat, energy intake and lipolysis.

Evidence suggests that the worldwide obesity epidemic is likely to continue its rise and several factors influence weight and risk of obesity [47]. Non-modifiable risk factors such as life style changes, healthy eating patterns, reducing caloric intake, and physical activity help to achieve long term weight loss. In the U.S. more than 20.60% women and 9.70% men are using weight loss dietary supplement at some point in their life and spend about $2 billion a year on weight loss dietary supplements in pill form (tablets, capsules, and soft gels). The use of multivitamin multi minerals decreased, and trends in use of individual supplements varied and were heterogeneous by population subgroups [48–50]. CAPs have shown effects on appetite, WHR [45], energy expenditure [15] and lipolysis [10, 11]. Capsaicinoids ingestion prior to a meal reduced ad libitum energy intake by 309.9 kJ (74.0 kcal) $p < 0.001$ during a meal. In a recent meta- analysis, suggest that capsaicin or capsaicinoids or capsiate could be a new therapeutic approach in obesity promoting a negative energy balance and increased fat oxidation [51]. Capsaicin/Capsaicinoids induces apoptosis and inhibits adipogenesis in pre-adipocytes and adipocytes. Activation of the transient receptor potential vanilloid-1 channels may prevent adipogenesis and improves visceral fat remodeling through the up-regulation of connexin [46] (Cx43) and regulates fat metabolism [52–57].

Conclusion

Overall, CAPs to be used as long-term, natural weight management aide. Further long-term placebo controlled randomized trials with high dose of CAPs are now needed to investigate these effects further.

Abbreviations

CAPs: Capsaicinoids; Cx43: Connexin; DEXA: Dual x-ray absorptiometry; FFMI: Fat free mass index; FMI: Fat mass index; LDL: Low-Density Lipoprotein; PBF: Percentage of body fat; QoL: Quality of life; SHU: Scoville heat units; TRP: Transient receptor potential; UCP: Uncoupling protein; VR1: Vanilloid receptor subtype 1

Acknowledgements

Authors are grateful to all volunteers for their participation in the study and thankful to all statisticians involved in statistical analysis for the study.

Funding

OmniActive Health Technologies Ltd., India.

Authors' contributions

JR prepared the data file for the statistical analyses, performed parts of the statistical analyses and drafted the manuscript. SU, CW and LT are responsible for the collection of the clinical data and prepared the data file for the statistical analyses. CW RJ and MP designed the main study, was responsible for the practical implementation, finalized the manuscript and is responsible for the integrity of the work. VJ involved as a scientist in study design, study initiation, discussions, manuscript review, reviewed valuable comments from all authors and opinions on the manuscript and all authors reviewed and approved the last version.

Competing interests

All authors listed had no conflict of interest. VJ is an employee of Omni Health Technologies Inc., NJ. JR is a consulting statistician for Omni Health Technologies Inc., NJ.

Author details

[1]Summit Analytical, LLC, 8354 Northfield Blvd., Building G, Suite 3700, Denver, CO 80238, USA. [2]Human Performance Laboratory, University of Mary Hardin-Baylor, Belton, TX 76513, USA. [3]Increnovo LLC, 2138 E Lafayette Pl, Milwaukee, WI 53202, USA. [4]OmniActive Health Technologies Inc., 67 East Park Place, Suite 500, Morristown, NJ 07950, USA.

References

1. http://www.aboutcapsinoids.com/pages/history.htm. Retrieved on 02/07/2017.
2. https://www.apcorganics.com/our-products/peppers. Retrieved on 02/07/2017.
3. Silva LR, Azevedo J, Pereira MJ, Valentao P, Andrade PB. Chemical assessment and antioxidant capacity of pepper (Capsicum annuum L.) seeds. Food Chem Toxicol. 2013;53:240–8.
4. https://www.accessdata.fda.gov/scripts/cdrh/cfdocs/cfcfr/CFRSearch.cfm?fr=182.10. Retrieved on 02/07/2017.
5. https://www.gpo.gov/fdsys/granule/CFR-2012-title21-vol3/CFR-2012-title21-vol3-sec182-20. Retrieved on 02/07/2017.
6. http://www.accessdata.fda.gov/scripts/cdrh/cfdocs/cfcfr/cfrsearch.cfm?fr=73.340. Retrieved on 02/07/2017.
7. Parrish M. Liquid chromatographic method of determining capsaicinoids in capsicums and their extractives: collaborative study. J Assoc Off Anal Chem Intern. 1996;79(3):738–45.
8. Thomas BV, Schreiber AA, Weisskopf CP. Simple method for quantitation of capsaicinoids in peppers using capillary gas chromatography. J Agric Food Chem. 1998;46:2655–63.
9. Govindarajan VS, Sathyanarayana MN. Capsicum-production, technology, chemistry, and quality. Part V. Impact on physiology, pharmacology, nutrition, and metabolism; structure, pungency, pain, and desensitization sequences. Crit Rev Food Sci Nutr. 1991;29:435–74.
10. Bloomer RJ, Canale RE, Fisher-Wellman KH. The potential role of capsaicinoids in weight management. Agro Food Industry Hi-tech. 2009;20(4):60–2.
11. Bloomer RJ, Canale RE, Shastri S, Suvarnapathki S. Effect of oral intake of capsaicinoid beadlets on catecholamine secretion and blood markers of lipolysis in healthy adults: a randomized, placebo controlled, double-blind, cross-over study. Lipids Health Dis. 2010;9:72.
12. Choi SE, Kim TH, Yi SA, Hwang YC, Hwang WS, Choe SJ, Han SJ, Kim HJ, Kim DJ, Kang Y, Lee KW. Capsaicin attenuates palmitate induced expression of macrophage inflammatory protein 1 and interleukin 8 by increasing palmitate oxidation and reducing c-Jun activation in THP-1 (human acute monocytic leukemia cell) cells. Nutr Res. 2011;31(6):468–78.
13. Henning SM, Zhang Y, Seeram NP, Lee RP, Wang P, Bowerman S. Antioxidant capacity and phytochemical content of herbs and spices in dry, fresh and blended herb paste form. Inter J Food Sci Nutr. 2011;62(3):219–25.
14. Yang ZH, Wang XH, Wang HP, Hu LQ, Zheng XM, Li SW. Capsaicin mediates cell death in bladder cancer T24 cells through reactive oxygen species production and mitochondrial depolarization. Urology. 2010;75(3):735–41.

15. Whiting S, Derbyshir E, Tiwari BK. Capsaicinoids and capsinoids. A potential role for weight management? A systematic review of the evidence. Appetite. 2012;59:341–8.

16. Heinonen I, Helajärvi H, Pahkala K, Heinonen OJ, Hirvensalo M, Pälve K, Tammelin T, Yang X, Juonala M, Mikkilä V, Kähönen M, Lehtimäki T, Viikari J, Raitakari OT. Sedentary behaviours and obesity in adults: the Cardiovascular Risk in Young Finns Study. BMJ Open. 2013;3(6)

17. Deshmukh-Taskar PR, O'Neil CE, Nicklas TA, Yang SJ, Liu Y, Gustat J, Berenson GS. Dietary patterns associated with metabolic syndrome, sociodemographic and lifestyle factors in young adults: the Bogalusa heart study. Public Health Nutr. 2009;12(12):2493–503.

18. Ghosh A, Das Chaudhuri AB. Explaining body composition by some covariate factors among the elderly Bengalee Hindu women of Calcutta, India. J Nutr Health Aging. 2005;9(6):403–6.

19. Popkin BM. Global nutrition dynamics: the world is shifting rapidly toward a diet linked with noncommunicable diseases. Am J Clin Nutr. 2006;84(2):289–98.

20. Urbina SL, Villa KB, Santos E, Olivencia A, Bennett H, Lara M, Foster C, Taylor L, Roberts M, Kephart W, Purpura M, Jaeger R, Wilborn C. Twelve weeks of capsaicinoid supplementation reduces appetite and self-reported caloric intake. Appetite: Submitted; 2016.

21. Sahai H, Ageel M. The Analysis of Variance: Fixed, Random and Mixed Models. Boston, Basel and Berlin: Birkhauser; 2000. p. 543–50.

22. Verbeke G, Molenberghs G. Linear Mixed Models for Longitudinal Data. New York: Springer-Verlag; 2000. p. 93–120.

23. NCSS 10 Statistical Software. Mixed Model – No Repeated Measures (). NCSS, LLC, Kaysville, Utah, USA, 2015; Chapter 221. ncss.com/software/ncss

24. Kang JH, Tsuyoshi G, Le Ngoc H, et al. Dietary capsaicin attenuates metabolic dysregulation in genetically obese diabetic mice. J Med Food. 2011;14:310–5.

25. Lejeune MP, Kovacs EM, Westerterp-Plantenga MS. Effect of capsaicin on substrate oxidation and weight maintenance after modest bodyweight loss in human subjects. Br J Nutr. 2003;90:651–9.

26. Kang JH, Goto T, Han IS, Kawada T, Kim YM, Yu R. Dietary capsaicin reduces obesity-induced insulin resistance and hepatic steatosis in obese mice fed a high-fat diet. Obesity. 2010;18:780–7.

27. Chularojmontri L, Suwatronnakorn M, Wattanapitayakul SK. Influence of capsicum extract and capsaicin on endothelial health. J Med Assoc Thail. 2010;93:S92–101.

28. Ahuja KDK, Ball MJ. Effects of daily ingestion of chili on serum lipoprotein oxidation in adult men and women. Br J Nutr. 2006;96(2):239–42.

29. Kawada T, Watanabe T, Takaishi T, Tanaka T, Iwai K. Capsaicin-induced beta-adrenergic action on energy metabolism in rats: influence of capsaicin on oxygen consumption, the respiratory quotient, and substrate utilization. Proc Soc Exp Biol Med. 1986;183:250–6.

30. Kawabata F, Inoue N, Yazawa S, Kawada T. Effects of Ch-19 sweet, a non-pungent cultivar of red pepper, in decreasing the body weight and suppressing body fat accumulation by sympathetic activation in humans. Biosci Biotechnol Biochem. 2006;70:2824–35.

31. Belza A, Frandsen E, Kondrup J. Body fat loss achieved by stimulation of thermogenesis by a combination of bioactive food ingredients: a placebo-controlled, double-blind 8-week intervention in obese subjects. Int J Obesity. 2007;31:121–30.

32. Yoshioka M, St-Pierre S, Drapeau V, et al. Effects of red pepper on appetite and energy intake. Br J Nutr. 1999;82:115–23.

33. Yoshioka M, Doucet E, Drapeau V, Dionne I, Tremblay A. Combined effects of red pepper and caffeine consumption on 24 h energy balance in subjects given free access to foods. Br J Nutr. 2001;85:203–11.

34. Westerterp-Plantenga MS, Smeets A, Lejeune MP. Sensory and gastrointestinal satiety effects of capsaicin on food intake. Int J Obes. 2005;29(6):682–8.

35. Yoshioka M, Lim K, Kikuzato S, et al. Effects of red-pepper diet on the energy metabolism in men. J Nutr Sci Vitaminol (Tokyo). 1995;41:647–56.

36. Yoshioka M, St-Pierre S, Suzuki M, Tremblay A. Effects of red pepper added to high-fat and high-carbohydrate meals on energy metabolism and substrate utilization in Japanese women. Br J Nutr. 1998;80:503–10.

37. Matsumoto T, Miyawaki C, Ue H, et al. Effects of capsaicin-containing yellow curry sauce on sympathetic nervous system activity and diet-induced thermogenesis in lean and obese young women. J Nutr Sci Vitaminol (Tokyo). 2000;46:309–15.

38. Mahmmoud YA. Capsaicin stimulates uncoupled ATP hydrolysis by the sarcoplasmic reticulum calcium pump. J Biol Chem. 2008;283:21418–26.

39. Inoue N, Matsunaga Y, Satoh H, Takahashi M. Enhanced energy expenditure and fat oxidation in humans with high BMI scores by the ingestion of novel and non-pungent capsaicin analogues [capsinoids]. Biosci Biotechnol Biochem. 2007;71:380–9.

40. Osaka T, Lee T-H, Kobayashi A. Thermogenesis mediated by a capsaicin-sensitive area in the ventrolateral medulla. Neuroreport. 2000;11:2425–8.

41. Ludy MJ, Moore GE, Mattes RD. The effects of capsaicin and capsiate on energy balance: critical review and meta-analyses of studies in humans. Chem Senses. 2012;37:103–21.

42. Story GM, Crus-Orengo L. Feel the burn. Am Scientist. 2007;95:326–33.

43. Caterina MJ, Leffler A, Malmberg AB, et al. Impaired nociception and pain sensation in mice lacking the capsaicin receptor. Science. 2000;288:306–13.

44. Szallasi A, Blumberg PM. Vanilloid (capsaicin) receptors and mechanisms. Pharmacol Rev. 1999;51:159–212.

45. Lee MS, Kim CT, Kim IH, Kim Y. Effects of capsaicin on lipid catabolism in 3T3-L1 adipocytes. Phytother Res. 2011;25:935–9.

46. Urbina SL, Villa KB, Santos E, Olivencia A, Bennett H, Lara M, Foster C, Taylor L, Roberts M, Kephart W, Purpura M, Jaeger R and Wilborn C. Capsaicinoids Supplementation Reduces Appetite and Body Circumferences in Healthy Men and Women A Placebo Controlled Randomized Double Blind Study. FASEB J 2016, 30 (1) Supplement lb 356.

47. Lenz TL, Hamilton WR. Supplemental products used for weight loss. J Am Pharm Assoc. 2004;44:59–67.

48. Blanck HM, Serdula MK, Gillespie C, Galuska DA, Sharpe PA, Conway JM, Khan LK, Ainsworth BE. Use of nonprescription dietary supplements for weight loss is common among Americans. J Am Diet Assoc. 2007;107(3):441–7.

49. Nutrition Business Journal. Is sports nutrition its own worst enemy?. NBJ. 2014, XI. http://www.newhope.com/news/sports-nutrition-its-own-worst-enemy.

50. Kantor ED, Rehm CD, Du M, White E, Giovannucci EL. Trends in Dietary Supplement Use Among US Adults From 1999-2012. JAMA. 2016;316(14):1464–74.

51. Zsiborás C, Mátics R, Hegyi P, Balaskó M, Pétervári E, Szabó I, Sarlós P, Mikó A, Tenk J, Rostás I, Pécsi D, Garami A, Rumbus Z, Huszár O, Solymár M. Capsaicin and capsiate could be appropriate agents for treatment of obesity: a meta-analysis of human studies. Crit Rev Food Sci Nutr. 2018; 58(9):1419-27.

52. Zhang LJ, et al. Activation of transient receptor potential vanilloid type-1 channel prevents adipogenesis and obesity. Circ Res. 2007;100:1063–70.

53. Leung FW. Capsaicin as an anti-obesity drug. Prog Drug Res. 2014;68:171–9.

54. Chen J, Li L, Li Y, Liang X, Sun Q, Yu H, Zhong J, Ni Y, Chen J, Zhao Z, Gao P, Wang B, Liu D, Zhu Z, Yan Z. Activation of TRPV1 channel by dietary capsaicin improves visceral fat remodeling through connexin43-mediated Ca2+ influx. Cardiovasc Diabetol. 2015;14:22.

55. Motter AL, Ahern GP. TRPV1-null mice are protected from diet-induced obesity. FEBS Lett. 2008;582(15):2257–62.

56. Szolcsányi J. Effect of capsaicin on thermoregulation: an update with new aspects. Temperature (Austin). 2015;2(2):277–96.

57. Szolcsányi J, Pintér E. Transient receptor potential vanilloid 1 as a therapeutic target in analgesia. Expert Opin Ther Targets. 2013;17(6):641–57.

18

Multi-sensor ecological momentary assessment of behavioral and psychosocial predictors of weight loss following bariatric surgery: study protocol for a multicenter prospective longitudinal evaluation

Stephanie P. Goldstein[1], J. Graham Thomas[1*], Sivamainthan Vithiananthan[2], George A. Blackburn[3], Daniel B. Jones[3], Jennifer Webster[1], Richard Jones[4], E. Whitney Evans[1], Jody Dushay[5], Jon Moon[6] and Dale S. Bond[1*]

Abstract

Background: Bariatric surgery is currently the most effective strategy for producing significant and durable weight loss. Yet, not all patients achieve initial weight loss success and some degree of weight regain is very common, sometimes as early as 1–2 years post-surgery. Suboptimal weight loss not fully explained by surgical, demographic, and medical factors has led to greater emphasis on patient behaviors evidenced by clinical guidelines for appropriate eating and physical activity. However, research to inform such guidelines has often relied on imprecise measures or not been specific to bariatric surgery. There is also little understanding of what psychosocial factors and environmental contexts impact outcomes. To address research gaps and measurement limitations, we designed a protocol that innovatively integrates multiple measurement tools to determine which behaviors, environmental contexts, and psychosocial factors are related to outcomes and explore how psychosocial factors/environmental contexts influence weight. This paper provides a detailed description of our study protocol with a focus on developing and deploying a multi-sensor assessment tool to meet our study aims.

Methods: This NIH-funded prospective cohort study evaluates behavioral, psychosocial, and environmental predictors of weight loss after bariatric surgery using a multi-sensor platform that integrates objective sensors and self-report information collected via smartphone in real-time in patients' natural environment. A target sample of 100 adult, bariatric surgery patients (ages 21–70) use this multi-sensor platform at preoperative baseline, as well as 3, 6, and 12 months postoperatively, to assess recommended behaviors (e.g., meal frequency, physical activity), psychosocial indicators with prior evidence of an association with surgical outcomes (e.g., mood/depression), and key environmental factors (e.g., type/quality of food environment). Weight also is measured at each assessment point.

(Continued on next page)

* Correspondence: jthomas4@lifespan.org; dbond@lifespan.org
Dale S. Bond and J. Graham Thomas are co-principle investigators.
Dale S. Bond and J. Graham Thomas are equal contributors.
[1]Weight Control and Diabetes Research Center, Department of Psychiatry and Human Behavior, The Miriam Hospital/Warren Alpert Medical School of Brown University, 196 Richmond Street, Providence, RI 02909, USA
Full list of author information is available at the end of the article

(Continued from previous page)
Discussion: This project has the potential to build a more sophisticated and valid understanding of behavioral and psychosocial factors contributing to success and risk after bariatric surgery. This new understanding could directly contribute to improved (i.e., specific, consistent, and validated) guidelines for recommended pre- and postoperative behaviors, which could lead to improved surgical outcomes. These data will also inform behavioral, psychosocial, and environmental targets for adjunctive interventions to improve surgical outcomes.

Keywords: Bariatric surgery, Weight loss, Obesity, Ecological momentary assessment, Diet, Physical activity, Technology

Background

Over the past 15 years, bariatric surgery has amassed a strong evidence base as a first-line treatment for severe obesity [1, 2]. Approximately 468,609 surgeries are performed worldwide each year [3]. The most common procedures are sleeve gastrectomy (SG) and Roux-en-Y gastric bypass (RYGB). Bariatric surgery involves anatomical changes, as well as neural and hormonal shifts that facilitate weight loss through changes in energy balance, metabolism, satiety and appetite, and disease processes [4]. As such, surgical procedures can also lead to remission or resolution of obesity co-morbidities (e.g., Type 2 diabetes) and restore health-related quality of life [5]. Bariatric surgery produces approximately 30% weight loss over a period of 6–7 years [6, 7]. However, there is substantial individual variability in short- and long-term weight loss [6, 7].

While several factors have been shown to influence weight loss outcomes (e.g., procedure, baseline weight, age, and race), energy balance behaviors and related psychosocial factors are of considerable interest given their amenability to change and potential to enhance surgical effects [8]. As such, various clinical guidelines have been put forth to describe recommended eating and physical activity behaviors to maximize surgical benefits [9]. Examples of dietary recommendations include ≥ 5 recommended meals/ snacks per day of ≤ 8 oz, ≥ 5 servings of fruits and vegetables daily, and ≥ 20-min duration of meals/ snacks. Guidelines also suggest ≥ 30 min of daily physical activity.

At present, development of evidence-based behavioral guidelines for the bariatric surgery population is challenging due to relative lack of prospective observational and experimental research and limitations associated with traditional measurement methodologies. Unfortunately, there is little research focused on bariatric surgery patients specifically, making the formation of consistent, empirically-supported behavioral guidelines for this population difficult. Compounding these concerns, there is a paucity of research examining compliance with recommended eating and physical activity behaviors. Moreover, the few published studies

have relied primarily on retrospective chart reviews, self-report questionnaires, and clinical interviews. These traditional methodologies are known for biases that reduce validity and reliability of information collected. For example, research comparing self-reported to objectively-measured physical activity and sedentary behavior revealed that bariatric surgery patients typically self-report postoperative increases in physical activity that are not supported by objective measurements [10, 11]. Additionally, traditional methodologies do not collect data with the level of detail, number of repeated observations, or environmental context that would allow for precise estimates of behavior and associated variability.

To this end, innovative measurement strategies that maximize data quality are needed to study behavioral, psychosocial, and environmental contributors to postoperative weight loss, thus providing a more rigorous evidence base for pre- and postoperative clinical guidelines and interventions [12]. One potential solution is ecological momentary assessment (EMA), a method by which participants are prompted to give in-the-moment reports on selected behaviors, cognitive/emotional states, and environmental conditions several times throughout the day (usually using mobile phones) [13]. Not only does EMA capitalize on external validity by assessing constructs in the environment as they occur naturally, but it also eliminates the need for retrospective self-report, thereby removing many sources of bias [14, 15]. The power of EMA data can be strengthened further using a multi-method measurement approach [12]. The recent rise of unobtrusive, wearable sensors that connect to smartphones in real-time makes it possible to obtain continuous, objective behavioral measurements in an individual's natural environment.

We have successfully employed both EMA and objective sensors (separately, but not in combination) to investigate adherence to postoperative guidelines. EMA of physical activity intentions and behavior demonstrated that participants are rarely fulfilling their intentions to exercise and these intentions are not consistent with established guidelines [16]. Our use of EMA to measure eating behavior revealed that participants refrained from drinking while eating and took vitamin supplements and medication as prescribed, but they were not generally adherent with the remainder of postoperative guidelines for eating [17]. These studies indicate that EMA and objective sensors can facilitate a deeper understanding of eating and physical activity behaviors, and the contexts in which they occur, that can better inform postoperative guidelines as well as behavioral interventions to improve adherence to such guidelines [18].

While our preliminary studies indicated that mobile health (mHealth) technology (i.e., use of smartphones for self-report surveys, wearable sensors) is a promising avenue to measure eating and physical activity behaviors of bariatric surgery patients, there remains several key areas for growth. First, the use of an *integrated* mHealth system is warranted, as research to date has only employed these methods separately within the bariatric population. By combining EMA with objective sensors, it is possible to obtain more valid and reliable estimates of behavioral patterns that can be further enriched by additional contextual information. For example, accelerometry, a well-accepted method for objectively assessing physical activity, can be enhanced with EMA questions delivered by smartphone to assess type of exercise, context, motivational factors, and barriers (all of which accelerometry alone cannot provide). Second, little attention has been devoted to examining whether compliance with published behavioral recommendations relates to postoperative weight loss outcomes overall, and specifically the intervals during which compliance may have the greatest impact. Third, there has been little consideration given to whether important psychosocial aspects (e.g., mood, disinhibition, cognitive restraint) and/or environmental factors (e.g., location of eating, availability of foods) may predict weight loss outcomes via influence on pre- and/or postoperative behavioral compliance.

Recognizing the aforementioned gaps in research on behavioral and psychosocial predictors of bariatric surgery outcomes, the NIH called for projects to address the problem and funded the project described herein to address the following aims: (1) assess the feasibility and acceptability of using a multi-sensor mHealth platform to collect data in real-time on behavioral and psychosocial predictors of weight loss outcomes; (2) evaluate which behavioral and psychosocial factors predict outcomes and the times at which each factor has the strongest effect; and (3) identify causal pathways by which psychosocial factors influence outcomes via effects on behavior, as well as moderators that explain for whom and under what conditions the influence is the strongest. The following sections describe the overall study design, with an emphasis on the multi-sensor mHealth platform, given its novelty and innovation. Additionally, challenges and considerations in developing and deploying the platform that are representative of those encountered in mHealth studies more broadly, are discussed.

Methods

The project involves a prospective cohort study designed to evaluate predictors of weight loss after bariatric surgery, including energy balance behaviors (i.e. physical activity, sedentary behavior, and eating behavior), psychosocial factors (e.g., appetite/motivation to eat, physical and social cues), and environmental factors (e.g., availability of food). In particular, we aim to improve our understanding of the associations between weight loss and behaviors targeted by postoperative guidelines so that the guidelines can be made more specific and consistent. Participants (target $n = 100$) with severe obesity (body mass index ≥ 35 kg/m^2) are recruited prior to undergoing bariatric surgery with predictor variables measured 3 to 8 weeks preoperatively (baseline) and at 3, 6, and 12 months postoperatively. As described in greater detail below, we configured an established EMA platform to allow for integration of: 1) direct, sensor-based measures of energy balance behaviors (i.e. ActiGraph Link (ActiGraph, LLC, Pensacola, FL, USA)) to measure physical activity, sedentary behavior and sleep; Bite Counter ((Bite Technologies, Pendleton SC, USA) to measure eating behavior), and 2) self-report surveys administered several times daily via smartphone to capture subjective reports of other behaviors and experiences. These data are further supplemented with phone-based 24-h dietary recalls, paper-and-pencil questionnaires, and chart reviews. Weight is measured at all assessment points.

Setting

This study is taking place at two university-based hospital bariatric surgery centers, The Miriam Hospital (Providence, Rhode Island, USA) and the Beth Israel Deaconess Medical Center (Boston, Massachusetts, USA).

Participants

A target sample of 100 participants is enrolled on a rolling basis. Eligibility is limited to individuals greater than 21 years of age with severe obesity (body mass index ≥ 35 kg/m^2) who are undergoing RYGB or SG at either study site. Individuals are excluded from participating if they: 1) are currently involved in a weight loss or related behavioral form of treatment outside the context of standard surgical care (patient support groups, education, and pre- and postoperative dietary counseling are considered standard surgical care); or 2) report a condition that in the opinion of the investigators would preclude adherence to the measurement protocol, primarily including plans to relocate geographically, substance abuse or other significant uncontrolled psychiatric problem, or terminal illness. The above inclusion/exclusion criteria are designed to identify a heterogeneous sample of patients, ensure maximum generalizability to the national bariatric surgery population, and provide data on behavioral and psychosocial outcomes of interest.

Procedure

This study was approved by The Miriam Hospital Institutional Review Board (Version 2.0 July 2017). Protocol modifications were submitted to this IRB for approval. The Miriam Hospital IRB requires that modifications include plans for notifying participants should the modification impact their study participation. There were no modifications of the current protocol requiring notice to participants, funding agency, or trial registries. An additional file details the informed consent protocol approved by The Miriam Hospital IRB (see Additional file 1).

See Fig. 1. Study Timeline for a study schematic. Patients from both sites are recruited 3 to 8 weeks preoperatively during a regularly scheduled clinic visit. At these visits, a surgeon or another provider and member of the surgical team provides patients with a flyer describing the study. Patients who wish to be contacted further about the study provide a signature and contact number to the staff. A bariatric surgery team member faxes this information to the appropriate research center so that research staff can conduct a brief screening by phone and schedule an in-person orientation/baseline study visit.

At the in-person initial orientation/baseline visit participants provide informed consent with a trained member of the study staff, have height, weight and waist circumference measured by trained research staff, complete questionnaires, are shown how the 24-h dietary recalls will be completed, and receive the EMA equipment described below (Android smartphone, Acti-Graph Link, and Bite Counter). Participants then receive training in how to wear the sensor devices and complete self-report surveys using electronic forms on the smartphone.

Upon completion of training, participants begin their first 10-day EMA assessment period. A 10-day period is consistent with prior EMA studies and balances participant burden with the need to measure each key construct multiple times at each assessment period over weekdays and weekends [13, 19]. At all subsequent postoperative assessments (i.e., 3, 6, and 12 months), participants return to the research centers to complete questionnaires, receive a refresher on the EMA protocol, and then complete the protocol for 10 days. Anthropometric measurements (i.e., height, weight, body mass index, waist circumference, weight loss) are obtained by

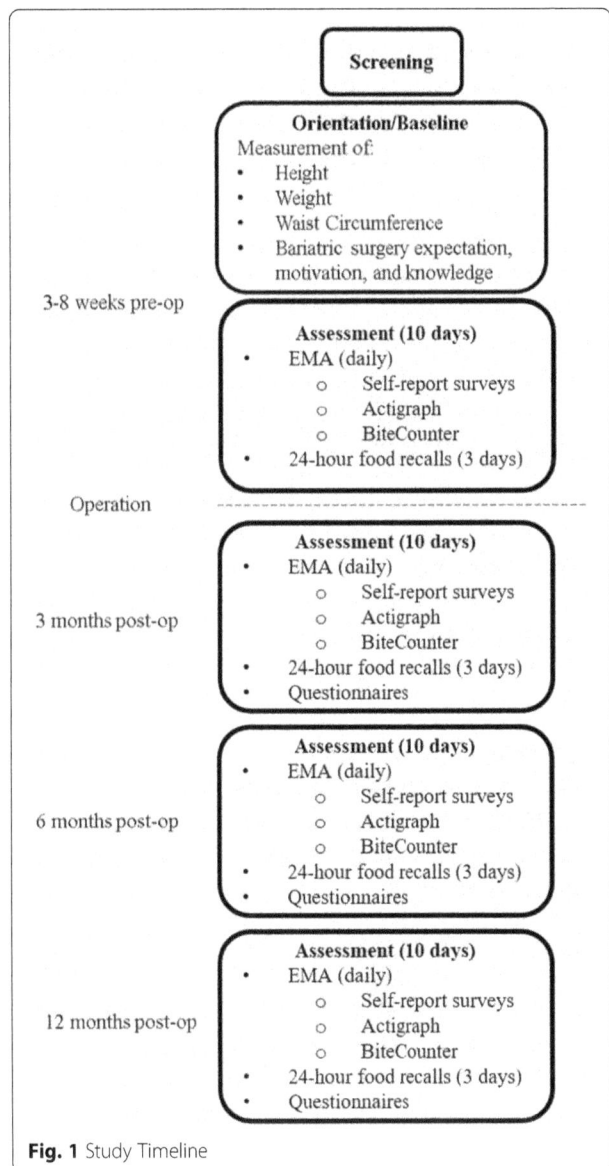

Fig. 1 Study Timeline

trained research staff at all the above time points. Participants receive $75 at the end of each assessment and can earn 50 cents for each survey completed via smartphone. This extra compensation of 50 cents per survey adds up to about $25 during each 10-day assessment if the participant completes about 80% of the surveys. Participants with good compliance are therefore expected to earn a total compensation of about $100 for each 10-day assessment. The smartphone used for EMA automatically tracks and displays participants' compliance with prompted self-report surveys, which is a novel and innovative method to encourage high compliance in a research setting. Real-time EMA data are supplemented with assessment of dietary intake, paper-and-pencil questionnaires, chart review, and anthropometric measures to establish a comprehensive record of pre- and postoperative patterns. Below, we first describe the PiLR Health System and procedure for delivering smartphone surveys. Then, we describe the study measures (i.e., the objective sensors and constructs assessed with smartphone self-report surveys).

PiLR EMA system

PiLR Health™ is a platform for mobile assessment and intervention that has been developed and is maintained by MEI Research, Ltd. through grants and contracts from multiple NIH institutes. We collaborated with MEI to customize the platform to execute the study procedures. The PiLR platform used for the current study consists of a smartphone-based application, or "hub", that operates on Android devices and cloud servers. Using its always-on Internet connection, the smartphone hub receives instructions from, and transmits its data to, a study server that coordinates EMA implementation and data integration for the study. The server is accessible via a Web-based interface that allows the research team to implement the EMA protocol (e.g., load surveys, define participant engagement periods, assign devices to participants, assign sensors), view summary reports (e.g., real-time participant compliance with the EMA protocol), and retrieve data files. The smartphone native app is configured for store-and-forward communications so that it functions independently if Internet connectivity is interrupted.

See Fig. 2. EMA System and Components for a depiction of the multi-sensor measurement tools. The EMA components used in the current study are a wrist-worn accelerometer (ActiGraph Link; ActiGraph, LLC, Pensacola, FL, USA) to detect physical activity,

sedentary behavior, and sleep; a wrist-worn device to monitor eating (Bite Counter; Bite Technologies, Pendleton SC, USA), and smartphone-based self-report surveys. These measurement tools were chosen based on their methodological rigor and feasibility for use in the bariatric surgery population.

The PiLR platform was chosen for this study for specific advantages related to maximizing data quality and assessment that allow us to achieve the study aims. First, we can check the quality of the data during collection to ensure compliance with the EMA protocol and detect any errors that could occur. In this project, research staff review the first 2 days of participants' smartphone self-report surveys and sensor data remotely to check adherence and confirm that data are being collected and received as expected. If adherence to prompted self-report surveys is less than 90% or there are problems with data collection from any of the devices (e.g., the participant is not wearing devices, or the data are not being received), the participant is contacted by phone to resolve the problem. Those first 2 days of EMA can then be excluded from analysis to account for reactivity (i.e., change in behavior occurring at EMA initiation, before it becomes routine). Second, the system automatically monitors data quality in real-time throughout the remainder of the study period. For example, PiLR Health alerts the research team and participant if cumulative adherence to prompted self-report surveys falls below 85%, or if the sensor devices are not worn during waking hours for ≥4 h. The research team can then contact the participant by phone to resolve the problem(s) if they persist beyond the end of the day.

To limit participant burden and improve data quality, EMA self-report surveys can be programmed so that

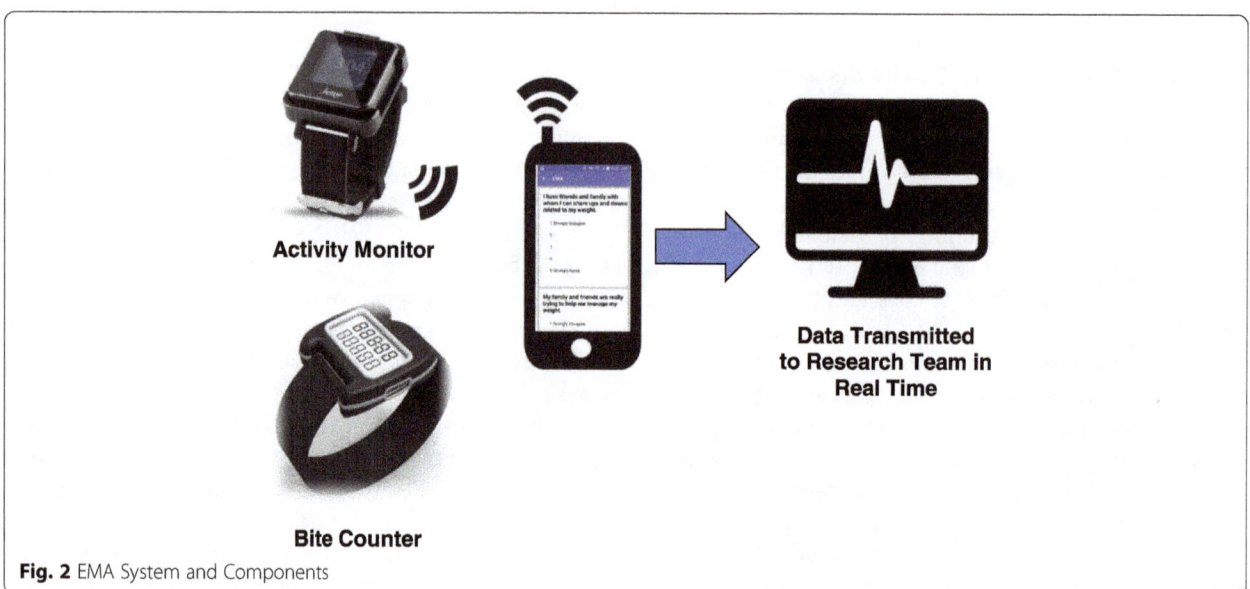

Activity Monitor

Bite Counter

Data Transmitted to Research Team in Real Time

Fig. 2 EMA System and Components

they are adaptive by selecting questions based on prior responses earlier in the survey (e.g., if participants indicate early in a survey that eating has not occurred recently, they are asked no more questions about eating in that survey and are instead asked about other, more relevant behaviors or experiences). The PiLR platform used in this study extends that concept by capitalizing on sensors data to determine when certain surveys are triggered. We use the objective sensors in the current project not only as assessment tools, but also to prompt completion of "in-the-moment" self-report surveys about experiences related to physical activity and sedentary behavior that cannot be measured via sensor (e.g., type of physical activity, location of activity).

Smartphone self-report surveys
All participants are provided with an Android device (Samsung Galaxy S7; Samsung Electronics, South Korea) running the mobile application described above. Participants are asked to respond to "in-the-moment" self-report surveys on this device for 10-day assessment periods. Participants are prompted via vibration, an audible tone, and a message on the smartphone screen to complete real-time self-report surveys several times per day. A beginning-of-day survey is initiated at 8:00 a.m. Prompts to rate eating, physical activity, and sedentary behavior are initiated when specific events are detected via objective monitoring, as described above. Key psychosocial and environmental variables are rated during these prompts and at 4 semi-random prompts anchored at 11:00 a.m., 2:00 p.m., 5:00 p.m., and 8:00 p.m. Participants are asked to self-initiate an end-of-day survey "before bed". All prompted surveys are capped at 12 per day to limit participant burden [13, 19]. Below we describe the content of self-report surveys.

Measures
See Table 1 for a summary of all behavioral, psychosocial and environmental predictors assessed in this study with related assessment methods.

Physical activity, sedentary behavior, and sleep
The ActiGraph GT9X Link (ActiGraph, LLC, Pensacola, FL, USA) objectively assesses daily time spent in physical activity, sedentary behaviors, and sleep. This device employs rigorously validated triaxial accelerometer and proprietary data filtering technology used in previous generation devices to reliably estimate free-living activity in adult populations, including those undergoing bariatric surgery [20, 21]. The ActiGraph Link is equipped with a sensor on the back of the device that automatically detects when the device has been removed to assist with compliance monitoring. The ActiGraph Link is also thought to be more tolerable to participants, as compared

Table 1 Behavioral, Psychosocial, and Environmental Predictors and Related Assessment Methods

Predictor	Assessment Method
Physical activity	
Level (light-vigorous), duration	ActiGraph Link
Total & active energy expenditure (kcal/d)	ActiGraph Link
Steps and total distance/day	ActiGraph Link
Types of PA	EMA
PA barriers and intentions	EMA
Sedentary behavior	
Total minutes/day and % time	ActiGraph Link
Types of sedentary behavior	EMA
Eating behavior	
Frequency, timing, duration, rate, and volume	Bite Counter
Total energy intake, diet composition, & quality	Dietary Recall
Hunger and satiety	EMA
Appetite/motivation to eat	EMA
Binge eating & loss of control	EMA
Planned eating	EMA
Grazing	EMA
Dietary restraint and disinhibition	EMA
Behavioral complications	EMA
Sleep habits (total time and efficiency)	ActiGraph Link
Other adherence behaviors	
Self-weighing	EMA
Attendance at clinical follow-ups	Chart Review
Adherence to medications/vitamins	EMA
Psychosocial factors	
Mood, stress, energy, fatigue	EMA
Health locus of control	EMA
Social support	EMA
Outcomes expectations	Questionnaires
Bariatric surgery motivation & satisfaction	Questionnaires
Understanding of behavioral recommendations	Questionnaires
Environmental factors	
Exposure to and availability of palatable foods	EMA
Cues for eating, activity, and sedentariness	EMA
Eating location/setting & behavior/proximity of others	EMA

to waist-worn monitors or armbands, because it is specifically designed to appear and feel like a wrist watch.

Participants are instructed to wear the ActiGraph Link on their non-dominant wrist 24 h per day, exclusive of bathing and swimming, for the 10-day EMA protocol at the 4 assessment periods. For each of the 10-day assessments, a participant's data is considered valid if he or she wears the device for ≥10 h on ≥ 5 days (including ≥1 weekend day). The number of minutes per day participants spend in sedentary behavior and physical activity of different intensities is being determined using metabolic equivalents (METs), with activities < 1.5 METs, activities1.5–2.9 METs, activities 3.0–5.9 METs, and activities ≥ 6.0 METs classified as sedentary, light, moderate, and vigorous, respectively. We are particularly interested in moderate-to-vigorous physical activity (MVPA) and bout-related MVPA (≥ 10 min of activity at a time) given that this level of physical activity is emphasized in recommendations for both bariatric surgery patients and the general adult population [22–24]. Additionally, we are examining sedentary behavior accumulated in bouts ≥ 30 min to capture the prolonged nature of sedentary behavior and associated health risks [25]. Finally, we also employ the ActiGraph Link as a sleep detection device to measure both duration and quality. Research in non-bariatric populations with obesity suggests that short sleep duration is a risk factor for weight gain and is improved via weight loss [26]; however, these relationships have received little attention in the bariatric population. The ActiGraph Link was chosen as a measurement tool for this project because it is tolerable to participants, unobtrusive, difficult to manipulate, and capable of wireless connectivity.

Smartphone surveys are used in conjunction with the ActiGraph Link to understand the context in which objectively measured physical activity and sedentary behaviors are occurring. When the ActiGraph Link detects that a MVPA bout lasting ≥10-min has concluded (as defined by ≥2 min below 3 METs), participants are prompted to self-report the type(s) of activities performed (walking, cycling, etc.) through PiLR. Likewise, participants are asked to self-report the type(s) of sedentary behaviors (watching TV, driving, etc.) performed. Four random prompts to complete a smartphone survey about sedentary behavior are administered per day between 10 a.m. – 12 p.m., 1 p.m.- 3 p.m., 4 p.m. – 6 p.m., and 7 p.m. – 9 p.m. If the participant is sedentary for 60 consecutive minutes (as defined by ≥2 min above 1.5 METs) without more than one minute of activity between sedentary minutes, then a random prompt is activated. However, if no prompt has been activated by the end of the window, then a survey is delivered at that time (e.g., 12 p.m., 3 p.m., 6 p.m., 9 p.m.). Smartphone surveys are also used to examine physical activity intentions and barriers through beginning- and end-of-day surveys.

Eating behavior

The Bite Counter (Bite Technologies, Pendelton SC, USA) is a wrist-worn device that detects bites of food using an on-board tri-axial accelerometer to sense an upward arcing motion from table to mouth (i.e., "wrist roll") thus tracking individual bites of food. The Bite Counter has been validated to detect bites taken during controlled eating in laboratory settings and free-living eating in adults [27, 28]. The number of bites determined by the Bite Counter has been well-correlated with estimated energy intake [29]. Using bite data, the device and accompanying software are validated to provide detailed information on patterns of eating (number, timing, duration, and rate of eating bouts) and approximate amount (in kilocalories) of food and drink ingested within and across daily eating bouts [28]. The Bite Counter has proven to be tolerable for participants to wear on a daily basis [30, 31].

Participants wear the Bite Counter on their dominant wrist for all waking hours during each 10-day assessment period (except time spent bathing, swimming, and charging the device). Participants are instructed to push a button on the device each time they begin eating to signal the device to begin collecting bite data. They push the same button when the eating episode has finished. For the current project, we sought to collect information in accordance with postoperative guidelines related to eating patterns [9]. As such, variables of interest are daily frequency, and duration of eating bouts, as well as bite count. The strengths of the Bite Counter are that it provides objective measurement on aspects of eating that are difficult to self-report (especially for individuals with overweight/obesity) [32], it is unobtrusive compared to other objective methods of assessing eating behavior, it was developed using sophisticated and systematic methods, and the display can be inactivated for assessment and activated for intervention purposes [33, 34].

For contextual factors related to eating that cannot be detected by sensor, questions regarding eating, appetitive experiences and attitudes are included in the 4 semi-random prompts to complete self-report surveys. The following factors are assessed: hedonic hunger (i.e., the drive to eat for pleasure rather than energy deficit), homeostatic hunger (i.e., the drive to eat due to prolonged food deprivation), satiety (i.e., the processes that inhibit further consumption in the postprandial period) and satiation (i.e., the processes that bring an eating episode to an end), dietary restraint (i.e., conscious efforts to restrict food intake to influence body weight and/or shape) [35], disinhibition (i.e., overeating in response to internal or external cues) [35], and grazing. End-of-day surveys include questions about binge eating, loss of control, consumption of high-fat/sugar foods, and bariatric complications (i.e., reflux, nausea, vomiting, diarrhea, cramping, bloating, dehydration, and fatigue).

Assessment of dietary intake

Dietary intake is measured during each assessment period via three non-consecutive, 24-h diet recalls representing two weekdays and one weekend day. During dietary recalls, participants are asked to recount all foods, beverages, and supplements consumed in the prior 24-h period. The first of the three recalls is collected at the in-person study visit, and the subsequent two recalls are collected over the phone. A trained interviewer collects the recalls using Nutrition Dietary Systems for Research (NDSR; Nutrition Coordinating Center, University of Minnesota, 2017). NDSR utilizes a multiple-pass interview approach, which provides the participant multiple opportunities to recall intake [36]. NDSR output files are used to characterize energy intake, percent energy from macronutrients, as well as micronutrient intake from the diet and supplements, separately. This output allows us to examine adherence to diet-specific surgical guidelines including: eating frequency, total energy intake, percent energy from macronutrients (protein, fat and carbohydrate), micronutrient intake (including supplements), and diet quality (as measured by the Healthy Eating Index, 2015 [37]). Regarding diet quality, the variable of interest for this particular population is the percent energy from empty calories (which includes calories from solid fats, added sugars and alcohol). As such, the percentage of empty calories is used to measure intake of "risky" foods. Dietary recalls are necessary as they are a valid and reliable method to study composition of dietary intake [38], which is not adequately measured by the Bite Counter alone.

Other behavioral recommendations
Self-weighing facilitates weight loss and maintenance for non-bariatric patients but its importance in bariatric patients is less established [39]. Medication and supplement use is a focus of bariatric surgery guidelines [9]. Both are assessed in end-of-day surveys per our prior research [17].

Psychosocial factors
These predictors are expected to relate to weight loss outcomes and may explain for whom and under what circumstances behaviors are related to weight loss outcomes due to prior evidence in the bariatric population and related health conditions. The following factors are being assessed during the 4 semi-random prompts: mood, stress, energy, and fatigue using items from the Profile of Mood States [40], Positive and Negative Affect Scale [41], and Daily Stress Inventory [42]; locus of control using items from the Multidimensional Health Locus of Control Scale [43]; and social support using items from the Multidimensional Scale of Perceived Social Support [44]. When possible, items were drawn from validated measures and adjusted for EMA administration if necessary.

Environmental factors
While not yet emphasized in bariatric surgery guidelines, environmental factors may explain variability in weight loss outcomes via effects on behavior [45]. In this study, random survey prompts query the number and types of high quality palatable foods available, and other environmental characteristics of eating episodes studied in previous EMA studies including where eating occurs, where the food originated (e.g., prepared by self/other at home, restaurant, fast food), and the presence of others [17, 45–47]. Cues for physical activity (e.g., availability of exercise equipment and apparel) are also assessed during semi-random prompts.

Paper and pencil questionnaires
Participants complete validated questionnaires to capture more general information on behaviors (e.g., physical activity, sedentary behavior, and eating) and clinical symptomatology (e.g., depression and anxiety symptoms). We also evaluate bariatric surgery expectations and perceptions (at baseline), as well as level of satisfaction with bariatric surgery outcomes (at each postoperative assessment) as these factors can impact adherence to dietary and health goals [48, 49].

Chart review
Medical charts are reviewed after the study period is complete to collect data about attendance at clinical follow-up visits and patient support groups, types of postoperative care attended, (e.g., nutritional counseling), and adherence to clinical care regimen. Pre- and postoperative medical comorbidities are also extracted. Participants who drop-out provide consent for the research team to retrieve these data after discontinuing the study.

Body weight and waist circumference
Participants' body weight and waist circumference are measured at pre- and all postoperative assessments through 12 months. Weight is measured to the nearest 0.1 kg using a calibrated digital scale. Height is measured in millimeters using a wall-mounted Harnpenden stadiometer. From these measures, body mass index (kg/m^2) is calculated. Postoperative weight loss is expressed in terms of kg and % weight loss. Waist circumference is measured at the midpoint between the highest point of the iliac crest and the lowest part of the costal margin in the mid-axillary line.

Data monitoring and management
Prior to the start of the trial, a data safety monitoring plan was developed and approved by a pre-appointed Safety Officer. The Safety Officer, approved by the funding agency, is an expert in working with weight loss and bariatric surgery populations and has familiarity with the assessment tools employed in the current study. In the first 6 months of the project period (and annually

thereafter), we have been submitting tables indicating our progress with recruitment, assessment retention, reasons for dropouts, and adverse events to the Safety Officer for review. After the review, the Safety Officer has provided written notice to the principle investigators and the funding agency as to whether the study is progressing appropriately and safely. Adverse events and serious adverse events are collected and reported from the beginning of study-related procedures to the end of the study follow-up period for each individual. At each visit, study staff specifically query participants for adverse events and participants are encouraged to report through telephone calls and emails as well. Should they occur, our policy is to report adverse events within 1–2 weeks to the IRB and serious adverse events are reported to the IRB and the funding agency within 24 h.

Our active data management plan involves cleaning the data, generating composite measures and performing data reduction activities with data collected via EMA, questionnaire, chart review and anthropomorphic measurement. Participant number identifies data collected and data is kept in locked files behind locked doors in the research centers. Additional safeguards are in place to protect participant data collected via sensor devices and electronic forms on smartphones. These data are stored temporarily on the smartphone but are regularly transmitted to encrypted secure storage on PiLR Health servers. Thus, if a study smartphone is lost or stolen, it is very unlikely that a participant's confidential data would be compromised. Data transmitted via smartphones is also heavily encrypted by mobile phone carriers to prevent interception (e.g., from the smartphone to PiLR Health servers). No personally identifiable information is stored or transmitted via the smartphone. All participant smartphone data is coded using a unique identifying number. Any electronic data collected by study staff is stored in an encrypted form (with a randomly generated 26-character key).

Statistical analysis

Aim 1 of this project seeks to develop and implement the EMA system and assess its feasibility and acceptability. The analytical plan for this aim is therefore descriptive in nature (e.g., examining compliance with wearing devices, completing survey prompts). Aim 2 seeks to examine which behavioral and psychosocial factors predict weight loss outcomes and the times at which each factor has the strongest effect on outcomes. Aim 2 will be evaluated using general longitudinal linear mixed effect models for weight loss and waist circumference as the dependent variables and baseline and time-varying behavioral, psychosocial, and environmental factors as predictors. Models will include the effect of control variables and covariates that are potential confounders

between psychosocial and behavioral factors and weight loss outcomes, including: sex, race, ethnicity, and age. Aim 3 seeks to identify causal pathways by which psychosocial factors influence outcomes via effects on behavior; and moderators that explain for whom and under what conditions the influence is the strongest. To evaluate Aim 3, we will use the counterfactual approach to mediation modeling with exposure-mediator interaction (i.e., moderation) as described by Valeri and VanderWeele [50].

In all models, we will consider EMA and in-person measures of the same construct separately, and only together with the use of composites, to avoid multicollinearity. Patterns and potential causes of missingness will be evaluated. We plan to treat missing data as missing at random, to be addressed in analysis with multiple imputation and/or maximum likelihood parameter estimation [51].

Given the novelty of the current study, the sample size was selected in collaboration with the NIH as adequate to assess the feasibility of the study protocol and to also obtain reliable estimates of effect sizes to inform preliminary estimates and future studies. As our analysis plan is primarily descriptive, we note that a sample size of 100 is suitable for the detection of correlation coefficients that are small to moderate in magnitude ($r > 0.28$) as statistically significant using conventional type-I and type-II error probabilities (5 and 20%, respectively), and similarly group mean differences of 0.56 standard deviation units under similar assumptions and balance in representation across group. Such minimally detectable effect sizes are subtle enough to fall below conventional thresholds for clinical significance.

Discussion

In line with the NIH focus on behavioral and psychosocial predictors of bariatric surgery outcomes, using a novel multi-sensor mHealth approach is expected to provide contextually rich data that can validate existing pre- and postoperative behavioral guidelines, inform new behavioral guidelines, and identify treatment targets for clinicians working with this population. The current study will be the first to capitalize on advancements in mHealth within the bariatric population by integrating multiple sensors and self-report methods to examine a variety of behavioral and psychosocial factors longitudinally over the pre- and postoperative period. As such, our methodology is expected to inform best practices in assessment for future studies of bariatric patients and produce data that will serve as a strong foundation for additional research within this population.

Our approach has many benefits over using solely traditional methodologies (i.e., chart review, self-report questionnaires) to study behavior in this population. EMA is, at present, one of the most valid and reliable tools for assessing individuals' behaviors, thoughts, and emotions throughout the course of their daily lives in their natural environments. Our project extends the value of EMA by *combining and integrating* several EMA measurement methods (i.e., self-report surveys, actigraphy, and passively sensed eating) to inform a nuanced understanding of the contexts in which behaviors and psychosocial factors occur. In addition to enhanced accuracy and contextual validity, using an mHealth approach provides a temporal granularity that is paramount to understanding complex relationships between stable traits, changing states, and their influence on health behaviors [52]. For example, continuous data on behaviors of interest (e.g., physical activity, eating behavior) and repeated measurements of psychosocial factors (e.g., mood, environment, hunger) will allow us to understand the quasi-causal and reciprocal within-person associations between specific psychosocial factors and behaviors that impact surgical outcomes. In this vein, our multi-sensory methods are expected to generate a substantial amount of outcome data from which to answer a myriad of research questions related to bariatric surgery outcomes.

Another major strength of this study is that it was conceived and executed by a highly multidisciplinary research team including experts in behavioral science, bariatric surgery, clinical patient care, computer science, engineering, and business. Just as a multidisciplinary medical team is recommended to optimize care for bariatric surgery patients, our team approach has allowed us to develop a protocol and utilize assessment tools that are particularly well-suited to the needs of studying this complex population. Further, the multi-faceted expertise within our research team allowed us to use the challenges of this research to form novel interdisciplinary collaborations. For example, the tool used to objectively assess eating behavior in the current study (i.e., Bite Counter) requires a button press to start and stop monitoring of eating. This method likely introduced complications such as non-compliance with the button press and, in some individuals, reactivity. These complications created a need and opportunity to explore the viability of other methods for objectively assessing eating behavior. Thus, our team is now conducting research to use the ActiGraph Link (the device used for measuring physical activity, sedentary behavior, and sleep in our study) for continuous eating detection without button press using similar algorithms to the Bite Counter. This innovation is thought to enhance data quality and will allow for a single device to measure four different health behaviors (i.e., eating, activity, sedentariness, and sleep), which could reduce user burden and increase acceptability of protocol. Moreover, using the ActiGraph Link to passively sense eating behavior will allow for surveys to

be triggered automatically when eating episodes are detected to better assess the physiological, psychological, and environmental factors related to eating (similar to the way in which the current protocol assesses physical activity). Finally, the combination of using both methods would allow for the validation of self-reported eating patterns collected via telephone dietary recalls.

There also have been general technical challenges to executing the current study that are inherent to any study utilizing mHealth methods. One major barrier was that our goal of continuously monitoring and integrating self-report surveys and sensor data is stretching the bounds of current technological capabilities. Much of a smartphone's functionality is governed by a mobile operating system that dictates resource allocation to enable consistent functioning of multiple systems such as the touchscreen, Global Positioning System, Bluetooth, Wi-Fi, and camera. Typically, mobile operating systems work to conserve battery life of the device by limiting the degree to which software applications are allowed to run "in the background" (i.e., when they are not actively in use by the user or when the phone is in standby mode waiting to be used). This function makes it challenging to continuously synchronize sensor devices such as the ActiGraph Link with a smartphone and subsequently trigger self-report surveys in a timely manner as the corresponding applications are not permitted by the mobile operating system to run in the background. Mobile operating systems and software on sensor devices also tend to be updated by the manufacturer at unpredictable intervals and such updates often occur automatically outside of the control of the researchers. Such updates can disrupt a research study by causing mobile data collection systems to function unpredictably or cease functioning altogether. For this reason, it is important for researchers to have a plan (i.e., extra devices, back-up servers, contact with information technology teams) to maintain data collection systems and address problems caused by software updates.

Another way that we sought to mitigate these challenges was to increase our control of the technology by giving each participant the same type of smartphone for answering the self-report surveys and using research-grade sensors. However, as studies include longer monitoring periods and smartphones become more ubiquitous, it is becoming evident that the field should work towards deploying multi-sensor assessment methods that capitalize on the smartphones that many participants already own. This strategy would reduce the cost of conducting the study and lessen participant inconvenience, for example by eliminating the need for a participant to carry a personal smartphone and a research smartphone. The trade-off is that using personal smartphones would diminish control that the research team has over the tools used for data collection. Given that there are now a variety of mobile operating systems, using personal devices would also necessitate that data collection software to be interoperable (i.e., functional on a wide range of smartphone of smartphone operating systems). Many of the challenges experienced by our team in implementing mHealth tools reflect common barriers to conducting technology-based research in the field and call for deeper integration of information systems and behavioral science fields.

Conclusion

As behavioral factors are increasingly recognized as contributors to bariatric surgery outcomes, the current study is critical for identifying factors and contexts that influence behavior among individuals who have undergone bariatric surgery. The project is designed to accumulate large quantities of data from both the pre- and postoperative period to evaluate a wide range of predictors of weight loss outcomes. Examples of potential research questions that will be tested using these data include: examining preoperative associations among behaviors and psychosocial factors; identifying preoperative predictors of outcome; demonstrating postoperative trajectories of weight and associated health behaviors; and systematically evaluating the that way in which various psychosocial factors can impact outcomes via changes in behavior. We plan to disseminate findings from the current study via peer-reviewed publication and conference presentations (no identifying participant information will be included in disseminated materials). Data and methods from the current study are also expected to provide a foundation for subsequent trials funded by NIH to examine behaviors that influence bariatric surgery outcomes. Overall, this program of research will contribute significantly to evidence-based clinical care for bariatric surgery patients.

Abbreviations

EMA: Ecological Momentary Assessment; IRB: Institutional Review Board; mHealth: Mobile health; MVPA: Moderate-to-vigorous physical activity; NDSR: Nutrition Data System for Research; RYGB: Roux-en-Y gastric bypass; SG: Sleeve gastrectomy

Funding

This project is funded by the National Institute of Diabetic and Digestive and Kidney Diseases (R01 DK108579; PIs: DB and JGT). The funding source collaborated with principle investigators on study design and had no additional roles on the project.

Authors' contributions

SPG, JGT, and DSB were major contributors in writing the manuscript. DSB and JGT obtained funding to conduct the study protocol described in the manuscript. JM, JGT, and DSB collaborated to develop/modify the multi-sensor platform described in this manuscript. SV, JW, RJ, EWE, DBJ, JD, and GAB are executing the study protocol and provided feedback on this manuscript. All authors read and approved the final manuscript.

Competing interests

JM is President of MEI Research, Ltd., which is the company that developed the PiLR Health system described in this manuscript. The remainder of the authors declare that they have no competing interests.

Author details

[1]Weight Control and Diabetes Research Center, Department of Psychiatry and Human Behavior, The Miriam Hospital/Warren Alpert Medical School of Brown University, 196 Richmond Street, Providence, RI 02909, USA. [2]Department of Surgery, The Miriam Hospital/Warren Alpert Medical School of Brown University, 195 Collyer Street, Providence, RI 02904, USA. [3]Beth Israel Deaconess Medical Center, Department of Surgery, Center for the Study of Nutrition Medicine, Feldberg 880, East Campus, 330 Brookline Avenue, Boston, MA 02215, USA. [4]Department of Psychiatry and Human Behavior, Warren Alpert Medical School of Brown University, Butler Hospital, 345 Blackstone Boulevard, Box G-BH, Providence, RI 02906, USA. [5]Department of Medicine, Division of Endocrinology, Beth Israel Deaconess Medical Center, Feldberg 880, East Campus, 330 Brookline Avenue, Boston, MA 02215, USA. [6]MEI Research, Ltd, 6016 Schaefer Road, Edina, MN 55436, USA.

References

1. Chang S-H, Stoll CR, Song J, Varela JE, Eagon CJ, Colditz GA. The effectiveness and risks of bariatric surgery: an updated systematic review and meta-analysis, 2003-2012. JAMA surgery. 2014;149(3):275–87.
2. le Roux CW, Heneghan HM. Bariatric surgery for obesity. Med Clin N Am. 2018;102(1):165–82.
3. Angrisani L, Santonicola A, Iovino P, Formisano G, Buchwald H, Scopinaro N. Bariatric surgery worldwide 2013. Obes Surg. 2015;25(10):1822–32.
4. Yarmush ML, D'Alessandro M, Saeidi N. Regulation of energy homeostasis after gastric bypass surgery. Annu Rev Biomed Eng. 2017;19:459–84.
5. Adams TD, Davidson LE, Litwin SE, Kolotkin RL, LaMonte MJ, Pendleton RC, Strong MB, Vinik R, Wanner NA, Hopkins PN. Health benefits of gastric bypass surgery after 6 years. Jama. 2012;308(11):1122–31.
6. Courcoulas AP, King WC, Belle SH, Berk P, Flum DR, Garcia L, Gourash W, Horlick M, Mitchell JE, Pomp A. Seven-year weight trajectories and health outcomes in the longitudinal assessment of bariatric surgery (LABS) study. JAMA surgery. 2018;153.5:427–34.
7. Adams TD, Davidson LE, Litwin SE, Kim J, Kolotkin RL, Nanjee MN, Gutierrez JM, Frogley SJ, Ibele AR, Brinton EA. Weight and metabolic outcomes 12 years after gastric bypass. N Engl J Med. 2017;377(12):1143–55.
8. Benoit SC, Hunter TD, Francis DM, De La Cruz-Munoz N. Use of bariatric outcomes longitudinal database (BOLD) to study variability in patient success after bariatric surgery. Obes Surg. 2014;24(6):936–43.
9. Mechanick JI, Youdim A, Jones DB, Garvey WT, Hurley DL, McMahon MM, Heinberg LJ, Kushner R, Adams TD, Shikora S. Clinical practice guidelines for the perioperative nutritional, metabolic, and nonsurgical support of the bariatric surgery patient—2013 update: cosponsored by American Association

of Clinical Endocrinologists, the Obesity Society, and American Society for Metabolic & bariatric surgery. Surg Obes Relat Dis. 2013;9(2):159–91.

10. Bond DS, Thomas JG, Unick JL, Raynor HA, Vithiananthan S, Wing RR. Self-reported and objectively measured sedentary behavior in bariatric surgery candidates. Surg Obes Relat Dis. 2013;9(1):123–8.

11. Bond DS, Jakicic JM, Unick JL, Vithiananthan S, Pohl D, Roye GD, Ryder BA, Sax HC, Wing RR. Pre-to postoperative physical activity changes in bariatric surgery patients: self report vs. Objective Measures Obesity. 2010;18(12):2395–7.

12. Thomas JG, Bond DS, Sarwer DB, Wing RR. Technology for behavioral assessment and intervention in bariatric surgery. Surg Obes Relat Dis. 2011; 7(4):548–57.

13. Shiffman S, Stone AA, Hufford MR. Ecological momentary assessment. Annu Rev Clin Psychol. 2008;4:1–32.

14. Engel SG, Crosby RD, Thomas G, Bond D, Lavender JM, Mason T, Steffen KJ, Green DD, Wonderlich SA. Ecological momentary assessment in eating disorder and obesity research: a review of the recent literature. Curr Psychiatry Rep. 2016;18(4):37.

15. Stone, AA, Shiffman, S. Ecological momentary assessment (EMA) in behavioral medicine. Ann Behav Med. 1994;16(3):199–202.

16. Bond DS, Thomas JG, Ryder BA, Vithiananthan S, Pohl D, Wing RR. Ecological momentary assessment of the relationship between intention and physical activity behavior in bariatric surgery patients. Int J Behav Med. 2013;20(1):82–7.

17. Thomas JG, Bond DS, Ryder BA, Leahey TM, Vithiananthan S, Roye GD, Wing RR. Ecological momentary assessment of recommended postoperative eating and activity behaviors. Surg Obes Relat Dis. 2011;7(2):206–12.

18. Bond DS, King WC. The role of physical activity in optimizing bariatric surgery outcomes. In: The ASMBS textbook of bariatric surgery. Edn: Springer; New York. 2014. p. 217–29.

19. Shiffman S. Designing protocols for ecological momentary assessment. The science of real-time data capture: self-reports in health research. New York: Oxford University Press, Inc; 2007. p. 27–53.

20. Berglind D, Willmer M, Eriksson U, Thorell A, Sundbom M, Uddén J, Raoof M, Hedberg J, Tynelius P, Näslund E. Longitudinal assessment of physical activity in women undergoing roux-en-Y gastric bypass. Obes Surg. 2015; 25(1):119–25.

21. Toth LP, Park S, Springer CM, Feyerabend M, Steeves JA, Bassett DR. Video-recorded validation of wearable step counters under free-living conditions. Med Sci Sports Exerc. 2018;50(6):1315–22.

22. Blackburn GL, Hutter MM, Harvey AM, Apovian CM, Boulton HR, Cummings S, Fallon JA, Greenberg I, Jiser ME, Jones DB. Expert panel on weight loss surgery: executive report update. Obesity. 2009;17(5):842–62.

23. Poirier P, Cornier M-A, Mazzone T, Stiles S, Cummings S, Klein S, McCullough PA, Fielding CR, Franklin BA. Bariatric surgery and cardiovascular risk factors: a scientific statement from the American Heart Association. Circulation. 2011;123(15):1683–701.

24. Haskell WL, Lee I-M, Pate RR, Powell KE, Blair SN, Franklin BA, Macera CA, Heath GW, Thompson PD, Bauman A. Physical activity and public health: updated recommendation for adults from the American College of Sports Medicine and the American Heart Association. Circulation. 2007;116(9):1081.

25. Kim Y, Welk GJ, Braun SI, Kang M. Extracting objective estimates of sedentary behavior from accelerometer data: measurement considerations for surveillance and research applications. PLoS One. 2015;10(2):e0118078.

26. Ford ES, Li C, Wheaton AG, Chapman DP, Perry GS, Croft JB. Sleep duration and body mass index and waist circumference among US adults. Obesity. 2014;22(2):598–607.

27. Scisco JL, Muth ER, Dong Y, Hoover AW. Slowing bite-rate reduces energy intake: an application of the bite counter device. J Am Diet Assoc. 2011; 111(8):1231–5.

28. Desendorf J, Bassett DR Jr, Raynor HA, Coe DP. Validity of the bite counter device in a controlled laboratory setting. Eat Behav. 2014;15(3):502–4.

29. Scisco JL, Muth ER, Hoover AW. Examining the utility of a bite-count–based measure of eating activity in free-living human beings. J Acad Nutr Diet. 2014;114(3):464–9.

30. Salley JN, Hoover AW, Wilson ML, Muth ER. Comparison between human and bite-based methods of estimating caloric intake. J Acad Nutr Diet. 2016; 116(10):1568–77.

31. Wilson ML, Kinsella AJ, Muth ER. User compliance rates of a wrist-worn eating activity monitor: the bite counter. In: Proceedings of the human factors and ergonomics society annual meeting: 2015. Los Angeles, CA: SAGE publications Sage CA; 2015. p. 902–6.

32. Lichtman SW, Pisarska K, Berman ER, Pestone M, Dowling H, Offenbacher E, Weisel H, Heshka S, Matthews DE, Heymsfield SB. Discrepancy between self-reported and actual caloric intake and exercise in obese subjects. N Engl J Med. 1992;327(27):1893–8.

33. Jasper PW, James MT, Hoover AW, Muth ER. Effects of bite count feedback from a wearable device and goal setting on consumption in young adults. J Acad Nutr Diet. 2016;116(11):1785–93.

34. Turner-McGrievy GM, Wilcox S, Boutté A, Hutto BE, Singletary C, Muth ER, Hoover AW. The dietary intervention to enhance tracking with mobile devices (DIET mobile) study: a 6-month randomized weight loss trial. Obesity. 2017;25(8):1336–42.

35. Stunkard AJ, Messick S. The three-factor eating questionnaire to measure dietary restraint, disinhibition and hunger. J Psychosom Res. 1985;29(1):71–83.

36. Johnson RK, Driscoll P, Goran MI. Comparison of multiple-pass 24-hour recall estimates of energy intake with total energy expenditure determined by the doubly labeled water method in young children. J Am Diet Assoc. 1996;96(11):1140–4.

37. Overview and Background of the Healthy Eating Index [https://epi.grants.cancer.gov/hei/]. Accessed 1 May 2018.

38. Subar AF, Freedman LS, Tooze JA, Kirkpatrick SI, Boushey C, Neuhouser ML, Thompson FE, Potischman N, Guenther PM, Tarasuk V. Addressing current criticism regarding the value of self-report dietary data, 2. J Nutr. 2015; 145(12):2639–45.

39. Van Wormer JJ, French SA, Pereira MA, Welsh EM. The impact of regular self-weighing on weight management: a systematic literature review. Int J Behav Nutr Phys Act. 2008;5(1):54.

40. McNair DM, Lorr M, Droppleman LF. Profile of mood states: manual: edits; 1992.

41. Watson D, Clark LA, Tellegen A. Development and validation of brief measures of positive and negative affect: the PANAS scales. J Pers Soc Psychol. 1988;54(6):1063.

42. Brantley PJ, Waggoner CD, Jones GN, Rappaport NB. A daily stress inventory: development, reliability, and validity. J Behav Med. 1987;10(1):61–73.

43. Wallston KA, Strudler Wallston B, DeVellis R. Development of the multidimensional health locus of control (MHLC) scales. Health Educ Monogr. 1978;6(1):160–70.

44. Zimet GD, Dahlem NW, Zimet SG, Farley GK. The multidimensional scale of perceived social support. J Pers Assess. 1988;52(1):30–41.

45. Thomas JG, Doshi S, Crosby RD, Lowe MR. Ecological momentary assessment of obesogenic eating behavior: combining person-specific and environmental predictors. Obesity. 2011;19(8):1574–9.

46. Carels RA, Douglass OM, Cacciapaglia HM, O'brien WH. An ecological momentary assessment of relapse crises in dieting. J Consult Clin Psychol. 2004;72(2):341.

47. Carels RA, Hoffman J, Collins A, Raber AC, Cacciapaglia H, O'Brien WH. Ecological momentary assessment of temptation and lapse in dieting. Eat Behav. 2001;2(4):307–21.

48. Foster GD, Wadden TA, Phelan S, Sarwer DB, Sanderson RS. Obese patients' perceptions of treatment outcomes and the factors that influence them. Arch Intern Med. 2001;161(17):2133–9.

49. Foster GD, Wadden TA, Vogt RA, Brewer G. What is a reasonable weight loss? Patients' expectations and evaluations of obesity treatment outcomes. J Consult Clin Psychol. 1997;65(1):79.

50. Valeri L, VanderWeele TJ. Mediation analysis allowing for exposure–mediator interactions and causal interpretation: theoretical assumptions and implementation with SAS and SPSS macros. Psychol Methods. 2013;18(2):137.

51. Ware JH, Harrington D, Hunter DJ, D'Agostino RB Sr. Missing data. In: Mass Medical Soc; 2012.

52. Riley WT. Behavioral and social sciences at the National Institutes of Health: adoption of research findings in health research and practice as a scientific priority. Translational behavioral medicine. 2017;7(2):380–4.

19

Improved physiology and metabolic flux after Roux-en-Y gastric bypass is associated with temporal changes in the circulating microRNAome: a longitudinal study in humans

Abdullah Alkandari[1,2]* iD, Hutan Ashrafian[1,3], Thozhukat Sathyapalan[4], Peter Sedman[5], Ara Darzi[1], Elaine Holmes[1], Thanos Athanasiou[1], Stephen L. Atkin[6] and Nigel J. Gooderham[1]

Abstract

Background: The global pandemic of obesity and the metabolic syndrome are leading causes of mortality and morbidity. Bariatric surgery leads to sustained weight loss and improves obesity-associated morbidity including remission of type 2 diabetes. MicroRNAs are small, endogenous RNAs that regulate gene expression post-transcriptionally, controlling most of the human transcriptome and contributing to the regulation of systemic metabolism. This preliminary, longitudinal, repeat sampling study, in which subjects acted as their own control, aimed to assess the temporal effect of bariatric surgery on circulating microRNA expression profiles.

Methods: We used Exiqon's optimized circulating microRNA panel (comprising 179 validated miRNAs) and miRCURY locked nucleic acid plasma/serum Polymerase Chain Reaction (PCR) to assess circulating microRNA expression. The microRNAome was determined for Roux-en-Y gastric bypass (RYGB) patients examined preoperatively and at 1 month, 3 months, 6 months, 9 months and 12 months postoperatively. Data was analysed using multivariate and univariate statistics.

Results: Compared to the preoperative circulating microRNA expression profile, RYGB altered the circulating microRNAome in a time dependent manner and the expression of 48 circulating microRNAs were significantly different. Importantly, these latter microRNAs are associated with pathways involved in regulation and rescue from metabolic dysfunction and correlated with BMI, the percentage of excess weight loss and fasting blood glucose levels.

Conclusions: The results of this pilot study show that RYGB fundamentally alters microRNA expression in circulation with a time-dependent progressive departure in profile from the preoperative baseline and indicate that microRNAs are potentially novel biomarkers for the benefits of bariatric surgery.

Keywords: MicroRNA, miRNA, Circulating, Bariatric, Gastric bypass, RYGB, Biomarker, Longitudinal, Temporal

* Correspondence: abdullah.alkandari@dasmaninstitute.org
[1]Department of Surgery and Cancer, Imperial College London, London, UK
[2]Clinical Trials Unit, Dasman Diabetes Institute, PO Box 1180, Dasman, 15462 Kuwait City, Kuwait
Full list of author information is available at the end of the article

Introduction

Bariatric surgery has been established as the most effective strategy for inducing sustained weight loss and enhancing metabolism to manage morbid obesity and its systemic co-morbidities. These procedures improve longevity and quality of life and lead to remission of type 2 diabetes mellitus (T2DM) and reduction in cardiovascular risk, often independent of weight loss [1]. The physiological effects of bariatric surgery include the BRAVE steps (bile flow alteration, reduction of gastric size, anatomical gut rearrangement and altered flow of nutrients, vagal manipulation and enteric gut hormone modulation) with the associated modulation of the gut microbiome and a multitude of downstream physiological and disease-modifying effects [2, 3]. However, the precise mechanism behind bariatric surgery remain poorly understood.

MicroRNAs are a family of endogenous, non-coding RNAs that regulate gene expression at the post-transcriptional level. These small, evolutionarily conserved RNA transcripts bind to target messenger RNA (mRNA) transcripts leading to mRNA cleavage or translational repression [4]. This enables each of the approximately 3000 distinct human microRNA sequences to fine-tune or silence several mRNA targets involved in a diverse array of cellular pathways. Thus, microRNAs form a complex network of gene 'super-regulators' controlling virtually every biological process. As such microRNAs have been implicated in the progression of obesity and its many co-morbidities. MicroRNAs regulate adipogenesis, insulin secretion, glucose uptake and lipid metabolism and many other biological processes linked with obesity [5].

While microRNAs act at the subcellular level, they are also found in the circulation within exosomes or complexed with high-density lipoproteins or argonaute proteins [6]. The mechanisms whereby microRNAs appear in the circulation and the biological implications of circulation expression are not understood. However, microRNAs are stable in circulation, not readily digested by ribonucleases and able to withstand repeated freeze-thaw cycles allowing for long-term storage of circulatory fluids without compromising the microRNA integrity [7]. They can also be measured with speed, ease and sensitivity through quantitative PCR and other platforms. This has given microRNAs rich clinical and therapeutic potential as novel biomarkers [8]. Recent studies have reported circulating microRNAs as biomarkers for cancer, obesity, diabetes and many other disorders [7, 9, 10].

Recently, single post-surgical timepoint studies have shown that bariatric surgery modulates circulating microRNA expression [9, 11, 12]. The objective of the present work was to complete a longitudinal repeat sampling study in which patients were their own preoperative controls, to assess the temporal effect of bariatric surgery on circulating microRNA expression profiles and to identify potential microRNA biomarkers.

Methods
Recruitment
Plasma samples were collected from 4 men and 5 women undergoing laparoscopic RYGB at Hull and East Yorkshire Hospitals NHS Trust in the United Kingdom under ethics approval 10/H1304/13. All patients were morbidly obese preoperatively and met qualifying criteria for bariatric surgery set out by NICE [13]. Plasma samples were collected in a fasting state and body mass index (BMI) and fasting blood glucose were measured immediately preoperatively and where possible at 1 month, 3 months, 6 months, 9 months and 12 months postoperatively. All participants provided informed written consent prior to the study.

Sample preparation and extraction
Plasma samples were acquired by standard venipuncture and centrifugation in EDTA-coated vacutainer tubes (Becton Dickinson) and frozen at -80 °C until use. RNA was extracted from plasma using the *mir*Vana PARIS Isolation Kit (Life Technologies), according to the manufacturer's instructions with one modification; prior to the addition of acid-phenol:chloroform, 150Amoles of c-elegans miR 39 (Life Technologies) was added as an internal standard and RNA carrier. RNA was extracted from 100 µl plasma and eluted in 100 µl nuclease free water. A 4 µl aliquot of RNA elute was reverse transcribed in 20 µl reactions using the Universal cDNA Synthesis Kit (Exiqon), according to the manufacturer's instructions.

Profiling of circulating microRNA
Plasma samples were profiled using Exiqon's miRCURY locked nucleic acid (LNA) platform and Serum/Plasma Focus microRNA PCR panels, according to the manufacturer's instruction. Panels comprised two 96-well plates coated with LNA microRNA primers for 179 microRNAs, selected and optimized by the manufacturer for their typical expression in circulation [14]. No template and UniSp3 spike-in primers were included for quality control. PCR was carried out on the StepOnePlus 7500 PCR system (Life Technologies) using the SYBR Green dye as instructed by the manufacturer.

Data analysis
Pre-processing and initial analysis of profiling data was performed with Exiqon's GenEx6 software. The threshold for expression was set as Cq < 37. MicroRNAs not detected in over 60% of samples were removed from consideration. Individual microRNA expression levels are expressed relative to preoperative expression. The miR-Walk (v.2) database of predicted and validated microRNA

targets and the PANTHER classification system were used to allocate regulated pathways as previously described [15]. To ensure confidence and accuracy, only mRNA targets predicted by 2 or more algorithms were included in the analysis. Statistical significance was determined by ANOVA and the Student's t test with Sidak-Bonferroni correction for multiple comparisons as appropriate. Expression of microRNAs was correlated with clinical parameters by the Pearson test. Principal component analysis (PCA) pattern recognition was applied to visualise differences in whole microRNA profiles prior to and following RYGB. All analysis was performed using GraphPad Prism 6.0 and R (www.r-project.org).

Results

As expected, all patients demonstrated substantial time-dependent reduction in weight following surgery (Table 1). Mean BMI decreased gradually and significantly from 49 kg/m^2 to 30.7 kg/m^2 and patients lost on average 72% of their mean preoperative excess weight 1 year following surgery. Although there were no significant changes in mean fasting blood glucose following surgery, only 2 out of the 9 patients in this study were diabetic and both demonstrated decreases in postoperative fasting blood glucose relative to their individual preoperative level.

Normalization

Profiling found 159 microRNAs that surpassed detection threshold. This offered multiple normalizing options to minimize technical variation. Five different approaches were assessed; microRNA expression was (a) not normalized, (b) normalized to the mean expression of all expressed microRNAs (global mean), (c) normalized to miR 223-3p and 26a, relatively stable microRNAs as determined by geNorm [16], (d) normalized to miR 101-3p and 19a, relatively stable microRNAs as determined by Normfinder [17] and (e) normalized to a combination of these 4 endogenous microRNAs. Overall variation was assessed through coefficient of variances (CV) and cumulative distribution as previously described

[18] (Additional file 1: Figure S1). The optimum method was normalization to the combination of miR 223-3p miR 26a, miR 101-3p and miR 19a which displayed significantly lower mean CVs of the 50% least variable microRNAs compared to all other assessed methods (Additional file 1: Figure S1B). As a result, all profiling data were normalized to these 4 endogenous microRNAs.

Multivariate analysis

Using an untargeted approach, multivariate statistical analysis with PCA scores plot demonstrated separation between the preoperative and 5 postoperative groups (Additional file 2: Figure S2A). There appeared to be discrete clustering according to time: preoperative profiles (pink); 1 month postoperative profiles (red); 3 months postoperative profile (green); 6 month postoperative profiles (light blue); 9 month postoperative profiles (blue); and 12 month postoperative profiles (black). This powerful untargeted approach was further demonstrated in the trajectory PCA, which plots the mean components of all 6 groups (Additional file 2: Figure S2B). The preoperative and 1 month postoperative microRNA profiles were similar but there is a notable shift of increasing separation with each sequential postoperative timepoint. This trajectory shift is also evident in the preoperative-postoperative comparative heatmap of microRNA expression and the associated group cluster dendrogram (Additional file 2: Figure S2C and D).

Univariate analysis

Since each patient served as their own control in this longitudinal study, we also used univariate analysis in a targetted approach for individual microRNAs. The majority of circulating microRNAs remained unaltered following RYGB. However, 48 out of the 159 detected microRNAs were differentially expressed in at least one postoperative timepoint compared to preoperative levels (Fig. 1). At 1 month following surgery circulating microRNA levels were largely unchanged, with only 1 microRNA significantly increased and 1 microRNA significantly decreased

Table 1 Summary of patient information and clinical outcomes of surgery[a]

Patients	Pre	1 m	3 m	6 m	9 m	12 m	ANOVA
n	9	6	8	7	7	4	
Age	46.1 (9.8)	–	–	–	–	–	–
Sex (Female)	5/9	–	–	–	–	–	–
Diabetics	2/9	–	–	–	–	–	–
BMI (kg/m^2)	49 (10)	41.2 (7.9)	37.5 (6.5)	36.4 (8.2)	33.7 (7.9)	30.7 (4.5)	0.0028 (**)
%EWL	0.0	33.7 (13.5)	48.2 (16.8)	55.9 (18.5)	68.9 (17.5)	71.7 (16.7)	0.0044 (**)
Fasting blood glucose (mmol/L)	7.5 (5.4)	4.2 (0)	6.9 (3.5)	5.7 (1.4)	5.6 (1.4)	5.9 (1.3)	0.733

[a]*BMI* body mass index, *EWL* excess weight lost. Parentheses indicate standard deviation. **p < 0.001 by ANOVA

Pre vs 1 Month	Fold change	p
miR-338-3p	-4.48213	0.0385
miR-574-3p	2.74287	0.049

Pre vs 3 Months	Fold change	p
let-7b-5p	-1.82723	0.0436
miR-93-5p	-11.42136	0.0481
miR-106b-5p	-2.24716	0.0277
miR-194-5p	-6.79215	0.0011
miR-374b-5p	4.93347	0.05

Pre vs 6 Months	Fold change	p
let-7i-5p	-1.92065	0.0392
miR-27a-3p	13.53321	0.0225
miR-33a-5p	4.73908	0.0236
miR-125b-5p	-7.14436	0.0077
miR-192-5p	-3.9763	0.0069
miR-301a-3p	5.37949	0.018
miR-320a	-4.93124	0.0367
miR-374b-5p	6.26218	0.0349
miR-378a-3p	-11.13685	0.0319
miR-590-5p	-2.72931	0.0223

Pre vs 9 Months	Fold change	p
let-7d-3p	-2.147	0.0379
let-7i-5p	-2.15403	0.0317
miR-15a-5p	-6.5224	0.0127
miR-16-2-3p	-4.05593	0.045
miR-21-5p	-2.99337	0.0262
miR-22-5p	-5.34766	0.0183
miR-28-3p	-3.38722	0.0271
miR-29c-3p	-4.36596	0.0111
miR-32-5p	-5.87211	0.025
miR-92a-3p	-4.50946	0.015
miR-99a-5p	-11.74445	0.0183
miR-125b-5p	-3.06655	0.0332
miR-148a-3p	-2.57524	0.0381
miR-148b-3p	-1.86248	0.0496
miR-192-5p	-3.68028	0.0158
miR-194-5p	-7.38657	0.0063
miR-320a	-5.05808	0.0072
miR-320b	-3.36266	0.0397
miR-363-3p	-4.16517	0.0389
miR-365a-3p	-14.39258	0.0004
miR-374b-5p	6.42042	0.0267
miR-378a-3p	-9.02419	0.0059
miR-423-3p	-4.64168	0.0211
miR-424-5p	-3.0694	0.0289
miR-502-3p	-5.75474	0.0379
miR-532-3p	-5.65122	0.0109
miR-629-5p	-34.77156	0.0006
miR-660-5p	-12.73778	0.0032

Pre vs 12 Months	Fold change	p
let-7d-3p	-2.76011	0.0354
miR-15a-5p	-84.90506	0.0192
miR-20b-5p	-5.5804	0.0497
miR-21-5p	-4.98989	0.0158
miR-22-5p	-19.12843	0.0017
miR-29a-5p	-5.74618	0.0101
miR-29b-3p	-3.09641	0.0352
miR-29c-3p	-7.43735	0.0045
miR-30e-3p	-4.25004	0.0211
miR-32-5p	-11.79701	0.0075
miR-92a-3p	-7.40402	0.0156
miR-93-3p	-5.51755	0.0072
miR-99a-5p	-6.78184	0.0471
miR-106b-5p	-3.74037	0.0402
miR-125b-5p	-3.70064	0.0481
miR-130b-3p	-13.8712	0.0055
miR-192-5p	-3.45762	0.0466
miR-194-5p	-8.75819	0.0032
miR-301a-3p	6.22679	0.046
miR-320a	-5.63933	0.0242
miR-339-3p	-11.9564	0.0157
miR-363-3p	-6.01488	0.0373
miR-378a-3p	-35.24316	0.0034
miR-423-3p	-4.01317	0.0169
miR-497-5p	-7.82366	0.0385
miR-502-3p	-13.22781	0.0036
miR-505-3p	-21.45293	0.042
miR-532-3p	-16.70047	0.007
miR-629-5p	-30.33645	0.0015
miR-660-5p	-16.14743	0.0089
miR-766-3p	-3.76456	0.0436

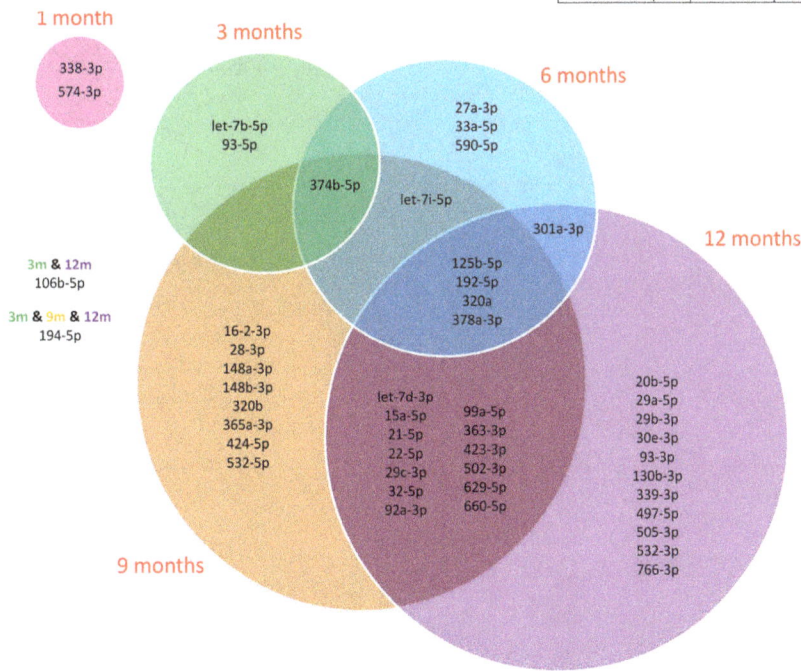

Fig. 1 Circulating microRNAs significantly deregulated following RYGB. (Top) Circulating microRNAs significantly differentiated at 1 month, 3 months, 6 months, 9 months and 12 months following RYGB. Statistical significance was determined by Student's t-test with Sidak-Bonferroni correction for multiple comparisons. (Bottom) A Venn diagram illustrating which significantly differentiated microRNAs are unique and shared between timepoints following RYGB

relative to preoperative levels. At 3 months only 1 microRNA was significantly increased and 4 microRNAs were significantly decreased relative to preoperative levels. The number of differentiated microRNAs continued to increase with each sequential timepoint following RYGB, rising to 10 at 6 months (4 increased, 6 decreased). At 9 months the expression of 28 microRNAs were significantly altered (1 increased, 27 decreased) and at 12 months 31 microRNAs were significantly altered (1 increased, 30 decreased) compared to preoperative expression. A series of volcano plots of circulating microRNA expression at each postoperative timepoint relative to preoperative levels can be found in Fig. 2.

These changes in circulating microRNA expression following RYGB were broadly characterized into 2 types of temporal response. The first early response was characterized by microRNAs whose expression was significantly different in the first months following RYGB before reverting to the preoperative baseline at the later months. MicroRNAs that followed this pattern included miR 338-3p, miR 93-5p and miR 590, whose levels significantly decreased in the early months following surgery, as well as miR 547-3p, miR 27a and mR 33a, whose levels increased (Fig. 3). However, most microRNAs differentially expressed following RYGB remained unchanged in the early months following surgery. Compared to preoperative levels of expression, their expression significantly altered 6 or 9 months following surgery and this was maintained and in some cases enhanced at 12 months. These microRNAs comprised the sustained late response. The most prominent microRNA that followed this pattern was miR 15a, whose expression at 3 months and 6 months remained comparable to preoperative levels but at 9 months miR 15a levels decreased significantly 6.52 fold and decreased further to 85 fold at 12 months. Similar patterns were found with circulating levels of miR 125b, miR 378a, miR 192, miR 629 and miR 22-5p, all were

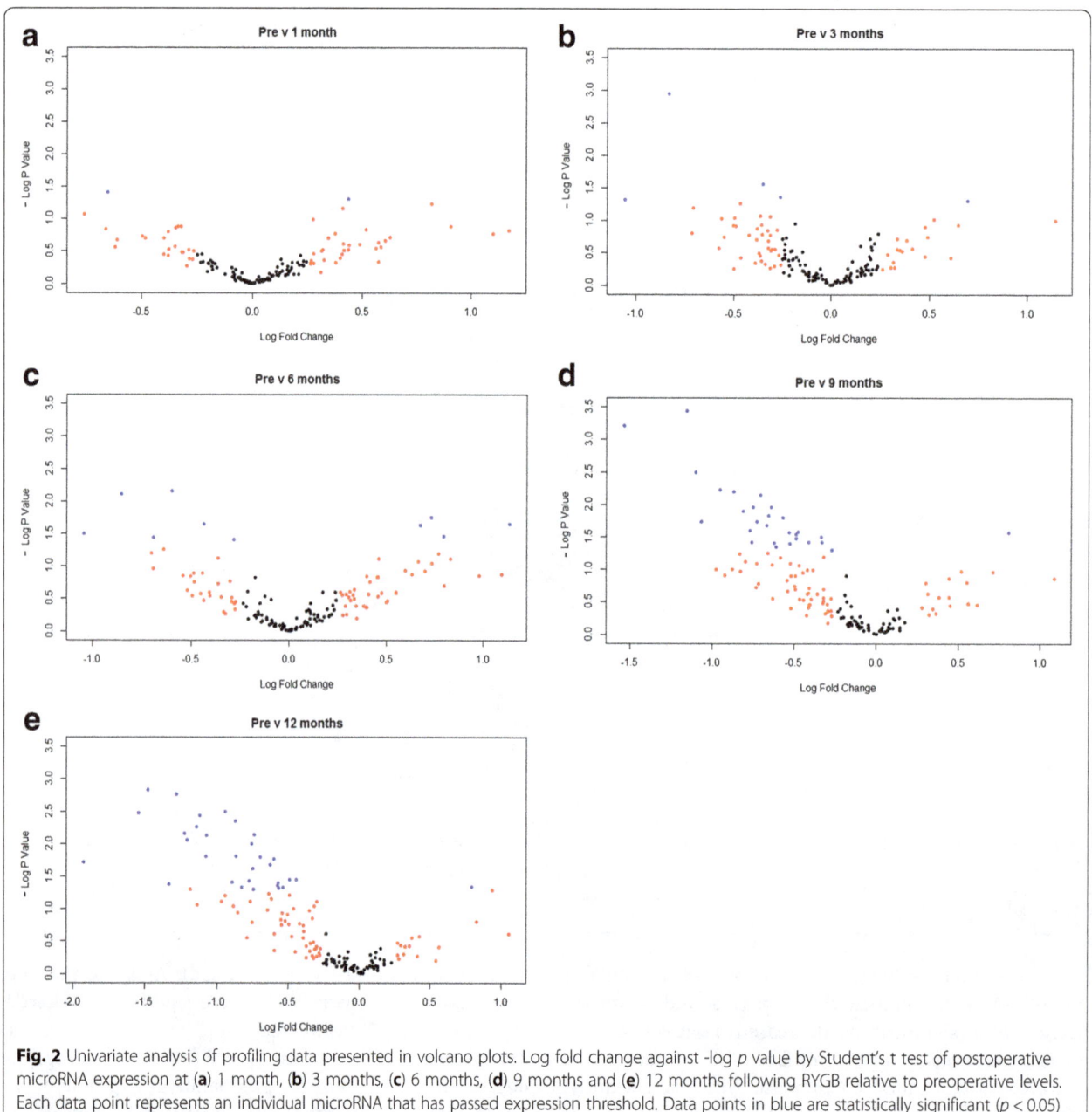

Fig. 2 Univariate analysis of profiling data presented in volcano plots. Log fold change against -log p value by Student's t test of postoperative microRNA expression at (a) 1 month, (b) 3 months, (c) 6 months, (d) 9 months and (e) 12 months following RYGB relative to preoperative levels. Each data point represents an individual microRNA that has passed expression threshold. Data points in blue are statistically significant ($p < 0.05$)

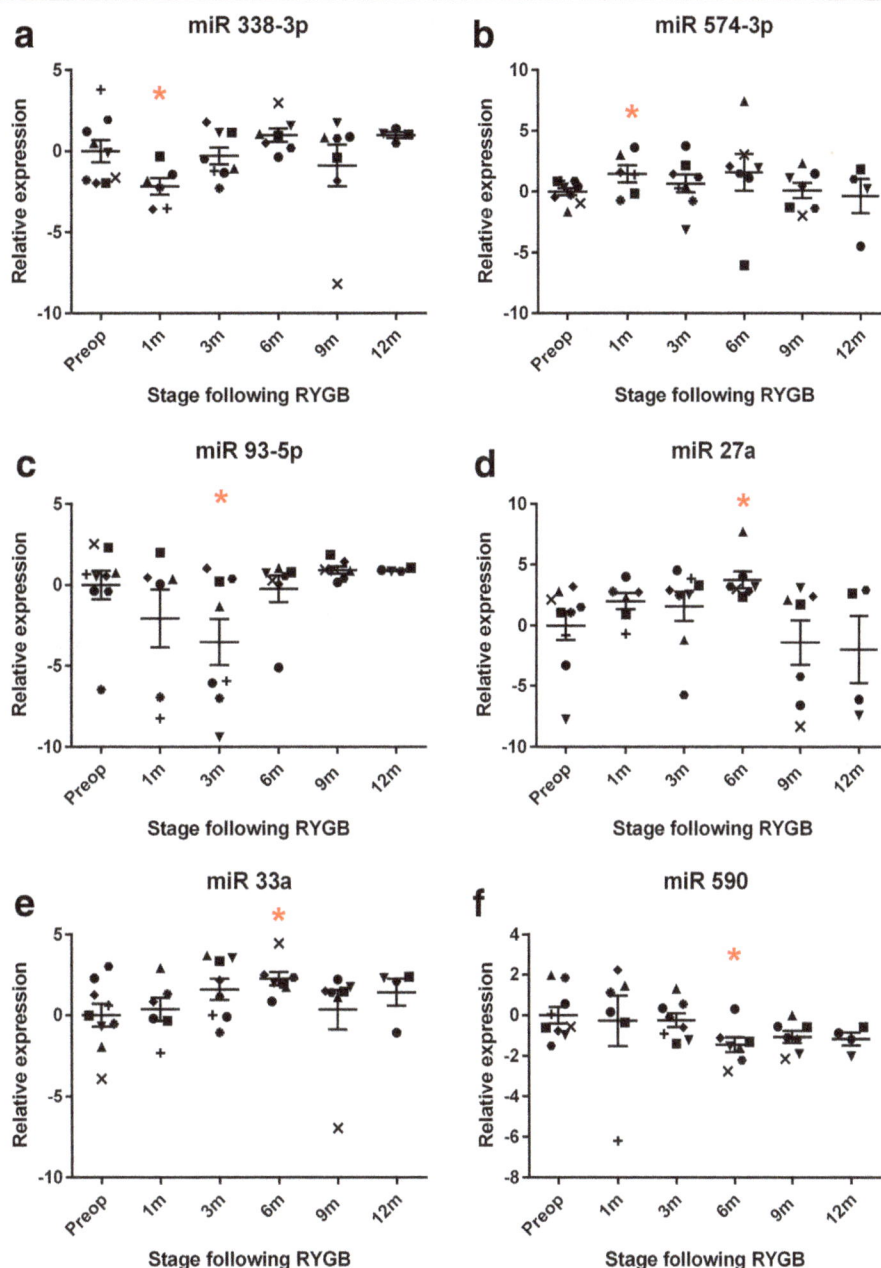

Fig. 3 The early bariatric circulating microRNA response showing temporal selectivity. Normalised logarithmic relative preoperative and postoperative expression of differentiated microRNAs. **a** miR 338-3p, (**b**) miR 574-3p, (**c**) miR 93-5p, (**d**) miR 27a, (**e**) miR 33a, (**f**) miR 590. Data represents mean ± standard error of mean. *$p < 0.05$ by Student's t test following Sidak-Bonferroni correction for multiple comparisons. Each patient is represented by a unique symbol

downregulated following RYGB (Fig. 4). All microRNAs whose expression was significantly different following RYGB are listed in Fig. 1 and all detected microRNA expression data is tabulated in Additional file 3: Table S1.

Correlations with clinical outcomes

Circulating microRNAs levels correlated with clinical measurements (Additional file 4: Table S2). A total of 16 microRNAs significantly correlated with BMI. Expression levels of seven microRNAs were positively correlated with BMI including miR 148a-3p and miR 125b. In contrast circulating levels of nine microRNAs demonstrated a negative correlation with BMI including miR 33a. The expression of 19 circulating microRNAs significantly correlated with the percentage of excess preoperative weight lost. All but two (miR 301a and miR 374b) correlated negatively. Nine microRNAs significantly correlated with fasting blood glucose, including miR 320a and miR

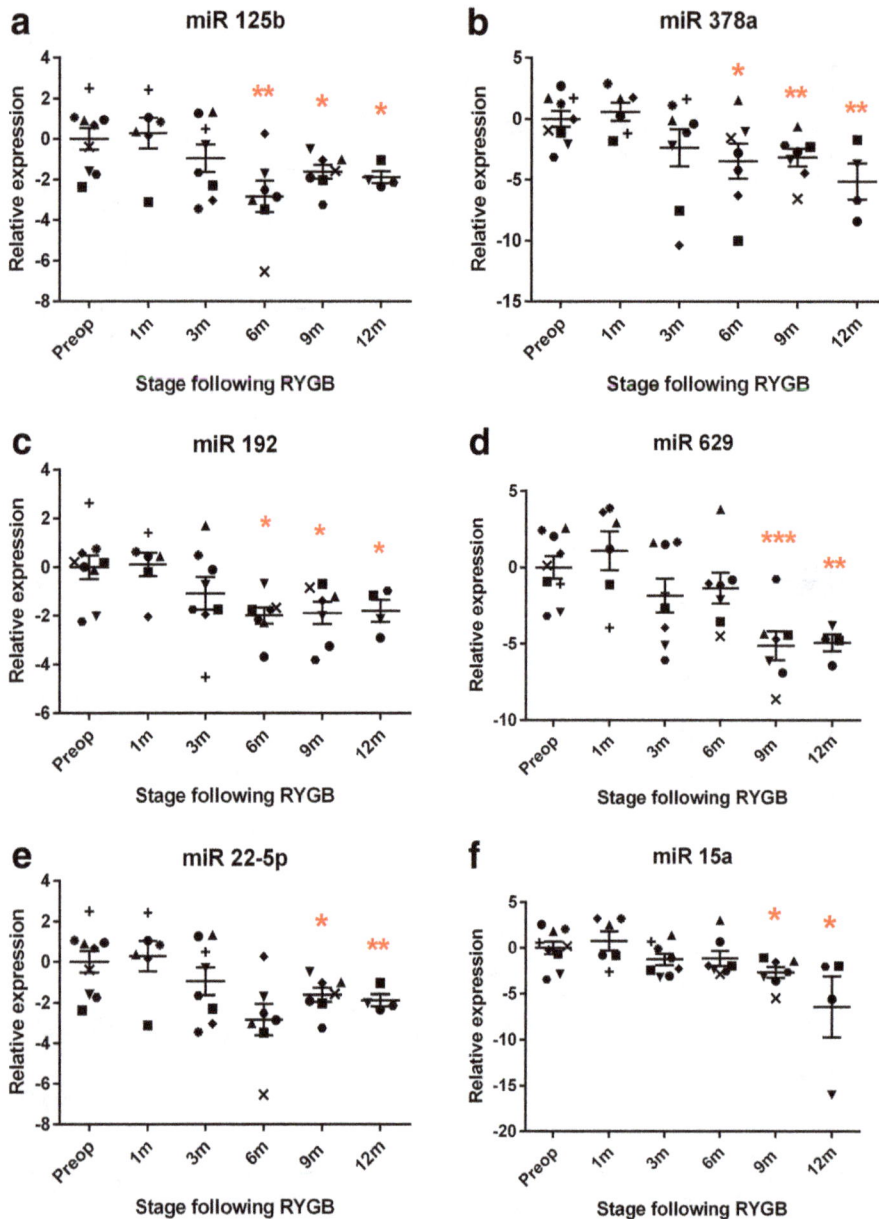

Fig. 4 The late bariatric circulating microRNA response showing progressive temporal selectivity. Normalised logarithmic relative preoperative and postoperative expression of differentiated microRNAs. **a** miR 125b, (**b**) miR 378a, (**c**) miR 192, (**d**) miR 629, (**e**) miR 22-5p and (**f**) miR 15a. Data represents mean ± standard error of mean. *$p < 0.05$, **$p < 0.01$, ***$p < 0.001$ by Student's t test following Sidak-Bonferroni correction for multiple comparisons. Each patient is represented by a unique symbol

590-5p. Only one microRNA (miR 346) correlated positively with fasting blood glucose levels. Additionally, 17 microRNAs significantly correlated with age.

Pathway analysis

To determine the potential biological consequences of changes in the expression of circulating microRNAs that made up the early and late post-bariatric responses, their mRNA targets and associated metabolic pathways were predicted using miRWalk and PANTHER bioinformatics (Fig. 5). The regulation of pathways involved in cell growth and proliferation, inflammation and neurological processes were predicted in both the early and late stages of response. The early response was also characterized by the predicted regulation of insulin/IGF pathways and the PI3 kinase pathway. Predicted pathways unique to the late stage of response were the cholecystokinin receptor pathway, α/β-adrenergic receptor pathway, cadherin signaling and the VEGF signaling pathway.

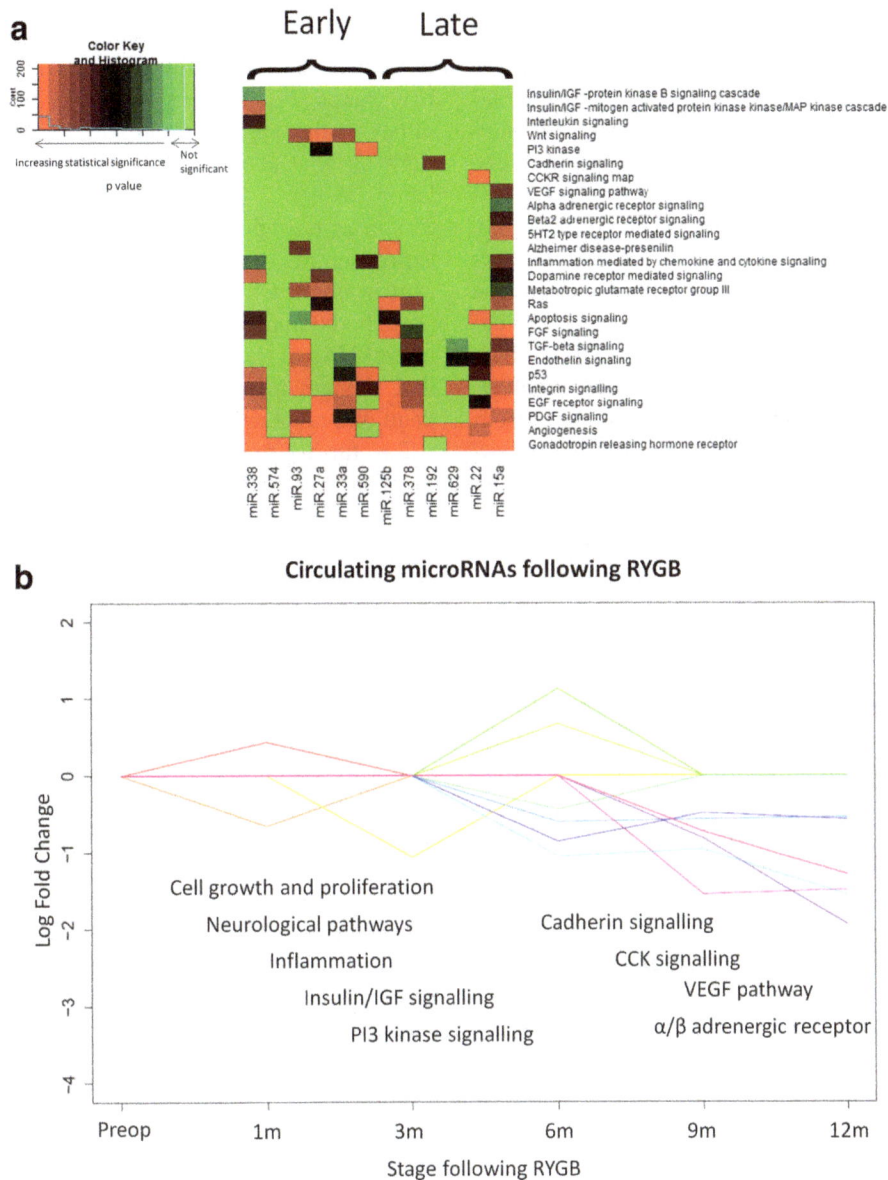

Fig. 5 Pathway analysis. **a** Comparative heatmap of p values of pathways predicted to be regulated by microRNAs in the early and late response following RYGB. Increasing statistical significance is indicated by the shift in colour from green to red. **b** The circulating microRNA response following RYGB and some of the biological processes they're predicted to regulate. Each line and shade of colour represents a circulating microRNA in the early and late microRNA responses following RYGB

Discussion

We have shown for the first time that RYGB persistently and progressively modulates circulating microRNA expression in a temporal manner with an increasing departure in profile from the preoperative obese state. In total, RYGB led to the differentiated expression of 48 circulating microRNAs typified by the selective, time-dependent differential expression of specific microRNAs. A temporary, immediate response is followed by a longer-lasting late response.

The circulating microRNAs whose expression is modified following RYGB are predicted to regulate cell growth, inflammation and neurological processes, and at the later months receptor pathways involved in gut hormone signaling, lipolysis and diabetic kidney disease. Although pathway analysis was largely predicted computationally, many of the circulating microRNAs whose expression is modified by RYGB have been experimentally linked with the metabolic syndrome. MiR 93, shown here to be decreased in the first few months following surgery, inhibits glucose transport and is overexpressed in insulin-resistant women with polycystic ovary syndrome [19]. MiR 27, another member of the early bariatric microRNA response, is a reported promoter of adipogenesis [20]. MiR 15a, decreased an astonishing 85 fold 1 year following surgery, also promotes adipogenesis [21] and miR 192 has a central regulatory role in diabetic nephropathy [22]. The altered expression of these microRNAs following RYGB may explain some of the mechanisms behind the health benefits associated with bariatric surgery.

The early postoperative months demonstrated the fewest changes in circulating microRNA expression, but the number increased longitudinally. Interestingly, as illustrated by the PCA scores plot of circulating microRNA profiles (Additional file 2: Figure S2), at 1 month following RYGB the microRNA circulating profile shifts from the preoperative profile, before a pronounced and gradual trajectory shift in the opposite direction from 3 months onwards. A possible explanation is that the initial physiological response to bariatric surgery was homeostatic as the body attempted to maintain the *status quo*. There is increasing evidence to suggest microRNAs help to maintain system robustness, fine-tuning or 'buffering' gene expression in response to subtle internal or external stimuli [23]. However, once a tipping point has been reached this homeostatic safety mechanism was adjusted and reset, moving the individual physiologically and phenotypically further from the morbidly obese state. In essence, this progressive timeline shift of circulating microRNA expression reveals a view of the physiological trajectory of bariatric surgery.

Many of the circulating microRNAs whose expression has been found to be altered by RYGB in the current study have also been reported as circulating biomarkers of T2DM, including of miR 15a, miR 192, miR 130b and miR 125b [24–26]. The loss of circulating miR 126 in particular is reportedly a strong selector for T2DM [25]. MiR 126 expression increased over 10 fold in each of the first 4 postoperative time points relative to preoperative levels, although none of the increases reached statistical significance (Additional file 3: Table S1). Importantly, fasting blood glucose levels positivity correlated with circulating miR 320a (Additional file 3: Table S2), consistent with previous findings [26] and supporting its candidacy as a novel diabetic biomarker. Circulating expression of miR 320a also correlated negatively with weight loss. In total, circulating levels of 9 microRNAs significantly correlated with fasting blood glucose levels. Correlations between circulating microRNAs levels and age were also found, supporting previous studies that show age impacts microRNA levels [27].

Although previous studies [9, 11, 12] have reported that bariatric surgery leads to changes in the expression of circulating microRNAs, these were time snapshots and lacked the temporal dependencies we have uncovered in the present longitudinal study. Lirun et al. looked at the effect of Roux-en-Y gastric bypass on circulating microRNAs 3 months postoperatively in diabetic patients, divided into a low BMI and high BMI preoperative groups [11]. They reported that 39 microRNAs were differentially expressed after surgery across both groups. Both *Lirun* et al. and our study reported the downregulation of let 7, miR 93 and miR 106b expression 3 months postoperatively, while the decrease in miR 16 expression at 3 months in *Lirun* et al. was only significant in our study after 9 months. Interestingly, they reported differences in the postoperative changes in microRNAs in the low and high BMI groups, suggesting that changes in microRNAs following surgery may depend on preoperative conditions.

Two further studies assessed circulating microRNA expression before and 12 months after RYGB. Ortega et al. [9] reported a significant modulation of 14 circulating microRNAs including decreases in miR 125b and miR 16 and an increase in miR 221, mirroring our findings (miR 211 increased across all postoperative timepoints, albeit not significantly). However, they also reported significant increases in the circulating levels of miR 130b and miR 21. The expression of both microRNAs were significantly decreased in our study 12 months following RYGB. Ortega et al. were also unable to detect a change in miR 15a following surgery. In another study, Hubal et al. reported the modified expression of 168 exosome-derived circulating microRNAs 1 year following RYGB and illustrated a correlation between altered microRNAs and improvements in insulin resistance [12]. Filtering for microRNAs with validated targets in insulin signaling or that correlated with changes insulin resistance, they identified several surgery-responsive microRNAs, including miR 125b and miR 122. However, it is important to reiterate that each of these previous studies measured circulating microRNAs at a single postoperative timepoint and are therefore merely snapshots of a dramatically altering physiology. Our longitudinal study emphasizes that the post-bariatric surgery circulating microRNAome and associated changes of physiology are both dynamic.

In rats, circulating levels of miR 122 decrease 60 fold following RYGB compared to sham-operated animals [15]. MiR 122 is a liver microRNA responsible for regulating lipid metabolism [28] and its decrease leads to increased glucose transportation, accelerated glycolysis and the inhibition of gluconeogenesis following RYGB [15]. This is consistent with the recent discovery that RYGB reprograms intestinal glucose metabolism by increasing glycolysis and glucose uptake [29], and suggests miR 122 could contribute to this effect. The present study also found a consistent decrease in circulating miR 122 in humans following RYGB from 3 months onwards, although this did not achieve statistical significance (Additional file 3: Table S1). Other microRNAs that decreased following RYGB in rats include miR 93, miR 30e and miR 320 [15] and we report significant decreases in the human orthologs of these microRNAs in our study.

The role of microRNAs following bariatric surgery remains relatively unexplored and offers potential insights into the dynamic physiological changes that follow surgical intervention. Our study, as with the few that have preceded it, was limited to a small number of participating individuals and should be considered a pilot study at this stage. Additionally, not all subjects provided samples at all post-operative timepoints. Nevertheless, our study confirms the proof of principle that analysis of circulating microRNAs offers insight into the dynamic physiological changes associated with bariatric intervention. Well-designed, multi-center studies with larger diabetes subsets, non-bariatric obese and lean control groups and more robust clinical follow-ups and endpoints would provide a clearer picture into the role microRNAs play following bariatric surgery. Although the field is still in its infancy, bariatric surgery has been consistently shown to significantly alter circulating microRNA levels. MicroRNA expression profiles offer a wealth of biological information and mechanistic insights, as the changes in the regulation of several core physiological processes are related to the expression of the microRNAs that regulate them. MicroRNAs can act as mediators or effectors in positive and negative feedback loops in wider regulation networks. Their presence in circulation in exosomes and high-density lipoprotein or argonaute complexes that can be taken up in an active form by recipient cells is also suggestive of a potential tissue-to-tissue communicative role and that microRNAs may have hormonal as well as biomarker potential [30].

Conclusions

We have shown here that RYGB fundamentally alters microRNA expression in the circulation in a temporal manner with an increasing departure from the preoperative state. These microRNAs correlate with the beneficial physiological and metabolic fluxes seen after these operations and they therefore represent potentially novel post-surgical biomarkers of surgical outcomes. There is ongoing debate on updating the criteria for bariatric surgery, in recognition of its ability to improve health beyond weight loss. MicroRNA expression profiles could potentially add another facet for consideration in the decision-pathway for bariatric operations and offer additional opportunity for developing the next generation of combined multi-modal metabolic interventions to enhance the treatment outcomes for obesity and its associated disorders.

Abbreviations
BMI: Body mass index; CV: Coefficient of variances; LNA: Locked nucleic acid; mRNA: Messenger ribonucleic acid; NICE: National Institute of Health and Care Excellence; PCA: Principal component analysis; RYGB: Roux-en-Y Gastric Bypass; T2DM: Type 2 diabetes mellitus

Funding
This study was financially supported by a PhD studentship awarded to A.A. funded by the State of Kuwait.

Authors' contributions
All authors contributed to the conceptual design of this study. AA performed the data collection and analysis. AA, HA and NJG contributed to the interpretation of the data and drafting the article. AA, HA, TS, PS, AD, EH, TA, SLA and NJG were all involved in the critical evaluation and final approval of the article.

Competing interests
The authors declare that they have no competing interests.

Author details
[1]Department of Surgery and Cancer, Imperial College London, London, UK. [2]Clinical Trials Unit, Dasman Diabetes Institute, PO Box 1180, Dasman, 15462 Kuwait City, Kuwait. [3]Department of Bariatric and Metabolic Surgery, Chelsea and Westminster NHS Foundation Trust, London, UK. [4]Department of Academic Endocrinology, Diabetes and Metabolism, Hull York Medical School, Hull, UK. [5]Division of Upper Gastrointestinal and Minimally Invasive Surgery, Hull and East Yorkshire Hospitals NHS Trust, Hull, UK. [6]Weill Cornell Medical College Qatar, Qatar Foundation, Doha, Qatar.

References
1. Sjöström L. Review of the key results from the Swedish obese subjects (SOS) trial – a prospective controlled intervention study of bariatric surgery. J Intern Med. 2013;273(3):219–34.
2. Ashrafian H, Bueter M, Ahmed K, Suliman A, Bloom SR, Darzi A, Athanasiou T. Metabolic surgery: an evolution through bariatric animal models. Obes Rev. 2010;11(12):907–20.
3. Li JV, Ashrafian H, Bueter M, Kinross J, Sands C, le Roux CW, Bloom SR, Darzi A, Athanasiou T, Marchesi JR, et al. Metabolic surgery profoundly influences gut microbial-host metabolic cross-talk. Gut. 2011;60(9):1214–23.
4. Krol J, Loedige I, Filipowicz W. The widespread regulation of microRNA biogenesis, function and decay. Nat Rev Genet. 2010;11(9):597–610.
5. Arner P, Kulyte A. MicroRNA regulatory networks in human adipose tissue and obesity. Nat Rev Endocrinol. 2015;11(5):276–88.
6. Creemers EE, Tijsen AJ, Pinto YM. Circulating MicroRNAs: novel biomarkers and extracellular communicators in cardiovascular disease? Circ Res. 2012; 110(3):483–95.

7. Mitchell PS, Parkin RK, Kroh EM, Fritz BR, Wyman SK, Pogosova-Agadjanyan EL, Peterson A, Noteboom J, O'Briant KC, Allen A, et al. Circulating microRNAs as stable blood-based markers for cancer detection. Proc Natl Acad Sci U S A. 2008;105(30):10513–8.

8. Sharkey JW, Antoine DJ, Park BK. Validation of the isolation and quantification of kidney enriched miRNAs for use as biomarkers. Biomarkers. 2012;17(3):231–9.

9. Ortega FJ, Mercader JM, Catalan V, Moreno-Navarrete JM, Pueyo N, Sabater M, Gomez-Ambrosi J, Anglada R, Fernandez-Formoso JA, Ricart W, et al. Targeting the circulating microRNA signature of obesity. Clin Chem. 2013;59(5):781–92.

10. Guay C, Regazzi R. Circulating microRNAs as novel biomarkers for diabetes mellitus. Nat Rev Endocrinol. 2013;9(9):513–21.

11. Lirun K, Sewe M, Yong W, Pilot Study A. The effect of roux-en-Y gastric bypass on the serum MicroRNAs of the type 2 diabetes patient. Obes Surg. 2015;25(12):2386–92.

12. Hubal MJ, Nadler EP, Ferrante SC, Barberio MD, Suh JH, Wang J, Dohm GL, Pories WJ, Mietus-Snyder M, Freishtat RJ. Circulating adipocyte-derived exosomal MicroRNAs associated with decreased insulin resistance after gastric bypass. Obesity (Silver Spring). 2017;25(1):102–10.

13. Obesity: NICE Clinical Guideline 43. 2015. [http://www.nice.org.uk/CG43].

14. miRCURY LNA Universal RT microRNA PCR. 2016. [https://www.exiqon.com/ls/Documents/Scientific/Universal-RT-microRNA-PCR-manual-serum.pdf].

15. Wu Q, Li JV, Seyfried F, le Roux CW, Ashrafian H, Athanasiou T, Fenske W, Darzi A, Nicholson JK, Holmes E, et al. Metabolic phenotype-microRNA data fusion analysis of the systemic consequences of Roux-en-Y gastric bypass surgery. Int J Obes (Lond). 2015;39:1126–34.

16. Vandesompele J, De Preter K, Pattyn F, Poppe B, Van Roy N, De Paepe A, Speleman F. Accurate normalization of real-time quantitative RT-PCR data by geometric averaging of multiple internal control genes. Genome Biol. 2002;3(7):RESEARCH0034.

17. Andersen CL, Jensen JL, Orntoft TF. Normalization of real-time quantitative reverse transcription-PCR data: a model-based variance estimation approach to identify genes suited for normalization, applied to bladder and colon cancer data sets. Cancer Res. 2004;64(15):5245–50.

18. Mestdagh P, Van Vlierberghe P, De Weer A, Muth D, Westermann F, Speleman F, Vandesompele J. A novel and universal method for microRNA RT-qPCR data normalization. Genome Biol. 2009;10(6):R64.

19. Chen YH, Heneidi S, Lee JM, Layman LC, Stepp DW, Gamboa GM, Chen BS, Chazenbalk G, Azziz R. miRNA-93 inhibits GLUT4 and is overexpressed in adipose tissue of polycystic ovary syndrome patients and women with insulin resistance. Diabetes. 2013;62(7):2278–86.

20. Sun L, Trajkovski M. MiR-27 orchestrates the transcriptional regulation of brown adipogenesis. Metabolism. 2014;63(2):272–82.

21. Dong P, Mai Y, Zhang Z, Mi L, Wu G, Chu G, Yang G, Sun S. MiR-15a/b promote adipogenesis in porcine pre-adipocyte via repressing FoxO1. Acta Biochim Biophys Sin. 2014;46(7):565–71.

22. Krupa A, Jenkins R, Luo DD, Lewis A, Phillips A, Fraser D. Loss of MicroRNA-192 promotes fibrogenesis in diabetic nephropathy. Journal of the American Society of Nephrology : JASN. 2010;21(3):438–47.

23. Ebert MS, Sharp PA. Roles for microRNAs in conferring robustness to biological processes. Cell. 2012;149(3):515–24.

24. Ortega FJ, Mercader JM, Moreno-Navarrete JM, Rovira O, Guerra E, Esteve E, Xifra G, Martinez C, Ricart W, Rieusset J, et al. Profiling of circulating microRNAs reveals common microRNAs linked to type 2 diabetes that change with insulin sensitization. Diabetes Care. 2014;37(5):1375–83.

25. Zampetaki A, Kiechl S, Drozdov I, Willeit P, Mayr U, Prokopi M, Mayr A, Weger S, Oberhollenzer F, Bonora E, et al. Plasma microRNA profiling reveals loss of endothelial miR-126 and other microRNAs in type 2 diabetes. Circ Res. 2010;107(6):810–7.

26. Karolina DS, Tavintharan S, Armugam A, Sepramaniam S, Pek SL, Wong MT, Lim SC, Sum CF, Jeyaseelan K. Circulating miRNA profiles in patients with metabolic syndrome. J Clin Endocrinol Metab. 2012;97(12):E2271–6.

27. Ameling S, Kacprowski T, Chilukoti RK, Malsch C, Liebscher V, Suhre K, Pietzner M, Friedrich N, Homuth G, Hammer E, et al. Associations of circulating plasma microRNAs with age, body mass index and sex in a population-based study. BMC Med Genet. 2015;8:61.

28. Esau C, Davis S, Murray SF, Yu XX, Pandey SK, Pear M, Watts L, Booten SL, Graham M, McKay R, et al. miR-122 regulation of lipid metabolism revealed by in vivo antisense targeting. Cell Metab. 2006;3(2):87–98.

29. Saeidi N, Meoli L, Nestoridi E, Gupta NK, Kvas S, Kucharczyk J, Bonab AA, Fischman AJ, Yarmush ML, Stylopoulos N. Reprogramming of intestinal glucose metabolism and glycemic control in rats after gastric bypass. Science. 2013;341(6144):406–10.

30. Cortez MA, Bueso-Ramos C, Ferdin J, Lopez-Berestein G, Sood AK, Calin GA. MicroRNAs in body fluids–the mix of hormones and biomarkers. Nat Rev Clin Oncol. 2011;8(8):467–77.

20

Association of Metabolic Markers with self-reported osteoarthritis among middle-aged BMI-defined non-obese individuals: a cross-sectional study

Kelsey H. Collins[1]*[†], Behnam Sharif[2]*[†] ⬤, Raylene A. Reimer[3], Claudia Sanmartin[4], Walter Herzog[1], Rick Chin[5] and Deborah A. Marshall[2]

Abstract

Background: Osteoarthritis (OA) is a chronic degenerative joint disease. While it is well-established that obesity affects OA through increased axial loading on the joint cartilage, the indirect effect of obesity through metabolic processes among the body mass index (BMI)-defined non-obese population, i.e., BMI < 30 kg/m^2, is less known. Our goal was to evaluate the association of metabolic markers including body fat percentage (BF%), waist circumference, maximum weight gain during adulthood and serum creatinine with self-reported OA to establish if such measures offer additional information over BMI among the non-obese population between 40 and 65 years of age.

Methods: Cross-sectional data from two cycles of the Canadian Health Measures Survey (CHMS) in 2007–2009 and 2009–2011 were analyzed. Sex-specific logistic regression models were developed to evaluate the association of self-reported OA with metabolic markers. Models were separately adjusted for age, BMI categories and serum creatinine, and a stratified analysis across BM categories was performed. In a secondary analysis, we evaluated the association of self-reported OA, cardiovascular diseases and hypertension across BF% categories.

Results: Of 2462 individuals, 217 (8.8%) self-reported OA. After adjusting for age and BMI, those within BF%-defined overweight/obese category had 2.67 (95% CI: 1.32–3.51) and 2.11(95% CI: 1.38–3.21) times higher odds of reporting self-reported OA compared to those within BF%-defined athletic/acceptable category for females and males, respectively. BF% was also significantly associated with self-reported OA after adjusting for age and serum creatinine only among females (OR: 1.47, 95%CI: 1.12–1.84). Furthermore, among the BMI-defined overweight group, the age-adjusted odds of self-reported OA was significantly higher for overweight/obese BF% compared to athletic/acceptable BF% in both females and males. In a secondary analysis, we showed that the association of self-reported OA and hypertension/cardiovascular diseases is significantly higher among BF% overweight/obese (OR: 1.37, 95%CI: 1.19–3.09) compared to BF% athletic/acceptable (OR: 1.13, 95%CI: 0.87–2.82).

Conclusion: Our results provide corroborating evidence for a relationship between body fat and OA in a population-based study, while no significant independent correlates were found between other metabolic markers and OA prevalence. Future investigation on the longitudinal relationship between BF and OA among this sub-population may inform targeted prevention opportunities.

Keywords: Osteoarthritis, Obesity, Adipose tissue, Metabolic markers, Body fat, Population-based survey

* Correspondence: Khmcolli@ucalgary.ca; behnam.sharif@ucalgary.ca
[†]Kelsey H. Collins and Behnam Sharif contributed equally to this work.
[1]Human Performance Laboratory, University of Calgary, Calgary, AB, Canada
[2]Department of Community Health Sciences, University of Calgary, 3280 Hospital Drive NW, Calgary, AB T2N 4Z6, Canada
Full list of author information is available at the end of the article

Introduction

Osteoarthritis (OA) is a multifactorial degenerative joint disease affecting more than 1 in 8 individuals worldwide [1]. OA is among the fastest growing causes of loss in Disability Adjusted Life Years (DALYs) [2] mainly because of the aging population and increasing incidence of obesity [1, 2]. Obesity is conventionally measured using body mass index (BMI), and several studies have shown that individuals with obesity according to a BMI ≥ 30 are at higher risk for developing radiographic and symptomatic OA [1, 3]. Previous studies have shown that measurements of body composition and fat distribution may offer no advantage over BMI in assessment of risk for severe radiographic knee OA among the obese population [4, 5]. However, there is a paucity of research evaluating the independent association of metabolic markers and OA prevalence among a non-obese population [6].

Previous studies suggested that the initiation and progression of OA results from a complex interaction between mechanical axial loading on joints and various lipid, metabolic, and humoral risk factors [7–10]. Furthermore, recent findings on the significant association of body fat distribution with OA in non-weight bearing joints suggests that obesity-associated systemic factors could play an important role in the development and progression of OA [11–15]. Brasnjevic et al. [16] showed that abdominal obesity was associated with radiographic progression of knee OA, and in a large Japanese cohort study, accumulation of metabolic syndrome components was related to the incidence and progression of knee OA components [17]. Preclinical models in rats also suggested a role of chronic inflammation, likely from metabolic stress, in OA onset and progression [18–22].

Muscle weakness has also been identified as a key factor affecting OA onset and progression that further emphasizes the role for body composition, body fat distribution and OA development [23–27]. In a population-based study, Ding et al. [24] noted a link between muscle weakness and body fat with OA, and found that the additive effects of muscle weakness and body fat increase the relative risk of OA compared to age and sex matched controls. Serum creatinine levels have been used as a surrogate measure for muscle mass in patients with chronic diseases [28, 29] and are also associated with lean mass in healthy individuals [30].

Several studies have also demonstrated that overweight (BMI between 25 to 30 kg/m^2) during middle adulthood may play an important role in OA's initiation and progression [31, 32]. Furthermore, OA management strategies and obesity prevention interventions [33] are most effective in the long-run when they are targeted to patients with overweight (BMI-defined non-obese) at early stages of the disease process [34]. As such, Manninen et al. [35] highlights the need to identify candidates for OA prevention and management strategies in the middle-aged and the non-obese.

The purpose of this study was to investigate the independent association between metabolic markers and self-reported OA among middle-aged BMI-defined non-obese individuals (40 to 65 years of age and BMI < 30 kg/m^2). As such, we focus on measurements that are low-cost, ready to be implemented, and widely used in large population-based study cohorts including skinfold measured body fat, waist circumference and weight gained since adulthood. As the study population may not be assessed for OA prevalence at this time, the use of such metrics may be a feasible approach to support data collection and potential screening for adiposity and OA prevalence in this population who may not otherwise be assessed [35].

Methods

Data source and population

The Canadian Health Measures Survey (CHMS) is a bi-annual survey of Canadians health and health habits [36]. In the CHMS, Statistics Canada collects data from a nationally representative sample of the Canadian population aged 6–79 years living in private households in which approximately 96% of Canadians were represented [37]. CHMS is the first comprehensive and representative direct health measures study in Canada since the 1978–1979 Canada Health Survey [37].

The survey involved two components: an interview in the respondent's home and a visit to a mobile examination center for a series of physical and clinical measurements. In all cycles of CHMS, data were collected at 15 sites across Canada. The interview included questions from respondents about a range of chronic conditions, defined as a condition diagnosed by a health professional and lasting, or expected to last, more than 6 months including OA, type 2 diabetes, and heart disease. Clinical and physical measures at an examination center included anthropometry, blood pressure, oral health examination, and blood and urine specimens [37]. Ethics approval to conduct the CHMS was obtained from Health Canada's Research Ethics Board. Informed written consent was obtained from all adult respondents.

Sample selection

In this study, we used two cycles of the CHMS: 2007–2009, and 2009–2011. Health measures were included from both cycles. As our aim was to evaluate the relationship between body composition measurements and OA in non-obese middle-aged individuals, we included individuals between ages 40 to 65 years with BMI < 30 kg/m^2. Individuals were not included if data were missing due to invalid BMI measurement, invalid skinfold measurements or if there were no body fat data collected. Figure 1 depicts the diagram of the sample selection from two cycles of CHMS included in this study.

Primary outcome

Osteoarthritis was determined from a patient reported response to the survey question about the physician-diagnosed arthritis: what kind of arthritis do you have? 1. Rheumatoid arthritis, 2. Osteoarthritis, 3. Rheumatism, or 4. Other. As a result, self-reported physician diagnosed OA was used as the outcome.

Metabolic markers

The measures used in this study were selected according to the metrics used in the literature for OA patients [4–7], which are low-cost, readily available and have been validated in population-based studies. Height was measured to the nearest 0.1 cm and weight was measured to the nearest 0.1 kg by standard devices on each mobile examination center [36]. BMI was calculated and classified according to standardized thresholds: normal (18.5 to 24.9 kg/m^2), overweight (25.0 to 29.9 kg/m^2) [36]. To determine the body fat, body density was first calculated using the summation of skinfold measures at four sites (triceps, biceps, subscapula, and iliac crest). Once body density was determined, body fat was calculated using a general sex-specific equation previously derived and validated by Durnin et al. [38]. Individual body fat percentages (BF%) were grouped into two body fat categories according to their distributions: athletic/acceptable (males:

≤20% females ≤30%), or overweight/obese (male > 20% females > 30%). This skinfold caliper technique is only validated for use in a population with BMI < 30 kg/m^2, and as such, evaluating it excludes individuals who are obese by BMI [7].

Waist circumference was measured between the last rib and the top of the iliac crest after an expiration to the nearest 0.1 cm [36]. Waist circumference categories was defined according to standard thresholds used for females (> 88 cm and < 88 cm) and those for males (> 102 cm and < 102 cm) [39]. Maximum weight gain during adulthood was derived by subtracting "most adult weight ever" from the "weight at 18 years of age". Previous studies have also examined maximum weight gain during adulthood in assessing risk of chronic diseases [40]. Laboratory Serum creatinine measures (μmol/L) were used as a surrogate for muscle mass [41]. Threshold for definition of high and low value of serum creatinine was used from [41] in which high values were defined as those with ≥65 μmol/L among males and ≥ 73 μmol/L among females.

Comorbidity assessments

We also extracted data on cardiovascular (CVD)-related comorbidities which included self-reported measures on history of heart disease, heart attack or high blood pressure. These were assessed using a response to three CHMS household questionnaire: (i) CCC_Q61: Do you have heart disease (1) Yes (0) No or (ii)CCC_Q63: Have you had a heart attack? (1) Yes (0) No, or (iii) CCC_Q64: Do you have high blood pressure?, (1) Yes (0) No.

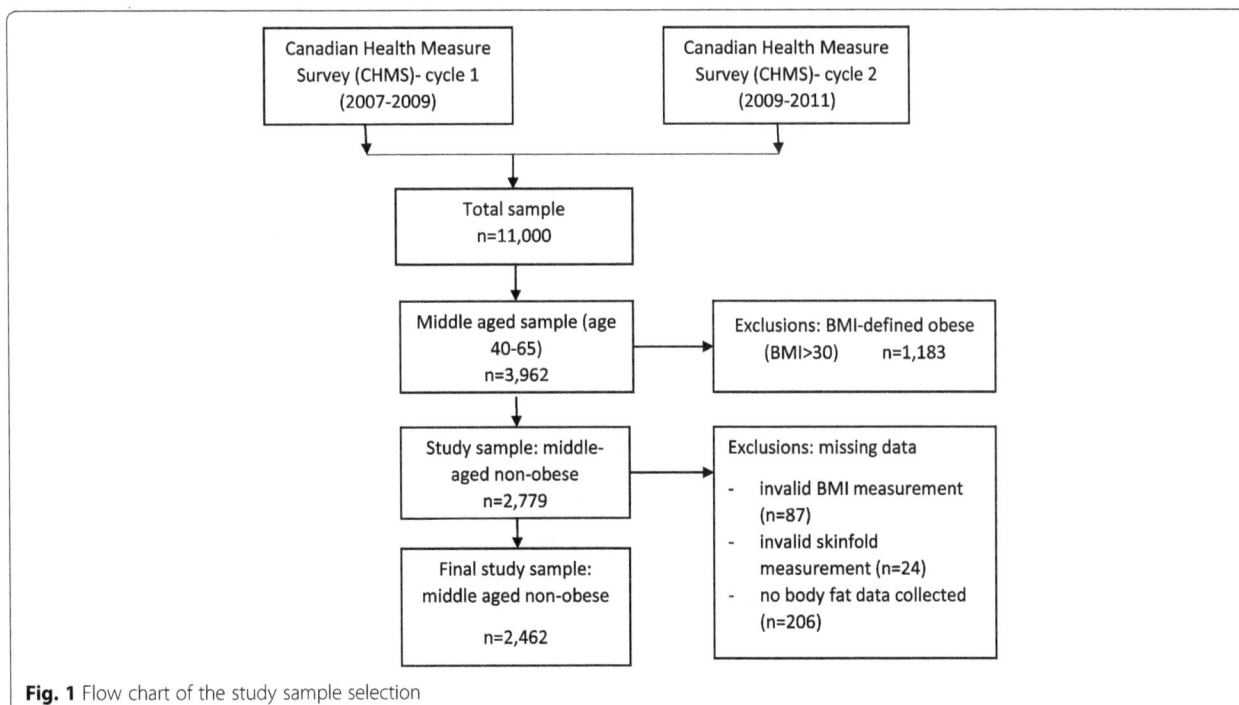

Fig. 1 Flow chart of the study sample selection

Clinical measurement for blood creatinine was also included as an indirect assessment of muscle mass (μmol/L). The sample size for responses to other chronic conditions including diabetes was small, and violated the minimal cell count prescribed by Statistics Canada, and therefore they were not included in the analysis.

Statistical analysis

All variables were assessed to ensure similarities in questions and responses. Cycles 1 and 2 were combined using methods described in the Statistics Canada documentation for combining the two CHMS datasets [36]. Quality assurance and quality control measures were previously performed independently on both CHMS datasets to minimize systematic bias [37]. Categorical variables were examined using frequency tables, and continuous variables were evaluated using summary statistics. If laboratory values were missing for blood creatinine, they were imputed using the level of detection limit divided by 2 [36]. Univariate analyses were conducted to investigate crude associations between the covariates and self-reported OA. In univariate analysis, p-values were based on an adjusted Pearson chi-squared test for independence (categorical variables), or a Bonferroni-adjusted Wald F-test (continuous variables). All results are weighted and standard errors are estimated using bootstrapping to account for the survey design effects of the CHMS. Kolmogorov–Smirnov tests were also performed to assess the normality of data for metabolic markers ($p < 0.05$). Multicollinearity diagnostics were performed by calculating variance inflation factor (VIF), which quantifies the severity of multicollinearity in an ordinary least squares regression analysis. VIF of BMI in all models were less than 2.6, which is below the threshold of 4 to represent multicollinearity.

Sex-stratified logistic regression models were developed to evaluate the association of self-reported OA with the five metabolic markers in this study. Models were separately adjusted for age, age and BMI, and age and blood creatinine levels in order to detect additional correlations that may exist between metabolic markers and self-reported OA. We further performed a stratified analysis across BMI groups to evaluate the independent association of BF% and self-reported OA among the BMI-defined overweight group and assess the additional information BF% could potentially provide other than those gained from BMI. In a secondary analysis, we developed logistic regression models to assess the association between OA and hypertension/CVD across BF% categories to identify the possible mediating role of the body fat on the association of OA and hypertension/CVD. Due to the small sample size within each cell for logistic regression modelling, and the limited age range in this sample of interest, no interactions with age or sex were included. All results were weighted according to

the survey weights to represent the population-based sampling scheme of the CHMS. To account for survey design effects of the CHMS, standard errors, coefficients of variation, and 95% confidence intervals were estimated using the bootstrap technique (500 replications) provided in the CHMS documentation[36].

Results

A total of 2462 individuals between 40 to 65 years of age with BMI < 30 were selected for the final analysis, of which 217 (8.8%) reported OA (Fig. 1). Kolmogorov–Smirnov tests revealed that BMI, BF%, waist circumference and maximum weight gain data were normally distributed ($p > 0.05$). As shown in Table 1, the proportion of females was significantly higher among the individuals with self-reported OA (77%, SE: 3.5) compared to the non-OA (49.5%, SE: 0.94). The average BF% of individuals with self-reported OA was also higher than those of the non-OA group among both men [28.1%, SE:0.5) vs. (23.2%, SE:0.3), $p < 0.01$] and women [30.2%, SE: 0.3) vs. 33.9%, SE:0.2, $p < 0.01$], while waist circumference was significantly higher only among men [89.0 cm (SE:0.5) vs. 93.0 cm (SE:1.1), $p < 0.01$]. Furthermore, higher proportion of the self-reported OA indicated at least one CVD-related comorbidity compared to that of the non-OA sample among males [12.4%, SE: 2. vs. 4.9%, SE: 0.6, p < 0.01] and females [9.1% (SE: 2.1) vs. 3.8% (SE:0.5)] and had lower blood creatinine among males [78.1 μmol/L (SE: 1.0) vs. 82.4 μmol/L (SE: 0.5), p = < 0.01] and females [67.3 μmol/L (SE:1.0) vs. 72.8 μmol/L (SE:0.5), $p = < 0.01$]. The detailed results for the count of individuals within each BF%, BMI and sex groups are provided in Additional file 1: Table S1.

As shown in Table 2 for the result of the multivariate analysis, higher BF% and waist circumference categories were significantly associated with self-reported OA, independent of age, for both males and females ($p < 0.05$). Those within the BF%-defined obese/overweight category had higher odds of self-reported OA compared to those within the BF%-defined athletic/acceptable category for females (OR: 3.2, 95% CI: 1.25–4.4) and males (OR: 1.82, 95% CI: 1.15–3.58) after adjusting for age. Similarly, those in the high waist circumference category had significantly higher odds of self-reported OA compared to those in the low category for both females (OR: 2.62, 95% CI: 1.51–3.01) and males (OR: 2.21, 95% CI:1.3–3.81) after adjusting for age. Furthermore, among males, each kilogram of maximum weight gained was associated with 3% higher odds of self-reported OA independent of the current age (OR: 1.04, 95% CI: 1.02–1.76).

As shown in Table 2, only the BF%-defined obese/overweight category was associated with self-reported OA independent of BMI and age. The adjusted odds of self-reported OA was higher among overweight/

Table 1 Characteristics of individuals with self-reported osteoarthritis (OA) compared to individuals without self-reported OA[a]

Characteristics [b]	Overall sample n = 2462	No Self-Reported OA n = 2245	Self-Reported OA n = 217	p-value[d]
Demographics				
Age (years), mean (SE[c])	52.6 (0.3)	52.2 (0.2)	57.3 (0.6)	< 0.001
Females, % (SE)	51 (1.2)	49.0 (0.9)	77.0 (3.5)	< 0.001
Metabolic Markers				
Females (n = 1267)				
Body Fat Percentage, mean (SE)	30.58 (0.3)	30.20 (0.2)	33.90 (0.3)	< 0.01
Body Mass Index (kg/m^2), mean (SE)	26.33 (0.5)	26.20(0.4)	27.25(1.0)	0.112
Waist Circumference (cm), mean (SE)	78.49(0.4)	78.23(0.4)	80.31(0.9)	0.08
Maximum Weight Change (kg), mean (SE)	19.06(0.4)	18.90(0.5)	20.70 (0.9)	0.12
Serum Creatinine (μmol/L), mean (SE)	71.6 (0.6)	72.8 (0.5)	67.3 (1.0)	< 0.01
Hypertension/CVD[e], % (SE)	3.9 (0.6)	3.8 (0.5)	9.1 (2.1)	< 0.01
Males (n = 1195)				
Body Fat Percentage, mean (SE)	23.67 (0.4)	23.2(0.3)	28.12(0.5)	< 0.01
Body Mass Index (kg/m^2), mean (SE)	27.47 (0.6)	27.10 (0.5)	28.90 (1.2)	0.318
Waist Circumference (cm), mean (SE)	89.53 (0.6)	89.00 (0.5)	93.00 (1.0)	< 0.05
Maximum Weight Change (kg), mean (SE)	16.46 (0.6)	16.30 (0.5)	18.10 (1.1)	0.231
Serum Creatinine (μmol/L), mean (SE)	80.3 (0.5)	82.4 (0.5)	78.1 (1.0)	< 0.01
Hypertension/CVD[e], % (SE)	5.1 (0.7)	4.9 (0.6)	12.4 (2.0)	< 0.01

[a] All results are weighted according to the sample weights of the Canadian Health Measure Survey (CHMS); [b] Anthropometric, laboratory values, and percentage with comorbidity for patients with and without self-reported OA. [c] Standard error estimates were generated using 500 bootstrap replications. All statistics were evaluated at α = 0.05. [d] P-values are used for comparing measures across self-reported OA and non-OA; for categorical variables, p-values were based on an adjusted Pearson chi-squared test for independence, and p-values for continuous variables were based on an adjusted Wald F test. [e] Maximum Weight Change as an adult from 18-years-old; [f]Hypertension/CVD: Self-reported hypertension or Cardiovascular Disease

obese BF% compared to athletic/acceptable category among females (OR: 2.67, 95%CI:1.32–3.51) and males (OR:2.11, 95%CI:1.38–3.21) after adjusting for age and BMI. Furthermore, BF% was significantly associated with self-reported OA after adjusting for age and serum creatinine only among females (OR: 1.47, 95%CI: 1.12–1.84).

BMI-stratified analysis in Table 3 revealed that among the BMI-defined overweight group, the age-adjusted odds of self-reported OA was significantly higher for overweight/obese BF% compared to athletic/acceptable BF% in both females (OR:1.84, 95% CI:1.18–3.19) and males (OR:1.32,95% CI:1.12–2.79). The association between OA and BF% categories was not significant among the BMI-defined underweight/ normal group.

According to our secondary analysis for association of OA and CVD across BF% categories, the age and sex–adjusted odds of self-reported OA was 37% (OR:1.37, 95%CI: 1.19–3.09) higher in those with CVD compared to those without CVD among the overweight/obese BF% category, while the OA and CVD association was not significant among those with athletic/acceptable BF% (OR: 1.13, 95% CI:0.87–2.82).

Discussion

In this study, BF% measured by skinfold calipers provides important information with respect to self-reported OA among a Canadian sample of middle-aged BMI-defined non-obese individuals (40 to 65 years of age and BMI < 30 kg/m^2) that is not necessarily captured by BMI alone. According to these results, BF% categories are independently associated with self-reported OA while adjusting for BMI and age, and there is a significant difference between the odds of OA across body fat categories for those within the BMI-defined overweight category (BMI between 25 and 30 kg/m^2) in both male and female models. No independent correlates were found between other metabolic markers used in this study and self-reported OA among the study population.

Our results, however, demonstrate a univariate relationship between decreased serum creatinine, an indirect measurement of muscle mass [29] with increased OA. Furthermore, in the female-specific model, the odds of self-reported OA was significantly higher among obese/overweight BF% compared to athletic/acceptable BF% when adjusting for age and blood creatinine. This suggests that body fat may provide independent information

Table 2 Odds ratios (and 95% confidence intervals) from logistic regressions for associations of metabolic markers with self-reported OA[a]

	Models	Categories	Adjusted models (by age)	Adjusted models (by age, BMI)	Adjusted models (by age, serum creatinine)
Female (n = 1267)	Model 1. BMI categories	Underweight/normal (< 25 kg/m²)	Ref	–	Ref
		Overweight (25–30 kg/m²)	1.53 (0.65, 2.13)	–	1.32 (0.87,2.21)
	Model 2. BF%[b] categories	Athletic/ Acceptable	Ref	Ref	Ref
		Overweight/obese	3.12 (1.25,4.4)*	2.67 (1.32,3.51)*	1.47 (1.12,1.84)*
	Model 3. Waist circumference (cm)	< 88 cm	Ref	Ref	Ref
		> 88 cm	2.62 (1.51,3.01)*	0.91 (0.80,2.64)	1.27 (0.91,2.14)
	Model 4. Maximum Weight change (kg)[c]	–	1.03 (0.91,1.43)	1.07 (0.96,2.46)	1.03 (0.82,2.68)
	Model 5. Serum Creatinine	≥65 µmol/L	Ref	Ref	–
		< 65 µmol/L	1.21 (0.87,2.45)	0.87 (0.45,1.97)	–
Male (n = 1195)	Model 1. BMI categories	Underweight/normal (< 25 kg/m²)	Ref	–	Ref
		Overweight (25–30 kg/m²)	0.92 (0.75,1.91)	–	1.43 (0.93,2.45)
	Model 2. BF%[b] categories	Athletic/ acceptable	Ref	Ref	Ref
		Overweight/obese	1.82 (1.15,3.58)*	2.11 (1.38,3.21)*	1.12 (0.78,1.93)
	Model 3. Waist circumference (cm)	< 102 cm	Ref	Ref	Ref
		> 102 cm	2.21 (1.3,3.81)*	0.91(0.83,1.54)	1.08 (0.91,1.72)
	Model 4. Maximum Weight change [c](kg)	–	1.04 (1.02,1.76)*	1.05 (0.87,2.32)	0.29 (0.12,2.16)
	Model 5. Serum Creatinine	≥73 µmol/L	Ref	Ref	–
		< 73 µmol/L	1.97 (0.91,2.89)	0.91 (0.35,2.1)	–

[a] All results are weighted according to the sample weights of the Canadian Health Measure Survey (CHMS); [b] Body Fat percentage (BF%);[c] Individual body fat percentages were grouped into three body fat categories: athletic/good (males: < 14% females < 23%), acceptable (males 15–20%, females 24–30%), or overweight/obese (male > 21% females > 31%).; [d] Maximum Weight change as an adult from 18-years-old (kg); * p-value< 0.05

other than that gained from serum creatinine regarding the relations between body composition and OA. Our findings suggest that both increased body fat and decreased lean mass may be characteristic of OA, but the causal contribution of these metabolic abnormalities to OA have yet to be directly tested and explored [29]. In a previous study, the combined effects of reduced lean mass with increased fat mass were shown to be associated with elevated risk of OA compared to obesity alone [42]. Results from the present study provide cross-sectional evidence for an association between obesity and OA among the

Table 3 Age-adjusted odds ratio (and 95% confidence intervals) for self-reported OA across BF% categories stratified by BMI groups and sex

	BMI Body Fat Percentage	Underweight/Normal (BMI < 25 kg/m²)	Overweight (BMI 25–29.99 kg/m²)
Female	Athletic/Acceptable	Reference	Reference
	Overweight/Obese	1.92 (0.81,2.87)	1.84 (1.18,3.19)*
		(n = 711)	(n = 556)
Male	Athletic/Acceptable	Reference	Reference
	Overweight/Obese	1.41 (0.61,2.39)	1.32 (1.12,2.79)*
		(n = 394)	(n = 801)

All four models were adjusted for age; Individual body fat percentages were grouped into three body fat categories: athletic/good (males: < 14% females < 23%), acceptable (males 15–20%, females 24–30%), or overweight/obese (male > 21% females > 31%).;* p-value< 0.05

middle-aged non-obese population. Longitudinal studies are needed to confirm these associations.

We further showed that the age and sex-adjusted association of self-reported OA and CVD was significantly higher in the obese/overweight BF% group compared to the association observed in athletic/acceptable BF% group. This highlights the importance of BF% in identifying those with multi-morbidity among OA population. Similar results were reported in a recent large Japanese cohort study [17] where accumulation of metabolic syndrome components were shown to be related to the incidence and progression of knee OA components. OA individuals with overweight or obesity have shown to demonstrate higher abdominal adiposity (waist circumference) [25], increased waist-to-height ratio, increased rates of high blood pressure, high cholesterol, and higher body fat compared to OA patients with athletic/acceptable BF% [43]. A recent study evaluated the cross-sectional association between metabolic markers and OA among the BMI-defined non-obese and showed that skinfold BF% is associated with higher OA prevalence [44] which corresponds to our results. Brasnjevic et al. [16] showed that abdominal obesity was associated with radiographic progression of knee OA.

While several studies showed that body fat distribution does not provide additional information other than those gained through BMI among individuals with severe knee OA [4, 5], there is a scarcity of research that individually assesses the non-obese population in this context. Our study demonstrates that measuring body fat may provide additional information that is supplementary to, or independent of, BMI with regards to OA prevalence among the middle-aged non-obese OA patients. Understanding the association of BF% and other metabolic markers with OA within a non-obese population may help improve the development of screening policies for prevention and management strategies in OA [33]. For instance, the discordance between BMI and body fat is predominantly observed in women with "healthy" BMIs (BMI ≤24.99) but who are overweight or obese based on metabolic markers such as levels of body fat (BF% ≥ 31%) [21, 23, 24] or abdominal obesity measured by waist circumference [8, 9]. Given that these metabolic markers have shown to be significantly associated with OA progression [16] and health outcomes [17], such women would traditionally be medically managed as healthy, and as such, and may miss OA prevention opportunities even though they may be at increased risk.

As our data are representative of the Canadian population, they are likely generalizable to other countries with population characteristics similar to that of Canada. There are known differences in body fat and body composition across races and ethnicities [45], and the predictability of body fat by the equations used by the CHMS dataset. The data presented in this study reflects the ethnic diversity of Canadians. OA affects more than 4.6 million Canadians [46], and it is estimated that 1 in 4 Canadians will have OA by 2040 due to aging, increased longevity of the population and the obesity epidemic [46]. Countries with a homogeneous racial or ethnic population should validate these findings in their given population, as differences in fat storage between races have been previously reported [47].

A body fat classification system from Durnin et al. [38] was used in this study that divided individuals into categories based on BF% and sex. Other body fat categorization schemes have been developed, but include age [48]. Specifically, the World Health Organization criteria incorporates increased BF% in the "acceptable" category for each increasing age group, which makes isolating the individual effect of body fat on OA challenging [49]. As the goal of this study was to evaluate the effects of discrete BF% values on OA, a fixed sex-specific classification of BF% was used. Body fat changes with age [50], and both age and sex are strongly associated with OA [1]. To compensate for this, our models were adjusted for age and stratified by sex.

There are several limitations to this work. One significant limitation of the CMHS dataset is that it does not include data on previous injury or family history of OA. However, as previously mentioned, there are several accepted primary risk factors calling for sub classification, or subtypes of OA to define a "profile" that describes each of these subtypes [25]. Therefore, we speculate that the trend toward an increased odds ratio of athletic/acceptable BF% individuals for OA demonstrated here may be related to these factors that were not measured. As all individuals included in this study had a BMI < 30 kg/m^2, it is possible that they demonstrate a "pre-metabolic syndrome" phenotype but may still have metabolic abnormalities contributing to their OA. Here, we were unable to evaluate all metabolic parameters of interest in the logistic regression models because of weighting limitations associated with combining fasted lab values from the CHMS Statistics Canada dataset. Due to the limited sample size of our study, we also did not adjust for a variety of risk factors that are known to be related to OA (socioeconomic status, ethnicity, smoking), but that would be useful to consider in future investigations. Additionally, the limited age group evaluated did not allow for us to evaluate these relations across the weight or age spectrum. There are also limitations associated with the use of skinfold anthropometry; it may underestimate BF% when compared to other methods such as dual energy x-ray absorptiometry as the former does not account for intra-abdominal or visceral adipose tissue stores [51]. Consequently, skinfold anthropometry lacks appropriate population-specific cut-off values to identify health risks among individuals with obesity [51]. Lastly, a substantial limitation of this work was the binary and self-reported nature of the primary outcome measure, OA. This analysis is based on an outcome variable acquired from self-report data. However, we suggest that the preliminary context of this study and information gained from this analysis justifies the use of this outcome.

Future work should longitudinally evaluate the association of body fat, lean mass, muscle strength, pain and structural graded MRI Osteoarthritis Knee Score [4] or radiographic Kellgren-Lawrence outcomes [4] to better understand implications of metabolic risk factors, adiposity, and osteoarthritis severity among the non-obese population. Clinically, better measures of body fat or body composition (e.g., DXA [47]) could be used to understand risk of developing OA according to body fat measurements in patients across the spectrum of body composition. The presence of an OA subtype may be supported by a relationship between increased body fat, indirect measures of body composition, elevated CVD risk, and OA.

Conclusion

This study demonstrates that measuring body fat may provide additional information over and above BMI with regards to OA prevalence among the middle-aged non-obese population. However, no independent correlate was found between other metabolic markers used in this study and the self-reported OA among the study population. Given the rise in prevalence of OA among the middle-aged population [46] and the increased effectiveness of prevention interventions among the BMI-defined non-obese population [34], this study highlights the need to better understand the interrelation of body fat and risk of OA among the BMI-defined non-obese population. Our results pave the way to further explore the use of low-cost, readily available, population-based metrics for metabolic markers as a primary care screening tool among younger non-obese individuals, who may not otherwise be assessed for OA risk or musculoskeletal compromise.

Abbreviations

BF: Body Fat; BMI: Body Mass Index; CHMS: Canadian Health Measures Survey; CVD: Cardiovascular diseases; OA: Osteoarthritis; SE: Standard Error

Acknowledgements

We wish to acknowledge the assistance of the Prairie Regional Research Data Centre, Statistics Canada, Dr. Cyril Frank, Sarah L. Lacny, and thoughtful conversations about data interpretation with fellow members and trainees from the Alberta Innovates Health Solutions Team in Osteoarthritis.

Funding

Alberta Innovates Health Solutions Team in Osteoarthritis. DM is supported by a Canada Research Chair in Health Systems and Services Research, and Arthur J.E. Child Chair in Rheumatology. KH is supported by an Izaak Walton Killam pre-doctoral scholarship. WH is supported by a Canada Research Chair in Applied Cellular and Molecular Biomechanics and a Killam Memorial Research Chair. The funding agencies listed here had no role in the project design, execution, analysis, or manuscript drafting.

Authors' contributions

Study concept and design: BS, KC, DM, CS, RR, RC, WH; Acquisition of data: CS,KC, RC, DM,CS; Analysis and interpretation of data: BS, KC, DM, RR, CS, WH; Statistical analysis: RC, BS; Drafting of the manuscript: KC, BS, DM, CS, RR, RC, WH, Critical revision of the manuscript for important intellectual content: BS, KC, RC, RR, CS, WH, DM. All authors read and approved the final manuscript.

Competing interests

The views expressed in this paper are solely those of the authors and do not reflect those of Statistics Canada. We thank Claudia Sanmartin for her contributions related to data access and analysis

Author details

[1]Human Performance Laboratory, University of Calgary, Calgary, AB, Canada. [2]Department of Community Health Sciences, University of Calgary, 3280 Hospital Drive NW, Calgary, AB T2N 4Z6, Canada. [3]Faculty of Kinesiology and Department of Biochemistry and Molecular Biology, University of Calgary, Calgary, AB, Canada. [4]Health Analysis Division, Statistics Canada, Ottawa, ON, Canada. [5]Department of Medicine, University of Calgary, Calgary, AB, Canada.

References

1. Oliveria SA, Felson DT, Cirillo PA, Reed JI, Walker AM. Body weight, body mass index, and incident symptomatic osteoarthritis of the hand, hip, and knee. Epidemiology. 1999 Mar 1;10(2):161–6.
2. Cross M, Smith E, Hoy D, Nolte S, Ackerman I, Fransen M, Bridgett L, Williams S, Guillemin F, Hill CL, Laslett LL. The global burden of hip and knee osteoarthritis: estimates from the global burden of disease 2010 study. Ann Rheum Dis 2014 Feb 19.
3. Blagojevic M, Jinks C, Jeffery A, Jordan KP. Risk factors for onset of osteoarthritis of the knee in older adults: a systematic review and meta-analysis. Osteoarthr Cartil. 2010 Jan 31;18(1):24–33.
4. Abbate LM, Stevens J, Schwartz TA, Renner JB, Helmick CG, Jordan JM. Anthropometric measures, body composition, body fat distribution, and knee osteoarthritis in women. Obesity. 2006 Jul 1;14(7):1274–81.
5. Lohmander LS, de Verdier MG, Rollof J, Nilsson PM, Engström G. Incidence of severe knee and hip osteoarthritis in relation to different measures of body mass: a population-based prospective cohort study. Ann Rheum Dis. 2009 Apr 1;68(4):490–6.
6. Sowers MR, Karvonen-Gutierrez CA. The evolving role of obesity in knee osteoarthritis. Curr Opin Rheumatol. 2010 Sep;22(5):533.
7. Velasquez MT, Katz JD. Osteoarthritis: another component of metabolic syndrome? Metab Syndr Relat Disord. 2010;8:295–305.

8. Wang Y, Simpson JA, Wluka AE, Teichtahl AJ, English DR, Giles GG, Graves S, Cicuttini FM. Relationship between body adiposity measures and risk of primary knee and hip replacement for osteoarthritis: a prospective cohort study. Arthritis research & therapy. 2009 Apr;11(2):R31.

9. Hart DJ, Doyle DV, Spector TD. Association between metabolic factors and knee osteoarthritis in women: the Chingford study. J Rheumatol. 1995;22:1118–23.

10. Conaghan PG, Kloppenburg M, Schett G, Bijlsma JW. Osteoarthritis research priorities: a report from a EULAR ad hoc expert committee. Ann Rheum Dis. 2014 Aug 1;73(8):1442–5.

11. Berenbaum F, Griffin TM, Liu-Bryan R. Metabolic regulation of inflammation in osteoarthritis. Arthritis & rheumatology. 2017 Jan 1;69(1):9–21.

12. Bliddal H, Leeds AR, Christensen R. Osteoarthritis, obesity and weight loss: evidence, hypotheses and horizons–a scoping review. Obes Rev. 2014 Jul 1; 15(7):578–86.

13. Gregor MF, Hotamisligil GS. Inflammatory mechanisms in obesity. Annu Rev Immunol. 2011 Apr 23;29:415–45.

14. Hotamisligil GS. Inflammation and metabolic disorders. Nature. 2006 Dec 14; 444(7121):860–7.

15. Visser AW, Ioan-Facsinay A, de Mutsert R, Widya RL, Loef M, de Roos A, le Cessie S, den Heijer M, Rosendaal FR, Kloppenburg M. Adiposity and hand osteoarthritis: the Netherlands epidemiology of obesity study. Arthritis research & therapy. 2014 Jan 22;16(1):1.

16. Vasilic-Brasnjevic S, Marinkovic J, Vlajinac H, Vasiljevic N, Jakovljevic B, Nikic M, Maksimovic M. Association of body mass index and waist circumference with severity of knee osteoarthritis. Acta reumatologica portuguesa. 2016;41(3):226–31.

17. Yoshimura N, Muraki S, Oka H, Tanaka S, Kawaguchi H, Nakamura K, et al. Accumulation of metabolic risk factors such as overweight, hypertension, dyslipidaemia, and impaired glucose tolerance raises the risk of occurrence and progression of knee osteoarthritis: a 3-year follow-up of the ROAD study. Osteoarthr Cartil. 2012;20:1217–26.

18. Gierman LM, van der Ham F, Koudijs A, Wielinga PY, Kleemann R, Kooistra T, Stoop R, Kloppenburg M, van Osch GJ, Stojanovic-Susulic V, Huizinga TW. Metabolic stress–induced inflammation plays a major role in the development of osteoarthritis in mice. Arthritis & Rheumatism. 2012 Apr 1; 64(4):1172–81.

19. Griffin TM, Huebner JL, Kraus VB, Yan Z, Guilak F. Induction of osteoarthritis and metabolic inflammation by a very high-fat diet in mice: effects of short-term exercise. Arthritis & Rheumatism. 2012 Feb 1;64(2):443–53.

20. Brunner AM, Henn CM, Drewniak EI, Lesieur-Brooks A, Machan J, Crisco JJ, Ehrlich MG. High dietary fat and the development of osteoarthritis in a rabbit model. Osteoarthr Cartil. 2012 Jun 30;20(6):584–92.

21. Louer CR, Furman BD, Huebner JL, Kraus VB, Olson SA, Guilak F. Diet-induced obesity significantly increases the severity of posttraumatic arthritis in mice. Arthritis & Rheumatism. 2012 Oct 1;64(10):3220–30.

22. Collins KH, Herzog W, MacDonald GZ, Reimer RA, Rios JL, Smith IC, Zernicke RF, Hart DA. Obesity, metabolic syndrome, and musculoskeletal disease: common inflammatory pathways suggest a central role for loss of muscle integrity. Front Physiol. 2018;9:112. https://www.frontiersin.org/article/10.3389/fphys.2018.00112.

23. Lee R, Kean WF. Obesity and knee osteoarthritis. Inflammopharmacology. 2012 Apr;20(2):53–8.

24. Ding C, Stannus O, Cicuttini F, Antony B, Jones G. Body fat is associated with increased and lean mass with decreased knee cartilage loss in older adults: a prospective cohort study. Int J Obes. 2013 Jun 1;37(6):822–7.

25. Karlsson MK, Magnusson H, Cöster M, Karlsson C, Rosengren BE. Patients with knee osteoarthritis have a phenotype with higher bone mass, higher fat mass, and lower lean body mass. Clin Orthop Relat Res. 2015 Jan 1;473(1):258–64.

26. World Health Organization. Obesity: Preventing and Managing the Global Epidemic [Internet]. Report of a WHO consultation on obesity. 1998 [cited 2016 June 18]. Available from: http://www.who.int/nutrition/publications/obesity/WHO_TRS_894/en/

27. Mokdad AH, Ford ES, Bowman BA, Dietz WH, Vinicor F, bales VS, et al. prevalence of obesity, diabetes, and obesity-related health risk factors, 2001. JAMA 2003 Jan 1;289(1):76–79.

28. Patel SS, Molnar MZ, Tayek JA, Ix JH, Noori N, Benner D, Heymsfield S, Kopple JD, Kovesdy CP, Kalantar-Zadeh K. Serum creatinine as a marker of muscle mass in chronic kidney disease: results of a cross-sectional study and review of literature. J Cachexia Sarcopenia Muscle. 2013 Mar 1;4(1):19–29.

29. Heymsfield S, Arteaga C, McManus C, Smith J, Moffitt S. Measurement of muscle mass in humans: validity of the 24-hour urinary creatinine method. Am J Clin Nutr. 1983 Mar 1;37(3):478–94.

30. Kim SW, Jung HW, Kim CH, Kim KI, Chin HJ, Lee H. A new equation to estimate muscle mass from creatinine and cystatin C. PLoS One. 2016 Feb 5; 11(2):e0148495.

31. Holliday KL, McWilliams DF, Maciewicz RA, Muir KR, Zhang W, Doherty M. Lifetime body mass index, other anthropometric measures of obesity and risk of knee or hip osteoarthritis in the GOAL case-control study. Osteoarthr Cartil. 2011;19:37–43.

32. Liu B, Balkwill A, Banks E, Cooper C, Green J, Beral V. Relationship of height, weight and body mass index to the risk of hip and knee replacements in middle-aged women. Rheumatology (Oxford). 2007;46:861–7.

33. Chan RS, Woo J. Prevention of overweight and obesity: how effective is the current public health approach. Int J Environ Res Public Health. 2010 Feb 26;7(3):765–83.

34. Collins KH. Association of body mass index (BMI) and percent body fat among BMI-defined non-obese middle-aged individuals: insights from a population-based Canadian sample. Canadian Journal of Public Health. 2016;107(6):E520.

35. Manninen P, Riihimaki H, Heliövaara M, Suomalainen O. Weight changes and the risk of knee osteoarthritis requiring arthroplasty. Ann Rheum Dis. 2004 Nov 1;63(11):1434–7.

36. Statistics Canada. Canadian Health Measures Survey (CHMS) Data User Guide: Cycle 1 [Internet]. 2011 [cited 2016 June 18]. Available from: http://www23.statcan.gc.ca/imdb-bmdi/pub/document/5071_D2_T1_V1-eng.htm.

37. Tremblay M, Wolfson M, Connor Gorber S. Canadian Health Measures Survey: rationale, background, and overview. Stat Canada Heal Reports. 2007;18 Supp:7–20.

38. Durnin JVG a, Womersley J. Body fat assessed from total body density and its estimation from skinfold thickness: measurements on 481 men and women aged from 16 to 72 years. Br J Nutr. 2007 Mar 9;32(01):77–97.

39. US Department of Health and Human Services. Clinical Guidelines on the Identification, Evaluation, and Treatment of Overweight and Obesity in Adults: An Evidence Report [Internet]. 1998. p.98–4083 [cited 2016 June 18]. Available from: https://www.ncbi.nlm.nih.gov/books/NBK2003/.

40. Lim S, Kim KM, Kim MJ, Woo SJ, Choi SH, Park KS, Jang HC, Meigs JB, Wexler DJ. The association of maximum body weight on the development of type 2 diabetes and microvascular complications: MAXWEL study. PLoS One. 2013 Dec 4;8(12):e80525.

41. Hjelmesæth J, Røislien J, Nordstrand N, Hofsø D, Hager H, Hartmann A. Low serum creatinine is associated with type 2 diabetes in morbidly obese women and men: a cross-sectional study. BMC Endocr Disord. 2010 Dec;10(1):6.

42. Patel SS, Molnar MZ, Tayek JA, Ix JH, Noori N, Benner D, et al. Serum creatinine as a marker of muscle mass in chronic kidney disease: results of a cross-sectional study and review of literature. J Cachexia Sarcopenia Muscle. 2013 Mar;4(1):19–29.

43. Lee S, Kim T-N, Kim S-H. Sarcopenic obesity is more closely associated with knee osteoarthritis than is nonsarcopenic obesity: a cross-sectional study. Arthritis Rheum. 2012 Dec;64(12):3947–54.

44. Sanghi D, Srivastava RN, Singh A, Kumari R, Mishra R, Mishra A. The association of anthropometric measures and osteoarthritis knee in non-obese subjects: a cross sectional study. Clinics. 2011;66(2):275–9.

45. Topp R, RN PD, Malkani AL. Self-reported chair-rise ability relates to stair-climbing readiness of total knee arthroplasty patients: a pilot study. J Rehabil Res Dev. 2007 Jul 1;44(5):751.

46. Arthrtiis Alliance of Canda. The Impact of Arthritis in Canada: Today and Over the Next 30 Years [internet]. 2011[cited 2016 June 18]. Available from: http://www.arthritisalliance.ca/images/PDF/eng/Initiatives/20111022_2200_impact_of_arthritis.pdf.

47. Davidson LE, Wang J, Thornton JC, Kaleem Z, Silva-Palacios F, Pierson RN, et al. Predicting fat percent by skinfolds in racial groups: Durnin and Womersley revisited. Med Sci Sports Exerc. 2011 Mar;43(3):542–9.

48. Gallagher D, Heymsfield SB, Heo M, Jebb SA, Murgatroyd PR, Sakamoto Y. Healthy percentage body fat ranges: an approach for developing guidelines based on body mass index. Am J Clin Nutr. 2000 Sep;72(3):694–701.

49. Woolf AD, Pfleger B. Burden of major musculoskeletal conditions. Bull World Health Organ. 2003 Jan;81(9):646–56.

50. Kuk JL, Saunders TJ, Davidson LE, Ross R. Age-related changes in total and regional fat distribution. Ageing Res Rev. 2009 Oct;8(4):339–48.

51. Garcia AL, Wagner K, Hothorn T, Koebnick C, Zunft H-JF, Trippo U. Improved prediction of body fat by measuring skinfold thickness, circumferences, and bone breadths. Obes Res. 2005;13(3):626–34.

21

Treatment fidelity in the Camden Weight Loss (CAMWEL) intervention assessed from recordings of advisor-participant consultations

Lorraine M Noble[1*] ⓘ, Emma Godfrey[2], Liane Al-Baba[3], Gabriella Baez[2], Nicki Thorogood[4] and Kiran Nanchahal[4]

Abstract

Background: Variations in the delivery of content and process can alter the effectiveness of complex interventions. This study examined the fidelity of a weight loss intervention (Camden Weight Loss) from recorded consultations by assessing advisors' delivery of content, use of motivational interviewing approach and therapeutic alliance.

Methods: A process evaluation was conducted of advisor-participant consultations in a 12-month randomised controlled trial of an intervention for adult volunteers with a body mass index categorised as overweight or obese. A convenience sample of 22 consultations (12% of 191 participants) recorded at the intervention mid-point were available for analysis. Consultations were independently rated by two observers independent of intervention or study delivery, using: a fidelity scale, the Motivational Interviewing Treatment Integrity Scale and the Primary Care Therapy Process Rating Scale. Raters were blind to participants' responses to the intervention and weight outcomes. Half the participants ($N = 11$) achieved significant weight loss ($\geq 5\%$ of baseline weight).

Results: A mean of 41% of prescribed content was delivered, with a range covered per session of 8–98%, falling below the 100% content expected per session. Tasks included most frequently were: taking weight and waist measurements (98%), scheduling next appointment (86%), review of general progress (85%) and reviewing weight change (84%). Individual items most frequently addressed were 'giving encouragement' and 'showing appreciation of participant's efforts' (95 and 88% respectively). Consultation length (mean 19 min, range 9–30) was shorter than the 30-min allocation. Quantity of content correlated with consultation length ($p < 0.01$). Advisors' use of motivational interviewing was rated at 'beginner proficiency' for Global Clinician Rating, Reflection to Question Ratio and Percent Open Questions. Therapeutic alliance scores were moderate. Affective aspects were rated highly (e.g. supportive encouragement, involvement and warmth).

Conclusions: Intervention fidelity varied in both content and process, emphasising the importance of ongoing fidelity checks in a complex intervention. Advisors focused on certain practical aspects of the intervention and providing an encouraging interpersonal climate. This concurs with other research findings, which have revealed the value participants in a weight loss intervention place on an empathic advisor-participant relationship.

Clinical trials registration: Registered with Clinicaltrials.gov, number NCT00891943.

Keywords: Obesity, Overweight, Weight loss, Trial, Intervention, Fidelity, Motivational interviewing, Therapeutic alliance, Communication

---

* Correspondence: lorraine.noble@ucl.ac.uk
[1]UCL Medical School, University College London, Royal Free Hospital, Rowland Hill Street, NW3 2PF, London, UK
Full list of author information is available at the end of the article

Background

The increasing impact of obesity on health has caused international alarm [1, 2]. It is estimated that 2.8 million people die annually due to overweight or obesity [2]. In the UK, 65% of men, 58% of women and 33% of children aged 10–11 are overweight or obese [3]. Health problems related to obesity are estimated to cost the UK National Health Service £5 billion per year [4].

Guidance recommends multi-component weight management interventions focusing on dietary intake, physical activity and behaviour change, and that behaviour modification addresses: *'problem solving; goal setting; how to carry out a particular task or activity; planning to provide social support or make changes to the social environment; self-monitoring of weight and behaviours that can affect weight; and feedback on performance'* [5]. Affective features of weight management interventions are also highlighted, emphasising empathy, support and encouragement, and a respectful and non-judgemental approach.

Guidance reflects the complexity of evidence about weight management and the theoretical basis for behaviour change [6–12]. Multi-component interventions are superior to single-component interventions and result in greater longer term weight loss than control conditions [7, 8]. However, intervention success varies, with variation not accounted for by participant characteristics or programme components (such as length, intensity or face-to-face contact). Long term weight loss remains a challenge [9, 12, 13].

Behaviour change interventions aim to encourage people to self-manage their weight in the long term. Motivational interviewing aims to support this by identifying and enhancing an individual's own motivation and self-efficacy. The health professional employs an empathic, supportive and collaborative approach, emphasising the individual's autonomy and encouraging the person to explore their own reasons for, and ambivalence about, changing the target behaviour [14].

Whilst motivational interviewing is effective in promoting behaviour change, many health professionals are 'generalists', using a variety of approaches rather than a single, 'pure' approach. 'Motivational interviewing-style' approaches, which employ some of the elements (such as empathy) without using the full range of techniques, have been investigated [15]. Weight management programmes including either pure or adapted forms of motivational interviewing improve outcomes relative to traditional behaviour change interventions or control conditions [16, 17]. However, in primary care consultations with patients who were overweight or obese, low levels of techniques consistent with a motivational interviewing approach were observed, specifically empathy and motivational interviewing 'spirit' [18].

The importance of the quality of the therapeutic relationship on outcomes of behaviour change interventions has also been recognised [19]. Therapeutic alliance includes affective aspects of the professional-patient relationship (such as empathy, rapport and warmth) and instrumental aspects (such as agreement on goals and tasks). Baldwin and colleagues highlighted the impact of therapeutic alliance in weight management outcomes, and noted importance of the professional's contribution to developing this alliance [20].

Weight management interventions require professionals to skilfully select and deliver elements in line with evidence and an individual's needs. The importance of initial training and continuing professional development has been highlighted [5]. Key features to promote fidelity (defined as the degree to which an intervention is delivered as intended) are staff training, supervision and an intervention manual [21]. Failure to implement the intervention as designed can result in a 'Type III error', where study results do not reflect the effects of the planned intervention [22]. Fidelity includes exposure, adherence to content and quality of delivery [21]. It is commonly assessed by trained observers, either live or from recordings [16, 21, 23]. For example, one study of fidelity in a behaviour change intervention for diabetes found that staff training improved motivational interviewing spirit [24].

In a 12-month weight loss intervention trial for obese and overweight volunteers, a third of the intervention group achieved clinically significant weight loss (5% or more of their baseline weight) [25]. The present study was designed to examine intervention fidelity, to explore whether differences in intervention delivery may have contributed to variability in intervention group outcome.

Study aim

To investigate weight loss intervention fidelity through assessing the content and process of advisor-participant consultations. Specifically, to establish whether: (i) intervention topics and activities were delivered as intended; (ii) advisors' consultation style was consistent with approaches to support lifestyle behaviour change, in particular, using a motivational interviewing approach and establishing a therapeutic alliance.

Method
Design

This was an independent evaluation examining fidelity of a multi-component weight loss intervention delivered by health advisors to participants with weight categorised as overweight and obese, in the intervention arm of a pragmatic randomised control trial in primary care. This was a descriptive, observational study, conducting a process evaluation using independent, blind ratings of recorded advisor-participant consultations. Fidelity of intervention content (scheduled topics and activities) and process (motivational interviewing and therapeutic alliance) were examined. Recordings were taken from the mid-point of the intervention to: (i) assess the therapeutic relationship that had developed, (ii) reduce the influence of participants' and advisors' awareness of intervention outcome (i.e. final weight change).

Participants

Participants were adults attending the 12-month Camden Weight Loss programme during a two year research period. Consultations were recorded during a five month period. Written consent was obtained from all participants. Out of 191 participants who received the intervention, 104 audio or video-recordings were obtained for 42 participants during the recording period. Including only participants for whom final weight outcomes were available resulted in 34 participants. Of these, recordings from the three mid-intervention sessions were available for 27 participants. Due to problems with sound quality, recordings from five participants were excluded, resulting in a total sample of 22 participants (12% of 191).

The 22 participants were 10 women and 12 men, predominantly White British/White Other (17 participants), with a mean age of 53 years (range 26–80 years) and a mean body mass index at baseline of 32.6 (range 25.2–45.1). At outcome (12 months), 11 had achieved clinically significant weight loss (5% or more of baseline weight) and 11 had not. The 22 participants did not significantly differ from the other 169 trial participants in the intervention arm for: age, baseline weight, waist or body mass index, or final weight loss, but were more likely to be male (12/22 compared to 42/169, $Chi^2(1) = 8.5$, $p < 0.01$) and to complete more sessions (mean 10.9 compared to 7.4, $t(158) = 3.5$, $p < 0.01$).

The weight loss intervention

The Camden Weight Loss programme was offered to adults with weight categorised as clinically overweight or obese in primary care practices in a research trial [25]. The trial aimed to develop a locally delivered weight loss intervention, in line with the National Health Service *Health Trainers Initiative* [26], drawing health advisors from local communities, who are trained to support people in adopting healthier lifestyles by using psychological techniques to promote behaviour change. These techniques include supporting others to: choose a behaviour to change, set 'SMART' goals, plan behaviour change, improve confidence, review behaviour change, and embed behaviour change into their lifestyle [26]. The intervention was devised as a multi-component programme to promote behaviour change in line with National Institute for Health and Care Excellence guidance [27] and based on

behaviour change models (Social Cognitive Theory, Goal Setting, Systems Thinking) [28–30]. Baseline and final weight were measured by research staff. The results of the randomised controlled trial of 381 participants, which included the 191 participants in the intervention arm, are published elsewhere [25].

Six advisors with a background in health care or exercise were trained to deliver a structured one-to-one intervention. The recordings included five of the advisors: one nurse, two osteopaths and two qualified personal fitness trainers, one of whom also had training in nutrition (CYQ Central YMCA Qualification Level 3 Award). Each participant was allocated to one advisor and were scheduled to attend 14 sessions, lasting 30 min per session, over 12 months in a primary care setting. The session length was intended to enable more in-depth discussion of weight management than is possible in a standard National Health Service primary care consultation (10 min), whilst being delivered to participants in their local practice. Sessions 9, 10 and 11 straddled the intervention mid-point (6 months).

Advisors attended two days of training, including:

(i)   the intervention design and rationale
(ii) effective behaviour change strategies and principles of motivational interviewing
(iii) simulated practice in setting weight loss goals, talking about weight and behaviour change and addressing difficult issues.

Advisors were given a detailed manual listing the goals and content of each session, including handouts for participants in some sessions, and a 20-page booklet on Helping People Change Behaviour, including worked examples of techniques for: motivational interviewing, agenda setting, assessing importance and confidence, listening and informing. During the intervention, advisors attended additional group meetings, including further training in motivational interviewing techniques, and met with research staff individually to discuss intervention progress and any issues in intervention delivery.

Each consultation included a review of progress, recording and reviewing pedometer counts, taking weight and waist measurements, reviewing weight loss progress, introducing a new topic, goal setting, making an action plan and confirming the next appointment. The review included discussing the participant's experience and success with the previous session's topic. The intervention schedule is shown in Table 1. Sessions were delivered on a regular schedule with tapering frequency: fortnightly for 12 weeks, 3-weekly to 27 weeks, 4-weekly to 35 weeks and a 12-week interval to the last session. Further details of the intervention are published elsewhere [25]. The topics addressed in sessions 9, 10 and 11 were: positive and

Table 1 CAMWEL weight loss programme sessions

Session	Week	Topic	Content
Pre-intervention: baseline measurements by researchers			
1	0	Getting started	Eliciting personal reasons for losing weight, commitment to programme
2	2	Changing habits	Importance of changing habits permanently
3	4	Healthy eating	Regular meals, portion sizes, easy food swaps
4	6	Let's get active	Incorporating physical activity into daily lifestyle
5	8	Taking charge of your environment	Acting on environmental cues
6	10	Eating when out and about	Making healthy choices, discuss alcohol if appropriate
7	12	Tip the calorie balance	Energy balance equation, and action planning
8	15	Positive thinking	Ways to stop negative thoughts
9	18	Getting off the slippery slope	Slips, and getting back on course
10	21	Social eating	Difficult social settings and how to control eating
6 month measurements by researchers			
11	27	Staying on course	Identify successes, and how to stay on course
12	31	Staying active	Additional physical activity to be added to the routine
13	35	Managing stress	How stress can affect weight, how to overcome
14	47	Reshaping habits	Review progress, how to continue in long term
12 month measurements by researchers			

negative thinking, responding to situations where you might 'slip up', social eating, and staying on course in the long term.

Measures
Treatment fidelity
Checklists were devised for the three sessions by itemising the session content from the manual, using the same wording for items repeated across sessions. Eight topics were included in every session: (1) reviewing overall progress, (2) reviewing previous topic and handouts, (3) reviewing pedometer counts and physical activity, (4) taking weight and waist measurements, (5) reviewing weight change, (6) presenting new topic, (7) setting goals, making action plans and assigning home activities, (8) setting date of next appointment. Due to the detail in the manual, the initial checklists contained 41, 40, and 52 items respectively for the three sessions. The final checklist for session 9 is shown in Table 2 as an example.

The checklist was piloted using a scoring key of 0 (not done), 1 (partially done) and 2 (completely done) for most of the items (e.g. 'feedback is given on performance'), with some simple items (e.g. 'waist circumference is measured') assessed on a binary scale of 0 (not done) and 1 (done). However, low frequency and brevity of advisor behaviours observed during piloting indicated that measurement was better suited to assessing the presence of behaviours in comparison to expected content, rather than a combination of presence and quality. The scoring key for all items was converted to a binary

scale (done/not done). An additional category ('not recorded') noted where items could not be rated due to poor sound quality. A rater crib sheet specified item content, including strategies or examples the advisors had been encouraged to use.

Motivational interviewing
The Motivational Interviewing Treatment Integrity Scale [31] assesses adherence to and competence in using motivational interviewing, with good inter-rater reliability reported [32, 33]. Global ratings are made for five dimensions: Evocation, Collaboration, Autonomy/ Support, Direction and Empathy on a 5-point scale, and a summary score: Spirit of Motivational Interviewing. Behaviour counts are made for seven aspects: Giving Information, Closed Questions, Open Questions, Simple Reflections, Complex Reflections, Motivational Interviewing Adherent Behaviours and Motivational Interviewing Non-adherent Behaviours. Further summary scores are also computed.

Therapeutic alliance
The 14-item Alliance scale of the Primary Care Therapy Process Rating Scale [34] assesses the quality of the professional-patient therapeutic bond in psychological interventions conducted in primary care settings. It was designed for research into treatment fidelity and process-outcome relationships and has good internal consistency (Cronbach's alpha 0.88). Items are scored

Table 2 Example treatment fidelity checklist: session 9

Item	Topic
1. Reviewing overall progress	
1	Previously set goals or intentions are reviewed
2	Feedback on performance is given
3	General encouragement is given
2. Reviewing previous topic and handouts	
4	Positive Thinking handout is reviewed
	The following questions are taken into consideration when reviewing the Positive Thinking handout
5	• What negative thoughts did you catch yourself thinking?
6	• When was this (in what situation)?
7	• Were you able to stop them?
8	• Did you talk back with positive thoughts?
9	• How did positive thinking help with eating a healthy diet?
10	• What about changes to your activity habits?
11	• Did you manage to go for a 30-min walk every day?
12	Any barriers are uncovered
	Usefulness of the other handouts is reviewed:
13	• CAMWEL walks handout
14	• Steps/Walks Chart handout
15	• Rate Your Plate handout
3. Reviewing pedometer counts and physical activity	
16	Pedometer counts are recorded
17	Participants are asked if they wore the pedometers every day
18	(a) If the participant did not wear the pedometer every day, they are asked what got in the way OR (b) If the participant did wear the pedometer every day, they are praised
19	Efforts made by the participant are appreciated
20	Advisor is positive and non-judgmental; good things are noticed
4. Taking weight and waist measurements	
21	Waist circumference is measured
22	Weight is measured
5. Reviewing weight change	
23	(a) If participant has lost weight they are congratulated OR (b) If the participant has not lost weight they are helped to develop a plan to address their particular problem
6. Presenting new topic – Avoiding The Slippery Slope of Changing Habits for Life	
24	'Slips' are defined in a manner that is relevant to the participant
25	Advisor discusses what to do after a 'slip' to get the participant back on their feet again
26	Advisor helps to identify some things or situations when the participant 'slips' from healthy eating and being active
7. Setting goals, making action plans and assigning home activities	
27	Participant is encouraged to continue to get back on track
	The following leaflets are given:
28	• Camden Change4Health Walks
29	• Recipe book (British Heart Foundation 'Healthy Meals, Healthy Hearts' or 'Food Should be Fun… And Healthy')
30	Participant is reminded to continue to wear their pedometer and record their steps
8. Confirming date of next appointment	
31	The appointment for the next session is confirmed

on a 7-point scale, with anchors at four points (not at all, somewhat, considerably, extensively).

Rater training

Raters were blind to participants' weight loss outcomes. The raters (LA and GB) practised using consultations not included in the analysis (five for treatment fidelity, 18 for motivational interviewing and 10 for therapeutic alliance) and discussed discrepancies. The raters independently rated consultations in batches of five and reconvened to discuss discrepancies. For motivational interviewing, a third rater (LN) independently rated six consultations and met with the raters to discuss discrepancies. For therapeutic alliance, a third rater (EG) independently rated three consultations and met with raters to discuss discrepancies and provide additional examples of ratings. Raters coded each consultation four times: once for treatment fidelity, twice for motivational interviewing (global ratings followed by behaviour counts) and once for therapeutic alliance.

Results

Treatment fidelity analysis

Inter-rater reliability

Overall and specific agreement, for positive and negative agreement, were calculated for each item [35, 36]. Overall agreement was 0.82 (i.e. for 770/937 decisions, the raters agreed that the item had been done or not done). Items with low inter-rater reliability (defined as agreement in less than 70% of decisions) or with too many missing (due to issues with sound in the recording) were excluded. The items deleted were: (1) initial items, as advisors did not necessarily start the recording immediately, (2) items that could not be reliably recorded from audio-only recordings, e.g. 'advisor shows acceptance of the participant' (which could have been communicated non-verbally) or 'showing the participant's weight change on a graph', (3) repeated items (e.g. 'reviewing previously set goals or intentions' appeared in two places in the session plan), and (4) items that could not be assessed without knowledge of the participant's perspective (e.g. 'uses analogies that are meaningful to the participant').

The resulting checklists contained 31, 32 and 35 items respectively for the three sessions. In the final versions, the proportion of overall agreement was 0.90 (0.88, 0.90 and 0.93 respectively). The proportions of specific agreement were 0.88 for positive agreement and 0.92 for negative agreement.

Fidelity identified from the recordings

Overall, a mean of 41% of scheduled content was addressed, with session totals of 39, 35 and 49% respectively (Table 3). The amount of content addressed per participant ranged from 24 to 54% (SD 10%).

Table 3 Percentage session content addressed by the advisors

Content of topics	Session 9 N = 10	Session 10 N = 6	Session 11 N = 6	Total N = 22
1. Review of general progress Discussing goals from previous session General feedback and encouragement Uncovering barriers	85%	71%	98%	85%
2. Review of previous topic and handouts Participant's use of information from last session (Positive Thinking/Avoiding the Slippery Slope/Social Eating) Uncovering barriers Participant's use of handouts	13%	0%	3%	8%
3. Review of pedometer counts and physical activity Pedometer use and step counts Appreciation of participant's efforts Use of handout about walks	42%	60%	12%	39%
4. Taking weight and waist measurements	100%	100%	92%[a]	98%
5. Reviewing weight change	75%	83%	100%	84%
6. Presenting new topic Discussing topic with examples (Avoiding the Slippery Slope, Social Eating, Staying on Course)	68%	21%	79%	60%
7. Setting goals, developing action plans and assigning home activities Encouragement to keep on track New information leaflets Reminder to use pedometer	11%	13%	39%	24%
8. Setting date of next appointment	80%[a]	83%	100%	86%
Totals	39%	35%	49%	41%

[a]2 data points missing due to problems with the recording

Content included most frequently was: taking weight and waist measurements (98%), setting date of next appointment (86%), reviewing general progress (85%), and reviewing weight change (84%). The most frequent items were 'giving encouragement' and 'showing appreciation of participant's efforts' (95% in reviewing general progress and 88% in reviewing pedometer counts and physical activity).

Topics with lower or more variable frequency were: reviewing participant's use of the previous session's topic and handouts (8%), reviewing pedometer use, reviewing step counts and physical activity (excluding the item about appreciation of participant's efforts) (19%), setting goals, developing action plans and assigning home activities (24%), and presenting the new topic, which varied from 21% for session 10 (Social Eating) to 79% for session 11 (Staying on Course).

Mean consultation length was 18.9 min (SD 7.6, range 9.0–30.4). Quantity of content correlated with consultation length (Spearman's rho 0.73, $p < 0.01$).

Motivational interviewing
Inter-rater reliability
For the global dimensions, using the categories described by Cicchetti [37] the intra-class correlation coefficients (two-way random, testing for consistency) were excellent for Direction, fair for Empathy, and poor for Evocation, Collaboration, Autonomy/Support and Spirit of Motivational Interviewing (Table 4).

For the behaviour counts, the intra-class correlation co-efficients showed excellent reliability for Giving Information, Simple Reflections, Complex Reflections and Motivational Interviewing Adherent, good reliability for Closed Questions, fair reliability for Open Questions and poor reliability for Motivational Interviewing Non-adherent.

Motivational interviewing identified from the recordings
The scale authors suggested that a mean score of 3.5 indicates 'beginning proficiency' and 4.0 indicates 'competency' for the global dimensions [31]. The mean scores for Evocation, Collaboration, Autonomy/Support and Spirit of Motivational Interviewing fell below the threshold for 'beginning proficiency', and Empathy was at 'beginning proficiency' (Table 5). The mean score for Direction was high, indicating that advisors maintained focus on the target topic of weight loss.

Mean total questions asked by the advisors was 4.8 (SD 3.0) and mean total reflections was 5.9 (SD 4.5). Summary scores for the behaviour counts fell between the scale authors' suggested scores for 'beginning proficiency' and 'competency' for Reflection to Question ratio and Percent Open Questions, and below the threshold for 'beginning proficiency' for Percent Complex Reflections and Percent MI-Adherent.

Therapeutic alliance
Inter-rater reliability and internal consistency
Excellent internal consistency was found (Cronbach's alpha 0.92). Intra-class correlation coefficients (Table 6) showed excellent reliability for two items (warmth and empathy), good reliability for four items (involvement, rapport, client self-discloses thoughts and feelings, and client and therapist agree on the kind of changes to make), fair reliability for five items (supportive encouragement, client expresses emotions, client works actively

Table 4 Motivational interviewing mean scores by rater and inter-rater reliability for global dimensions and behaviour counts

Global dimensions	Rater 1 Mean (SD)	Rater 2 Mean (SD)	ICC(2,2)	95% CI Lower	95% CI Upper
Evocation	3.2 (1.0)	3.5 (0.7)	0.34	−0.58	0.73
Collaboration	3.3 (0.9)	3.2 (0.6)	0.37	−0.52	0.74
Autonomy/Support	3.1 (0.7)	3.4 (0.6)	Scale not reliable[a]		
Direction	4.2 (1.2)	3.8 (1.1)	0.83	0.59	0.93
Empathy	3.6 (0.7)	3.6 (0.6)	0.53	−0.14	0.80
Spirit of Motivational Interviewing	3.2 (0.8)	3.3 (0.5)	0.33	−0.62	0.72
Behaviour counts					
Giving Information	12.3 (5.5)	9.1 (4.1)	0.86	0.67	0.94
Closed Questions	3.0 (3.0)	2.3 (2.6)	0.65	0.16	0.85
Open Questions	2.0 (1.7)	2.4 (1.4)	0.53	−0.13	0.81
Simple Reflections	5.1 (3.9)	5.4 (4.4)	0.83	0.59	0.93
Complex Reflections	0.9 (1.2)	0.4 (1.0)	0.63	0.11	0.85
Motivational Interviewing Adherent	6.5 (4.3)	7.8 (5.1)	0.81	0.53	0.92
Motivational Interviewing Non-adherent	8.2 (6.9)	4.8 (3.5)	0.37	−0.52	0.74

[a]Landers [39]

Table 5 Motivational interviewing summary scores for behaviour counts and thresholds for proficiency

Summary score	Mean (SD)	Thresholds for proficiency from Moyers et al. 2010	
		Beginning proficiency	Competency
Reflection to Question ratio	1.8% (2.3)	1%	2%
Percent Open Questions	54.6% (27.4)	50%	70%
Percent Complex Reflections	9.3% (9.2)	40%	50%
Percent Motivational Interviewing Adherent	53.1% (17.2)	90%	100%

with therapist's comments, client and therapist share same sense about how to proceed, and client and therapist agree on salient themes), and poor reliability for the remaining three items.

Therapeutic alliance identified from the recordings
Mean total score was 4.1 (SD 0.8) indicating that the consultations were being rated around the mid-point, between the anchor points of 'somewhat' and 'considerably'. Of the 11 items with fair to excellent reliability, items with a mean score above the mid-point were: supportive encouragement (mean 5.0, SD 1.3), involvement (mean 4.8, SD 1.1), warmth (mean 4.7, SD 1.2), client self-discloses thoughts and feelings (mean 4.5, SD 1.5), rapport (mean 4.4, SD 1.3) and empathy (mean 4.2, SD 1.3).

Relationship of process measures to weight outcome
Using independent t-tests to compare the 11 participants who had lost 5% or more of their baseline weight with the 11 participants who had not, there was no difference between the groups for: (i) consultation length, (ii) percentage of total content covered, (iii) motivational

interviewing: Motivational Interviewing Spirit, percentage open questions, percentage complex reflections, percentage Motivational Interviewing Adherent, (iv) therapeutic alliance total score (Table 7).

Discussion
Intervention fidelity should be improved by providing advisors with training, supervision and supporting materials [21]. Nonetheless, observed adherence to intervention content was lower than expected. Paradoxically, having detailed session content may cause a conflict between achieving an intervention that can be *consistently* delivered and one that can be *realistically* delivered. The development of the fidelity measure revealed a relatively high number of items for the intended consultation length. However, advisors were not routinely using the full time allocation, with the average duration of the consultations being a third less than the time scheduled. This suggests that health advisors were selective in delivering content. Certain elements were performed consistently, such as reviewing general progress and taking weight and waist measurements, whilst others were

Table 6 Alliance mean scores by rater and inter-rater reliability

Scale items	Rater 1 Mean (SD)	Rater 2 Mean (SD)	ICC(2,2)	95% CI Lower	95% CI Upper
1. Supportive encouragement	4.9 (1.8)	5.1 (1.3)	0.58	−0.01	0.83
2. Convey expertise	4.1 (1.5)	4.5 (1.0)	Scale not reliable[a]		
3. Therapist's communication style	4.4 (1.3)	4.6 (0.6)	0.07	−1.26	0.61
4. Involvement	4.8 (1.4)	4.8 (1.1)	0.73	0.34	0.89
5. Warmth	4.8 (1.4)	4.6 (1.3)	0.81	0.54	0.92
6. Rapport	4.3 (1.7)	4.6 (1.2)	0.73	0.35	0.89
7. Empathy	3.8 (1.6)	4.6 (1.3)	0.79	0.50	0.91
8. Client self-discloses thoughts and feelings	4.6 (2.1)	4.5 (1.3)	0.67	0.21	0.86
9. Client expresses emotions	2.9 (1.6)	2.6 (1.5)	0.56	−0.07	0.82
10. Client works actively with therapist's comments	3.1 (1.6)	4.0 (1.0)	0.52	−0.17	0.80
11. Client shows confidence in therapy and therapist	3.7 (1.6)	4.0 (1.3)	0.36	−0.55	0.73
12. Client and therapist agree on the kind of changes to make	3.2 (1.9)	3.8 (1.4)	0.65	0.17	0.86
13. Client and therapist share same sense about how to proceed	3.6 (1.4)	3.5 (1.4)	0.51	−0.19	0.80
14. Client and therapist agree on salient themes	4.0 (1.2)	3.8 (0.9)	0.55	−0.09	0.81
Total score	4.0 (1.1)	4.2 (0.8)	0.72	0.33	0.89

[a]Landers [39]

Table 7 Comparison of consultations by participants' final weight change

Mean (SD) score	Lost 5% or more of baseline weight (N = 11)	Did not lose 5% or more of baseline weight (N = 11)	Statistic	Significance	95% CI Lower	95% CI Upper
Fidelity						
Consultation length (minutes)	21.7 (7.5)	16.1 (6.9)	t(20) = 1.8	p > 0.05	−0.81	11.98
Percentage total content	40.3 (15.1)	38.9 (10.6)	t(20) = 0.2	p > 0.05	−10.23	33.43
Motivational interviewing						
Motivational Interviewing Spirit	3.4 (0.4)	3.1 (0.6)	t(20) = 1.3	p > 0.05	−0.18	0.73
Percentage open questions	59.0 (30.3)	50.3 (24.7)	t(20) = 0.7	p > 0.05	−15.83	33.43
Percentage complex reflections	8.2 (9.5)	10.4 (9.1)	t(20) = −0.6	p > 0.05	−10.48	6.06
Percentage Motivational Interviewing Adherent	55.8 (15.6)	50.5 (19.0)	t(20) = 0.7	p > 0.05	−10.15	20.75
Therapeutic alliance						
Alliance total score	4.3 (0.7)	3.9 (1.0)	t(20) = 1.0	p > 0.05	−0.39	1.01

performed inconsistently, such as reviewing participants' use of information from the previous session and goal-setting. The findings indicated that advisors focused more on practical elements and education than on exploring participants' perspectives. The latter is potentially more challenging, despite the availability of time and relationship continuity. Notwithstanding the detailed guide to content, differing levels of skill are required across intervention components. This may highlight a limitation of interventions designed to be delivered by trained advisors rather than by traditionally trained health professionals, in that elements of the intervention requiring more advanced psychological consultation techniques were not delivered, despite the availability of time.

The advisors knew they were being recorded, indeed, they switched on the recording equipment, as is common in UK primary care settings. During the five-month recording period, all consultations were recorded (whether or not at the mid-point of the intervention), to 'normalise' the routine of recording, of which a fifth (22/104) were analysed. The raters reported that the advisors appeared to have a 'routine' for the consultations and that the language used (for example, in beginning the consultation and initiating the 'taking measurements' task) indicated that this was a routine familiar to the participants. This suggests that the aim of capturing a well-developed relationship and consultation routine was achieved by recording at the intervention mid-point. Whilst it cannot be ruled out, there was no evidence to suggest that the advisors were behaving differently whilst being recorded.

Higher inter-rater reliabilities were achieved for 'basic' and specific skills in motivational interviewing (e.g. whether the advisor maintains a focus on the target topic, demonstrates an empathic approach, or asks closed questions). The authors of the scale noted that it performs better for rating 'entry level' than expert therapeutic behaviours, and specifically, for measuring empathy and

micro-skills (such as using open and closed questions) rather than advanced skills (such as creating a discrepancy between client values and behaviours or eliciting change talk) [32]. The findings of the present study are consistent with this. It is, however, easier to code a behaviour reliably when it is present, as behaviours which appear to meet the criteria can be scrutinised and any discrepancies between raters discussed.

The findings suggested that the advisors were operating at 'entry level' proficiency in motivational interviewing, which is consistent with the advisors' level of experience and skill. Advisors consistently demonstrated an empathic approach and maintained a focus on the topic of weight loss. This concurs with the results about fidelity, which also found the advisors to be consistently encouraging and supportive. However, more advanced therapeutic skills in motivational interviewing were not observed. This 'layering' of skills in motivational interviewing, with increasing complexity requiring considerable experience and training, is consistent with other research [24].

In terms of therapeutic alliance, higher inter-rater reliability was achieved for affective qualities of the relationship (e.g. involvement, warmth, rapport and empathy) than specific skills (e.g. client works actively with therapist's comments). Consistent with the findings from the other two measures, advisors demonstrated 'entry level' proficiency, achieving higher ratings for aspects of the quality of the interpersonal climate, such as supportive encouragement, involvement, warmth, rapport and empathy.

Overall, the findings demonstrated that certain aspects of the intervention were consistently delivered. Participants' weight was checked, information was provided, and sessions maintained a focus on the target outcome. Furthermore, these tasks were conducted in the context of a warm and supportive advisor-participant relationship. Interviews with participants in the Camden Weight Loss trial reported elsewhere revealed that the most valued aspects of the intervention were the relationship they formed with the advisor, followed by regularity of meetings [38].

The aim of the trial was to examine the feasibility and effectiveness of a weight management programme which was centrally organised but locally delivered in a primary care setting. Other research examining consultations in primary care in which weight management is discussed has demonstrated the importance of training health professionals in weight management interventions [18]. The results of the present study, however, highlight the importance of ongoing training and supervision. Multi-component weight management interventions comprise a spectrum of tasks and skills at varying levels of sophistication, which take time to acquire and develop.

An important determinant of intervention delivery is the congruence between the aims of the intervention and the experience and skill of the provider. One solution may be to use recorded consultations during supervision to provide feedback about fidelity and discuss strategies the advisor might use to achieve the intervention aims. In addition to providing ongoing training and supervision, another solution might be to alter the complexity of the intervention over time, as advisors' experience and skill increase.

This study had several limitations. Consultation recordings were not available for all participants in the study, as they were gathered during a five-month period and participants varied in their start date for the 12-month intervention. Recordings were also subject to the vagaries of the primary care settings, including technical failure. The present sample attended a greater number of sessions compared to others in the intervention group, as those included necessarily continued to at least session 9, and were more likely to be male, although there is no clear explanation for this (there was no gender difference in the number of sessions completed). The small sample size made it difficult to assess the impact of variation in fidelity on intervention outcome (final weight change). Nonetheless, the observed consultations appeared to provide a representative picture of the intervention as delivered in practice.

The health advisors in the study were recruited and trained as recommended by the National Health Service *Health Trainers Initiative* [26]. However, the study did not examine delivery of the intervention by other types of advisors, such as professionals trained in primary care or psychological interventions. Advisors with different backgrounds and experience may have delivered the intervention differently.

Conclusions

The results of randomised controlled trials and the effectiveness of complex interventions addressing behaviour change are dependent on the fidelity of the intervention delivered. Obesity statistics indicate that weight management interventions will continue to be required for the foreseeable future, emphasising the need for effective intervention delivery. This study has demonstrated that an independent process evaluation can identify the components of a complex intervention which are and are not reliably delivered. As these interventions are complex and layered, advisors delivering such interventions require considerable support, training and ongoing supervision to support those attempting to achieve significant weight loss.

Abbreviations
CAMWEL: Camden Weight Loss; CI: confidence interval; EG: Emma Godfrey; GB: Gabriella Baez; ICC: intra-class correlation coefficient; KN: Kiran Nanchahal; LA: Liane Al-Baba; LN: Lorraine Noble; N: number; NHS: National Health Service; NICE: National Institute for Health and Care Excellence; NT: Nicki Thorogood; SD: standard deviation; UCL: University College London; UK: United Kingdom

Funding
Camden Primary Care Trust (NHS Camden) funded the intervention from which the data were gathered. The funding source had no role in the design or conduct of the study; collection, management, analysis or interpretation of the data and preparation, review or approval of the manuscript.

Authors' contributions
LN, EG, KN and NT conceived and designed the study, KN and NT contributed to acquisition of data, LN, EG, LA and GB contributed to analysis of the data; LN drafted the article, all authors contributed to the interpretation of the data, preparation of the manuscript and have read and approved the manuscript.

Competing interests
The authors declare they have no competing interests.

Author details
[1]UCL Medical School, University College London, Royal Free Hospital, Rowland Hill Street, NW3 2PF, London, UK. [2]Department of Psychology, Institute of Psychiatry, Psychology and Neuroscience, King's College London, London, UK. [3]UCL Research Department of Epidemiology and Public Health, UCL, London, UK. [4]Department of Social and Environmental Health Research, London School of Hygiene and Tropical Medicine, London, UK.

References

1. The LancetUrgently needed: a framework convention for obesity control. Lancet. 2011;378(9793):741.
2. World Health Organization. Global Health Observatory (GHO) data: Obesity; 2016 http://www.who.int/gho/ncd/risk_factors/obesity_text/en/#. Accessed 17 Jan 2017.
3. Health and Social Care Information Centre. Statistics on obesity, physical activity and diet, England; 2016. ISBN 978-1-78386-698-4.
4. Department of Health. Policy paper. 2010 to 2015 government policy: obesity and healthy eating; 2015. https://www.gov.uk/government/publications/2010-to-2015-government-policy-obesity-and-healthy-eating/2010-to-2015-government-policy-obesity-and-healthy-eating. Accessed 17 Jan 2017.
5. NICE National Institute for Health and Social Care Excellence. Weight management: lifestyle services for overweight or obese adults. NICE public health guidance 53; 2014. https://www.nice.org.uk/guidance/ph53. Accessed 17 Jan 2017.
6. Buckroyd J. Psychological interventions for people with a BMI ≥ 35. In: Obesity in the UK: a psychological perspective. Obesity Working Group, Professional Practice Board, The British Psychological Society; 2011. https://www1.bps.org.uk/system/files/Public%20files/Policy/obesity_in_the_uk_-_a_psychological_perspective.pdf. Accessed 17 Jan 2017.
7. Hartmann-Boyce J, Johns D, Aveyard P, Onakpoya I, Jebb S, Phillips D et al. Managing overweight and obese adults: update review. The clinical effectiveness of long-term weight management schemes for adults. Review 1a. University of Oxford; 2013a. https://www.nice.org.uk/guidance/ph53/evidence/evidence-review-1a-431707933. Accessed 17 Jan 2017.
8. Hartmann-Boyce J, Johns D, Aveyard P, Onakpoya I, Jebb SA, Phillips D et al. How components of behavioural weight management programmes affect weight change. Review 1b. University of Oxford; 2013b. https://www.nice.org.uk/guidance/ph53/evidence/evidence-review-1b-431707934. Accessed 17 Jan 2017.
9. Johns D, Hartmann-Boyce J, Aveyard P, Onakpoya I, Jebb S, Phillips D et al. Weight regain after behavioural weight management programmes. Review 1c. University of Oxford; 2013a. https://www.nice.org.uk/guidance/ph53/evidence/evidence-review-1c-431707935. Accessed 17 Jan 2017.
10. Johns D, Hartmann-Boyce J, Aveyard P, Lewis A, Jebb SA, Phillips D et al. Managing overweight and obese adults: evidence review. Review 2. University of Oxford; 2013b. https://www.nice.org.uk/guidance/ph53/evidence/evidence-review-2-431707936. Accessed 17 Jan 2017.
11. Marchant D. Exercise for obese individuals. In obesity in the UK: a psychological perspective. Obesity working group, professional practice board, the British psychological society; 2011. https://www1.bps.org.uk/system/files/Public%20files/Policy/obesity_in_the_uk_-_a_psychological_perspective.pdf. Accessed 17 Jan 2017.
12. Sniehotta FF, Simpson SA, Greaves CJ. Weight loss maintenance: an agenda for health psychology. Br J Health Psychol. 2014;19(3):459–64.
13. Jeffery RW, Epstein LH, Wilson GT, Drewnowski A, Stunkard AJ, Wing RR. Long-term maintenance of weight loss: current status. Health Psychol. 2000;19(1S):5–16.
14. Miller W, Rollnick S. Motivational interviewing: preparing people for change. 2nd ed. New York: Guilford Press; 2002.
15. Burke BL, Arkowitz H, Menchola M. The efficacy of motivational interviewing: a meta-analysis of controlled clinical trials. J Consult Clin Psychol. 2003;71(5):843–61.
16. Armstrong MJ, Mottershead TA, Ronksley PE, Sigal RJ, Campbell TS, Hemmelgarn BR. Motivational interviewing to improve weight loss in overweight and/or obese patients: a systematic review and meta-analysis of randomized controlled trials. Obes Rev. 2011;12(9):709–23.
17. van Dorsten B. The use of motivational interviewing in weight loss. Current Diabetes Reports. 2007;7(5):386–90.
18. Cox ME, Yancy WS, Coffman CJ, Østbye T, Tulsky JA, Alexander SC, et al. Effects of counseling techniques on patients' weight-related attitudes and behaviors in a primary care clinic. Patient Educ Couns. 2011;85(3):363–8.
19. Wampold BE. How important are the common factors in psychotherapy? An update. World Psychiatry. 2015;14(3):270–7.
20. Baldwin SA, Wampold BE, Imel ZE. Untangling the alliance-outcome correlation: exploring the relative importance of therapist and patient variability in the alliance. J Consult Clin Psychol. 2007;75(6):842–52.
21. Dane AV, Schneider BH. Program integrity in primary and early secondary prevention: are implementation effects out of control? Clin Psychol Rev. 1998;18(1):23–45.
22. Sánchez V, Steckler A, Nitirat P, Hallfors D, Cho H, Brodish P. Fidelity of implementation in a treatment effectiveness trial of reconnecting youth. Health Educ Res. 2007;22(1):95–107.
23. Appel LJ, Clark JM, Yeh HC, Wang NY, Coughlin JW, Daumit G, et al. Comparative effectiveness of weight-loss interventions in clinical practice. N Engl J Med. 2011;365(21):1959–68.
24. van Eijk-Hustings YJ, Daemen L, Schaper NC, Vrijhoef HJ. Implementation of motivational interviewing in a diabetes care management initiative in the Netherlands. Patient Educ Couns. 2011;84(1):10–5.
25. Nanchahal K, Power T, Holdsworth E, Hession M, Sorhaindo A, Griffiths U, et al. A pragmatic randomised controlled trial in primary care of the Camden weight loss (CAMWEL) programme. BMJ Open. 2012;2(3):e000793.
26. Michie S, Rumsey N, Fussell A, Hardeman W, Johnston M, Newman S et al. Improving health: changing behaviour. NHS health trainer handbook. London: Department of Health Publications (Best Practice Guidance: Gateway Ref 9721); 2008. http://eprints.uwe.ac.uk/12057. Accessed 17 Jan 2017.
27. NICE National Institute for Health and Social Care Excellence. Obesity prevention. Clinical guideline CG43; 2006. https://www.nice.org.uk/Guidance/cg43. Accessed 17 Jan 2017.
28. Bandura A. Social foundations of thought and action: a social cognitive theory. Englewood Cliffs, NJ: Prentice-Hall; 1986.
29. Locke EA. Latham GP. A theory of goal setting and task performance. Englewood Cliffs, NJ: Prentice-Hall; 1990.
30. Alemi F, Neuhauser D, Ardito S, Headrick L, Moore S, Hekelman F, et al. Continuous self-improvement: systems thinking in a personal context. Jt Comm J Quality and Patient Saf. 2000;26(2):74–86.
31. Moyers TB, Martin T, Manuel JK, Miller WR, Ernst D. Revised global scales: Motivational interviewing treatment integrity 3.1. 1 (MITI 3.1. 1). Unpublished manuscript, University of New Mexico, Albuquerque, NM; 2010. http://casaa.unm.edu/download/miti3_1.pdf. Accessed 17 Jan 2017.
32. Moyers TB, Martin T, Manuel JK, Hendrickson SM, Miller WR. Assessing competence in the use of motivational interviewing. J Subst Abus Treat. 2005;28(1):19–26.
33. Carels RA, Darby L, Cacciapaglia HM, Konrad K, Coit C, Harper J, et al. Using motivational interviewing as a supplement to obesity treatment: a stepped-care approach. Health Psychol. 2007;26(3):369–74.
34. Godfrey E, Chalder T, Ridsdale L, Seed P, Ogden J. Investigating the active ingredients of cognitive behaviour therapy and counselling for patients with chronic fatigue in primary care: developing a new process measure to assess treatment fidelity and predict outcome. Br J Clin Psychol. 2007;46(3):253–72.
35. Fleiss JL, Levin, Paik MC. The measure of inter-rater agreement. In: Fleiss JL, Levin B, Paik MC, Statistical methods for rates and proportions, New Jersey: John Wiley & Sons; 2013. p. 598–626.
36. Uebersax J. Raw agreement indices; 2014. http://www.john-uebersax.com/stat/raw.htm. Accessed 17 Jan 2017.
37. Cicchetti DV. Guidelines, criteria, and rules of thumb for evaluating normed and standardized assessment instruments in psychology. Psychol Assess. 1994;(4):284–90.
38. Holdsworth E, Thorogood N, Sorhaindo A, Nanchahal K. A qualitative study of participant engagement with a weight loss intervention. Health Promot Pract. 2016;1524839916659847
39. Landers R. Computing intra-class correlations as estimates of inter-rater reliability in SPSS. The Winnower, 2015;3:e143518.81744. https://thewinnower.com/papers/1113-computing-intraclass-correlations-icc-as-estimates-of-interrater-reliability-in-spss. Accessed 17 Jan 2017.

22

Prevalence and associated factors of overweight/obesity among children and adolescents in Ethiopia: a systematic review and meta-analysis

Alemu Gebrie[1*], Animut Alebel[2], Abriham Zegeye[1], Bekele Tesfaye[2] and Aster Ferede[3]

Abstract

Background: Overweight and obesity can be defined as excessive and abnormal fat depositions in our body. They have become one of the emerging and serious public health concerns of the twenty-first century in low income countries like Ethiopia. Hence, the aim of this study was to determine the pooled prevalence and review associated risk factors of overweight/obesity among children and adolescents in Ethiopia.

Method: The articles were identified through explicit and reproducible electronic search of reputable databases (PubMed, Google scholar, Science Direct, EMBASE, Cochrane library), and the hand search of reference lists of previous prevalence studies to retrieve more related articles. The 18 studies were selected based on a comprehensive list of inclusion and exclusion criteria. Data were extracted using a standardized and pre-tested data extraction checklist, and the analysis was done using STATA 14 statistical software. To assess heterogeneity, the Cochrane Q test statistic and I^2 tests were used. Since the included studies exhibited considerable heterogeneity, a random effect model was used to estimate the pooled prevalence of overweight/obesity. Moreover, the risk factors of overweight/obesity were reviewed.

Results: The combined pooled prevalence of overweight and obesity among children and adolescents in Ethiopia was 11.30% (95% CI: 8.71, 13.88%). Also, the separate pooled prevalence of overweight and obesity were 8.92 and 2.39%, respectively. Subgroup analysis revealed that the highest overweight/obesity prevalence among children and adolescents was observed in Addis Ababa, 11.94 (95% CI: 9.39, 14.50). Female gender of the children: 3.23 (95% CI 2.03,5.13), high family socioeconomic status: 3.16 (95% CI 1.87,5.34), learning in private school: 3.22 (95% CI 2.36,4.40), physical inactivity: 3.36 (95% CI 1.68,6.72), sweet nutriments preference: 2.78 (95% CI 1.97,3.93) and less use of fruits/vegetables: 1.39 (95% CI 1.10,1.75) have shown a positive association with the development of overweight/obesity among children and adolescents.

Conclusion: The pooled prevalence of overweight/obesity among children and adolescents in Ethiopia is substantially high, and has become an emerging nutrition linked problem. Female gender, high family socioeconomic status, learning in private school, physical inactivity, sweet nutriments preference and less use of fruits/vegetables were found to be significantly associated with overweight/obesity.

Keywords: Overweight, Obesity, Associated factors, Children, Adolescents, Ethiopia

* Correspondence: alemugebrie2@gmail.com
[1]Department of Biomedical Science, School of Medicine, Debre Markos University, P.O. Box 269, Debre Markos, Ethiopia
Full list of author information is available at the end of the article

Background

Overweight and obesity can be defined as excessive and abnormal fat depositions in our body. They are major risk factors for several diet-linked non-communicable diseases like dyslipidemia, cardiovascular diseases (CVD), and type II diabetes mellitus [1–4]. Worldwide, overweight/ obesity is becoming one of the most challenging current health concerns with the worrisome rise in children and adolescents. Contemporary evidence revealed that the worldwide prevalence of overweight / obesity among children and adolescents were 13.5% [5]. In Africa, under-nutrition is the major nutritional problem affecting both children and adolescents. However, overweight/obesity is noticeably high with a prevalence of 8.5% in 2010 and predicted to be 12.7% by 2020. This situation pinpoints a double burden of malnutrition, and epidemiological as well as nutrition transition by virtue of several socioeconomic and demographic changes [5–7].

Studies showed that many factors can potentially be associated with overweight/obesity in children and adolescents [8, 9]. Those factors that are of maternal origin were socioeconomic status, education level, marital status, and smoking status during pregnancy. Gender of the children and adolescents, weight at birth, their birth rank, and residence were also the factors associated with overweight /obesity among them [10, 11]. Children and adolescents in developing countries are prone to sugar, high fat salts, energy rich foods and micronutrient-poor foods that are less costly and lower in nutrient quality. These dietary habits in combination with other factors result in substantial upsurge of overweight/obesity [12].

School based health education and promotion tactics such as enhancing physical activity among the children and adolescents, vegetables and fruits intake have been helpful to minimize overweight/obesity [13]. To solve this emerging health problem, Ethiopia incorporated the concern of overweight/obesity into the national nutrition program and launched an initiative to promote physical activity in the population [6]. Nevertheless, the efforts do not target children and adolescents in particular.

In different regions of Ethiopia, several independent and fragmented studies [14–30] were conducted in children and adolescents to assess the prevalence and associated factors of overweight / obesity, but there was a great variation and inconsistency of the findings among the studies. Hence, the aim of this review was to determine the pooled prevalence and associated factors of overweight/obesity in children and adolescents in Ethiopia. The results of the present study will elevate the need for policy makers, program planners, guardians or parents, clinicians as well as concerned stakeholders to give more emphasis for childhood overweight / obesity in the country. The review question is: What is the best

available evidence on the prevalence and associated factors of overweight and/or obesity among children and adolescents in Ethiopia?

Methods

Literature search approach and study design

For its rigor, this study was guided by Preferred Reporting Items for Systematic Reviews and Meta-Analyses (PRISMA) [31]. The articles for this study were identified through comprehensive and reproducible electronic search of reputable databases (PubMed, Google scholar, Science Direct, EMBASE, Cochrane library), and the hand search of reference lists of previous prevalence studies to retrieve more related articles. The researchers also used the "related articles" option of PubMed and checked the reference lists of the original and review articles to detect more relevant publications. The search was independently performed by the two authors (AG, AA) using the following key terms: (a) population (preschool, children, schoolchildren, school aged, childhood, schooler, preadolescent, adolescent); (b) outcome (body composition, overweight, over nutrition, obesity, body constitution, weight status, body mass index, anthropometry; (c) study design (cross-sectional, prevalence, epidemiology, observational, pattern); and (d) location (Ethiopia and regions of Ethiopia) both in separation and in combination using the Boolean operator like "OR", "AND" or "NOT". Before searching the databases, the appropriateness of searching words was verified for retrieving the relevant articles. The literature search was limited to English language, and human study category. The literature records were managed using the EndNote X7 reference manager. The articles were searched from September, 2017 to November, 2017 and all the articles accessed until November, 2017 were included in this systematic review and meta-analysis.

Selection of studies
Inclusion criteria

The two investigators independently and reproducibly assessed the contents of each of the identified studies (AG and AA). Those articles which met the following criteria were included in the study.

Population: Articles conducted among children and adolescents (age < 20 years) were considered.

Study area: Only articles conducted in Ethiopia were considered.

Study design: Original studies that reported the prevalence and associated risk factors of overweight and/ or obesity, measured objectively by trained personnel, among children in Ethiopia were considered.

Language: Only articles published in English language were considered.

Publication condition: Studies that fulfilled the eligibility criteria were included regardless of their publication status (published, unpublished and grey literature, etc.)

Exclusion criteria

After screening the abstracts and the full texts of the articles, the three researchers (AG, AA and AF) carried out the data extraction independently and blindly. Articles with methodological problems were excluded by the three independent researchers after reading the full text as well as abstracts. The articles the full texts of which we were not able to fully access or failed to contact their primary authors were excluded from this review because of incomplete data.

Data abstraction and critical appraisal of the studies

The two researchers independently extracted all the necessary data using a standardized and pre-tested data extraction checklist. The necessary data extracted from the articles included: first author of the study, region in Ethiopia where the study was carried out, the particular area where the study was conducted, study design, publication year of the study, sample size, response rate, and prevalence of overweight/obesity. Any sort of discrepancies between the researchers on the data extracted were solved through discussion and consensus as well as through involvement of the third reviewer (AZ).

The reviewers employed the Newcastle-Ottawa quality assessment tool Scale adapted for cross-sectional studies so as to appraise the qualities of the studies [32]. The tool is composed of three important indicators. The first part is graded from five points (stars) and evaluates the methodological qualities of the studies. The second part has three stars and assesses the comparability of the studies. The last section of the tool is graded from two points and measures the quality of the original studies in terms of their statistical analyses. By using the tool as a guiding protocol, the two authors (AG and AA) appraised the qualities of the primary studies independently.

The qualities of the studies were assessed by using the following indicators; those with medium (fulfilling 50% of quality assessment criteria) or high quality (≥ 6 out of 10 scales) were considered for inclusion in the meta-analysis. Taking the mean score of the two reviewers, differences of their assessment results were determined.

Operationalization of the outcomes of the review

Firstly, the percentage of overweight/obesity among children and adolescents was the foremost outcome of the meta-analysis. The second outcome of the study was to examine the factors that are associated with overweight/obesity among the study subjects. The prevalence was obtained by dividing the number of children and/or adolescents who are either overweight or obese to the total

number of children and/or adolescents who have been included in the study (sample size) then multiplied by 100. The association between overweight/obesity and the factors were quantified by odds ratio. The odds ratio was calculated from the two by two table reports of the primary studies.

Data analysis/synthesis of results

After the relevant data had been extracted from the studies by using Microsoft excel 2016 format, the authors then analyzed the results by using STATA version 14.0 (STATA Corporation, College Station Texas) software. The original studies were summarized and presented by using a table and the forest plot. The authors computed the standard error of prevalence of overweight/obesity for each original study by using binomial distribution formula. We explored the potential heterogeneity among the reported prevalence of the studies using I^2 test and Cochrane Q statistics [33]. Since the test statistics revealed that there was a considerable heterogeneity [34] among the studies ($I^2 = 96.9\%$, $p = 0.000$), a random effects model was used to estimate the Der Simonian and Laird's pooled effect. We also undertook univariate meta-regression analysis taking publication year of the studies and the sample size to detect the potential source(s) of variation but both of them were found to be statistically insignificant, ($p = 0.65$ and $p = 0.45$ respectively). Possible publication bias was also objectively examined using Egger's weighted correlation and Begg's regression intercept tests at 5% significant level respectively [35, 36]. The test results showed there is a significant publication bias ($p = 0.000$), and therefore the final effect size was determined by applying Duval and Tweedie's Trim and Fill analysis in the Random-effects model. In addition, to minimalize the random variations between the point estimates of the original studies, subgroup analysis was carried out based on region of studies and publication year.

Results

Identification of eligible studies

From the outset, we searched a total of 602 records by the electronic search through a search engine of MEDLINE/PubMed, Google scholar, science direct, EMBASE, Cochrane Library and reference lists of previous related studies to retrieve more related articles. Since there were duplications in the records, 195 of them were removed from the inclusion. After assessing the abstracts and titles, the remaining 407 retrievals, 371 records were excluded since they were not relevant for this meta-analysis in terms of outcome the study is interested. Then, 36 full text studies were considered and assessed for eligibility based on the pre-set eligibility criteria. Finally, 18 studies were considered to be eligible and included in this systematic review and meta-analysis (Fig. 1).

From a total of 36 full text studies accessed, we removed twelve of them because they were review articles, and /or conducted in other nations which are not the location of interest of the study like: USA [37, 38], Russia [39], Japan [40], Yemen [41], Nigeria [42–45], South Africa [46], Egypt [47] and Morocco [48]. Moreover, six full text studies [49–54] that have been carried out from different parts of Ethiopia were excluded because their outcome measures were not prevalence of overweight/obesity in children and they were conducted in the adult population which is not the population of interest of the this study.

Description of original studies

Table 1 summarizes the descriptive characteristics of the 18 studies included in this systematic review and meta-analysis. All the studies were cross sectional by design, and conducted in different parts of Ethiopia with a sample size ranging from 174 in Adama, Oromia region [26] to 9880 in a national survey [55]. The included

studies have been conducted from 2010 to 2017. In the current systematic review and meta-analysis, a total of 19,031 children and adolescents were included to estimate the pooled prevalence of overweight/obesity.

The 18 studies have been conducted in the six regions of Ethiopia: about one third (six) of the included studies were carried out in Addis Ababa: Addis Ababa [19, 21–23, 29, 30], Dire dawa [14], Amhara [17, 18, 21, 24], Harari [28], Oromia [15, 25, 26], Southern Nations, Nationalities and peoples' region (SNNPR) [20, 27] and one nationwide survey study [55]. Whereas the highest prevalence of overweight/obesity (20.54%) was reported in Dire dawa [14], the nationwide survey study [55] reported the lowest prevalence (3%) of the problem. Furthermore, the original studies included in this meta-analysis and reporting response rate had a response rate that ranges from 91 to 100% showing that all the studies had good response rate.

Concerning the quality of the articles: only one [29] of the 18 studies was unpublished article and the studies included in the meta-analysis were identified by exhaustive search from reputable journals like PubMed. Blinded

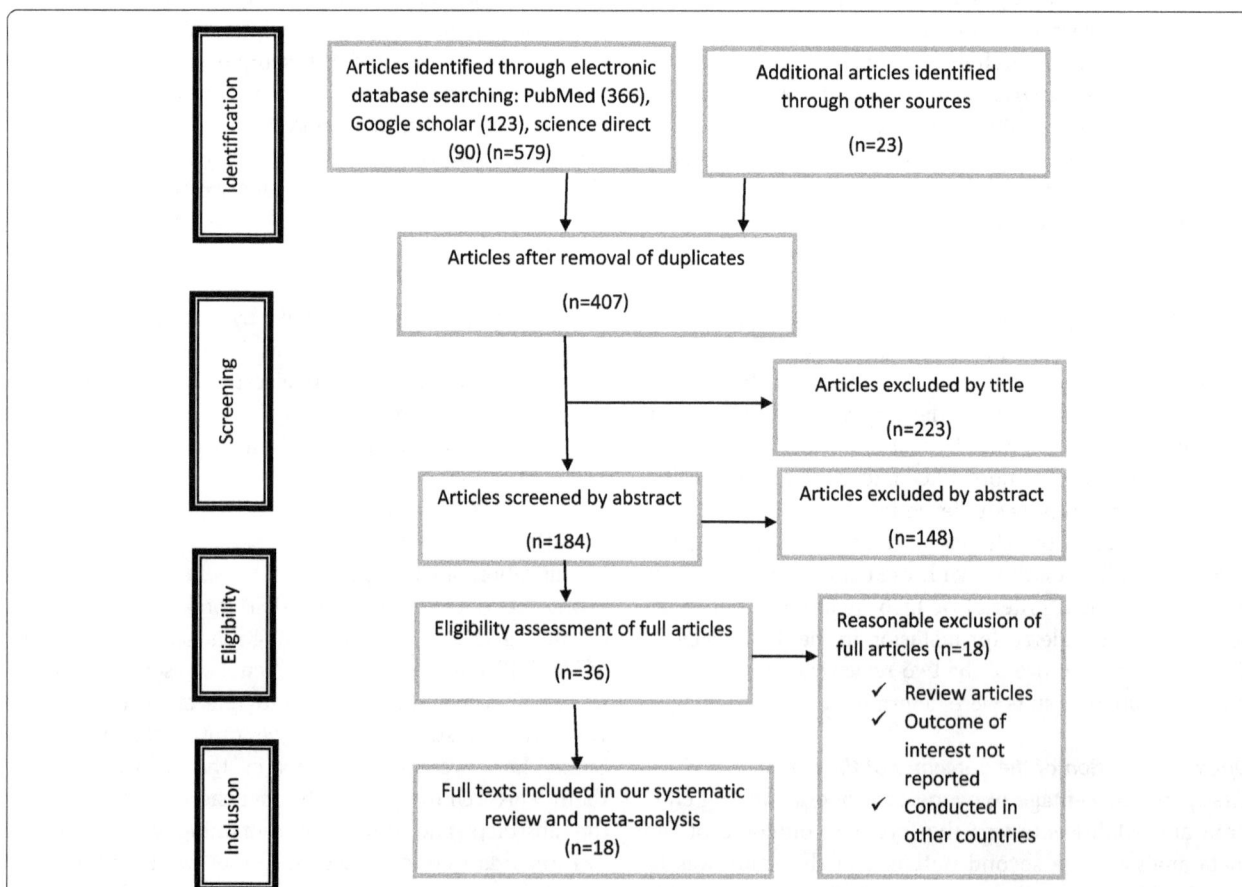

Fig. 1 Flow chart diagram describing selection of studies for the systematic review and meta-analysis of prevalence and associated factors of overweight/obesity among children and adolescents in Ethiopia, 2018 (identified, screened, eligible and included studies). Articles may have been excluded for more than one reason

Table 1 Characteristics of 18 studies reporting the prevalence of overweight/obesity among children and adolescents in Ethiopia included in the current systematic review and meta-analysis, 2018

Region	Area	Author	Publication year	Sample size	Response rate (%)	Quality score (10 pts)	Prevalence (95% CI)
Addis Ababa	Addis Ababa	Gebremichael et al. [22]	2017	463	96.9	6	12.74 (9.71,15.78)
	Bole subcity	Askal et al. [19]	2015	828	97.9	7	9.78 (7.76,11.81)
	Addis Ababa	Dessalegn and Robel [29]	2016	390	96.3	6	18.21 (14.38,22.03)
	Addis Ababa	Mulugeta et al. [30]	2016	446	97.8	6	15.25 (11.91,18.58)
	Arada subcity	Alemu et al. [23]	2014	800	100	7	9.38 (7.36,11.39)
	Addis Ababa	Yoseph et al. [16]	2014	1024	100	6	8.50 (6.79,10.20)
Amhara	Bahirdar	Tadesse et al. [21]	2017	462	97	8	6.93 (4.61,9.24)
	Gondar	Sorrie et al. [18]	2017	500	99.2	8	13.80 (10.78,16.82)
	Gondar	Gebremedhin et al. [17]	2013	791	98.9	7	5.94 (4.29,7.59)
	Bahirdar	Zelalem et al. [24]	2015	431	95.6	8	16.71 (13.18,20.23)
Dire dawa	Dire dawa	Desalew et al. [14]	2017	448	98.2	7	20.54 (16.80,24.28)
Ethiopia	Ethiopia	EDHS [55]	2011	9880	NR	7	3.00 (2.66,3.33)
Harari	Babile	Kedir Teji et al. [28]	2016	547	91	6	5.85 (3.88,7.82)
Oromia	Ambo	Mesert Yetubie et al. [25]	2010	425	NR	7	8.71 (6.03,11.39)
	Jimma	Dessalegn et al. [15]	2017	510	93.4	8	13.33 (10.38,16.28)
	Adama	Wakayo et al. [26]	2016	174	98	7	10.92 (6.29,15.55)
SNNP	Hawasa	Woldie and Belachew [20]	2014	358	100	7	10.61 (7.42,13.81)
	Hawasa	Teshome et al. [27]	2013	554	97	5	15.70 (12.67,18.73)

reviewers re-evaluated all the studies before analysis and the articles were found fit for their quality (quality score ranged from 5 to 8 out of 10 points).

Meta-analysis and meta-regression

As it is depicted in the forest plot of 18 included studies below (Fig. 2a), the combined pooled prevalence of overweight and obesity among children and adolescents in Ethiopia was 11.30% (95% CI: 8.71, 13.88%). Also, from the 16 studies, the separate pooled prevalence of overweight and obesity were 8.92 and 2.39%, respectively (Fig. 2b and c). Considerable heterogeneity [34] was observed among the 18 studies and detected by I^2 statistic ($I^2 = 96.9$, p value < 0.000). As a result, the DerSimonian and Laird random-effects method, which gives more conservative estimate, was used to estimate the overall pooled prevalence of overweight and obesity among children and adolescents. To determine the likely sources for the variation, we checked the potential factors associated with the prevalence variation, publication year and sample size by using univariate meta-regression models but both of them were found to be statistically insignificant for the variation (Table 2). Egger's and Begg's tests showed that there is a statistically significant publication bias, ($p = 0.000$) and ($p = 0.002$) respectively. Hence, we performed Trim and Fill analysis so as to adjust the final pooled prevalence of overweight/obesity among the subjects.

Subgroup analysis

We have also performed subgroup analysis based on the region where the studies were carried out and year of publication of the studies to assess possible causes of considerable heterogeneity. As per the result, the highest prevalence of overweight/obesity among children and adolescents was observed in Addis Ababa, where most of the studies have been conducted, with a prevalence of 11.94 (95% CI: 9.39, 14.50) followed by regions classified (in this study) as others, 10.97% (95% CI: 5.09, 16.85) and Oromia region 10.94% (95% CI: 7.86, 14.02) (Table 3). Regarding year of publication, the prevalence of childhood overweight/obesity was significantly higher in studies which have been published since 2014, 12.95% (95% CI: 10.17, 15.73) compared to those articles published before 2014, 8.70% (95% CI: 5.40, 11.99) (Table 3).

Associated factors of overweight/obesity among children and adolescents

We have comprehensively reviewed and meta-analyzed the associated risk factors of overweight/obesity among children and adolescents by using thirteen relevant studies [14–20, 23, 24, 26, 27, 29, 30] from the eligible articles included in this study. Sex of the children, family income, family educational status, type of school the children attend, physical activity status, habit of using sweet nutriments, use of fruits and vegetables were found to be worth reviewing and meta-analyzable. They

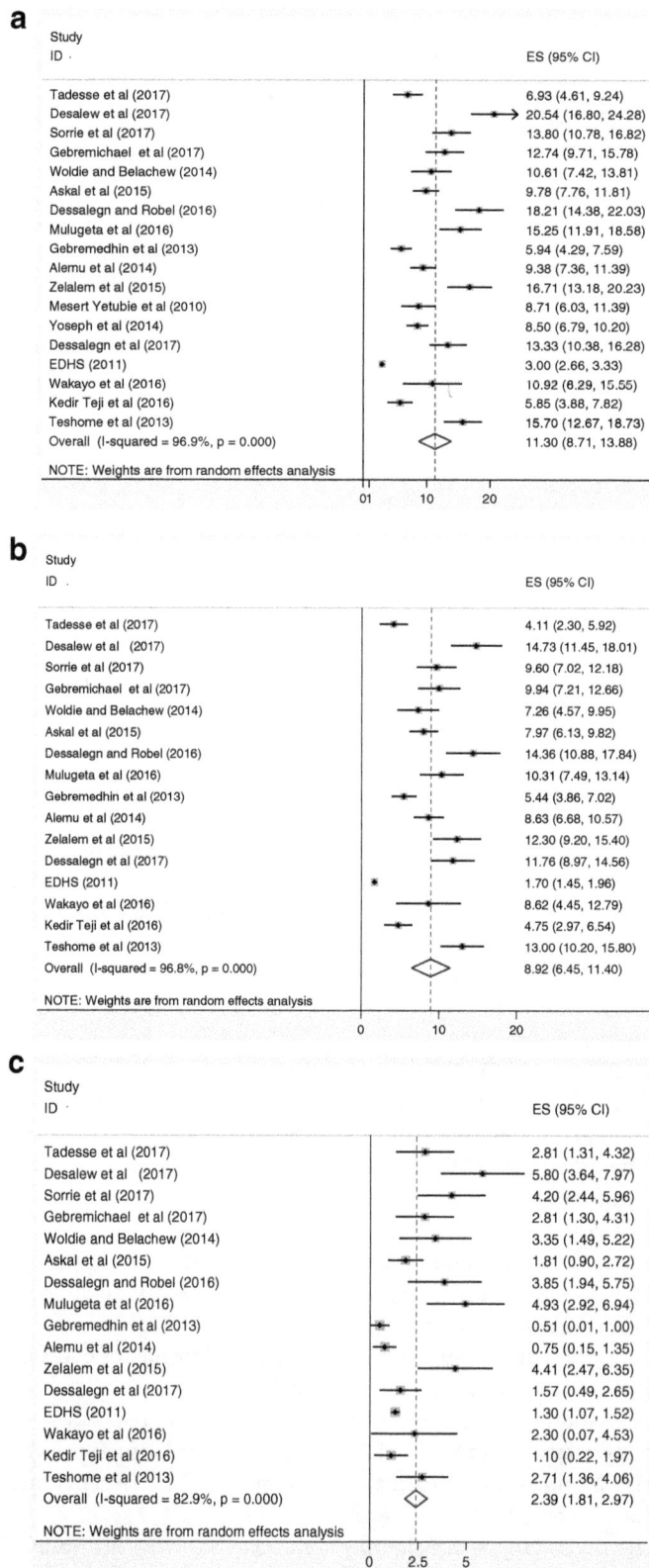

Fig. 2 Forest plot of the pooled prevalence of overweight and obesity in children and adolescents, 2018 (**a**: The combined pooled prevalence of overweight/obesity; **b**: The pooled prevalence of overweight; **c**: The pooled prevalence of obesity)

Table 2 Related factors with the heterogeneity of overweight/obesity prevalence among children and adolescents in Ethiopia in the meta-analysis (univariate meta-regression)

Variables	Coefficient	P-value
Year of publication studies	0.2866022	0.817
Sample sizes of the studies	−0.0005473	0.411

were associated with overweight/obesity among children and adolescents in Ethiopia (Fig. 3). We have also performed sensitivity analysis for each of the factors but none of the studies revealed significant difference.

The pooled effect size of six studies showed that female children and adolescents were 3.23 times more likely to be overweight/obese than their male counterparts, odds ratio 3.23 (95% CI 2.03,5.13) (Fig. 3a). The pooled result of ten studies also revealed that children and adolescents from high income families were 3.16 times more likely to be overweight/obese as compared to those children with middle and low-income families, odds ratio 3.16 (95% CI 1.87,5.34) (Fig. 3b). Those children and adolescents whose families are not illiterate (educated) were 1.57 times more likely to have overweight or obesity compared to those whose families are illiterate, odds ratio 1.57 (95% CI 0.93,2.64) (Fig. 3c).

We have also found that children and adolescents attending at private schools were 3.22 times more likely to develop overweight/obesity as compared to those attending at governmental schools, odds ratio 3.22 (95% CI 2.36,4.40) (Fig. 3d). Physically inactive children and adolescents were also 3.36 times more to be overweight/obese than those children who were physically active, odds ratio 3.36 (95% CI 1.68,6.72) (Fig. 3e). In addition, children and adolescents who had the habit of using sweet food stuffs were 2.78 times more likely to suffer from the emerging nutritional problem of overweight and obesity as compared to those children who have seldom used sweet food items, odds ratio 2.78 (95% CI 1.97,3.93) (Fig. 3f). Moreover, the results of three studies showed that infrequent consumption of fruits and vegetables was a risk factor for the development of overweight/obesity among children, odds ratio 1.39 (95% CI 1.10,1.75) (Fig. 3g).

Discussion

Overweight/obesity, an emerging nutritional problem in developing countries, increases the burden of nutrition related diseases and have far-reaching consequences on economic growth of countries [4–6, 12]. Evidences have revealed that nutrition-linked non-communicable diseases are significantly in upsurge over time. In contrary to previous concerns that mainly focused on the issue of under nutrition, overweight/obesity is now emerging as a nutrition related public health burden. The problem is debilitating and a double burden in low income communities in different parts of Africa most importantly in Ethiopia. Therefore, the result of the present study is of paramount importance in pinpointing the emerging problems of nutrition-linked concerns particularly among children and adolescents in the country.

A systematic review and meta-analysis has not yet been carried out to estimate the pooled prevalence of overweight/obesity, and review its associated factors among children and adolescents in Ethiopia. However, about 18 cross sectional studies, which are relevant for this research question, have been conducted in different parts of Ethiopia. Hence, the aim of this study was to estimate the pooled prevalence of overweight/obesity as well as to identify and review the risk factors that are associated with it among the study subjects. Using those relevant studies, the result of this meta-analysis showed that the combined overall prevalence of overweight and obesity, as per WHO 2007 definition, was 11.30% (95% CI: 8.71, 13.88%) among children and adolescents in the country. This prevalence is substantially high even comparable with the results reported for some developed countries (8.7%) a couple of years ago, and higher than the global prevalence (7%) [56, 57]. Despite methodological differences, nutritional patterns and the availability of recreational facilities may be attributed for the variation in the results, the findings of this study clearly indicate that there is a nutrition transition, and overweight/obesity is becoming a growing problem and a double burden in the country.

Also, the subgroup analysis of this meta-analysis revealed that the prevalence of childhood overweight/obesity varies across the regions of Ethiopia. The prevalence

Table 3 Results from subgroup analysis of the prevalence of overweight/obesity among children and adolescents in Ethiopia, 2018 (n = 18)

Variables	Characteristics	Number of studies	Prevalence with 95%
Region	Addis Ababa	6	11.94 (9.39, 14.50)
	Amhara	4	10.66 (5.92, 15.41)
	Oromia	3	10.94 (7.86, 14.02)
	Others	5	10.97 (5.09, 16.85)
Year of publication	≤ 2014	7	8.70 (5.40, 11.99)
	> 2014	11	12.95 (10.17, 15.73)

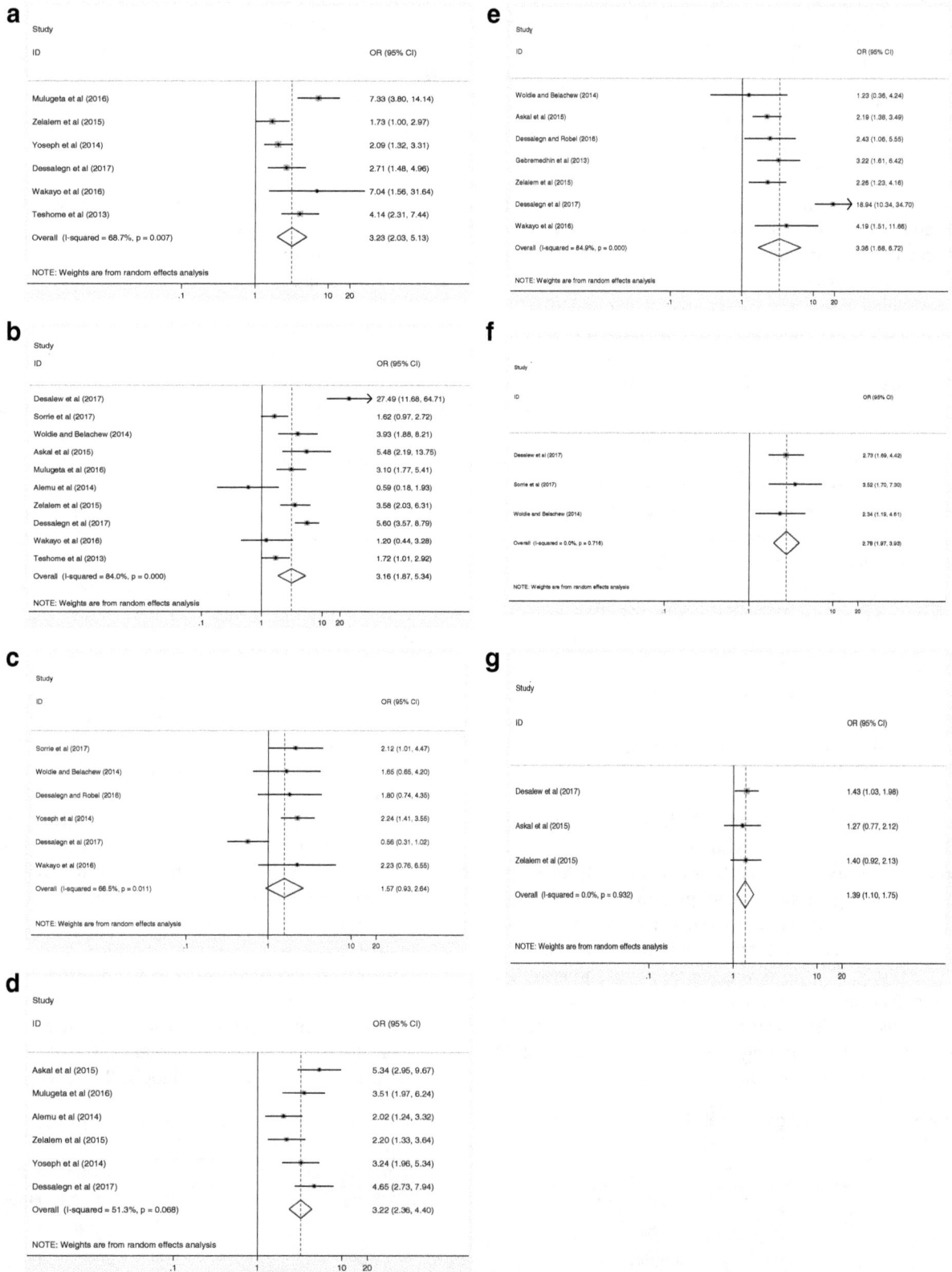

Fig. 3 Forest plot showing the pooled odds ratio of the associations between overweight/obesity and its purported associated risk factors among children and adolescents in Ethiopia (**a**: Sex, **b**: Family income, **c**: Family education, **d**: School type of children, **e**: Physical activity, **f**: Use of sweet food, **g**: use of fruits and vegetables)

was highest in children and adolescents of Addis Ababa as compared to other regions of the country. This could be due to better access to high calorie diets because of better socioeconomic status of the population in the capital compared to other regions of the country [4]. The prevalence of overweight/obesity was also significantly higher in those studies published since 2014 as compared to studies published before 2014. This shows that childhood overweight/obesity is increasing alarmingly in the country [57].

We reviewed and meta-analyzed the risk factors related with overweight/obesity among children and adolescents that have been addressed by the relevant studies. The risk of developing childhood overweight/obesity among females was higher than males in this review. Though they are not reviews, the result was congruent with studies conducted in African countries that female subjects were more likely to be at risk of having overweight/obesity compared to the male ones [58, 59]. But the result is in contrary to studies conducted from other countries [60–62] in which overweight/obesity was more prevalent in males than females. However, the prevalence in most developing countries is more in females which is true for this meta-analysis too. This may be explained that there is a biological difference in energy need for males and females in relation to rate of growth and timing of sexual maturation [63]. Males are also more physically active than females particularly during childhood [64]. In addition, in developing countries such as Ethiopia, girls usually stay at home for long period and there is a cultural influence not to move much from place to place than boys leading to physical inactivity and ultimately the development of overweight and obesity.

Children and adolescents from families with high monthly income were more likely to be overweight/obese as compared to those from families with low and moderate income. This is in line with a study done in Saudi Arabia [65], but in contrary to studies conducted in Germany and Korea [66, 67] where lower income was found to significantly increase the risk of being overweight/obese in the study subjects. This could be due to the reason that adolescents from socioeconomic status families have access for fat rich foods and follow sedentary life style. On the other hand, patterns of high expenditure of energy among the poor families and cultural attitude towards a larger body size tendency could also contribute to the positive relations observed. In lower-income countries like Ethiopia childhood overweight/obesity has been considered as a sign of better social status, and healthiness [68].

In contrast to cross sectional studies conducted in developed countries like Brazil and Iran [69, 70], the educational level of families was positively associated with overweight/obesity in the subjects but not statistically significant. Those children and adolescents whose mothers had primary educational level and above were more likely to be overweight/obese as compared to mothers with no education. This shows that educated mothers in developing countries fail to make healthy choices regarding food stuffs like the incorporation of fruits and vegetables in the diet.

There was a remarkable difference in the prevalence of overweight/obesity between government and private schools where children attended. The odds of having overweight/obesity was higher among children attending at private schools than those at governmental schools. This is in trajectory with studies conducted in India [71], Yemen [72], Saudi Arabia [73], Kenya [74] and Burkina Faso [66]. Often, children attending private schools are from families of higher socioeconomic status. Therefore, they are exposed to unhealthy nutritional patterns such as highly-processed and fast foods, more animal products as well motorized lifestyle compared to those children attending government schools.

In addition, adolescents not engaged in physical activities were more likely to be overweight and obese compared to those who were doing physical activities. The finding is concordant to other cross-sectional studies [75, 76]. The possible explanation could be because doing physical exercise burns off body fat (negative energy balance) leads to less risk of overweight/obesity. Children who consumed sweetened foods were more likely to be overweight/obese compared to those who didn't consumed. This was congruent with WHO report of different studies done in Europe [77], Egypt [78], Kenya [79]. This could be reasoned out that sweet food products are calorie rich and have a greater acceptance by children and adolescents resulting in a positive energy balance to them. Moreover, the results of three studies showed that infrequent consumption of fruits and vegetables was a risk factor for the development of overweight/obesity among children and adolescents.

Strengths and limitations of the study

The strengths of this study were the use of multiple reputable databases to exhaustively and explicitly search eligible literatures as well as uniform and reproducible extraction of data using a preset and pretested checklist so as to minimize errors. This systematic review and meta-analysis also included studies from different regions of the country. However, the study may have some potential limitations for it is restricted to articles published in English language. In addition, by virtue of the cross-sectional nature of the studies reviewed, temporal relationship cannot be established between the factors and overweight/obesity. Despite the incorporation of studies from different parts of the country, the representativeness of the population is not so strong as it could have been. Therefore, one had better interpret the findings of this systematic review and meta-analysis in context of the inherent limitations of both the original studies and the present review.

Conclusions

This meta-analysis revealed that the prevalence of overweight/obesity among children and adolescents in Ethiopia is substantially high, and has become an emerging nutrition linked problem. Unless successful preventive measures are taken, the problem may continue on upsurge in the future. Female gender of the children, high family socioeconomic status, learning in private school, physical inactivity, sweet nutriments preference and less use of fruits/vegetables were found to be significantly associated with overweight/obesity among the study subjects. We have recommended that integrated nutrition education program has to be successfully implemented in schools as well as in communities with existing health extension programs. Healthcare providers and policymakers should also give more emphasis on the design and implementation of preventive policies to control the rising prevalence of childhood overweight/ obesity in Ethiopia.

Abbreviations

PRISMA: Preferred Reporting Items of Systematic Reviews and Meta-Analysis; SNNPE: Southern Nations, Nationalities and peoples of Ethiopia; USA: United States of America

Funding
We have not obtained any fund for this study.

Authors' contributions

AG: Conception of research protocol, study design, literature review, data extraction, data analysis, interpretation and drafting the manuscript. AA, AZ, AF and BT: Data extraction, analysis and reviewing the manuscript and quality assessment. All authors read and approved the manuscript.

Competing interests

The authors declare that they have no competing interests.

Author details

[1]Department of Biomedical Science, School of Medicine, Debre Markos University, P.O. Box 269, Debre Markos, Ethiopia. [2]Department of Nursing, College of Health Sciences, Debre Markos University, Debre Markos, Ethiopia. [3]Department of Public Health, College of Health Sciences, Debre Markos University, Debre Markos, Ethiopia.

References

1. Organization WH: Global strategy on diet, physical activity and health. 2004 H ttp. wwwwho, Int/dietphysicalactivlty/en.
2. Van Der Sande MA, Ceesay SM, Milligan PJ, Nyan OA, Banya WA, Prentice A, McAdam KP, Walraven GE. Obesity and undernutrition and cardiovascular risk factors in rural and urban Gambian communities. Am J Public Health. 2001;91(10):1641–4.
3. WHo J, Organization WH: Diet, nutrition and the prevention of chronic diseases: report of a joint WH. 2003.
4. WHO. Diet, nutrition and the prevention of chronic diseases. World Health Organ Tech Rep Ser. 2003;916:i–viii–1–149.
5. Berman ML. From health care reform to public health reform. J Law Med Ethics. 2011;39(3):328–39.
6. Demissie T, Ali A, Mekonen Y, Haider J, Umeta M. Food Nutr Bull. 2010;31(2): 234–41.
7. Overseas-Development-Institute: Future diets: obesity rising to alarming levels around the world. 2014 . http://www.odi.org/future-diets. 2015 [cited 05 May 2015]
8. Roberts KC, Shields M, de Groh M, Aziz A, Gilbert J-A. Overweight and obesity in children and adolescents: results from the 2009 to 2011 Canadian health measures survey. Health Rep. 2012;23(3):37–41.
9. Vohra R, Bhardwaj P, Srivastava JP, Srivastava S, Vohra A. Overweight and obesity among school-going children of Lucknow city. J Family Community Med. 2011;18(2):59.
10. Toselli S, Zaccagni L, Celenza F, Albertini A, Gualdi-Russo E. Risk factors of overweight and obesity among preschool children with different ethnic background. Endocrine. 2015;49(3):717–25.
11. Rossen LM, Talih M. Social determinants of disparities in weight among US children and adolescents. Ann Epidemiol. 2014;24(10):705–13. e702
12. World Health Organization. Obesity and Overweight, Fact Sheet No 311. 2011.
13. Langford R, Bonell C, Jones H, Campbell R. Obesity prevention and the health promoting schools framework: essential components and barriers to success. Int J Behav Nutr Phys Act. 2015;12(1):15.
14. Desalew A, Mandesh A, Semahegn A. Childhood overweight, obesity and associated factors among primary school children in Dire Dawa, eastern Ethiopia; a cross-sectional study. BMC obesity. 2017;4(1):20.
15. Gali N, Tamiru D, Tamrat M. The emerging nutritional problems of school adolescents: overweight/obesity and associated factors in Jimma town, Ethiopia. J Pediatr Nurs. 2017;35:98–104.
16. Gebreyohannes Y, Shiferaw S, Demtsu B, Bugssa G. Nutritional status of adolescents in selected government and private secondary schools of Addis Ababa, Ethiopia. Adolescence. 2014;10:11.
17. Gebregergs G, Yesuf M, Beyen T. Overweight and obesity, and associated factors among high school students in Gondar town, north West Ethiopia. J Obes Wt Loss Ther. 2013;3(2):1–5.
18. Sorrie MB, Yesuf ME, GebreMichael TG. Overweight/obesity and associated factors among preschool children in Gondar City, Northwest Ethiopia: a cross-sectional study. PLoS One. 2017;12(8):e0182511.
19. TG G. Prevalence and associated factors of overweight and/or obesity among primary school children in bole Sub-City, Addis Ababa, Ethiopia. Nutrition & Food Sciences. 2015;
20. Wolde T, Belachew T. Prevalence and determinant factors of overweight and obesity among preschool children living in Hawassa City, South Ethiopia. Prevalence. 2014;29
21. Tadesse Y, Derso T, Alene KA, Wassie MM. Prevalence and factors associated with overweight and obesity among private kindergarten school children in Bahirdar town, Northwest Ethiopia: cross-sectional study. BMC Res Notes. 2017;10(1):22.
22. Gebremichael B, Chere A. Prevalence of childhood overweight and obesity and its determinant factors among elementary school children in Addis Ababa, Ethiopia: a cross sectional study. J Nutr Disorders Ther S. 2015;1: 2161–0509.
23. Alemu E, Atnafu A, Yitayal M, Yimam K. Prevalence of overweight and/or obesity and associated factors among high school adolescents in Arada sub city, Addis Ababa, Ethiopia. J Nutr Food Sci. 2014;4(2):1.
24. Anteneh ZA, Gedefaw M, Tekletsadek KN, Tsegaye M, Alemu D. Risk factors of overweight and obesity among high school students in Bahir Dar City, north West Ethiopia: school based cross-sectional study. Adv Prev Med 2015. 2015

25. Yetubie M, Haidar J, Kassa H, Fallon F. Socioeconomic and demographic factors affecting body mass index of adolescents students aged 10–19 in Ambo (a rural town) in Ethiopia. Int J Biomed Sci : IJBS. 2010;6(4):321.

26. Wakayo T, Whiting SJ, Belachew T. Vitamin D deficiency is associated with overweight and/or obesity among schoolchildren in Central Ethiopia: a cross-sectional study. Nutrients. 2016;8(4):190.

27. Teshome T, Singh P, Moges D. Prevalence and associated factors of overweight and obesity among high school adolescents in urban communities of Hawassa, southern Ethiopia. Current Research in Nutrition and Food Science Journal. 2013;1(1):23–36.

28. Teji K, Dessie Y, Assebe T, Abdo M. Anaemia and nutritional status of adolescent girls in Babile District, Eastern Ethiopia. Pan Afr Med J. 2016;24(1)

29. Robel Da. Assessment of sleep duration and overweight/obesity among high school adolescents in Addis Ababa, Ethiopia. In: Unpublished; 2016.

30. Mulugeta S, Mekitie W, Alemayehu A, Sshikur M, Zewdu S, Mukerem A, Gebresillasea G. Magnitude and determinants of overweight and obesity among adolescent students at Addis Ababa. International Journal of Medical and Health Sciences. 2016;10(4)

31. Liberati A, Altman DG, Tetzlaff J, Mulrow C, Gøtzsche PC, Ioannidis JP, Clarke M, Devereaux PJ, Kleijnen J, Moher D. The PRISMA statement for reporting systematic reviews and meta-analyses of studies that evaluate health care interventions: explanation and elaboration. PLoS Med. 2009;6(7):e1000100.

32. Modesti PA, Reboldi G, Cappuccio FP, Agyemang C, Remuzzi G, Rapi S, Perruolo E, Parati G. Panethnic differences in blood pressure in Europe: a systematic review and meta-analysis. PLoS One. 2016;11(1):e0147601.

33. Rücker G, Schwarzer G, Carpenter J, Schumacher M. Undue reliance on I 2 in assessing heterogeneity may mislead. BMC Med Res Methodol. 2008;8(79)

34. Higgins J, Thompson S. Quantifying heterogeneity in a metaanalysis. Stat Med. 2002;21:1539–58.

35. Sterne J, Egger M. Funnel plots for detecting bias in meta-analysis guidelines on choice of axis. J Clin Epidemiol. 2001;54:1046–55.

36. Egger M, Smith GD, Schneider M, Minder C. Bias in meta-analysis detected by a simple, graphical test. BMJ Open. 1997;315:629–34.

37. Fryar CD, Carroll MD, Ogden C. Prevalence of Overweight and Obesity Among Children and Adolescents Aged 2–19 Years: United States, 1963–1965 Through 2013–2014. Health E-Stats. 2016;

38. Cheung PC, Cunningham SA, Narayan KV, Kramer MR. Childhood obesity incidence in the United States: a systematic review. Childhood Obesity. 2016;12(1):1–11.

39. Jahns L, Adair L, Mroz T, Popkin BM. The declining prevalence of overweight among Russian children: income, diet, and physical activity behavior changes. Econ Hum Biol. 2012;10(2):139–46.

40. Nakano T, Sei M, Ewis AA, Munakata H, Onishi C, Nakahori Y. Tracking overweight and obesity in Japanese children; a six years longitudinal study. J Med Investig. 2010;57(1, 2):114–23.

41. Raja'a YA, Mohanna MAB. Overweight and obesity among schoolchildren in Sana'a City, Yemen. Ann Nutr Metab. 2005;49(5):342–5.

42. Adegoke S, Olowu W, Adeodu O, Elusiyan J, Dedeke I. Prevalence of overweight and obesity among children in Ile-ife, South-Western Nigeria. West Afr J Med. 2009;28(4):216–21.

43. Senbanjo I, Adejuyigbe E. Prevalence of overweight and obesity in Nigerian preschool children. Nutr Health. 2007;18(4):391–9.

44. Ejike CE. Child and adolescent obesity in Nigeria: a narrative review of prevalence data from three decades (1983-2013). Journal of Obesity and Metabolic Research. 2014;1(3):171.

45. Yusuf S, Mijinyawa M, Musa B, Gezawa I, Uloko A. Overweight and obesity among adolescents in Kano Nigeria. J Metab Syndr. 2013;2:126.

46. Pienaar AE. Prevalence of overweight and obesity among primary school children in a developing country: NW-CHILD longitudinal data of 6–9-yr-old children in South Africa. BMC obesity. 2015;2(1):2.

47. Talat MA, El Shahat E. Prevalence of overweight and obesity among preparatory school adolescents in urban Sharkia governorate, Egypt. Egyptian Pediatric Association Gazette. 2016;64(1):20–5.

48. Belahsen R, Mziwira M, Fertat F. Anthropometry of women of childbearing age in Morocco: body composition and prevalence of overweight and obesity. Public Health Nutr. 2004;7(4):523–30.

49. Abrha S, Shiferaw S, Ahmed KY. Overweight and obesity and its socio-demographic correlates among urban Ethiopian women: evidence from the 2011 EDHS. BMC Public Health. 2016;16:636.

50. Hassen K, Gizaw G, Belachew T. Dual burden of malnutrition among adolescents of smallholder coffee farming households of Jimma zone, Southwest Ethiopia. Food Nutr Bull. 2017;38(2):196–208.

51. Moges B, Amare B, Fantahun B, Kassu A. High prevalence of overweight, obesity, and hypertension with increased risk to cardiovascular disorders among adults in Northwest Ethiopia: a cross sectional study. BMC Cardiovasc Disord. 2014;14:155.

52. Tadewos A, Egeno T, Amsalu A. Risk factors of metabolic syndrome among hypertensive patients at Hawassa university comprehensive specialized hospital Southern Ethiopia. BMC Cardiovasc Disord. 2017;17(1):218.

53. Tebekaw Y, Teller C, Colon-Ramos U. The burden of underweight and overweight among women in Addis Ababa, Ethiopia. BMC Public Health. 2014;14:1126.

54. Worede A, Alemu S, Gelaw YA, Abebe M. The prevalence of impaired fasting glucose and undiagnosed diabetes mellitus and associated risk factors among adults living in a rural Koladiba town, Northwest Ethiopia. BMC Res Notes. 2017;10(1):251.

55. Gebremedhin S. Prevalence and differentials of overweight and obesity in preschool children in sub-Saharan Africa. BMJ Open. 2015;5(12):e009005.

56. De Onis M, Blössner M, Borghi E. Global prevalence and trends of overweight and obesity among preschool children. Am J Clin Nutr. 2010;92(5):1257–64.

57. Wang Y, Lim H. The global childhood obesity epidemic and the association between socio-economic status and childhood obesity. In: Taylor & Francis. 2012;

58. Peltzer K, Pengpid S. Overweight and obesity and associated factors among school-aged adolescents in Ghana and Uganda. Int J Environ Res Public Health. 2011;8(10):3859–70.

59. Baalwa J, Byarugaba B, Kabagambe E, Otim A. Prevalence of overweight and obesity in young adults in Uganda. Afr Health Sci. 2010;10(4)

60. Tremblay M, Katzmarzyk P, Willms J. Temporal trends in overweight and obesity in Canada, 1981-1996. International journal of obesity and related metabolic disorders: journal of the International Association for the Study of Obesity. 2002;26(4):538–43.

61. Krassas G, Tzotzas T, Tsametis C, Konstantinidis TPrevalence and trends in overweight and obesity among children and adolescents in Thessaloniki, Greece. Journal of pediatric endocrinology & metabolism: JPEM 2001, 14:1319–1326; discussion 1365.

62. Vignolo M, Pistorio A, Torrisi C, Parodi A, Grassi S, Aicardi G. Overweight and obesity in a group of Italian children and adolescents: prevalence estimates using different reference standards. Ital J Pediatr. 2004;30:53–7.

63. Wisniewski AB, Chernausek SD. Gender in childhood obesity: family environment, hormones and genes. Gend Med. 2009;6:76–85.

64. Kruger R, Kruger H, Macintyre U. The determinants of overweight and obesity among 10-to 15-year-old schoolchildren in the north West Province, South Africa–the THUSA BANA (transition and health during urbanisation of south Africans; BANA, children) study. Public Health Nutr. 2006;9(3):351–8.

65. Dupuy M, Godeau E, Vignes C, Ahluwalia N. Socio-demographic and lifestyle factors associated with overweight in a representative sample of 11-15 year olds in France: results from the WHO-collaborative health behaviour in school-aged children (HBSC) cross-sectional study. BMC Public Health. 2011;11(1):442.

66. Daboné C, Delisle HF, Receveur O. Poor nutritional status of schoolchildren in urban and peri-urban areas of Ouagadougou (Burkina Faso). Nutr J. 2011;10(1):34.

67. Freedman DS, Dietz WH, Srinivasan SR, Berenson GS. The relation of overweight to cardiovascular risk factors among children and adolescents: the Bogalusa heart study. Pediatrics. 1999;103(6):1175–82.

68. Monteiro CA, Moura EC, Conde WL, Popkin BM. Socioeconomic status and obesity in adult populations of developing countries: a review. Bull World Health Organ. 2004;82(12):940–6.

69. RCEd M, PlCd L, Oliveira JS, Leal VS, SCdS S, SLLSd A. Prevalence and determinants of overweight in preschool children. J Pediatr. 2011;87(3):231–7.

70. Do LM, Tran TK, Eriksson B, Petzold M, Nguyen CT, Ascher H. Preschool overweight and obesity in urban and rural Vietnam: differences in prevalence and associated factors. Glob Health Action. 2015;8(1):28615.

71. Jagadesan S, Harish R, Miranda P, Unnikrishnan R, Anjana RM, Mohan V. Prevalence of overweight and obesity among school children and adolescents in Chennai. Indian Pediatr. 2014;51(7):544–9.

72. Badi MAH, Triana BEG, Martínez RS. Overweight/obesity and socioeconomic status in children from Aden governorate, Yemen, 2009. Revista Habanera de Ciencias Médicas. 2013;12(3):1–7.

73. El-Hazmi MA, Warsy AS. A comparative study of prevalence of overweight and obesity in children in different provinces of Saudi Arabia. J Trop Pediatr. 2002;48(3):172–7.
74. Kyallo F, Makokha A, Mwangi AM. Overweight and obesity among public and private primary school children in Nairobi, Kenya. Health (N Y). 2013;5(08):85.
75. Santos DA, Silva AM, Baptista F, Santos R, Gobbo LA, Mota J, Sardinha LB. Are cardiorespiratory fitness and moderate-to-vigorous physical activity independently associated to overweight, obesity, and abdominal obesity in elderly? Am J Hum Biol. 2012;24(1):28–34.
76. Badawi NE-S, Barakat AA, El Sherbini SA, Fawzy HM. Prevalence of overweight and obesity in primary school children in port said city. Egyptian Pediatric Association Gazette. 2013;61(1):31–6.
77. Goyal RK, Shah VN, Saboo BD, Phatak SR, Shah NN, Gohel MC, Raval PB, Patel SS. Prevalence of overweight and obesity in Indian adolescent school going children: its relationship with socioeconomic status and associated lifestyle factors. J Assoc Physicians India. 2010;58:151–8.
78. Jain G, Bharadwaj S, Joglekar A: To study the prevalence of overweight and obesity among school children (13-17yrs) in relation to their socioeconomic status and Eating habits. Int J Sci Res Publ 2012, 2:1–4.
79. Börnhorst C, Wijnhoven TM, Kunešová M, Yngve A, Rito AI, Lissner L, Duleva V, Petrauskiene A, Breda J. WHO European childhood obesity surveillance initiative: associations between sleep duration, screen time and food consumption frequencies. BMC Public Health. 2015;15(1):442.

23

Use of various obesity measurement and classification methods in occupational safety and health research: a systematic review of the literature

Mahboobeh Ghesmaty Sangachin[1], Lora A. Cavuoto[1*] and Youfa Wang[2]

Abstract

Background: This study systematically examined obesity research in occupational safety and health regarding the use of various obesity measurement and classification methods.

Methods: A systematic search of the PubMed database on English language publications from 2000 to 2015 using related keywords and search of citations resulted in selection of 126 studies. They were categorized into two groups based on their main research question: 1) general physical or mental work-related functioning; and 2) task or body part specific functioning.

Results: Regardless of the study group, body mass index (BMI) was the most frequently used measure. Over 63% of the studies relied solely on BMI to define obesity. In only 22% of the studies, body fat was directly measured by methods such as dual energy x-ray absorptiometry. Abdominal obesity was defined using waist circumference in recent years, and waist-hip ratio in earlier years. Inconsistent cut-offs have also been used across studies investigating similar topics.

Conclusions: Few authors acknowledged the limitations of using indirect obesity measures. This is in part due to the limited understanding of some occupational safety and health researchers regarding the complex issues surrounding obesity classification and also the mixed recommendations over the past 2–3 decades and across populations. Efforts need to be made to promote appropriate obesity measurement and reporting in this field.

Keywords: Obesity, Overweight, Body mass index, Occupational safety and health, Ergonomics

Background

Obesity affects over 600 million adults worldwide and the number continues to grow [1]. Along with the rise in its worldwide prevalence [2, 3], the evidence for its adverse effects on individuals' health has been accumulating. Obesity has been identified as a risk factor for cardiovascular disease [4], pulmonary embolism [5], large joint osteoarthritis (OA) [6], and certain types of cancer [7]. It has also been associated with a decrease in general physical function [8], as well as cognitive abilities [9]. The diversity in the adverse outcomes attributed to

obesity, the complexity in the mechanisms leading to them, and the multi-factorial nature of this disease require the joint effort of different scientific disciplines to better understand the scope of the problem and to limit its detrimental effects.

With the prevalence of obesity among the workforce being equal to that of the general population [10], the occupational safety and health discipline has shown interest and effectively contributed to obesity research. The effects of obesity on work performance, physical capacity, and physical and cognitive function have been the research focus of many ergonomists, work analysts, and occupational health experts. As such, employees who are obese have been found to have higher rates of sick leave [11] and workplace injuries [12], along with

* Correspondence: loracavu@buffalo.edu
[1]Department of Industrial and Systems Engineering, University at Buffalo, 324 Bell Hall, Buffalo, NY 14260, USA
Full list of author information is available at the end of the article

increased employer-paid healthcare costs [13]. As these efforts expand to evaluate the relation between obesity and work [14], it is essential to explore how obesity status is measured in this field (e.g., body mass index (BMI) and body fat percentage (%BF)) as well as the basis for classifying individuals into distinct risk groups (e.g., types I and II obesity). In general, the issue of obesity measurement is two-fold: 1) selection of the appropriate measurement and 2) properly carrying out the measurement process to minimize measurement error.

Measurement selection

The World Health Organization (WHO) defines obesity as abnormal or excessive fat accumulation that may impair health [15], and this definition should serve as the basis for measurement selection. While underwater weighing and dual energy x-ray absorptiometry (DEXA) directly measure body fat, many indirect measures of adiposity have been used to measure obesity status. Anthropometric measures such as the weight-for-height index, BMI, waist circumference (WC), waist–hip ratio (WHR), and body fat percentage estimated by skinfold thickness (ST) are widely accepted indirect measures. Since the 1990s, BMI has been widely used to classify overweight and obesity, both in adults and children [16]. BMI has been suggested as an ideal measure of adiposity since it is easy to measure and is closely associated with obesity related health risks [17].

However, indirect measures such as BMI, fail to distinguish between fat, muscle or bone mass and are prone to misclassification, particularly among muscular subjects [18]. Mullie et al. [19] compared %BF, measured by bipolar bioelectrical impedance analysis (BIA), and BMI, for a cohort of 448 male military candidates and found a statistically significant difference between classifications of normal weight versus overweight. Almost 40% of the subjects classified as overweight with BMI > 25 kg/m^2 had a %BF corresponding to normal weight. Similarly, Deurenberg et al. [20] observed a higher rate of misclassification with BMI compared to DEXA in 416 European individuals. This study showcased how individual results based on a single classification method should be interpreted with caution.

Reliance only on BMI can also lead to misclassification of those with excess body fat, but BMIs corresponding to normal weight. These "metabolically obese but normal weight" [21] individuals share many health risks with those categorized as obese both based on BMI and %BF [22]. The elevated visceral fat observed in this category is accompanied by increased levels of both liver and muscle fat [23]. In a workplace study, comparing new industry hires from 1990 to 1992 and from 2000 to 2002, there was no significant difference in BMI but a significant difference in %BF, measured by ST [24].

There were also significant differences in physical fitness as measured by timed sit-ups and squats, suggesting that employers would miss information regarding their employees' fitness with reliance on BMI only. BMI is also not independently representative of body fatness. Significant dependencies on age and sex were observed in the relation between %BF and BMI in a study of 706 adult men and women [25]. BMI also overlooks the distribution of fat, which is an important factor in disease risk. For instance, android fat distribution (also referred to as abdominal, central, visceral, or upper body fat distribution) causes increased risk of diseases such as cardiovascular disease and type 2 diabetes [26], while gynoid fat distribution (i.e. larger hip and thigh circumferences) does not seem to have similar effects [27]. Indices such as WC and WHR are useful in characterizing the obesity morphology, particularly for studies where a difference in anthropometry among subjects is relevant to consider.

Misclassification and measurement error may be exacerbated in small sample sizes, which are common in exploratory laboratory-based occupational safety and health studies. Piers et al. [28] showed that despite the significant correlation between BMI and %BF (measured by underwater weighing method) of the 117 healthy samples, BMI only explained, on average, 50% of the variance in %BF. The reported poor sensitivity (47.7%) and positive predictive value (67.7%) of BMI makes it an unreliable measure of obesity in individuals. These findings not only suggest the inadequacy of BMI in classification of obesity status, particularly for individuals near the cutoff values, but also point out the importance of a rigorous obesity classification in studies with small sample sizes.

Measurement process and method

After selection of the suitable and hypothesis-relevant obesity measure, it is the researchers' responsibility to ensure that the measurement guidelines are thoroughly followed to reduce measurement error. For instance, WC is widely accepted as a simple and reliable measure of obesity in general, and abdominal obesity, in particular. There exist guidelines to ensure WC is appropriately measured [29, 30]. However, Agarwal et al. [31] found significant differences in the measured WC across varying anatomical sites, phases of respiration, and time since last meal, when following either the WHO or the National Institute of Health (NIH) guidelines. Overlooking these details can lead to an increase in the measurement error and the steps taken to control them should be acknowledged in publications.

Similarly, the cut-off values used to classify subjects into distinct risk groups are also worth scrutiny. For instance, WHO identifies 25 and 30 kg/m^2 as BMI cut points for overweight and obesity respectively. However, it has been shown that among certain populations (e.g., individuals of

Asian descent) cardio-metabolic risk is increased at lower body mass indexes [32]. While some researchers advocate using international cut-offs [33], some find nationally and ethnically selected cut points, when available, more advantageous [34]. Overall, inconsistency in the cut-offs used across studies with similar topics is detrimental to the strength of the body of evidence.

This study aims to examine the obesity-related research in occupational health and safety regarding obesity measurement methods. The findings will show how researchers in the aforementioned fields are conducting obesity research and will inform future obesity research in the occupational safety and health domain.

Methods

Research strategy and study inclusion criteria

A systematic review of the PubMed database was undertaken with the following MeSH terms: ('Work 'or 'Ergonomics' or 'Biomechanics\Biomechanical' or 'Occupational' or 'Motion' or 'Movement') and ('Obesity' or 'Skinfold Thickness'). In addition, a keyword search using Google Scholar and manual search of citations from relevant papers and literature reviews was done. The search was limited to journal articles dated between January 1, 2000 and December 31, 2014, published in English and studied human adults. An initial search was performed on 3 March 2015, and repeated on 24 September 2015 to update the search and results.

The study inclusion criteria were: (a) publication contributed to occupational health and safety rather than health promotion and (b) weight status was the independent variable or the major covariate included in the analysis and not the dependent variable. Review papers, simulation-based studies [35], and studies including normal weight subjects loaded with excess weight [36] were also excluded.

The initial search resulted in 3283 studies. The first author assessed all search outcomes by title and/or abstract, out of which 950 were selected based on relevance of the topic. A review of the abstracts reduced the number of studies to 111. Manual searches of the references from these studies and Google Scholar added 15 studies that were not initially captured. Overall, 126 studies were selected (see Fig. 1).

Selected studies review process and data extraction

Selected articles were reviewed and the following information was extracted: publication year, country of origin (based on the first author), main research question, design, outcomes measures, subject population, primary method of obesity measurement and the corresponding cut-offs used, whether or not subjects' weight status was self-reported, additional obesity classification methods applied, the statistical method used, sample size and number of subjects in overweight/obese (OW/OB) subgroup, whether or not the study included women in the

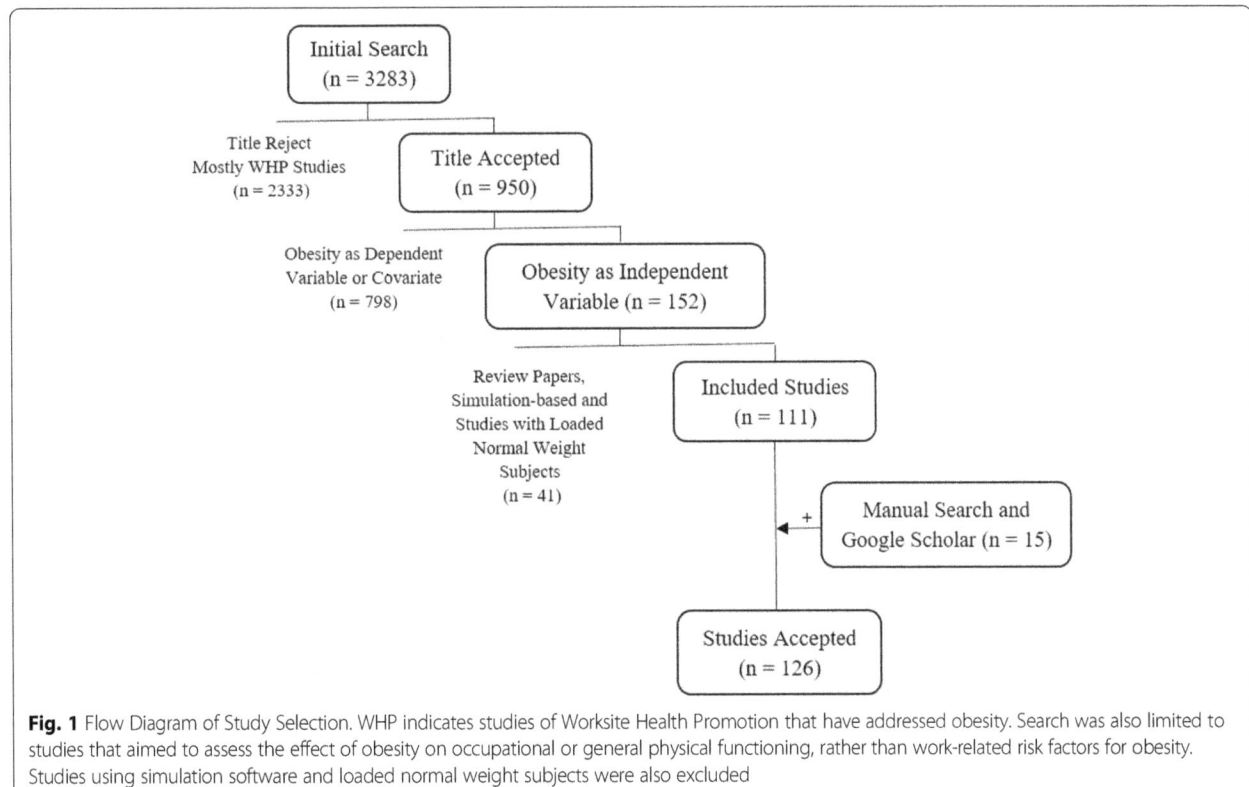

Fig. 1 Flow Diagram of Study Selection. WHP indicates studies of Worksite Health Promotion that have addressed obesity. Search was also limited to studies that aimed to assess the effect of obesity on occupational or general physical functioning, rather than work-related risk factors for obesity. Studies using simulation software and loaded normal weight subjects were also excluded

sample, the main finding and if the results indicated significance of the obesity (and overweight if applicable) effect, and finally if the authors mentioned any potential limitations of the obesity measurement method they have used. For studies carried out in a controlled lab setting where normal weight and overweight/obese subjects were compared, the mean BMI (or any other primary obesity classification measurement) of the overweight/obese group was extracted.

Analysis

The main research question was categorized into two types: 1) general physical or mental work-related functioning (GF) and 2) task or body part specific functioning (TBS). The summary of all included studies, together with details about the study relevant to obesity classification are presented in Tables 1 and 2.

Results

Within the selected time period (2000–2015), there has been an increasing trend in the number of studies published (see Fig. 2), with 2013 having the maximum number of publications ($n = 23$). This increase is mostly owed to the expanding interest in the specific effects of obesity rather than the general effects, which have been steadily studied by, on average, $n = 2.4$(SD = 1.9) studies per year. Overall, among all included studies, 63% relied solely on BMI to distinguish obese from non-obese and further classify them into distinct obesity status sub-groups (see Fig. 4). This is particularly concerning because some of these were lab-based studies with sample sizes as small as 12 or used young adults or older adults enrolled in aging research as subjects. In the following sections, studies focused on general vs. specific effects of obesity are discussed separately.

Category 1: General physical or mental work-related functioning

Among the 126 reviewed studies, 37 were related to the general effects of obesity as they pertain to occupationally-relevant outcomes such as performance, disability and discharge rate, healthcare cost, and overall well-being (see Table 1). The majority (64%) of the studies were from North America (see Fig. 3). Over the period of the review, the topic of general studies has gradually moved from work performance and workplace costs associated with obesity to the potential reasons behind elevated costs and poor performance, such as musculoskeletal symptoms and mental health issues. These studies applied a wide range of designs, with cross-sectional being the most frequent (15), followed by longitudinal prospective studies (13). Participants in 10 studies were army personnel, police officers, or career firefighters and the rest were either civilian labor force

(20) or their occupational status was not reported or relevant to the topic (7).

With regard to the measurement of obesity and group classification, in over 71% of these studies BMI was the only obesity measure used to distinguish obese from non-obese (see Fig. 4), with about 57% of these studies using self-reported weight and height to calculate BMI. About 13% of general studies used additional anthropometric measures such as WC and WHR to enhance obesity measurement accuracy. Finally, of the 6 studies using a direct adiposity measure, 5 were studies of army personnel, fire fighters, or police officers. Four studies reported using cut-off values other than 25 and 30 kg/m^2 to categorize subjects into distinct BMI subgroups, out of which two were army studies, one included Asian participants, and one provided no justification to use BMI ≤ 26 kg/m^2 as the cutoff for grouping. The median sample size was 1284 (14–69,515). With the exclusion of two studies that did not report the number of obese/overweight subjects included in their sample, on average 55.7(0.2) % of the samples consisted of OW/OB. Only 5 studies in this category provided information regarding the mean body mass index (or any other primary obesity classification measurement) of the OW/OB group. Overall, in 11 studies, the authors discussed the possibility of subject misclassification due to a reliance on BMI as the sole indicator of obesity status, either as a justification to use additional measures (2 studies) or as a limitation.

Category 2: Task or body part specific functioning

The majority of the reviewed studies (89) investigated a wide range of specific effects of obesity (see Table 2). North America and Europe contributed by 45 and 39% of such studies, respectively (see Fig. 3). Authors from Italy in particular contributed 16% of the publications, ranking higher than Asia and Australia, with five and six studies respectively. It should be noted that region of origin did not systematically affect the measurement approach used. Although the majority of the studies in this category were laboratory-based observational studies, BMI was still the most frequently used measure, with 59% of the studies relying solely on it to distinguish obese from non-obese. Study topics varied broadly, however, they were categorized in seven groups based on their main hypothesis and research focus (shown in Table 2). These groups, ordered based on number of studies, are discussed in more details as follows.

Twenty-three studies (~ 26%) discussed how obesity alters outcomes related to gait, such as metabolic cost, preferred speed, spatio-temporal parameters, and joint moments. From 2006 to 2014, at least one study related to the effects of obesity on gait was published each year. All of the studies in the gait category were lab-based observational studies. While other studies recruited

Table 1 The 37 studies that explored effects of obesity on general job-related outcomes, ordered chronologically

	Author, Year, Origin	Study Focus	Study Design	Subjects	Sample size (%OW/OB)	Outcome Variable(s)	Primary Obesity Measure / Other Measure(s)	Significant Obesity Effect	Significant Overweight Effect	Acknowledging Limitations of Obesity Measures
General physical or mental work-related functioning	Lee et al.,2001, Australia [48]	Asbestos exposure	Secondary data analysis	Former Australian mine workers	693 (68%)	Pleural thickening	**BMI**	+	–	+
	Clark et al.,2002, USA [49]	Duty fitness	Cross-sectional	Active firefighters(white)	218 (81%)	EKG, VO2 max, METS	**BMI**	+	+	+
	Poston et al.,2002, USA [50]	Discharge from training	Prospective cohort	Airmen	32,144 (19%)	Discharge status	*BMI	–	+	+
	Arbabi et al.,2003, USA [51]	Crash injury patterns	Secondary data analysis	Hospital admits of car crash	189 (57%)	Injury Scale and max AIS score, injury severity	BMI	+	–	+
	Bungum et al.,2003, USA [52]	Healthcare costs, absenteeism	Cross-sectional	Permanent employees	506 (74%)	Annual healthcare cost, absent days	BMI	+	NA	–
	Moreau et al.,2004, Belgium [53]	Sick leave	Prospective cohort	Belgium workers	20,463 (57%)	Sick leave	BMI / WC	+	+	–
	Pronk et al.,2004, USA [54]	Work performance	Cross-sectional	Current active employees	683 (43%)	# of work loss days, job performance, extra effort exerted, interpersonal relationships	**BMI**	+	–	–
	Laitinen et al.,2005, Finland [55]	Working ability	Prospective cohort	Young adults	11,637 (19%)	Perceived work ability	BMI / WHR	+	+	+
	Ricci & Chee,2005, USA [56]	Lost productive time	Cross-sectional	Employed adults	7472 (58%)	Self-reported lost productive time in past 2 weeks, lost labor costs	BMI	+	–	+
	Arena et al.,2006, USA [57]	Short-term disability	**Retrospective cohort**	White collar employees	1690 (37%)	Frequency + duration of short term disability	BMI	+	+	–
	Cormier & Israel-Assayag,2006, Canada [58]	Inflammatory response	Retrospective + experimental	Pig farmers + general population	14 (57%)	Inflammation biomarkers: C-reactive protein, interleukin 6,soluble adhesion molecules,	BMI / *Girth Size	NA	+	–
	Nishitani & Sakakibara,2006, Japan [59]	Job stress	Cross-sectional	Japanese manufacturing workers	208 (32%)	Job characteristics, eating behavior,	**BMI**	+	NA	–
	Wang et al.,2006, USA [60]	Healthcare costs	**Cross-sectional**	Manufacturing company employee & spouses	35,932 (74%)	Medical and pharmaceutical claims	BMI	+	+	–
	Østbye et al.,2007, USA [61]	Compensation claims, costs, lost workdays	Retrospective cohort	Health care and university employees	11,728 (56%)	Workers' compensation claims, associated costs, and lost workdays	BMI	+	+	–
	Charles et al., 2007, USA [62]	Hemato-logic parameters	**Cross-sectional**	Police officers	104 (78%)	White blood cell and platelet counts	BMI / WC,WHR, hip circumference,	+	+	–

Table 1 The 37 studies that explored effects of obesity on general job-related outcomes, ordered chronologically (Continued)

Author, Year, Origin	Study Focus	Study Design	Subjects	Sample size (%OW/OB)	Outcome Variable(s)	Primary Obesity Measure / Other Measure(s)	Significant Obesity Effect	Significant Overweight Effect	Acknowledging Limitations of Obesity Measures
Finkelstein et al.,2007, USA [63]	Injuries/ treatment costs	Cross-sectional	General population	42,304 (62%)	Medically attended injury rates by mechanism and nature and related treatment costs	BMI; abdominal height, waist to height ratio	+	+	–
Jans et al.,2007, Netherlands [64]	Absenteeism	Prospective cohort	Employees in industrial, administrative, and service sectors	1284 (40%)	Company-reported absenteeism	BMI	+	–	–
Gates et al., 2008, USA [65]	Presenteeism	Cross-sectional	Manufacturing company employees	341 (78%)	Work Limitations Questionnaire	BMI	+	–	–
Soteriades et al.,2008, USA [66]	Job disability	Prospective cohort	Firefighters	329 (88%)	Job disability	BMI	+	–	+
Claessen et al.,2009, Germany [67]	Work disability	Prospective cohort	Construction workers	16,875 (63%)	# of cases	BMI	+	–	–
Vissers et al.,2009, Belgium [68]	Whole body vibration	Lab-based	Premenopausal women	20 (100%)	Ventilation of oxygen, carbon dioxide, heart rate	*BMI / %BF: skinfold thickness	+	+	+
Bedno et al., 2010, USA [69]	Heat Illness/ healthcare utilization	Prospective cohort	Active duty US army members	9667 (57%)	Heat illness incidence	weight for height / %BF, BMI	+	–	–
Robroek et al.,2010, Netherlands [70]	Productivity loss /sick leave	Cross-sectional	Workers	10,624 (49%)	Sick leave, self-reported productivity loss	BMI	+	–	–
Vincent et al., 2010, USA [71]	Fear of movement	Cross-sectional	Patients with knee pain diagnoses	278 (73%)	Fear of movement, knee function	*BMI	+ (only morbid obesity)	–	–
Cowan et al., 2011, USA [72]	Training-related overuse injuries	Cross-sectional	Active duty US army members	7323 (47%)	Musculoskeletal injuries incidence and healthcare utilization	Weight for height / %BF, BMI	+	NA	–
Poston et al., 2011, USA [73]	Absenteeism	Cross-sectional	Career firefighters	478 (19%)	Injury, and injury-related absenteeism	BMI / %BF: BIA, WC	+	+	–
Haukka et al., 2012, Finland [74]	Multisite musculoskeletal pain	Prospective cohort	Kitchen workers	385 (46%)	Multisite musculoskeletal pain (3 and above out of 7)	BMI	+	–	–
	Musculoskeletal pain	Cross-sectional	Obesity treatment patients	95 (100%)	Musculoskeletal symptoms	*BMI	+	NA	–

Table 1 The 37 studies that explored effects of obesity on general job-related outcomes, ordered chronologically *(Continued)*

Author, Year, Origin	Study Focus	Study Design	Subjects	Sample size (%OW/OB)	Outcome Variable(s)	Primary Obesity Measure / Other Measure(s)	Significant Obesity Effect	Significant Overweight Effect	Acknowledging Limitations of Obesity Measures
Caberlon et al.,2013, Brazil [75]									
Gubata et al., 2013, USA [76]	Mental disorders	**Prospective cohort**	Active duty US army members	11,369 (40%)	Onset of mental disorder	*Circumference taping / BMI, weight-for-height standard, %BF	–	–	–
Jahnke et al., 2013, USA [77]	(Musculoskeletal) injury	Prospective cohort	Firefighters	301 (0%)	Incident injury, MS injury	BMI / %BF: BIA, WC	+	+	+
Kouvonen et al.,2013, UK [78]	Occupational injury	Prospective cohort	Finnish hospital workers	69,515 (0%)	Occupational injury incident	BMI	+	+	–
Lin et al.,2013, USA [79]	Occupational injury	Prospective cohort	Civilian labor force	~7000 (50%)	Injury at work	BMI	+	–	+
Roos et al.,2013, Finland [80]	Disability retirement	Prospective cohort	Middle aged employees	6542 (50%)	Pensions register data & questionnaire	BMI	+	NA	–
Van der Starre et al.,2013, Netherlands [81]	Need for recovery	Cross-sectional	Office workers	412 (42%)	Need for recovery after work	BMI	+	–	+
Viester et al.,2013, Netherlands [82]	Musculoskeletal symptoms/ recovery	Cross-sectional + longitudinal	Dutch workforce	44,793, 2nd phase: 7909, (43%)	Musculoskeletal symptoms	BMI	+	+/–	+
Gonzales et al.,2014, USA [83]	Cognitive functionality	**Lab-based**	General population	73 (67%)	Blood oxygen level-dependent response	WC / BMI	+	NA	–
Smith et al.,2014, USA [84]	Mental disorders	Secondary data analysis	Military personnel	15,195 (61%)	Mental health disorders	BMI	+	+	–

For primary obesity measure, * indicates that the study reported mean of obesity measure for obese group. Bolded measure indicates that measurement has been based on self-reported data. For study subjects, bolded indicates that only females were included as subjects and underlined shows that males were the only subjects. A bolded study design indicates that obesity status had been considered as continuous variable while underlined bolded indicates that it had been considered both as a continuous and categorical variable.

Table 2 The 89 studies that explored effects of obesity on task or body part specific functioning, are categorized into 7 groups based on their main focus and ordered chronologically within groups

	Author, Year, Origin	Study Focus	Subjects	Sample size (%OW/OB)	Outcome Variable(s)/Method	Primary Obesity Measure / Other Measure(s)	OB BMI: mean(SD)/ range	Significant Obesity Effect	Significant Overweight Effect	Acknowledging Limitations of Obesity Measures
Gait Characteristics	DeVita et al., 2003, USA [85]	Lower extremity joint kinetics & energetics	General population	39 (54%)	Motion analysis, force platform	BMI	42.3(2.9)	+	NA	–
	Browning et al., 2006, USA [86]	Metabolic rates & energy cost	General population	39 (49%)	Oxygen consumption, preferred walking speed	BMI / WHR, %BF: DEXA	M:33(2).1 F:33.8(3.3)	+	NA	–
	Browning & Kram., 2007, USA [87]	Walking biomechanics (knee-joint loads)	Young adults	20 (50%)	Ground reaction force, gait kinematics	BMI / *segment mass	M:34.1(3.7), F: 37(6)	+	NA	–
	Lafortuna et al., 2008, Italy [88]	Energetics and cardiovascular responses of walking & cycling	**Lean: hospital staff, OB: hospital admits (body mass reduction)**	21 (71%)	HR, Vo2 max, metabolic rate	BMI / %BF: BIA	41.1(5)	+	NA	–
	Lai et al., 2008, China [89]	Three-dimensional gait characteristics	General population	28 (50%)	Motion analysis	**BMI**	33.06(4.2)	+	NA	–
	Browning et al., 2009, USA [90]	External mechanical work	Young adults	20 (50%)	Ground reaction force	BMI	M:34.1(3.7), F:37(6)	–	NA	+
	Malatesta et al., 2009, Switzerland [91]	Mechanical external work	General population	49 (61%)	Center of mass displacement, mechanical external work, kinetic energy transduction	BMI	39.6(0.6)	–	NA	–
	Ko et al., 2010, USA [92]	Characteristics of gait	Older adults enrolled in aging research	164 (66%)	Motion analysis, force platform	BMI		+	+/–	–
	Russell et al., 2010, USA [93]	Energy expenditure & biomechanical risk factors for knee OA	**Young adults**	20 (50%)	O2 uptake, peak impact shock, peak external knee adduction moment knee adduction angular impulse	BMI	33.09(4.22)	–	NA	–
	Blaszczyk et al., 2011, Poland [94]	Basic spatiotemporal gait measures	**General population + outpatient obesity treatment clinic**	136 (74%)	Stance & swing time, stride length	BMI	37.2(5.2)	+	NA	+
	Ehlen et al., 2011, US [95]	Energetics and biomechanics of gait	General population	12 (100%)	Oxygen consumption, ground reaction	BMI / %BF: DEXA	33.4(2.4)	NA	NA	–

Table 2 The 89 studies that explored effects of obesity on task or body part specific functioning, are categorized into 7 groups based on their main focus and ordered chronologically within groups (Continued)

Author, Year, Origin	Study Focus	Subjects	Sample size (%OW/OB)	Outcome Variable(s)/Method	Primary Obesity Measure / Other Measure(s)	OB BMI: mean(SD)/ range	Significant Obesity Effect	Significant Overweight Effect	Acknowledging Limitations of Obesity Measures
				forces, & three-dimensional lower-extremity kinematics					
Cimolin et al., 2011, Italy [96]	Gait pattern	**Obese: admits to obesity multidisciplinary rehabilitation program**	28 (64%)	Gait Spatio-temporal parameters & kinematics	BMI / WC	OB + LBP: 42.4(5.5), OB - LBP: 39.3	+	NA	–
Russell & Hamill, 2011, US [97]	Obesity × laterally wedged insole effect on gait kinetic and kinematic	**Young females**	28 (50%)	Peak joint angles, external knee adduction moment & angular impulse	BMI / %BF: DEXA	37.2(6.1)	+	NA	–
Wu et al., 2012, USA [98]	Gait adaptations & implication on risk of slip initiations	Young male students	10 (50%)	Motion analysis, force plate	%BF from BIA / BMI	33.7(2.8)	+/–	NA	–
Harding et al., 2012, Canada [99]	Knee OA × obesity effect on knee joint mechanics	General population + orthopedic clinic admits	244 (72%)	Knee joint angles, joint moment	BMI / *thigh and calf circumference	34.9(4)	+	+	+
Russell et al., 2013, USA [100]	Laterally wedged insoles × obesity effect on knee joint contact force	**General population**	28 (50%)	Center of pressure on the tibial plateau	BMI / %BF: DEXA	37.2(6.1)	NA	NA	–
Browning et al., 2013, USA [101]	Metabolic rate, stride kinematics & external mechanical work	**young females**	37 (49%)	Oxygen uptake, ground reaction force, lower extremity kinematics	BMI / %BF: DEXA, *Trunk-to-leg fat mass ratio	33.9(3.6)	–	NA	–
Ranavolo et al., 2013, Italy [102]	Walking coordination during walking	General population	50 (50%)	**Motion analysis**	BMI / WC, %BF: Siri equation	Range(33.8–44)	+	NA	–
Vismara et al., 2014, Italy [103]	Changes in gait	General population	32 (44%)	Motion analysis	BMI	40.2(3.3)	+	NA	–
Haight et al., 2014, USA [104]	Compressive tibio-femoral forces	General population	19 (47%)	Motion analysis (lower extremity biomechanics), EMG	BMI / %BF: DEXA	35(3.8)	+/–	NA	–
Glave et al., 2014, USA [105]	Gait alterations	**General population**	22 (50%)	Gait variables	BMI / %BF: DEXA	31.42(7.3)	+	NA	+
	Gait strategy		35 (57%)		BMI	43(4.9)	+	NA	–

Table 2 The 89 studies that explored effects of obesity on task or body part specific functioning, are categorized into 7 groups based on their main focus and ordered chronologically within groups (Continued)

	Author, Year, Origin	Study Focus	Subjects	Sample size (%OW/OB)	Outcome Variable(s)/Method	Primary Obesity Measure / Other Measure(s)	OB BMI: mean(SD)/ range	Significant Obesity Effect	Significant Overweight Effect	Acknowledging Limitations of Obesity Measures
	Cau et al., 2014, Italy [106]		Hospital patients for weight reduction programs & staff		Center of pressure parameters					
	Lerner et al., 2014, USA [107]	Joint kinematics & individual muscle forces during gait	General population	19 (47%)	Motion analysis, EMG data, ground reaction force	BMI / lean mass (kg): DEXA	35(3.78)	+	NA	-
Disease Prevalence/ Incidenc	Kouyoumdjian et al., 2000, Brazil [108]	Severity of Carpal tunnel syndrome	Carpel tunnel syndrome patients	384 (13%)	Case - control study	BMI		+	NA	-
	Young et al., 2001, USA [109]	Asthma risk	Military population and their families (17-69 yrs)	38,924 (53%)	Case - control study	BMI		+	+	-
	J. D. Bland, 2005, UK [110]	Age × body mass index effect on carpal tunnel syndrome risk	Hospital admits	4166 (14%)	Self-report CTS diagnosis	BMI		+	+	-
	Liuke et al., 2005, Finland [111]	Prevalence and progression of lumbar disc degeneration	Employed middle-aged men	129 (50%)	Prospective cohort: MRI imaging	BMI		NA	+	-
	Dagan et al., 2006, Israel [112]	BMI as a screening method for detection of excessive daytime sleepiness	Professional drivers	153 (100%)	Sleep characteristics	BMI	36.78(7.32)	+	NA	-
	Zhao et al., 2007, USA [113]	Osteoporosis	Chinese general population + US Caucasian general population	6477 (0%)	Bone mass at the lumbar spine, total body bone mineral content	BMI / %BF: DEXA		+	+	+
	Sharifi-Mollayousefi et al., 2008, Iran [114]	BMI as independent risk determinants in the development and severity of Carpal tunnel syndrome	Patients with carpal tunnel syndrome (cases) and their relatives (controls)	262 (50%)	Case-control study	BMI		+	NA	-
	Grotle et al., 2008, Norway [115]	OA incident in hip, knee, and hand	General population	1675 (35%)	Prospective cohort: OA diagnosis	BMI		+	+/-	-
	Noorloos et al., 2008,	Obesity × whole body vibration	Occupational vehicle drivers	214 (69%)	Low back pain	BMI		-	-	-

Table 2 The 89 studies that explored effects of obesity on task or body part specific functioning, are categorized into 7 groups based on their main focus and ordered chronologically within groups *(Continued)*

Author, Year, Origin	Study Focus	Subjects	Sample size (%OW/OB)	Outcome Variable(s)/Method	Primary Obesity Measure / Other Measure(s)	OB BMI: mean(SD)/ range	Significant Obesity Effect	Significant Overweight Effect	Acknowledging Limitations of Obesity Measures
Netherlands [116]	effect on risk of LBP								
Toivanen et al., 2010, Finland [117]	Knee OA risk	Finnish adults aged 530 years	823 (39%)	Prospective cohort: OA diagnosis	BMI		+	+	–
Vismara et al., 2010, Italy [118]	LBP incidence	**General population**	37 (70%)	Trunk angle during standing, forward flexion & lateral bending	BMI	LBP:41.9(5.3), Non39.2(3.6)	+	NA	–
Wood et al., 2011, USA [119]	Pain experienced by persons with chronic back pain	Patients with lower back pain of over 3 months	198 (62%)	**Blood pressure, pain level**	BMI		–	–	–
Ackerman & Osborne., 2012, Australia [120]	Burden of hip & knee joint disease	General population	1157 (55%)	OA diagnosis	<u>BMI</u>		+	+	–
Jensen et al., 2012, Denmark [121]	LBP risk factor	**Newly educated health care helpers**	1355 (41%)	Prospective cohort: Self-reported levels of LBP	<u>BMI</u>	34.8(6.08)	–	–	–
Silvernail et al., 2013, USA [122]	Biomechanical risk factor for knee OA	Yong university and community members	30 (67%)	Gait kinetic & kinematics	BMI / %BF: BIA	34.4(3.9)	–	–	–
Seror & Seror., 2013, France [123]	Incidence of idiopathic median nerve lesion at the wrist	Patients with carpal tunnel syndrome	676 (25%)	Electrophysiological evaluation outcomes	BMI		+	+	–
Martin et al., 2013, USA [124]	Knee OA risk factor	British birth cohort participants	2957 (0%)	Knee Osteoarthritis	BMI (z-score)		+	NA	–
Romero-Vargas et al., 2013, Mexico [125]	Modifications on spino-pelvic parameters & type of lumbar lordosis	General population	200 (80%)	**Spino-pelvic values**	BMI / WC		–	–	+
Messier et al., 2014, USA [126]	Frontal plane alignment × obesity effect on knee joint loads in knee OA	Community dwelling older adults (age > 55 yrs)	157 (100%)	knee osteoarthritis: X-ray at baseline	BMI	33.4(3.7)	+	+	–
Urquhart et al., 2014, Australia [127]	Occupational activities × obesity effect on LBP	**General population + weight loss clinic attendees**	145 (61%)	Low back pain intensity & disability	<u>BMI</u>		+	NA	–

Table 2 The 89 studies that explored effects of obesity on task or body part specific functioning, are categorized into 7 groups based on their main focus and ordered chronologically within groups (Continued)

Author, Year, Origin	Study Focus	Subjects	Sample size (%OW/OB)	Outcome Variable(s)/Method	Primary Obesity Measure / Other Measure(s)	OB BMI: mean(SD)/ range	Significant Obesity Effect	Significant Overweight Effect	Acknowledging Limitations of Obesity Measures
Evanoff et al., 2014, France [128]	Physical occupational exposures × obesity effect on post-retirement shoulder/knee pain	French national power utility employees	9415 (52%)	Retrospective cohort: self-administered questionnaires	BMI		+	–	–
Functional Capacity									
Hulens et al, 2001, Belgium [129]	Submaximal & maximal exercise capacity	General population	306 (74%)	Oxygen uptake, carbon dioxide production, respiratory quotient, breathing efficiency, mechanical efficiency & anaerobic threshold	BMI / %BF: BIA	38.1(5.6)	+	NA	–
Hulens et al, 2002, Belgium [130]	Peripheral muscle strength	Outpatient Endocrinology Clinic patients	241 (100%)	Trunk strength, peak oxygen consumption	BMI / Fat free and fat mass: BIA	37.5(5.4)	NA	NA	–
Maffiuletti et al., 2007, Switzerland [131]	Voluntary & stimulated fatigue of the quadriceps femoris muscle	Lean: hospital staff, obese: hospital admits for body mass reduction	20 (50%)	Maximal voluntary isometric & isokinetic torque, torque loss	BMI / Fat free mass: BIA	41.3(5.4)	+	NA	–
Segal et al, 2009, USA [132]	Forces on the medial compartment of the knee joint	General population	59 (68%)	knee joint forces	BMI / WHR	Central: 35(4), lower body: 36.4 (5.4)	+/–	NA	+
Capodaglio et al., 2009, Italy [133]	Lower limb muscle function	General population	40 (50%)	Isokinetic strength during knee flexion & extension	BMI	38.1(3.1)	+	NA	+
Singh et al., 2009, USA [134]	Maximum acceptable weights of lift	General population	60 (67%)	MAWL	BMI / WC,WHR,%BF estimated: ST	II: 37.13(1.58) III:47.84(9.85)	–	NA	–
Faria et al., 2009, Portugal [135]	Muscle–tendon unit stiffness	General population	105 (77%)	Ankle muscle–tendon unit stiffness at 30% MVC	BMI	32.1(1.3)	+	+	–
Park et al., 2010, USA [136]	Joint RoM	Young and university affiliated	40 (50%)	RoM	BMI	44(7.4)	+/–	NA	–
			96 (38%)		BMI	35.3(3.9)	+	NA	–

Table 2 The 89 studies that explored effects of obesity on task or body part specific functioning, are categorized into 7 groups based on their main focus and ordered chronologically within groups (Continued)

	Author, Year, Origin	Study Focus	Subjects	Sample size (%OW/OB)	Outcome Variable(s)/Method	Primary Obesity Measure(s) / Other Measure(s)	OB BMI: mean(SD)/ range	Significant Obesity Effect	Significant Overweight Effect	Acknowledging Limitations of Obesity Measures
	Blazek et al., 2013, USA [137]	Age × obesity effect on knee adduction and flexion moments	General population		Ground reaction force magnitude, knee alignment, step width, toe-out angle, limb position					
	Cavuoto & Nussbaum,, 2013, USA [138]	Age × obesity effect on shoulder capacity	Young: students, old: retired or employed in non-physically demanding jobs	32 (50%)	Endurance, discomfort, motor control, task performance	BMI / WC, WHR	Young: 34.1(2.8), Old: 36.4(3.3)	+	NA	+
	Hamilton et al., 2013, USA [139]	BMI × workstation configuration effect on joint angles	General population	30 (80%)	Joint angle, forward functional reach	**BMI**	I: 32(1.26) II:37(1.73) III:44(4.97)	–	–	–
	Mignardot et al., 2013, France [140]	Motor control behavior	General population	20 (60%)	Kinematic variables, Center of mass displacement characteristics	BMI	36.6(3.3)	+	NA	–
	Wearing et al., 2013, Australia [141]	Resistance exercise × obesity effect on immediate transverse strain of the Achilles tendon	University faculty	20 (50%)	Sonographic examinations	**BMI**	30(3.1)	+	+	+
	Cavuoto & Nussbaum,, 2013, USA [142]	Strength and functional performance	Local community	36 (50%)	Endurance time, strength	BMI / WC,WHR	33.6(3.1)	+/–	NA	+
	Cavuoto & Nussbaum,, 2014, USA [143]	Age × obesity effect on functional performance	General population	32 (50%)	endurance, discomfort, motor control, task performance	BMI / WC,WHR	Young: 34.3(4), Old: 35.9(3.6)	+	NA	+
	Mehta & Cavuoto., 2015, USA [144]	Obesity × age effects on handgrip endurance	**General population**	45 (44%)	hand grip endurance	BMI	Young: 33.1(3.6),Old:36.1(8.1)	+/–	NA	–
Balance & Plantar Pressure	Hills et al., 2001, Australia [145]	Plantar pressure	General population	70 (50%)	**Pressure distribution**	BMI	38.75(5.97)	+	NA	+
	Gravante et al., 2003, Italy [146]	Centre of pressure location & plantar pressures	General population	72 (53%)	Centre of pressure location, plantar ground contact surface areas & pressures	BMI / WHR	M:36(7.4), F:38(6.8)	+/–	NA	–
		Plantar pressure distribution	General population	50 (50%)	**Pedobarographic evaluations**	BMI	32.2(2)	+	NA	–

Table 2 The 89 studies that explored effects of obesity on task or body part specific functioning, are categorized into 7 groups based on their main focus and ordered chronologically within groups (Continued)

Author, Year, Origin	Study Focus	Subjects	Sample size (%OW/OB)	Outcome Variable(s)/Method	Primary Obesity Measure / Other Measure(s)	OB BMI: mean(SD)/ range	Significant Obesity Effect	Significant Overweight Effect	Acknowledging Limitations of Obesity Measures
Birtane & Tuna, 2004, Turkey [147]									
Berrigan et al., 2006, Canada [148]	Balance control constraint during accurate and rapid arm movement	General population	17 (53%)	Body kinematics, center of pressure, displacement, reaction time, movement time	**BMI**	37(6.6)	+	NA	–
Teh et al., 2006, Singapore [149]	Pressure distribution under the feet	General population	120 (42%)	Plantar pressure distribution	BMI	I: 34.3 II: 38.9(3.6)	+/–	NA	–
Singh et al., 2009, USA [150]	obesity × task duration effect on postural sway and functional reach	Students & sedentary office workers	20 (50%)	Posture sway, functional reach	BMI / WHR	45.96(7.85)	+	NA	–
Blaszczyk et al., 2009, Poland [151]	Postural control	**Obesity treatment clinic patients**	133 (75%)	**CP measures: voluntary displacement, path, range**	BMI / %BF: BIA, WC,HC	37.2(5.2)	–	NA	–
Park et al., 2009, USA [152]	Postural stress during static posture maintenance	General population	40 (50%)	Rated perceived exertion	BMI / WHR,%BF estimated: ST	46.26(4.99)	+	NA	–
Menegoni et al., 2009, Italy [153]	Static posture variability	Orthopedic Rehabilitation Unit patients and staff (control)	54 (81%	**Center of pressure velocity & displacements along the antero-posterior & medio-lateral axis**	BMI	M:40.2(5), F: 41.1(4.1)	+	NA	+
Monteiro et al., 2010, Portugal [154]	Plantar pressure	**Postmenopausal women**	239 (79%)	Foot-scan pressure plate	%BF from BIA / **BMI**	29.6(3.2), 36.4(3.8)	+/–	NA	–
Miller et al., 2011, USA [155]	Balance recovery from small forward postural perturbations	Young adults (22 years old)	20 (50%)	Peak COM displacement, peak COM velocity, peak ankle torque	BMI	33.2(2.3)	–	NA	–
Matrangola & Madigan, 2011, USA [156]	Balance recovery using an ankle strategy	Young males	20 (50%	Body angle, ground reaction force	BMI	32.2(2.2)	+/–	NA	–
Peduzzi de Castro et al.,	Pressure relief insoles	General population	31 (32%)	Ground reaction force, plantar pressure	BMI	36.5(4.51)	+	NA	–

Table 2 The 89 studies that explored effects of obesity on task or body part specific functioning, are categorized into 7 groups based on their main focus and ordered chronologically within groups (*Continued*)

	Author, Year, Origin	Study Focus	Subjects	Sample size (%OW/OB)	Outcome Variable(s)/Method	Primary Obesity Measure / Other Measure(s)	OB BMI: mean(SD)/ range	Significant Obesity Effect	Significant Overweight Effect	Acknowledging Limitations of Obesity Measures
	2014, Portugal [157]									
Task Functionality	Galli et al., 2000, Italy [158]	Motion strategies: sit-to-stand	General population + obese subjects suffering from chronic lower back pain	40 (75%)	Movement kinetics & kinematics	BMI	40(5.9)	+	NA	–
	Sibella et al., 2003, Italy [159]	Biomechanical model: sit-to-stand	Hospital recovers	50 (80%)	Trunk flexion, feet movement, knee & hip joint torques	BMI	37.9(4.9)	+	NA	–
	Lafortuna et al., 2006, Italy [160]	Energy cost of submaximal cycling	Lean: hospital staff, obese: hospital admits for body mass reduction	18 (50%)	Oxygen uptake, Vo2 max, anaerobic threshold, mechanical efficiency	BMI / %BF: BIA	40(1.2)	+	NA	–
	Gilleard & Smith, 2007 [161]	Postural adaptations: trunk forward flexion motion in sitting and standing	**General Population**	20 (50%)	**Trunk flexion motion during forward flexion, trunk posture, hip joint moment**	WC / BMI	38.9(6.6)	+/–	NA	–
	Xu et al., 2008, USA [162]	Lifting kinematics & kinetics	College students	12 (50%)	Motion analysis	BMI	33.28 (30.4–38.8)	–	NA	+
	Taboga al., 2012, Italy [163]	Mechanical work, energy cost of transport, and efficiency: running	Hospital admits- adults from metabolic disorders	25 (40%)	Oxygen uptake, kinematics, center of mass location	BMI / %BF: BIA	41.5(5.3)	+	NA	–
	Hendrick et al., 2012, USA [164]	Neural processes of cognitive control: stop signal test	**General population**	43 (30%)	**Functional magnetic resonance imaging**	**BMI**	33.2(2.6)	+	NA	+
	Singh et al., 2013, USA [165]	Contact forces & moments exerted by the abdomen on the thigh: seated reaching	Older adults	10 (100%)	**Motion analysis, force plate**	BMI / WC	39.04(5.02)	+/–	NA	+
	Schmid et al., 2013, Switzerland [166]	Kinetic & kinematic variables: sit-to-stand test.	**Going to attend a weight loss program at hospital**	36 (72%)	Vertical ground reaction forces, rising velocity (motion analysis)	BMI	I: 32.68(1.53), II: 39.42(2.71)	+/–	NA	–
				45 (49%)		BMI / WHR, WC	36.2(5.9)	+	NA	+

Table 2 The 89 studies that explored effects of obesity on task or body part specific functioning, are categorized into 7 groups based on their main focus and ordered chronologically within groups *(Continued)*

	Author, Year, Origin	Study Focus	Subjects	Sample size (%OW/OB)	Outcome Variable(s)/Method	Primary Obesity Measure / Other Measure(s)	OB BMI: mean(SD)/ range	Significant Obesity Effect	Significant Overweight Effect	Acknowledging Limitations of Obesity Measures
Pysiological Responses	Willenberg et al., 2010, Switzerland [167]	Venous flow parameters of the lower limbs	Students and medical staff		**Venous hemodynamics: Diameter, flow volume, peak, mean, & minimum velocities**					
	Engelberger et al., 2014, Switzerland [168]	Diurnal leg volume increase	Obese subjects: weight management clinic patients, general population	39 (62%)	Common femoral vein diameter, peak flow velocity, mean velocity & minimal velocity	BMI / WHR	40.2(5.9)	+	NA	–
	Yang et al., 2015, China [169]	Acute high-altitude exposure	Chinese railroad construction workers	262 (46%)	Acute mountain sickness	**BMI**	29.9(3.8)	–	NA	–
Miscellaneous	Menegoni et al., 2007, Italy [170]	Clinical protocol to characterize the trunk movements	**Lean: hospital staff, obese: hospital admits for diet therapy and exercise classes**	20 (50%)		BMI	38.7(3.5)	NA	NA	–
	Forman et al., 2009, USA [171]	Restraint of automobile occupants	**Post mortem human surrogates**	5 (40%)	Chest deformation, acceleration, tension in the restraint system, etc.	BMI	40	+	NA	–
	Lerner et al., 2014, USA [172]	Obesity-specific kinematic marker set to account for subcutaneous adiposity	General population	18 (50%)	Ground reaction force, walking kinematics, EMG	BMI	35(3.78)	NA	NA	–
	Thorp et al., 2014, Australia [173]	Standing workstations effect on fatigue, musculoskeletal discomfort & work productivity	Middle-aged sedentary employees	23 (100%)	Self-reported fatigue, musculoskeletal discomfort, work productivity	BMI	33.7(4.3)	+	+	–

For primary obesity measure, Bolded measure indicates that a cut-off other than the common cut-offs are used and underlined measure indicates that measurement has been based on self-reported data. For study subjects, bolded indicates that only females were included as subjects and underlined shows that males were the only subjects. A bolded outcome variables/method indicates that obesity status had been considered as continuous variable while underlined bolded indicates that it had been considered both as a continuous and categorical variable

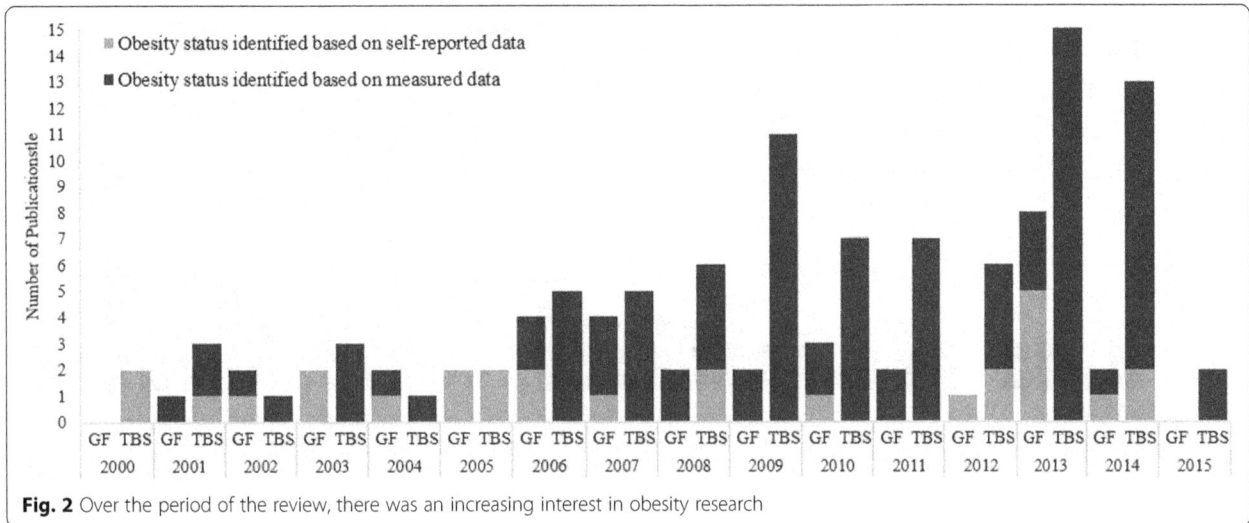

Fig. 2 Over the period of the review, there was an increasing interest in obesity research

subjects from a general population, obese subjects in three European studies were females, sampled from obesity clinics. The median sample size was 28 (10–244). More than half of the included subjects (56.7%) were categorized as OW/OB (only two had an overweight group). There were 11 studies which used BMI only (see Fig. 5). With the exclusion of the studies which reported sex or condition-stratified averages (4), the average BMI for nine studies were ≤ 35 kg/m^2, four were ≤ 40 kg/m^2 and four were > 40 kg/m^2. All but four studies reported a significant main effect for obesity or overweight on their outcomes of interest. It is noted that three of the

studies reporting non-significant results used BMI as the sole obesity measure.

The next largest group focused on the prevalence, incidence, burden, and changes in symptoms of diseases such as carpel tunnel syndrome, osteoarthritis, low back pain (LBP), asthma, and sleep disorders in association with obesity. This category included some large scale public health studies, hence there was more diversity in terms of study design. The median sample size was 384 (30–38,924). With the exclusion of two studies that did not report the proportion of OW/OB, on average 54 (24) % of the samples were obese or overweight. Six studies used patients and hospital admits as participants and six studies reported subjects belonging to a certain occupation. Eighteen studies relied solely on BMI, two added %BF and one added WC. Sixteen studies failed to report the obesity class of the obese group. In the four that did, all but one had mean BMI ≤ 35 kg/m^2. Only two studies, which both had one additional obesity measure, mentioned the inadequacy of BMI.

Changes in functional capacity were the topic of 16 studies. Functional capacity encompasses all topics related to muscle strength, endurance, functional reach, range of motion (RoM), and motor control behavior. Participants in two studies were outpatient clinic or hospital patients (endocrinology and body mass reduction admits) and the rest were recruited from the general population. Eight studies used BMI as the primary and only obesity measure, while three studies also measured body fat. Four studies augmented BMI with other anthropometric measures and one study reported using four obesity measures including both direct and indirect. While no studies relied on self-reported height and weight data, three studies used cut-offs other than 25 kg/m^2 and 30 kg/m^2 to classify subjects into distinct groups. Only three studies had an overweight sample as

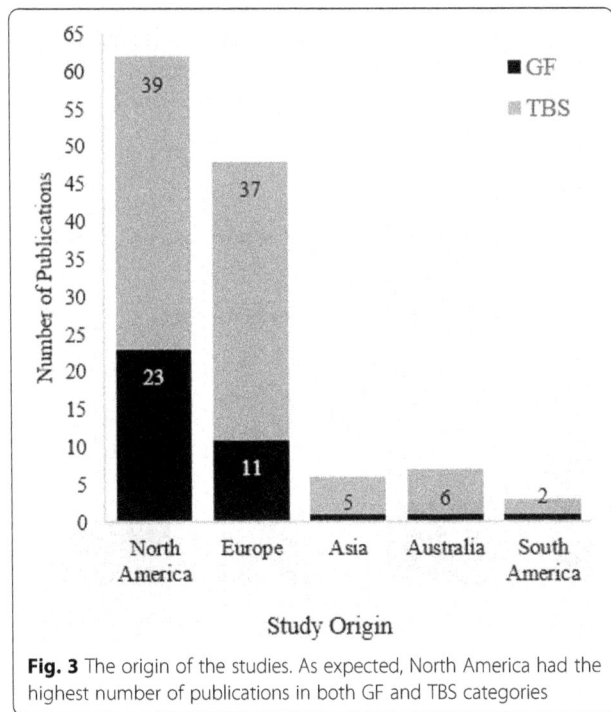

Fig. 3 The origin of the studies. As expected, North America had the highest number of publications in both GF and TBS categories

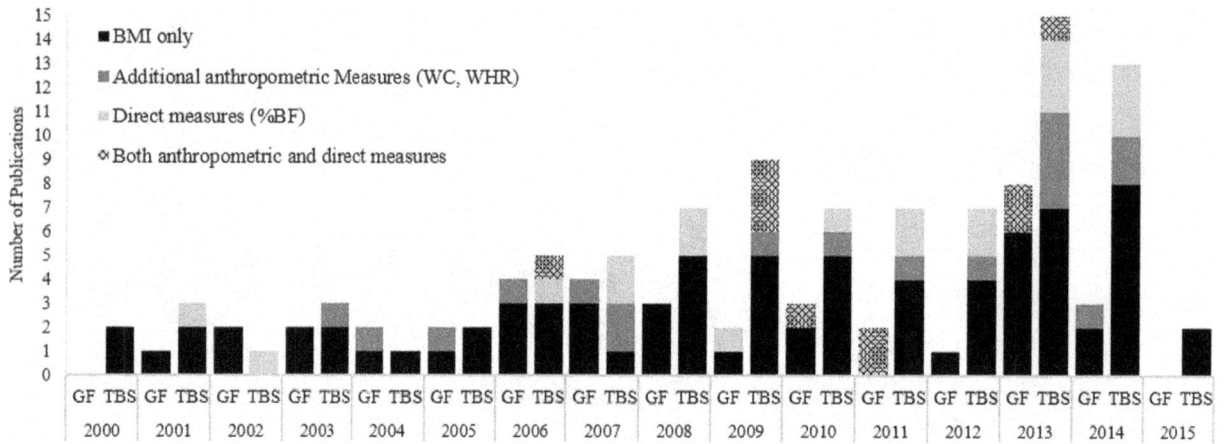

Fig. 4 The obesity measurement methods used in studies. Regardless of the study category, BMI was the most frequently used method of obesity measurement

well as obese. The median sample size was 40 (20–306). On average ~ 60% of the sample were OW/OB and the majority of reported mean BMI values were in the range of 35–40 kg/m². One Australian study in particular, which used BMI and cut-off values of 23 kg/m² and 27.5 kg/m², had mean BMI of 30 kg/m² for obese. All but three studies reported some significant obesity effect and two reported significant overweight effect. Authors of six studies, out of which five had used multiple anthropometric measures, included a mention of BMI's limitation as a measure of obesity.

Issues related to balance, postural stability, and plantar pressure were discussed by 13 lab-based studies. Subjects were recruited from the general population in all but three studies, two of which had sampled from orthopedic rehabilitation and obesity treatment clinic patients. In one study, %BF was the primary obesity measurement

used, but eight studies used BMI as the primary and only measure. Two other studies used both %BF and other anthropometric measures, and two studies used both BMI and WHR. It is noted that the two studies with the largest sample sizes used %BF measured by BIA. One included obesity clinic patients and the subjects in the other were part of a health promotion program for postmenopausal women. The median sample size among studies using only BMI was 40.5 (17–120) out of which on average 51(14) % were obese. No study in this sub-category included overweight subjects. Two studies, one testing Canadian and one testing Portuguese subjects reported using BMI cut-offs other than 25 and 30 kg/m². With the exception of three studies, the average BMI reported for subjects was above > 35 kg/m² and in four studies the mean BMI was > 40 kg/m². In terms of significance of the obesity effect, two study reported

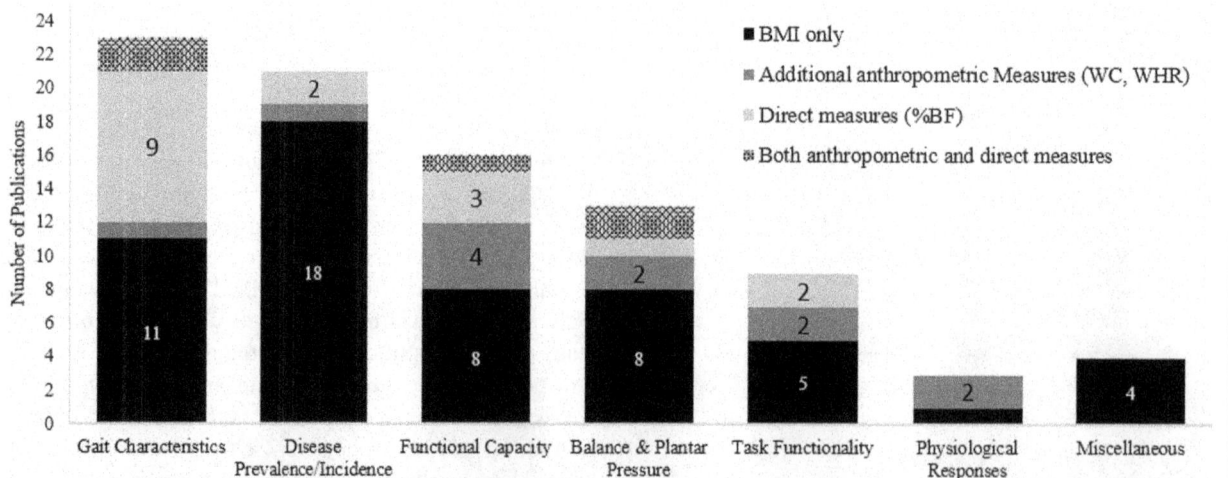

Fig. 5 The obesity measurement methods used across the 7 sub-categories of studies that explored effects of obesity on task or body part specific functioning. With the exception of studies in gait categories, anthropometrics, in particular BMI, were still the most frequently used measures of obesity

no significant effect and four reported some but not all outcome measures to be significantly affected by obesity. Only two studies had a mention of inadequacy of BMI, and they both used BMI only.

The effects of obesity on functionality while performing specific occupationally-relevant tasks was investigated by nine lab-based studies. All but one study tested physical tasks such as the sit-to-stand movement, lifting, seated reach, cycling, and running. The remaining study focused on cognitive control. Three studies published by Italian authors tested hospital admits or recovering patients for body mass reduction or metabolic disorders. One study from Switzerland also recruited from individuals who were going to participate in a weight loss program at a hospital. Five studies relied on BMI only, while two added %BF measured by BIA and two added WC. The average sample size was 28.2 (SD = 14.5) and 60% of the included sample were obese. Only one study had an overweight group as well as obese. With the exception of two studies, the reported mean BMI for obese group was > 35 kg/m². Five studies observed a significant effect of obesity on the performance of the specific tasks tested, while four reported no or partial effect. Three authors discussed how BMI is not the ideal obesity measure although only one used WC in addition.

Three studies discussed changes in physiological responses by obesity and the topics of four studies were not closely pertinent to the above mentioned subgroups. Details of these studies were reported in Table 2.

Discussion

Researchers worldwide have investigated the effect of obesity (sometimes including overweight) on a wide range of occupationally-relevant outcomes. Experts from diverse disciplines, including but not limited to, public health, medicine, health sciences and engineering, have contributed to our current understanding of the magnitude of an effect of obesity at work [37]. The diversity of scientific disciplines involved in obesity research has both advantages and disadvantages. It allows for more complex aspects of the obesity effect to be revealed by diverse methodologies. However, it increases the risk of misuse of methods due to unfamiliarity. In particular, the investigators' understanding of obesity and the methods to measure it and classify individuals into distinct risk groups can affect the quality of the findings.

The present study focused primarily on examining the use of various obesity measurement methods and secondarily on sampling strategies. Two categories of publications were considered: those investigating the effect of obesity on occupational disease development or business outcomes and those studying how obesity alters task-level performance or functional capacity. As expected, studies in the first category had large sample sizes and were mostly public health studies, carried out by public health professionals. While the samples mostly consisted of participants from the general population or a certain occupation, the large sample sizes justified the use of BMI as the sole obesity measure in over 70% of these studies. It is noted that the vast majority of the publications in this category failed to report descriptive statistics regarding the obesity status of the obese group included in the sample. This could serve as a critical source of information for comparative analyses. The WHO expert consultation [38] suggests that wherever possible, researchers should use all BMI categories for reporting purposes, in order to facilitate international comparisons (i.e., 18.5, 20, 23, 25, 27.5, 30, 32.5 kg/m², and in many populations, 35, 37.5, and 40 kg/m²).

Another issue with studies in the general category is in regard to abdominal obesity. It is often defined using waist circumference, especially in recent years, while waist-hip ratio was often used in earlier years. However, various cut points have been recommended over time, by different health organizations and across countries, and used across studies. Abdominal obesity is a major component of metabolic syndrome, a cluster of metabolic abnormalities that carry an increased risk of cardiovascular diseases and diabetes [39]. However, there is a subset of the obese population that are metabolically healthy and their inclusion in study samples can confound the results. Ortega et al., [40] studied a large cohort of 43,265 individuals and reported that when adjusting for fitness and other confounders, metabolically healthy but obese individuals had lower risk of all-cause mortality, non-fatal and fatal cardiovascular disease, and cancer mortality than their metabolically unhealthy obese counterparts. In their study, over 46% of the obese sample were metabolically healthy. From the reported exclusion criteria in the studies reported here, it cannot be decided whether obesity would have the same effects in the absence of other components of metabolic syndrome, particularly for outcomes such as healthcare cost, job disability, absenteeism, and presenteeism.

The studies in the second category focused on task-level performance or functional capacity. There are three main points of discussion identified for these studies: 1) selection of obesity measurement(s) (e.g. BMI, WC, %BF) and the corresponding cut-points to distinguish obese from non-obese, 2) the study participants, both in terms of sample size and the population targeted (e.g. young adults, certain occupation groups, hospital admits), and 3) measurement considerations (e.g. site of measurement for WC). While these factors are all individually important, their interaction may also present a challenge to studies. For instance, when using BMI in a study with a small sample size, recruiting only young adults may be more problematic [41, 42] than when a larger group of older adults are classified based on BMI.

In this category, BMI was still the most frequently used obesity classification measure. Overall, the selection of an obesity measure should depend on the hypothesized mechanism by which the obesity effect would manifest. While obesity presents by both changes in anthropometry and metabolic function, acknowledgement of the considered causal pathway is advantageous to study rigor. Also, while obesity morphology may not be as crucial to the outcomes in the studies of the previous category, it is highly relevant to the dependent variables investigated by the studies in this category. In particular, balance and gait parameters are likely to be affected by the distribution of weight in the body, therefore not only obesity status, but also fat distribution needs to be taken into account. BMI by itself fails to do so, however other anthropometric measures such as WC and WHR are able to distinguish central obesity from lower body and general obesity. Across the 36 studies in the two aforementioned sub-categories, only 10 studies used additional anthropometric measures.

Caution should be made in the use of BMI in studies with small samples that include young adults. Statistically significant age dependencies have been reported in the relation between %BF and BMI, such that older adults have higher %BF compared with younger adults with comparable BMIs [25]. WHO expert consultation acknowledges the issue by stating that most studies show the relation between BMI and %BF to be dependent on age and sex, and also different across ethnic groups. Experts affirmed that Asian populations have different associations between BMI and percentage of body fat than do Western populations [38], however, due to lack of comprehensive data from all Asians, they suggested retaining WHO BMI cut-off points as international classifications. Using ethnic-specific cut-offs may come at the expense of consistency among studies. As such, we observed two studies from Portugal in the balance sub-category that participants were recruited from the general population, one using a BMI cut-off of 25.5 kg/m^2 and the other using 30 kg/m^{2}to distinguish obese from non-obese. Arbitrary grouping of subjects, not backed up by ethnic or other expected underlying differences, as was the case in these two studies, should also be minimized. Overall, it is alarming that only 20% of the studies in this category acknowledged the aforementioned shortcomings of BMI as the obesity measure.

The majority of studies in this category (~ 80%) were observational studies. To isolate an obesity effect, and in contrast to the majority of studies in the first category, subjects were selected such that they were mostly otherwise healthy. The representativeness of this group and the extent to which the findings based from them can be generalized to the overall obese population is concerning. This exclusion of obese with comorbidities from the study samples in this category and their possible inclusion in samples of the first category may contribute to the higher proportion of publications in the first category to report a significant obesity effect in comparison to the second category.

Another issue with the sample representativeness is including only severe obesity (classes II (BMI 35–39.9 kg/m^2) and III (BMI ≥ 40 kg/m^2). While this practice may be statistically sound and increase the likelihood of capturing the obesity effect, it again limits the generalizability of the result. For instance, in the United States the prevalence of obesity is estimated to be over 35% but less than 15% of the obese population (~ 5% of the total population) are categorized as class II and less than 7% (~ 2.5%) as class III [43].

There are considerations for proper use of each measurement as well. WC for instance is shown to be significantly different across sites of measurement, postures, phases of respiration, and time since last meal [31]. By following the existing measurement guidelines [44] studies are less prone to error and consistency across subjects and studies is also warranted. Also, practices such as having a single trained staff doing all the measurements when possible, keeping the measurement conditions homogenous across all subjects and using multiple measurements are beneficial for internal validity and worthy of report in research manuscripts.

Overall, we assessed obesity research in the occupational health field and showcased the practices of obesity measurement since 2000. The present study has many strengths, but also some limitations. While obesity has become a global epidemic, this review was limited to PubMed database as well as Google Scholar journal articles available in English, primarily due to the authors' time and language proficiency constraints. Also, studies related to health promotion at work were excluded [45, 46]. Health risk assessment is a common part of these programs in which obesity status is commonly assessed as a health risk, however the topic of these studies were beyond the scope of this review. Moreover, although the effect of certain work types, such as shift work on the onset of obesity among workers is of importance and has been widely studied [47], this review focused on the obesity effect on occupationally-relevant outcomes.

Conclusion

Obesity is a serious global public health threat. In order to build up a comprehensive profile of its effects, it is crucial to have easy-to-use yet reliable measures that allow for classification of individuals into distinct risk groups. A large body of research has been conducted in the occupational health field regarding obesity. Use of indirect measures such as BMI may be justifiable in large scale public health studies due to their ease of use and low cost. However, due to limitations of these measures, cautious use of them is suggested as the sole obesity measure in small-scale observational studies.

Abbreviations
%BF: Body Fat Percentage; BIA: Bioelectrical Impedance Analysis; BMI: Body Mass Index; DEXA: Energy X-ray Absorptiometry; GF: General Physical or Mental Work-Related Functioning; LBP: Low Back Pain; NIH: National Institute of Health; OA: Osteoarthritis; OW/OB: Overweight/Obese; RoM: Range of Motion; ST: Skinfold Thickness; TBS: Task or Body Part Specific Functioning; WC: Waist Circumference; WHO: World Health Organization; WHR: Waist–Hip Ratio

Funding
Funding provided by the Grant or Cooperative Agreement Number, 1 R03 OH 010547–01, funded by the Centers for Disease Control and Prevention. YW's related effort in this study was supported in part by research grants from the National Institute of Health (NIH, U54 HD070725; 1R01HD064685-01A1). Its contents are solely the responsibility of the authors and do not necessarily represent the official views of the funders.

Authors' contributions
MGS participated in the design of the study and all the phases of the systematic review and drafted of the manuscript. LAC participated in the design of the study and provided oversight of the review and reviewed the draft of the manuscript. YW provided insight on the analysis of the results and reviewed the draft of the manuscript. All authors read and approved the final manuscript.

Competing interests
The authors declare that they have no competing interests.

Author details
[1]Department of Industrial and Systems Engineering, University at Buffalo, 324 Bell Hall, Buffalo, NY 14260, USA. [2]Department of Nutrition and Health Sciences, College of Health, Ball State University, Muncie, IN, USA.

References
1.	World Health Organization. Obesity and overweight. Fact sheet N 311. http://www.who.int/mediacentre/factsheets/fs311/en/ (2015). Accessed 8 May 2017.
2.	Ng M, Fleming T, Robinson M, Thomson B, Graetz N, Margono C, Mullany EC, Biryukov S, Abbafati C, Abera SF, Abraham JP. Global, regional, and national prevalence of overweight and obesity in children and adults during 1980–2013: a systematic analysis for the global burden of disease study 2013. Lancet. 2014;384:766–81.
3.	Wang Y, Beydoun MA. The obesity epidemic in the United States—gender, age, socioeconomic, racial/ethnic, and geographic characteristics: a systematic review and meta-regression analysis. Epidemiol Rev. 2007;29:6–28.
4.	Hubert HB, Feinleib M, McNamara PM, Castelli WP. Obesity as an independent risk factor for cardiovascular disease: a 26-year follow-up of participants in the Framingham heart study. Circulation. 1983;67:968–77.
5.	Goldhaber SZ, Grodstein F, Stampfer MJ, Manson JE, Colditz GA, Speizer FE, Willett WC, Hennekens CH. A prospective study of risk factors for pulmonary embolism in women. JAMA. 1997;277:642–5.
6.	Powell A, Teichtahl AJ, Wluka AE, Cicuttini FM. Obesity: a preventable risk factor for large joint osteoarthritis which may act through biomechanical factors. Br J Sports Med. 2005;39:4–5.
7.	Carroll KK. Obesity as a risk factor for certain types of cancer. Lipids. 1998 Nov 1;33:1055–9.
8.	Gilleard W. Functional task limitations in obese adults. Curr Obes Rep. 2012;1:174–80.
9.	Cournot MC, Marquie JC, Ansiau D, Martinaud C, Fonds H, Ferrieres J, Ruidavets JB. Relation between body mass index and cognitive function in healthy middle-aged men and women. Neurology. 2006;67:1208–14.
10.	Luckhaupt SE, Cohen MA, Li J, Calvert GM. Prevalence of obesity among US workers and associations with occupational factors. Am J Prev Med. 2014;46: 237–48.
11.	Neovius K, Johansson K, Kark M, Neovius M. Obesity status and sick leave: a systematic review. Obes Rev. 2009;10:17–27.
12.	Pollack KM, Sorock GS, Slade MD, Cantley L, Sircar K, Taiwo O, Cullen MR. Association between body mass index and acute traumatic workplace injury in hourly manufacturing employees. Am J Epidemiol. 2007;166:204–11.
13.	Schmier JK, Jones ML, Halpern MT. Cost of obesity in the workplace. Scand J Work Environ Health. 2006;1:5–11.
14.	Sangachin MG, Cavuoto LA. Obesity research in occupational safety and health: a mapping literature review. Proc Human Factors Ergon Soc Ann Meeting. 2016; doi: https://doi.org/10.1177/1541931213601237.
15.	World Health Organization. Obesity: preventing and managing the global epidemic. 2000. http://www.who.int/nutrition/publications/obesity/WHO_TRS_894/en/. Accessed 8 May 2017.
16.	World Health Organization. Physical status: The use of and interpretation of anthropometry, Report of a WHO Expert Committee. 1995. http://www.who.int/childgrowth/publications/physical_status/en/. Accessed 8 May 2017.
17.	Wang Y. Epidemiology of childhood obesity—methodological aspects and guidelines: what is new? Int J Obes. 2004;28:S21–8.
18.	Rothman KJ. BMI-related errors in the measurement of obesity. Int J Obes. 2008;32:S56–9.
19.	Mullie P, Vansant G, Hulens M, Clarys P, Degrave E. Evaluation of body fat estimated from body mass index and impedance in Belgian male military candidates: comparing two methods for estimating body composition. Mil Med. 2008;173:266–70.
20.	Deurenberg P, Andreoli A, Borg P, Kukkonen-Harjula K, de Lorenzo A, van Marken Lichtenbelt WD, Testolin G, Vigano R, Vollaard N. The validity of predicted body fat percentage from body mass index and fromimpedance in samples of five European populations. Eur J Clin Nutr. 2001;1:973–9.
21.	Ruderman NB, Schneider SH, Berchtold P. The" metabolically-obese," normal-weight individual. Am J Clin Nutr. 1981;34:1617–21.
22.	Dvorak RV, DeNino WF, Ades PA, Poehlman ET. Phenotypic characteristics associated with insulin resistance in metabolically obese but normal-weight young women. Diabetes. 1999;48:2210–4.
23.	Karelis AD, St-Pierre DH, Conus F, Rabasa-Lhoret R, Poehlman ET. Metabolic and body composition factors in subgroups of obesity: what do we know? J Clin Endocrinol Metab. 2004;89:2569–75.
24.	Harbin G, Shenoy C, Olson J. Ten-year comparison of BMI, body fat, and fitness in the workplace. Am J Ind Med. 2006;49:223–30.
25.	Gallagher D, Visser M, Sepulveda D, Pierson RN, Harris T, Heymsfield SB. How useful is body mass index for comparison of body fatness across age, sex, and ethnic groups? Am J Epidemiol. 1996;143:228–39.
26.	Wang Y, Rimm EB, Stampfer MJ, Willett WC, Hu FB. Comparison of abdominal adiposity and overall obesity in predicting risk of type 2 diabetes among men. Am J Clin Nutr. 2005;81:555–63.
27.	Després JP, Lemieux I, Prud'Homme D. Treatment of obesity: need to focus on high risk abdominally obese patients. Br Med J. 2001;322:716.
28.	Piers LS, Soares MJ, Frandsen SL, O'dea K. Indirect estimates of body composition are useful for groups but unreliable in individuals. Int J Obes. 2000;24:1145–52.
29.	Ross R, Berentzen T, Bradshaw AJ, Janssen I, Kahn HS, Katzmarzyk PT, Kuk JL, Seidell JC, Snijder MB, Sørensen TI, Després JP. Does the relationship between waist circumference, morbidity and mortality depend on measurement protocol for waist circumference? Obes Rev. 2008;9:312–25.

30. Lohman TJ, Roache AF, Martorell R. Anthropometric standardization reference manual. Med Sci Sports Exerc. 1992;24:952.

31. Agarwal SK, Misra A, Aggarwal P, Bardia A, Goel R, Vikram NK, Wasir JS, Hussain N, Ramachandran K, Pandey RM. Waist circumference measurement by site, posture, respiratory phase, and meal time: implications for methodology. Obesity. 2009;17:1056–61.

32. Pan WH, Yeh WT, Weng LC. Epidemiology of metabolic syndrome in Asia. Asia Pac J Clin Nutr. 2008;17:37–42.

33. Misra A. Revisions of cutoffs of body mass index to define overweight and obesity are needed for the Asian-ethnic groups. Int J Obes. 2003;27:1294–6.

34. Stevens J. Ethnic-specific cutpoints for obesity vs country-specific guidelines for action. Int J Obes. 2003;27:287–8.

35. Sangachin M, Samadi M, Cavuoto L. Modeling the spread of an obesity intervention through a social network. J Healthcare Eng. 2014;5:293–312.

36. Lee M, Roan M, Smith B. An application of principal component analysis for lower body kinematics between loaded and unloaded walking. J Biomech. 2009;42:2226–30.

37. Khan A, Choudhury N, Uddin S, Hossain L, Baur LA. Longitudinal trends in global obesity research and collaboration: a review using bibliometric metadata. Obes Rev. 2016; https://doi.org/10.1111/obr.12372.

38. World Health Organization Expert Consultation. Appropriate body-mass index for Asian populations and its implications for policy and intervention strategies. Lancet (London, England). 2004;363:157–63.

39. Eckel RH, Grundy SM, Zimmet PZ. The metabolic syndrome. Lancet. 2005; 365:1415–28.

40. Ortega FB, Lee DC, Katzmarzyk PT, Ruiz JR, Sui X, Church TS, Blair SN. The intriguing metabolically healthy but obese phenotype: cardiovascular prognosis and role of fitness. Eur Heart J. 2013;34:389–97.

41. Sangachin MG, Cavuoto LA. Obesity-related changes in prolonged repetitive lifting performance. Appl Ergon. 2016;56:19–26.

42. Pajoutan M, Mehta RK, Cavuoto LA. The effect of obesity on central activation failure during ankle fatigue: a pilot investigation. Fatigue Biomed Health Behavior. 2016;4:115–26.

43. Ogden CL, Carroll MD, Kit BK, Flegal KM. Prevalence of childhood and adult obesity in the United States, 2011-2012. JAMA. 2014;311:806–14.

44. National Institute of Health; National Heart, Lung, and Blood Institute. Joint National Committee on Prevention, Detection, Evaluation, and Treatment of High Blood Pressure. North American Association for the Study of Obesity. The Practical Guide: Identification, Evaluation, and Treatment of Overweight and Obesity in Adults. 2000. https://www.nhlbi.nih.gov/files/docs/guidelines/prctgd_c.pdf. Accessed 8May 2017.

45. Sangachin MG, Cavuoto LA. Worksite exercise programs why do employees participate? Proc Human Factors Ergon Soc Ann Meet. 2015; https://doi.org/10.1177/1541931215591187.

46. Sangachin MG, Gustafson WW, Cavuoto LA. Effect of active workstation use on workload, task performance, and postural and physiological responses. IIE Trans Occup Ergon Hum Factors. 2016;4:67–81.

47. Proper KI, van de Langenberg D, Rodenburg W, Vermeulen RC, van der Beek AJ, van Steeg H, van Kerkhof LW. The relationship between shift work and metabolic risk factors: a systematic review of longitudinal studies. Am J Prev Med. 2016;50:e147–57.

48. Lee YC, Runnion CK, Pang SC, de Klerk NH, Musk AW. Increased body mass index is related to apparent circumscribed pleural thickening on plain chest radiographs. Am J Ind Med. 2001;39:112–6.

49. Clark S, Rene A, Theurer WM, Marshall M. Association of body mass index and health status in firefighters. J Occup Environ Med. 2002;44:940–6.

50. Poston WS, Haddock CK, Talcott GW, Klesges RC, Lando HA, Peterson A. Are overweight and obese airmen at greater risk of discharge from the United States air Force? Mil Med. 2002;167:585–8.

51. Arbabi S, Wahl WL, Hemmila MR, Kohoyda-Inglis C, Taheri PA, Wang SC. The cushion effect. J Trauma. 2003;54:1090–3.

52. Bungum T, Satterwhite M, Jackson AW, Morrow JR. The relationship of body mass index, medical costs, and job absenteeism. Am J Health Behav. 2003;27:456–62.

53. Moreau M, Valente F, Mak R, Pelfrene E, de Smet P, De Backer G, et al. Obesity, body fat distribution and incidence of sick leave in the Belgian workforce: the Belstress study. Int J Obes Relat Metab Disord. 2004;28:574–82.

54. Pronk NP, Martinson B, Kessler RC, Beck AL, Simon GE, Wang P. The association between work performance and physical activity, cardiorespiratory fitness, and obesity. J Occup Environ Med. 2004;46:19–25.

55. Laitinen J, Nayha S, Kujala V. Body mass index and weight change from adolescence into adulthood, waist-to-hip ratio and perceived work ability among young adults. Int J Obes. 2005;29:697–702.

56. Ricci JA, Chee E. Lost productive time associated with excess weight in the US workforce. J Occup Environ Med. 2005;47:1227–34.

57. Arena VC, Padiyar KR, Burton WN, Schwerha JJ. The impact of body mass index on short-term disability in the workplace. J Occup Environ Med. 2006; 48:1118–24.

58. Cormier Y, Israel-Assayag E. Adiposity affects human response to inhaled organic dust. Am J Ind Med. 2006;49:281–5.

59. Nishitani N, Sakakibara H. Relationship of obesity to job stress and eating behavior in male Japanese workers. Int J Obes. 2006;30:528–33.

60. Wang F, McDonald T, Bender J, Reffitt B, Miller A, Edington DW. Association of healthcare costs with per unit body mass index increase. J Occup Environ Med. 2006;48:668–74.

61. Østbye T, Dement JM, Krause KM. Obesity and workers' compensation: results from the Duke health and safety surveillance system. Arch Intern Med. 2007;167:766–73.

62. Charles LE, Fekedulegn D, McCall T, Burchfiel CM, Andrew ME, Violanti JM. Obesity, white blood cell counts, and platelet counts among police officers. Obesity (Silver Spring). 2007;15:2846–54.

63. Finkelstein EA, Chen H, Prabhu M, Trogdon JG, Corso PS. The relationship between obesity and injuries among US adults. Am J Health Promot. 2007; 21:460–8.

64. Jans MP, van den Heuvel SG, Hildebrandt VH, Bongers PM. Overweight and obesity as predictors of absenteeism in the working population of the Netherlands. J Occup Environ Med. 2007;49:975–80.

65. Gates DM, Succop P, Brehm BJ, Gillespie GL, Sommers BD. Obesity and presenteeism: the impact of body mass index on workplace productivity. J Occup Environ Med. 2008;50:39–45.

66. Soteriades ES, Hauser R, Kawachi I, Christiani DC, Kales SN. Obesity and risk of job disability in male firefighters. Occup Med. 2008;58:245–50.

67. Claessen H, Arndt V, Drath C, Brenner H. Overweight, obesity and risk of work disability: a cohort study of construction workers in Germany. Occup Environ Med. 2009;66:402–9.

68. Vissers D, Baeyens JP, Truijen S, Ides K, Vercruysse CC, Van Gaal L. The effect of whole body vibration short-term exercises on respiratory gas exchange in overweight and obese women. Phys Sportsmed. 2009;37:88–94.

69. Bedno SA, Li Y, Han W, Cowan DN, Scott CT, Cavicchia MA, et al. Exertional heat illness among overweight US Army recruits in basic training. Aviat Space Environ Med. 2010;81:107–11.

70. Robroek SJ, Van den Berg TI, Plat JF, Burdorf A. The role of obesity and lifestyle behaviours in a productive workforce. Occup Environ Med. 2011;68: 134–9.

71. Vincent HK, Lamb KM, Day TI, Tillman SM, Vincent KR, George SZ. Morbid obesity is associated with fear of movement and lower quality of life in patients with knee pain-related diagnoses. PM R. 2010;2:713–22.

72. Cowan D, Bedno S, Urban N, Yi B, Niebuhr D. Musculoskeletal injuries among overweight army trainees: incidence and health care utilization. Occup Med. 2011;61:247–52.

73. Poston WS, Jitnarin N, Haddock CK, Jahnke SA, Tuley BC. Obesity and injury-related absenteeism in a population-based firefighter cohort. Obesity (Silver Spring). 2011;19:2076–81.

74. Haukka E, Ojajarvi A, Takala EP, Viikari-Juntura E, Leino-Arjas P. Physical workload, leisure-time physical activity, obesity and smoking as predictors of multisite musculoskeletal pain. A 2-year prospective study of kitchen workers. Occup Environ Med. 2012;69:485–92.

75. Caberlon CF, Padoin AV, Mottin CC. Importance of musculoskeletal pain in work activities in obese individuals. Obes Surg. 2013;23:2092–5.

76. Gubata ME, Urban N, Cowan DN, Niebuhr DW. A prospective study of physical fitness, obesity, and the subsequent risk of mental disorders among healthy young adults in army training. J Psychosom Res. 2013;75:43–8.

77. Jahnke SA, Poston WS, Haddock CK, Jitnarin N. Obesity and incident injury among career firefighters in the Central United States. Obesity (Silver Spring). 2013;21:1505–8.

78. Kouvonen A, Kivimaki M, Oksanen T, Pentti J, De Vogli R, Virtanen M, Vahtera J. Obesity and occupational injury: a prospective cohort study of 69,515 public sector employees. PLoS One. 2013;8:e77178.

79. Lin TC, Verma SK, Courtney TK. Does obesity contribute to non-fatal occupational injury? Evidence from the National Longitudinal Survey of youth. Scand J Work Environ Health. 2013;39:268–75.

80. Roos E, Laaksonen M, Rahkonen O, Lahelma E, Lallukka T. Relative weight and disability retirement: a prospective cohort study. Scand J Work Environ Health. 2013;39:259–67.

81. Van der Starre RE, Coffeng JK, Hendriksen IJ, van Mechelen W, Boot CR. Associations between overweight, obesity, health measures and need for recovery in office employees: a cross-sectional analysis. BMC Public Health. 2013;13:1207.

82. Viester L, Verhagen EA, Oude Hengel KM, Koppes LL, van der Beek AJ, Bongers PM. The relation between body mass index and musculoskeletal symptoms in the working population. BMC Musculoskelet Disord. 2013;14:238.

83. Gonzales MM, Kaur S, Eagan DE, Goudarzi K, Pasha E, Doan DC, et al. Central adiposity and the functional magnetic resonance imaging response to cognitive challenge. Int J Obes. 2014;38:1193–9.

84. Smith TJ, White A, Hadden L, Young AJ, Marriott BP. Associations between mental health disorders and body mass index among military personnel. Am J Health Behav. 2014;38:529–40.

85. DeVita P, Hortobagyi T. Obesity is not associated with increased knee joint torque and power during level walking. J Biomech. 2003;36:1355–62.

86. Browning RC, Baker EA, Herron JA, Kram R. Effects of obesity and sex on the energetic cost and preferred speed of walking. J Appl Physiol. 2006;100:390–8.

87. Browning RC, Kram R. Effects of obesity on the biomechanics of walking at different speeds. Med Sci Sports Exerc. 2007;39:1632–41.

88. Lafortuna CL, Agosti F, Galli R, Busti C, Lazzer S, Sartorio A. The energetic and cardiovascular response to treadmill walking and cycle ergometer exercise in obese women. Eur J Appl Physiol. 2008;103:707–17.

89. Lai PP, Leung AK, Li AN, Zhang M. Three-dimensional gait analysis of obese adults. Clin Biomech (Bristol, Avon). 2008;23:S2–6.

90. Browning RC, McGowan CP, Kram R. Obesity does not increase external mechanical work per kilogram body mass during walking. J Biomech. 2009;42:2273–8.

91. Malatesta D, Vismara L, Menegoni F, Galli M, Romei M, Capodaglio P. Mechanical external work and recovery at preferred walking speed in obese subjects. Med Sci Sports Exerc. 2009;41:426–34.

92. Ko S, Stenholm S, Ferrucci L. Characteristic gait patterns in older adults with obesity–results from the Baltimore longitudinal study of aging. J Biomech. 2010;43:1104–10.

93. Russell EM, Braun B, Hamill J. Does stride length influence metabolic cost and biomechanical risk factors for knee osteoarthritis in obese women? Clin Biomech (Bristol, Avon). 2010;25:438–43.

94. Blaszczyk JW, Plewa M, Cieslinska-Swider J, Bacik B, Zahorska-Markiewicz B, Markiewicz A. Impact of excess body weight on walking at the preferred speed. Acta Neurobiol Exp (Wars). 2011;71:528–40.

95. Ehlen KA, Reiser RF 2nd, Browning RC. Energetics and biomechanics of inclined treadmill walking in obese adults. Med Sci Sports Exerc. 2011;43:1251–9.

96. Cimolin V, Vismara L, Galli M, Zaina F, Negrini S, Capodaglio P. Effects of obesity and chronic low back pain on gait. J Neuroeng Rehabil. 2011;8:55.

97. Russell EM, Hamill J. Lateral wedges decrease biomechanical risk factors for knee osteoarthritis in obese women. J Biomech. 2011;44:2286–91.

98. Wu X, Lockhart TE, Yeoh HT. Effects of obesity on slip-induced fall risks among young male adults. J Biomech. 2012;45:1042–7.

99. Harding GT, Hubley-Kozey CL, Dunbar MJ, Stanish WD, Astephen Wilson JL. Body mass index affects knee joint mechanics during gait differently with and without moderate knee osteoarthritis. Osteoarthr Cartil. 2012;20:1234–42.

100. Russell EM, Miller RH, Umberger BR, Hamill J. Lateral wedges alter mediolateral load distributions at the knee joint in obese individuals. J Orthop Res. 2013;31:665–71.

101. Browning RC, Reynolds MM, Board WJ, Walters KA, Reiser RF 2nd. Obesity does not impair walking economy across a range of speeds and grades. J Appl Physiol. 2013;114:1125–31.

102. Ranavolo A, Donini LM, Mari S, Serrao M, Silvetti A, Iavicoli S, et al. Lower-limb joint coordination pattern in obese subjects. Biomed Res Int. 2013; https://doi.org/10.1155/2013/142323.

103. Cimolin V, Vismara L, Galli M, Grugni G, Cau N, Capodaglio P. Gait strategy in genetically obese patients: a 7-year follow up. Res Dev Disabil. 2014;35:1501–6.

104. Haight DJ, Lerner ZF, Board WJ, Browning RC. A comparison of slow, uphill and fast, level walking on lower extremity biomechanics and tibiofemoral joint loading in obese and nonobese adults. J Orthop Res. 2014;32:324–30.

105. Page Glave A, Di Brezzo R, Applegate DK, Olson JM. The effects of obesity classification method on select kinematic gait variables in adult females. J Sports Med Phys Fitness. 2014;54:197–202.

106. Cau N, Cimolin V, Galli M, Precilios H, Tacchini E, Santovito C, Capodaglio P. Center of pressure displacements during gait initiation in individuals with obesity. J Neuroeng Rehabil. 2014;11:82.

107. Lerner ZF, Board WJ, Browning RC. Effects of obesity on lower extremity muscle function during walking at two speeds. Gait Posture. 2014;39:978–84.

108. Kouyoumdjian JA, Morita MD, Rocha PR, Miranda RC, Gouveia GM. Body mass index and carpal tunnel syndrome. Arq Neuropsiquiatr. 2000;58:252–6.

109. Young SY, Gunzenhauser JD, Malone KE, McTiernan A. Body mass index and asthma in the military population of the northwestern United States. Arch Intern Med. 2001;161:1605–11.

110. Bland JD. The relationship of obesity, age, and carpal tunnel syndrome: more complex than was thought? Muscle Nerve. 2005;32:527–32.

111. Liuke M, Solovieva S, Lamminen A, Luoma K, Leino-Arjas P, Luukkonen R, Riihimaki H. Disc degeneration of the lumbar spine in relation to overweight. Int J Obes. 2005;29:903–8.

112. Dagan Y, Doljansky JT, Green A, Weiner A. Body mass index (BMI) as a first-line screening criterion for detection of excessive daytime sleepiness among professional drivers. Traffic Inj Prev. 2006;7:44–8.

113. Zhao LJ, Liu YJ, Liu PY, Hamilton J, Recker RR, Deng HW. Relationship of obesity with osteoporosis. J Clin Endocrinol Metab. 2007;92:1640–6.

114. Sharifi-Mollayousefi A, Yazdchi-Marandi M, Ayramlou H, Heidari P, Salavati A, Zarrintan S, Sharifi-Mollayousefi A. Assessment of body mass index and hand anthropometric measurements as independent risk factors for carpal tunnel syndrome. Folia Morphol (Warsz). 2008;67:36–42.

115. Grotle M, Hagen KB, Natvig B, Dahl FA, Kvien TK. Obesity and osteoarthritis in knee, hip and/or hand: an epidemiological study in the general population with 10 years follow-up. BMC Musculoskelet Disord. 2008;9:132.

116. Noorloos D, Tersteeg L, Tiemessen IJ, Hulshof CT, Frings-Dresen MH. Does body mass index increase the risk of low back pain in a population exposed to whole body vibration? Appl Ergon. 2008;39:779–85.

117. Toivanen AT, Heliovaara M, Impivaara O, Arokoski JP, Knekt P, Lauren H, Kroger H. Obesity, physically demanding work and traumatic knee injury are major risk factors for knee osteoarthritis–a population-based study with a follow-up of 22 years. Rheumatology (Oxford). 2010;49:308–14.

118. Vismara L, Menegoni F, Zaina F, Galli M, Negrini S, Capodaglio P. Effect of obesity and low back pain on spinal mobility: a cross sectional study in women. J Neuroeng Rehabil. 2010;7:3.

119. Wood D, Goodnight S, Haig AJ, Nasari T. Body mass index, but not blood pressure is related to the level of pain in persons with chronic pain. J Back Musculoskelet Rehabil. 2011;24:111–5.

120. Ackerman IN, Osborne RH. Obesity and increased burden of hip and knee joint disease in Australia: results from a national survey. BMC Musculoskelet Disord. 2012;13:254.

121. Jensen JN, Holtermann A, Clausen T, Mortensen OS, Carneiro IG, Andersen LL. The greatest risk for low-back pain among newly educated female health care workers; body weight or physical work load? BMC Musculoskelet Disord. 2012;13:87.

122. Freedman Silvernail J, Milner CE, Thompson D, Zhang S, Zhao X. The influence of body mass index and velocity on knee biomechanics during walking. Gait Posture. 2013;37:575–9.

123. Seror P, Seror R. Prevalence of obesity and obesity as a risk factor in patients with severe median nerve lesion at the wrist. Joint Bone Spine. 2013;80:632–7.

124. Martin KR, Kuh D, Harris TB, Guralnik JM, Coggon D, Wills AK. Body mass index, occupational activity, and leisure-time physical activity: an exploration of risk factors and modifiers for knee osteoarthritis in the 1946 British birth cohort. BMC Musculoskelet Disord. 2013;14:219.

125. Romero-Vargas S, Zarate-Kalfopulos B, Otero-Camara E, Rosales-Olivarez L, Alpizar-Aguirre A, Morales-Hernandez E, et al. The impact of body mass index and central obesity on the spino-pelvic parameters: a correlation study. Eur Spine J. 2013;22:878–82.

126. Messier SP, Pater M, Beavers DP, Legault C, Loeser RF, Hunter DJ, DeVita P. Influences of alignment and obesity on knee joint loading in osteoarthritic gait. Osteoarthr Cartil. 2014;22:912–7.

127. Urquhart DM, Phyomaung PP, Wluka AE, Sim MR, Forbes A, Jones G, Davies M, Cicuttini FM. Is there a relationship between occupational activities and low back pain in obese, middle-aged women? Climacteric. 2014;17:87–91.

128. Evanoff A, Sabbath EL, Carton M, Czernichow S, Zins M, Leclerc A, et al. Does obesity modify the relationship between exposure to occupational factors and musculoskeletal pain in men? Results from the GAZEL cohort study. PLoS One. 2014;9:e109633.

129. Hulens M, Vansant G, Lysens R, Claessens A, Muls E. Exercise capacity in lean versus obese women. Scand J Med Sci Sports. 2001;11:305–9.

130. Hulens M, Vansant G, Lysens R, Claessens AL, Muls E. Assessment of isokinetic muscle strength in women who are obese. J Orthop Sports Phys Ther. 2002;32:347–56.

131. Maffiuletti NA, Jubeau M, Munzinger U, Bizzini M, Agosti F, De Col A, et al. Differences in quadriceps muscle strength and fatigue between lean and obese subjects. Eur J Appl Physiol. 2007;101:51–9.

132. Segal NA, Yack HJ, Khole P. Weight, rather than obesity distribution, explains peak external knee adduction moment during level gait. Am J Phys Med Rehabil. 2009;88:180–8. quiz 9–91, 246

133. Capodaglio P, Vismara L, Menegoni F, Baccalaro G, Galli M, Grugni G. Strength characterization of knee flexor and extensor muscles in Prader-Willi and obese patients. BMC Musculoskelet Disord. 2009;10:47.

134. Singh D, Park W, Levy MS. Obesity does not reduce maximum acceptable weights of lift. Appl Ergon. 2009;40:1–7.

135. Faria A, Gabriel R, Abrantes J, Bras R, Moreira H. Triceps-surae musculotendinous stiffness: relative differences between obese and non-obese postmenopausal women. Clin Biomech (Bristol, Avon). 2009;24:866–71.

136. Park W, Ramachandran J, Weisman P, Jung ES. Obesity effect on male active joint range of motion. Ergonomics. 2010;53(1):102–8.

137. Blazek K, Asay JL, Erhart-Hledik J, Andriacchi I. Adduction moment increases with age in healthy obese individuals. J Orthop Res. 2013;31:1414–22.

138. Cavuoto LA, Nussbaum MA. Differences in functional performance of the shoulder musculature with obesity and aging. Int J Ind Ergon. 2013;43:393–9.

139. Hamilton MA, Strawderman L, Babski-Reeves K, Hale B. Effects of BMI and task parameters on joint angles during simulated small parts assembly. Int J Ind Ergon. 2013;43:417–24.

140. Mignardot JB, Olivier I, Promayon E, Nougier V. Origins of balance disorders during a daily living movement in obese: can biomechanical factors explain everything? PLoS One. 2013;8:e60491.

141. Wearing SC, Hooper SL, Grigg NL, Nolan G, Smeathers JE. Overweight and obesity alters the cumulative transverse strain in the Achilles tendon immediately following exercise. J Bodyw Mov Ther. 2013;17:316–21.

142. Cavuoto LA, Nussbaum MA. Obesity-related differences in muscular capacity during sustained isometric exertions. Appl Ergon. 2013;44:254–60.

143. Cavuoto LA, Nussbaum MA. The influences of obesity and age on functional performance during intermittent upper extremity tasks. J Occup Environ Hyg. 2014;11:583–90.

144. Mehta RK, Cavuoto LA. The effects of obesity, age, and relative workload levels on handgrip endurance. Appl Ergon. 2015;46:91–5.

145. Hills AP, Hennig EM, McDonald M, Bar-Or O. Plantar pressure differences between obese and non-obese adults: a biomechanical analysis. Int J Obes Relat Metab Disord. 2001;25:1674–9.

146. Gravante G, Russo G, Pomara F, Ridola C. Comparison of ground reaction forces between obese and control young adults during quiet standing on a baropodometric platform. Clin Biomech (Bristol, Avon). 2003;18:780–2.

147. Birtane M, Tuna H. The evaluation of plantar pressure distribution in obese and non-obese adults. Clin Biomech. 2004;19:1055–9.

148. Berrigan F, Simoneau M, Tremblay A, Hue O, Teasdale N. Influence of obesity on accurate and rapid arm movement performed from a standing posture. Int J Obes. 2006;30:1750–7.

149. Teh E, Teng LF, Acharya R, Ha TP, Goh E, Min LC. Static and frequency domain analysis of plantar pressure distribution in obese and non-obese subjects. J Bodyw Mov Ther. 2006;10:127–33.

150. Singh D, Park W, Levy MS, Jung ES. The effects of obesity and standing time on postural sway during prolonged quiet standing. Ergonomics. 2009;52:977–86.

151. Blaszczyk JW, Cieslinska-Swider J, Plewa M, Zahorska-Markiewicz B, Markiewicz A. Effects of excessive body weight on postural control. J Biomech. 2009;42:1295–300.

152. Park W, Singh DP, Levy MS, Jung ES. Obesity effect on perceived postural stress during static posture maintenance tasks. Ergonomics. 2009;52:1169–82.

153. Menegoni F, Galli M, Tacchini E, Vismara L, Cavigioli M, Capodaglio P. Gender-specific effect of obesity on balance. Obesity (Silver Spring). 2009;17:1951–6.

154. Monteiro M, Gabriel R, Aranha J, Neves e Castro M, Sousa M, Moreira M. Influence of obesity and sarcopenic obesity on plantar pressure of postmenopausal women. Clin Biomech (Bristol, Avon). 2010;25:461–7.

155. Miller EM, Matrangola SL, Madigan ML. Effects of obesity on balance recovery from small postural perturbations. Ergonomics. 2011;54:547–54.

156. Matrangola SL, Madigan ML. The effects of obesity on balance recovery using an ankle strategy. Hum Mov Sci. 2011;30:584–95.

157. Peduzzi de Castro M, Abreu S, Pinto V, Santos R, Machado L, Vaz M, Vilas-Boas JP. Influence of pressure-relief insoles developed for loaded gait (backpackers and obese people) on plantar pressure distribution and ground reaction forces. Appl Ergon. 2014;45:1028–34.

158. Galli M, Crivellini M, Sibella F, Montesano A, Bertocco P, Parisio C. Sit-to-stand movement analysis in obese subjects. Int J Obes Relat Metab Disord. 2000;24:1488–92.

159. Sibella F, Galli M, Romei M, Montesano A, Crivellini M. Biomechanical analysis of sit-to-stand movement in normal and obese subjects. Clin Biomech. 2003;18:745–50.

160. Lafortuna CL, Proietti M, Agosti F, Sartorio A. The energy cost of cycling in young obese women. Eur J Appl Physiol. 2006;97:16–25.

161. Gilleard W, Smith T. Effect of obesity on posture and hip joint moments during a standing task, and trunk forward flexion motion. Int J Obes. 2007;31:267–71.

162. Xu X, Mirka GA, Hsiang SM. The effects of obesity on lifting performance. Appl Ergon. 2008;39:93–8.

163. Taboga P, Lazzer S, Fessehatsion R, Agosti F, Sartorio A, di Prampero PE. Energetics and mechanics of running men: the influence of body mass. Eur J Appl Physiol. 2012;112:4027–33.

164. Hendrick OM, Luo X, Zhang S, Li CS. Saliency processing and obesity: a preliminary imaging study of the stop signal task. Obesity (Silver Spring). 2012;20:1796–802.

165. Singh B, Brown TD, Callaghan JJ, Yack HJ. Abdomen-thigh contact during forward reaching tasks in obese individuals. J Appl Biomech. 2013;29:517–24.

166. Schmid S, Armand S, Pataky Z, Golay A, Allet L. The relationship between different body mass index categories and chair rise performance in adult women. J Appl Biomech. 2013;29:705–11.

167. Willenberg T, Schumacher A, Amann-Vesti B, Jacomella V, Thalhammer C, Diehm N, Baumgartner I, Husmann M. Impact of obesity on venous hemodynamics of the lower limbs. J Vasc Surg. 2010;52:664–8.

168. Engelberger RP, Indermuhle A, Baumann F, Fahrni J, Diehm N, Kucher N, Egermann U, Laederach K, Baumgartner I, Willenberg T. Diurnal changes of lower leg volume in obese and non-obese subjects. Int J Obes. 2014;38:801–5.

169. Yang B, Sun Z, Cao F, Zhao H, Li C, Zhang J. Obesity is a risk factor for acute mountain sickness: a prospective study in Tibet railway construction workers on Tibetan plateau. Eur Rev Med Pharmacol Sci. 2015;19:119–22.

170. Menegoni F, Vismara L, Capodaglio P, Crivellini M, Galli M. Kinematics of trunk movements: protocol design and application in obese females. J Appl Biomater Biomech. 2007;6:178–85.

171. Forman J, Lopez-Valdes FJ, Lessley D, Kindig M, Kent R, Bostrom O. The effect of obesity on the restraint of automobile occupants. Ann Adv Automot Med. 2009;53:25–40.

172. Lerner ZF, Board WJ, Browning RC. Effects of an obesity-specific marker set on estimated muscle and joint forces in walking. Med Sci Sports Exerc. 2014;46:1261–7.

173. Thorp AA, Kingwell BA, Owen N, Dunstan DW. Breaking up workplace sitting time with intermittent standing bouts improves fatigue and musculoskeletal discomfort in overweight/obese office workers. Occup Environ Med. 2014;71:765–71.

Permissions

All chapters in this book were first published in OBESITY, by BioMed Central; hereby published with permission under the Creative Commons Attribution License or equivalent. Every chapter published in this book has been scrutinized by our experts. Their significance has been extensively debated. The topics covered herein carry significant findings which will fuel the growth of the discipline. They may even be implemented as practical applications or may be referred to as a beginning point for another development.

The contributors of this book come from diverse backgrounds, making this book a truly international effort. This book will bring forth new frontiers with its revolutionizing research information and detailed analysis of the nascent developments around the world.

We would like to thank all the contributing authors for lending their expertise to make the book truly unique. They have played a crucial role in the development of this book. Without their invaluable contributions this book wouldn't have been possible. They have made vital efforts to compile up to date information on the varied aspects of this subject to make this book a valuable addition to the collection of many professionals and students.

This book was conceptualized with the vision of imparting up-to-date information and advanced data in this field. To ensure the same, a matchless editorial board was set up. Every individual on the board went through rigorous rounds of assessment to prove their worth. After which they invested a large part of their time researching and compiling the most relevant data for our readers.

The editorial board has been involved in producing this book since its inception. They have spent rigorous hours researching and exploring the diverse topics which have resulted in the successful publishing of this book. They have passed on their knowledge of decades through this book. To expedite this challenging task, the publisher supported the team at every step. A small team of assistant editors was also appointed to further simplify the editing procedure and attain best results for the readers.

Apart from the editorial board, the designing team has also invested a significant amount of their time in understanding the subject and creating the most relevant covers. They scrutinized every image to scout for the most suitable representation of the subject and create an appropriate cover for the book.

The publishing team has been an ardent support to the editorial, designing and production team. Their endless efforts to recruit the best for this project, has resulted in the accomplishment of this book. They are a veteran in the field of academics and their pool of knowledge is as vast as their experience in printing. Their expertise and guidance has proved useful at every step. Their uncompromising quality standards have made this book an exceptional effort. Their encouragement from time to time has been an inspiration for everyone.

The publisher and the editorial board hope that this book will prove to be a valuable piece of knowledge for researchers, students, practitioners and scholars across the globe.

List of Contributors

Lindsay Fernández-Rhodes
Department of Epidemiology, UNC Gillings School of Global Public Health, University of North Carolina at Chapel Hill, 123 W Franklin St, Building C, Chapel Hill, NC, USA
Carolina Population Center, University of North Carolina at Chapel Hill, 123 W Franklin St, Building C, Chapel Hill, NC, USA

Annie Green Howard
Carolina Population Center, University of North Carolina at Chapel Hill, 123 W Franklin St, Building C, Chapel Hill, NC, USA
Department of Biostatistics, UNC Gillings School of Global Public Health, University of North Carolina at Chapel Hill, Chapel Hill, NC, USA

Mariaelisa Graff, Heather M. Highland, Kristin L. Young and Kari E. North
Department of Epidemiology, UNC Gillings School of Global Public Health, University of North Carolina at Chapel Hill, 123 W Franklin St, Building C, Chapel Hill, NC, USA

Carmen R. Isasi, Qibin Qi and Robert C. Kaplan
Department of Epidemiology and Population Health, Albert Einstein College of Medicine, Bronx, NY, USA

Esteban Parra
Department of Anthropology, University of Toronto at Mississauga, Mississauga, ON, Canada

Jennifer E. Below
Department of Medicine, Vanderbilt University Medical Center, Nashville, TN, USA

Anne E. Justice
Biomedical and Translational Informatics Institute, Geisinger Health System, Danville, PA, USA

George Papanicolaou
Epidemiology Branch, National Heart Lung and Blood Institute, Bethesda, MD, USA

Cathy C. Laurie
Department of Biostatistics, School of Public Health, University of Washington, Seattle, WA, USA

Struan F. A. Grant
Divisions of Human Genetics and Endocrinology, Children's Hospital of Philadelphia Research Institute, Philadelphia, PA, USA

Christopher Haiman
Department of Preventive Medicine, Norris Comprehensive Cancer Center, Keck School of Medicine, University of Southern California, Los Angeles, CA, USA

Ruth J. F. Loos
Charles R. Bronfman Instituted for Personalized Medicine, Icahn School of Medicine at Mount Sinai, New York, NY, USA

Eva O. Melin
Department of Clinical Sciences, Section Endocrinology and Diabetes, Lund University, Lund, Sweden
Department of Research and Development, Region Kronoberg, SE-35112 Växjö, Sweden Primary Care, Region Kronoberg, Växjö, Sweden

Hans O. Thulesius
Department of Research and Development, Region Kronoberg
Primary Care, Region Kronoberg, Växjö, Sweden
Department of Clinical Sciences, Section of Family Medicine, Lund University, Malmö, Sweden

Magnus Hillman
Department of Clinical Sciences, Diabetes Research Laboratory, Faculty of Medicine, Lund University, Lund, Sweden

Mona Landin-Olsson
Department of Clinical Sciences, Section Endocrinology and Diabetes, Lund University, Lund, Sweden
Department of Clinical Sciences, Diabetes Research Laboratory, Faculty of Medicine, Lund University, Lund, Sweden
Department of Endocrinology, Skane University Hospital, Lund, Sweden

Maria Thunander
Department of Research and Development, Region Kronoberg

Department of Clinical Sciences, Diabetes Research Laboratory, Faculty of Medicine, Lund University, Lund, Sweden
Department of Internal Medicine, Central Hospital, Växjö, Sweden

Akinlolu Gabriel Omisore
Department of Community Medicine, Osun State University, Osogbo, Nigeria

Bridget Omisore and Ibrahim Sebutu Bello
Department of Family Medicine, Obafemi Awolowo University Teaching Hospitals Complex, Ile-Ife, Nigeria

Emmanuel Akintunde Abioye-Kuteyi
Department of Family Medicine, Obafemi Awolowo University Teaching Hospitals Complex, Ile-Ife, Nigeria
Department of Community Health, Obafemi Awolowo University Ile-Ife, Ile-Ife, Nigeria

Samuel Anu Olowookere
Department of Family Medicine, Obafemi Awolowo University Teaching Hospitals Complex, Ile-Ife, Nigeria

Derek Anamaale Tuoyire
Department of Community Medicine, School of Medical Sciences, College of Health and Allied Sciences, University of Cape Coast, Cape Coast, Ghana

Cindy George
Non-Communicable Diseases Research Unit, South African Medical Research Council, Francie van Zijl Drive, Parow Valley,

Juliet Evans
Health Impact Assessment, Western Cape Department of Health, Cape Town, South Africa

Lisa K. Micklesfield
South African Medical Research Council/University of the Witwatersrand Developmental Pathways for Health Research Unit, Department of Pediatrics, Faculty of Health Sciences, University of Witwatersrand, Johannesburg, South Africa
Department of Human Biology, Division of Exercise Science and Sports Medicine, University of Cape Town, Cape Town, South Africa.

Tommy Olsson
Department of Medicine, Umeå University, Umeå, Sweden

Julia H. Goedecke
Non-Communicable Diseases Research Unit, South African Medical Research Council, Francie van Zijl Drive, Parow Valley, Cape Town, South Africa
Department of Human Biology, Division of Exercise Science and Sports Medicine, University of Cape Town, Cape Town, South Africa

Laurie K. Twells
Faculty of Medicine, Memorial University, Medical Education Building, 300 Prince Philip Drive, St. John's, NL A1B 3V6, Canada
School of Pharmacy, Memorial University, Health Sciences Centre, 300 Prince Philip Drive New found land and Labrador, St. John's A1B 3V6, Canada

Shannon Driscoll, Deborah M. Gregory and Kendra Lester
Faculty of Medicine, Memorial University, Medical Education Building, 300 Prince Philip Drive, St. John's, NL A1B 3V6, Canada

John M. Fardy and Dave Pace
Faculty of Medicine, Memorial University, Medical Education Building, 300 Prince Philip Drive, St. John's, NL A1B 3V6, Canada
Eastern Health, Health Sciences Centre, 300 Prince Philip Drive, St. John's, NL A1B 3V6, Canada

Karin Haby and Åsa Premberg
Primary Health Care, Research and Development Unit, Närhälsan, Region Västra Götaland, Gothenburg, Sweden
Institute of Health and Care Sciences, Sahlgrenska Academy, University of Gothenburg, Gothenburg, Sweden

Marie Bergand Hanna Gyllensten
Institute of Health and Care Sciences, Sahlgrenska Academy, University of Gothenburg, Gothenburg, Sweden
GPCC – University of Gothenburg Centre for Person-centred Care, Gothenburg, Sweden

Ragnar Hanas
Department of Pediatrics, NU Hospital Group, Region Västra Götaland, Uddevalla, Sweden.
Institute of Clinical Sciences, Sahlgrenska Academy, University of Gothenburg, Gothenburg, Sweden

Laura Otterbach, Noereem Z. Mena, Geoffrey Greene and Alison Tovar
Department of Nutrition and Food Sciences, University of Rhode Island, Fogarty Hall, 41 Lower College Rd, Kingston, RI 02881, USA

Colleen A. Redding
Cancer Prevention Research Center and Department of Psychology, University of Rhode Island, Chafee Hall, 142 Flagg Road, Kingston, RI 02881, USA

Annie De Groot
Institute for Immunology and Informatics, University of Rhode Island, Shepard Building, 80 Washington Street, Providence, RI 02903, USA

Seung Yong Han, Gina Agostini and Alexandra A.
Mayo Clinic/Arizona State University Obesity Solutions, 1000 Cady Mall Suite 164, Tempe, AZ 85287, USA

Amber Wutich
School of Human Evolution and Social Change, Arizona State University, 900 Cady Mall, Tempe, AZ 85287, USA

Brewis
Mayo Clinic/Arizona State University Obesity Solutions, 1000 Cady Mall Suite 164, Tempe, AZ 85287, USA
School of Human Evolution and Social Change, Arizona State University, 900 Cady Mall, Tempe, AZ 85287, USA

Joachim Westenhoefer
Competence Center Health, Department Health Sciences, Hamburg University of Applied Science, Ulmenliet 20, 21033 Hamburg, Germany

Robert von Katzler, Hans-Joachim Jensen, Volker Harth and Marcus Oldenburg
Institute for Occupational and Maritime Medicine (ZfAM) Hamburg, University Medical Center Hamburg-Eppendorf, Hamburg, Germany

Birgit-Christiane Zyriax
Preventive Medicine and Nutrition, Institute for Health Services Research in Dermatology and Nursing (IVDP), University Medical Center Hamburg-Eppendorf, Hamburg, Germany

Bettina Jagemann
I. Medical Clinic and Polyclinic, University Medical Center Hamburg-Eppendorf, Hamburg, Germany

Richmond Aryeetey
School of Public Health, University of Ghana, Accra, Ghana

Anna Lartey Helena Nti and Esi Colecraft
Department of Nutrition and Food Science, University of Ghana, Accra, Ghana

Grace S. Marquis
School of Dietetics and Human Nutrition, McGill University, 21,111 Lakeshore Road, Ste-Anne de-Bellevue, Montreal, QC H9X 3V9, Canada

Patricia Brown
Department of Biochemistry and Biotechnology, Kwame Nkrumah University of Science and Technology, Kumasi, Ghana

Jeffrey Wilkins
Biomedical Biotechnology Research Institute, North Carolina Central University, 1801 Fayetteville Street, Durham, NC 27707, USA

Palash Ghosh and Bibhas Chakraborty
Centre for Quantitative Medicine, Duke-NUS Medical School, 8 College Road, Singapore 169857, Singapore

Juan Vivar
Center for Tobacco Products, Food and Drug Administration, 10903 New Hampshire Avenue, Silver Spring, MD 20993, USA

Sujoy Ghosh
Program in Cardiovascular and Metabolic Disorders and Centre for Computational Biology, Duke-NUS Medical School, 8 College Road, Singapore 169857, Singapore

Samantha B. van Beurden, Sally I. Simmons, Charles Abraham and Colin J. Greaves
University of Exeter Medical School, University of Exeter, Exeter, UK

Avril J. Mewse
Psychology, University of Exeter, Exeter, UK

Jason C. H. Tang
School of Medicine, University of Dundee, Dundee, UK

Robert Winther
Department of Research, Innlandet Hospital Trust, PB 104, N-2381 Brumunddal, Norway

Faculty of Medicine, University of Aalborg, DK-9100 Aalborg, Denmark

Per G. Farup
Department of Research, Innlandet Hospital Trust, PB 104, N-2381 Brumunddal, Norway
Unit for Applied Clinical Research, Department of Clinical and Molecular Medicine, Faculty of Medicine and Health Sciences, Norwegian University of Science and Technology, N-7491 Trondheim, Norway

Martin Aasbrenn
Department of Surgery, Innlandet Hospital Trust, N-2819 Gjøvik, Norway
Unit for Applied Clinical Research, Department of Clinical and Molecular Medicine, Faculty of Medicine and Health Sciences, Norwegian University of Science and Technology, N-7491 Trondheim, Norway

Marisol Perez, Tara K. Ohrt and Amanda B. Bruening
Department of Psychology, Arizona State University, 950 S McAllister Avenue, Tempe, AZ 85287-1104, USA

Jeffrey Liew
Department of Educational Psychology, Texas A&M University, College Station, TX 77843-4225, USA

Ashley M. W. Kroon Van Diest
Nationwide Children's Hospital Department of Pediatric Psychology and Neuropsychology, The Ohio State University Department of Pediatrics, Cleveland, OH 44195, USA

Aaron B. Taylor and Tatianna Ungredda
Department of Psychology, Texas A&M University, College Station, TX 77843-4235, USA

Sara N. Bleich
Department of Health Policy and Management, Harvard T.H. Chan School of Public Health, Boston, MA, USA

Kelsey A. Vercammen
Department of Epidemiology, Harvard T.H. Chan School of Public Health, Boston, USA

James Rogers
Summit Analytical, LLC, 8354 Northfield Blvd., Building G, Suite 3700, Denver, CO 80238, USA

Stacie L. Urbina, Lem W. Taylor and Colin D. Wilborn
Human Performance Laboratory, University of Mary Hardin-Baylor, Belton, TX 76513, USA

Martin Purpura and Ralf Jäger
Increnovo LLC, 2138 E Lafayette Pl, Milwaukee, WI 53202, USA

Vijaya Juturu
Omni Active Health Technologies Inc., 67 East Park Place, Suite 500, Morristown, NJ 07950, USA

Stephanie P. Goldstein, E. Whitney Evans, Jennifer Webster, J. Graham Thomas and Dale S. Bond
Weight Control and Diabetes Research Center, Department of Psychiatry and Human Behavior, The Miriam Hospital/Warren Alpert Medical School of Brown University, 196 Richmond Street, Providence, RI 02909, USA

Sivamainthan Vithiananthan
Department of Surgery, The Miriam Hospital/Warren Alpert Medical School of Brown University, 195 Collyer Street, Providence, RI 02904, USA

George A. Blackburn and Daniel B. Jones
Beth Israel Deaconess Medical Center, Department of Surgery, Center for the Study of Nutrition Medicine, Feldberg 880, East Campus, 330 Brookline Avenue, Boston, MA 02215, USA

Richard Jones
Department of Psychiatry and Human Behavior, Warren Alpert Medical School of Brown University, Butler Hospital, 345 Blackstone Boulevard, Providence, RI 02906, USA

Jody Dushay
Department of Medicine, Division of Endocrinology, Beth Israel Deaconess Medical Center, Feldberg 880, East Campus, 330 Brookline Avenue, Boston, MA 02215, USA

Jon Moon
MEI Research, Ltd, 6016 Schaefer Road, Edina, MN 55436, USA

Abdullah Alkandari
Department of Surgery and Cancer, Imperial College London, London, UK
Clinical Trials Unit, Dasman Diabetes Institute, Dasman, 15462Kuwait City, Kuwait

Hutan Ashrafian
Department of Surgery and Cancer, Imperial College London, London, UK
Department of Bariatric and Metabolic Surgery, Chelsea and Westminster NHS Foundation Trust, London, UK

Thozhukat Sathyapalan
Department of Academic Endocrinology, Diabetes and Metabolism, Hull York Medical School, Hull, UK

Peter Sedman
Division of Upper Gastrointestinal and Minimally Invasive Surgery, Hull and East Yorkshire Hospitals NHS Trust, Hull, UK

Ara Darzi, Elaine Holmes, Thanos Athanasiou and Nigel J. Gooderham
Department of Surgery and Cancer, Imperial College London, London, UK

Stephen L. Atkin
Weill Cornell Medical College Qatar, Qatar Foundation, Doha, Qatar

Kelsey H. Collins and Walter Herzog
Human Performance Laboratory, University of Calgary, Calgary, AB, Canada

Behnam Sharif and Deborah A. Marshall
Department of Community Health Sciences, University of Calgary, 3280 Hospital Drive NW, Calgary, AB T2N 4Z6, Canada

Raylene A. Reimer
Faculty of Kinesiology and Department of Biochemistry and Molecular Biology, University of Calgary, Calgary, AB, Canada

Claudia Sanmartin
Health Analysis Division, Statistics Canada, Ottawa, ON, Canada

Rick Chin
Department of Medicine, University of Calgary, Calgary, AB, Canada

Lorraine M Noble
UCL Medical School, University College London, Royal Free Hospital, Rowland Hill Street, NW3 2PF, London, UK

Emma Godfrey and Gabriella Baez
Department of Psychology, Institute of Psychiatry, Psychology and Neuroscience, King's College London, London, UK

Liane Al-Baba
UCL Research Department of Epidemiology and Public Health, UCL, London, UK

Nicki Thorogood and Kiran Nanchahal
Department of Social and Environmental Health Research, London School of Hygiene and Tropical Medicine, London, UK

Alemu Gebrie and Abriham Zegeye
Department of Biomedical Science, School of Medicine, Debre Markos University

Animut Alebel and Bekele Tesfaye
Department of Nursing, College of Health Sciences, Debre Markos University, Debre Markos, Ethiopia

Aster Ferede
Department of Public Health, College of Health Sciences, Debre Markos University, Debre Markos, Ethiopia

Mahboobeh Ghesmaty Sangachin and Lora A. Cavuoto
Department of Industrial and Systems Engineering, University at Buffalo, 324 Bell Hall, Buffalo, NY 14260, USA

Youfa Wang
Department of Nutrition and Health Sciences, College of Health, Ball State University, Muncie, IN, USA.

Index

N
Naproxen, 114
Non-nutritive Sweeteners, 133-134, 136-138, 140-141

O
Oral Glucose Tolerance Test, 3, 7
Osteoarthritis, 52, 54, 56, 215-217, 219, 222-223, 247, 257, 263, 267, 269
Oxidative Stress, 112, 183

P
Pcr, 204-205, 214
Physical Activity, 14, 24-34, 39-45, 50, 62-63, 65-66, 68-69, 71-73, 75-77, 79-80, 82, 84-92, 103-110, 112, 128, 132-137, 139-140, 142, 183, 190, 196-199, 227-230, 236, 239, 242, 268-269

R
Roux-en-y Gastric Bypass, 58, 60, 85, 202-204, 212, 214

S
Serum Creatinine, 215-217, 219-220, 223
Serum Lipids, 15, 42-43, 47
Sleep Apnea, 52, 54, 56
Sleeve Gastrectomy, 52-53, 60, 85, 193, 202
Sugar-sweetened Beverages, 80, 105, 155, 179-181
Systolic Blood Pressure, 13-14, 16-21, 24, 27, 30, 45, 72, 187

T
Tcf7l2, 1-3, 6-12
Triglycerides, 13-14, 16-22, 42, 45-49
Type 2 Diabetes, 1-3, 8, 10-12, 14, 22, 41, 43, 51, 54, 56, 112, 121, 124, 139-140, 155, 177, 179, 193, 204-205, 213-214, 216, 223, 248, 267

W
Weight Bias Internalization Scale, 84, 91-92

www.ingramcontent.com/pod-product-compliance
Lightning Source LLC
Chambersburg PA
CBHW061314190326

41458CB00011B/3807